Medical Physiology

Medical Physiology

Editor: Johnny Carrey

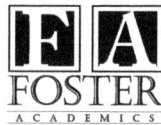

FOSTER
ACADEMICS

www.fosteracademics.com

www.fosteracademics.com

FA
FOSTER
ACADEMICS

Cataloging-in-Publication Data

Medical physiology / edited by Johnny Carrey.
    p. cm.
Includes bibliographical references and index.
ISBN 978-1-63242-782-3
1. Human physiology. 2. Medical sciences. 3. Physiology. 4. Human body. I. Carrey, Johnny.
QP34.5 .M43 2019
612--dc23

© Foster Academics, 2019

Foster Academics,
118-35 Queens Blvd., Suite 400,
Forest Hills, NY 11375, USA

ISBN 978-1-63242-782-3 (Hardback)

Contents

Preface

Medical physiology is a clinical specialty in medical science, which is concerned with the application of an understanding of human physiology to patients in a healthcare setting. Evaluation of the functions of the heart, lungs, kidneys, blood vessels, gastrointestinal tract, etc. is done to form a diagnosis of the underlying condition. Some of the diagnostic techniques for evaluating these include an electrocardiogram of the heart, pulmonary function testing using spirometry and ankle brachial pressure index measurement. Physiologists use imaging techniques such as MRI, ultrasonography, echocardiography, X-ray computed tomography, etc. to measure velocities, movements and metabolic processes. This book elucidates new techniques and applications of medical physiology in a multidisciplinary manner. It presents researches and studies performed by experts across the globe. It will serve as a valuable source of reference for graduate and post-graduate students.

This book has been the outcome of endless efforts put in by authors and researchers on various issues and topics within the field. The book is a comprehensive collection of significant researches that are addressed in a variety of chapters. It will surely enhance the knowledge of the field among readers across the globe.

It gives us an immense pleasure to thank our researchers and authors for their efforts to submit their piece of writing before the deadlines. Finally in the end, I would like to thank my family and colleagues who have been a great source of inspiration and support.

Editor

Mechanisms of pressure-diuresis and pressure-natriuresis in Dahl salt-resistant and Dahl salt-sensitive rats

Daniel A Beard* and Muriel Mescam

Abstract

Background: Data on blood flow regulation, renal filtration, and urine output in salt-sensitive Dahl S rats fed on high-salt (hypertensive) and low-salt (prehypertensive) diets and salt-resistant Dahl R rats fed on high-salt diets were analyzed using a mathematical model of renal blood flow regulation, glomerular filtration, and solute transport in a nephron.

Results: The mechanism of pressure-diuresis and pressure-natriuresis that emerges from simulation of the integrated systems is that relatively small increases in glomerular filtration that follow from increases in renal arterial pressure cause relatively large increases in urine and sodium output. Furthermore, analysis reveals the minimal differences between the experimental cases necessary to explain the observed data. It is determined that differences in renal afferent and efferent arterial resistances are able to explain all of the qualitative differences in observed flows, filtration rates, and glomerular pressure as well as the differences in the pressure-natriuresis and pressure-diuresis relationships in the three groups. The model is able to satisfactorily explain data from all three groups without varying parameters associated with glomerular filtration or solute transport in the nephron component of the model.

Conclusions: Thus the differences between the experimental groups are explained solely in terms of difference in blood flow regulation. This finding is consistent with the hypothesis that, if a shift in the pressure-natriuresis relationship is the primary cause of elevated arterial pressure in the Dahl S rat, then alternation in how renal afferent and efferent arterial resistances are regulated represents the primary cause of chronic hypertension in the Dahl S rat.

Background

Animal models of salt- and/or angiotensin II-induced chronic hypertension have revealed shifts in the observed pressure-natriuresis and pressure-diuresis relationships to higher pressures, as well as altered renal blood flow regulation [1-6]. The salt-sensitive Dahl S (SS) rat is a widely studied example of an animal that develops hypertension, associated with a shift of the pressure-natriuresis relationship (relationship between sodium excretion and arterial pressure) to higher pressures, when fed a high-salt diet. When maintained on high salt (e.g., 8% NaCl in chow) the kidneys of these animals are found to excrete a given amount of sodium per unit time at a higher input arterial pressure than the kidneys of control animals fed low-salt diets and of strains, such as the salt-resistant Dahl R (SR) rat, that do not exhibit salt-induced hypertension. Thus sodium balance (dietary sodium input minus sodium excretion) is achieved in hypertensive animals at higher pressures than in normotensive animals [7].

Guyton and Coleman and coworkers hypothesize that a shift in the pressure-natriuresis relationship to higher pressures is one of the central causal mechanisms of chronic hypertension in salt-sensitive hypertension [8]. Other investigators suggest that angiotensin II- and salt-induced increases in sympathetic nervous activity in the vasculature may be a primary causal factor in salt-sensitive hypertension while the shift in the renal

* Correspondence: beardda@gmail.com
Center for Computational Medicine, Biotechnology and Bioengineering Center, Department of Physiology, Medical College of Wisconsin, Milwaukee, WI, USA

pressure-natriuresis relationship may not [9-11]. Not only is it unclear whether and when the observed changes in the pressure-natriuresis relationship are causes or consequences of chronic hypertension (or in some way both), it remains unclear what specific aspects of renal physiology are altered in salt-sensitive hypertension, underlying the observed changes in the pressure-natriuresis and pressure-diuresis relationships.

Here we analyze data on blood flow regulation, renal filtration, and urine output in SS rats fed on high-salt (hypertensive) and low-salt (prehypertensive) diets and salt-resistant SR rats fed on high-salt diets. We use a simple mathematical model of renal blood flow regulation, glomerular filtration, and solute transport in a nephron to reveal the minimal differences between the three cases necessary to explain the observed data. It is found that the differences in renal blood flow, glomerular filtration, and pressure-diuresis and pressure-natriuresis relationships may be explained based solely on differences in afferent and efferent arteriole regulation in the hypertensive (high-salt) SS compared to the salt-resistant SR and the low-salt SS controls.

Sources of data

Data from the SS and SR rats used for model identification are obtained from Roman [12]. Additional independent data from SS and SR rats for model comparison were obtained from Roman and Kaldunski [13]. For these data sets measurements were made in denervated kidneys perfused *in vivo* with plasma levels of vasopressin, aldosterone, corticosterone, and norepinephrine clamped. Data from three experimental groups are analyzed: high-salt fed hypertensive SS rats with baseline pressure of 158 ± 2 mmHg, low-salt fed prehypertensive SS rats with baseline pressure of 133 ± 1 mmHg, and high-salt fed SR rats with baseline pressure of 124 ± 1 mmHg. Additional data for comparison to model predictions are obtained from Thompson and Pitts [14] and were obtained in normal dogs in which glomerular filtration rate was modulated by varying renal arterial pressure. (Data from Thompson and Pitts on adrenalectomized and sympathectomized dogs show similar trends.)

Methods

The mathematical model of renal blood flow, glomerular filtration, and mass transport in nephrons (diagrammed in Figure 1) is composed of two main components, a model for renal blood flow and glomerular filtration and a model for mass transport in a representative nephron. Both components are based on modifications made to models presented in Chapter 20 of Keener and Sneyd [15]. The blood flow and filtration model predicts glomerular filtration rate, glomerular pressure, and renal blood flow as functions of input arterial pressure. The predicted glomerular

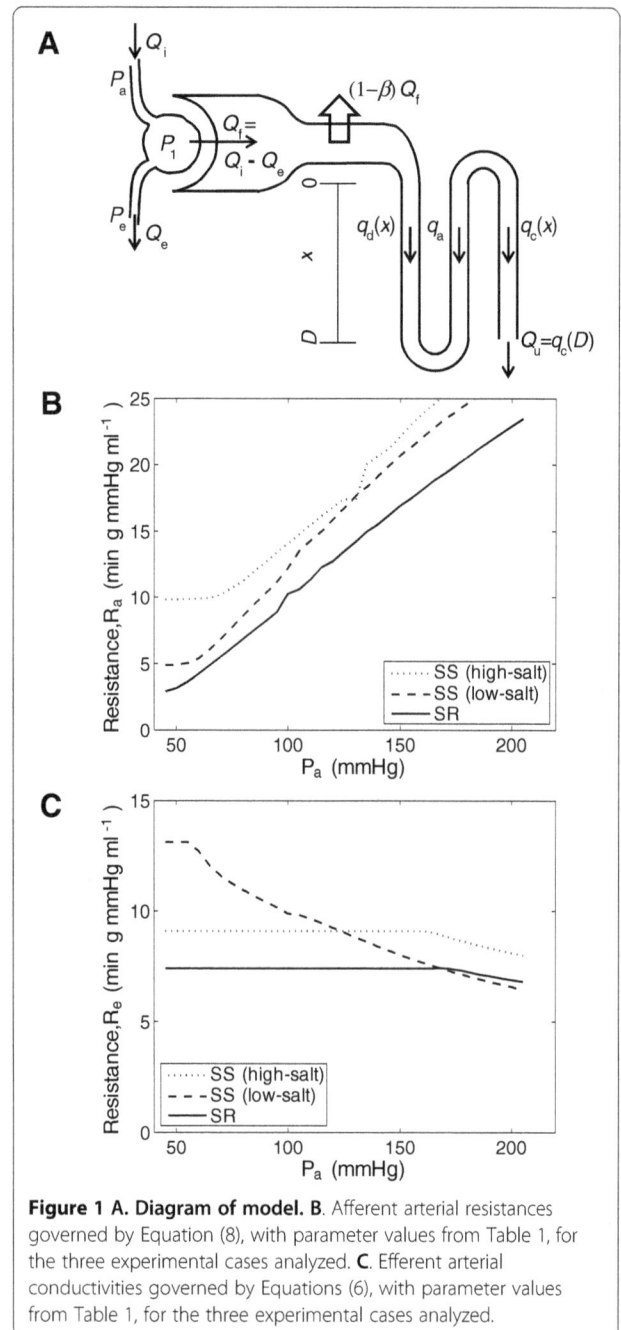

Figure 1 A. Diagram of model. B. Afferent arterial resistances governed by Equation (8), with parameter values from Table 1, for the three experimental cases analyzed. **C.** Efferent arterial conductivities governed by Equations (6), with parameter values from Table 1, for the three experimental cases analyzed.

filtration rate and pressure serve as inputs to the nephron model, which predicts concentrations of sodium and flows in the descending and ascending limbs of the loop of Henle and a combined intersitium/ascending vasa recta space. Predictions of the overall model are compared to data on renal blood flow, glomerular filtration, glomerular pressure, efferent capillary pressure, urine flow, and sodium excretion in low-salt fed prehypertensive and high-salt fed hypertensive SS and high-salt fed SR rats.

While the treatment of a single nephron as representative of whole kidney is a gross simplification compared to models that capture heterogeneities in loop length and the three-dimensional architecture of the tubules and vasculature [16-19], the model developed here is appropriate to capture the physiological function analyzed here. Models of renal flow regulation and tubuloglomerular feedback [20-22], transport in the proximal tubule and cortex [23-25], medulla [17,18,26-35], collecting duct [34,36], and other components [16] have been developed to capture much more biophysical detail than the whole-kidney model developed here. Yet we are aware that no previously developed model, however simplified, combines renal hemodynamics, filtration, and tubular transport to simulate and analyze data on whole-kidney pressure-natriuresis function.

Previous models of renal system that capture overall kidney function, including the pressure-natriuresis and pressure- diuresis phenomena, have been developed [37-40]. However, these models do not capture spatially distributed transport in kidney, even at the simplified level of the model developed here.

Governing equations for blood flow and filtration

Flow and filtration along glomerular capillaries is governed by the conservation equation for flow in a glomerular capillary, $q_1(y)$:

$$\frac{dq_1}{dy} = K_f(P_2 - P_1 + \Pi_c), y \in (0, L),$$ (1)

where y is the distance along the glomerular capillary, K_f is the hydraulic permeability, $\Pi_c(y)$ is the oncotic pressure in the plasma, and P_1 and P_2 are hydrostatic pressures in the capillary and Bowman's capsule, respectively. This expression assumes that the rate of fluid loss from the capillary is linearly proportional to the pressure difference driving force and that pressure remains effectively constant along the length of the glomerular capillary. Blood enters the capillary at $y = 0$ with an input oncotic pressure $\Pi_c(y = 0) = \Pi_i = 28$ mmHg and input flow $q_1(y = 0) = Q_i$. Assuming a linear relationship between concentration and oncotic pressure, we have

$$\Pi_c(y)q_1(y) = \Pi_i Q_i.$$ (2)

Combining Equations (1) and (2) yields

$$\frac{dq_1}{dy} = K_f\left(P_2 - P_1 + \Pi_i\frac{Q_i}{q_1}\right),$$ (3)

which is a separable equation that can be solved to yield the following relationship between input flow q_1 $(y = 0) = Q_i$ and output flow $q_1(y = L) = Q_e$:

$$\frac{Q_e}{Q_i} + \alpha\ln\left(\frac{Q_e/Q_i - \alpha}{1 - \alpha}\right) = 1 - \frac{K_f L \Delta P}{Q_i},$$ (4)

where $\Delta P = P_1 - P_2$, and $\alpha = \Pi_i/\Delta P$. The filtrate flow (glomerular filtration rate) is computed from the

difference between input and output blood flows, $Q_f = Q_i - Q_e$.

Blood flow into the glomerulus satisfies the Ohm's Law relationship

$$P_a - P_1 = Q_i \cdot R_a,$$ (5)

where P_a is the input arterial pressure and R_a is the afferent arterial resistance, which is phenomenologically modeled using the following increasing function of filtration

$$R_a(Q_i) = R_a^o\frac{Q_i^{n_i}}{Q_i^{n_i} + Q_{i0}^{n_i}} \cdot \frac{c_a(0)}{C_{TGF} + c_a(0)} + R_a^{\min},$$ (6)

where R_a^o, $R_a^{\min}$, n_i, Q_{a0}, and C_{TGF} are adjustable parameters, and $c_a(0)$ is the sodium concentration in the ascending limb at the location where it feeds into the distal tubule. The factor $Q_i^{n_i}/(Q_i^{n_i} + Q_{i0}^{n_i})$ increases smoothly with increasing blood flow, representing an autoregulatory vasoconstriction. The factor $c_a(0)/(C_{TGF} + c_a(0))$ is employed to account for tubular-glomerular feedback: increasing salt concentration in the distal tubule stimulates vasoconstriction. (The concentration $c_a(0)$ is obtained from the transport component of the model, detailed below.)

Similarly blood flow out of the glomerulus satisfies the Ohm's Law relationship

$$P_1 - P_e = Q_e \cdot R_e,$$ (7)

where P_e is the efferent capillary pressure and R_e is the efferent arterial resistance, which is phenomenologically modeled using the following decreasing function of P_1, the input pressure into the arteriole.

$$R_e(P_1) = \begin{cases} R_e^{\max}, & P_1 \leq (b - R_e^{\max})/m \\ b - mP_1, & P_1 > (b - R_e^{\max})/m \end{cases}$$ (8)

where $R_e^{\max}$, b, and m are adjustable parameters. Thus the efferent arteriole is assumed to contribute to the decreasing behavior of the resistance in direct response to increases in pressure beyond a certain cutoff value of P_1. Equations (6) and (8) predict that afferent resistance increases and efferent resistance decreases as renal perfusion pressure is increased, as illustrated in Figure 1. The tubular-glomerular feedback component of the model acts in the same direction as the autoregulatory factor in Equation (6). As pressure increases, filtration rate increases, leading to higher concentrations in the distal tubule, decreasing afferent conductivity.

Roman [12] reported measurements of pressures in peritubular capillaries (capillaries downstream of outer cortical glomeruli). As the model described here does not distinguish between corticomedullary and juxtamedullary glomeruli, the reported peritubular capillary pressures are compared to the model variable P_e, efferent capillary pressure. Data on P_e as a function of arterial pressure are used to fit representative function for $P_e(P_a)$:

$$P_e = P_{e0} + P_{e1} \frac{P_a^{n_{pe}}}{P_a^{n_{pe}} + P_{e2}^{n_{pe}}}, \tag{9}$$

which invokes four additional adjustable parameters, P_{e0}, P_{e1}, P_{e2}, and n_{pe}.

Filtrate flow satisfies the Ohm's Law relationship

$$P_2 - P_d = R_d Q_f, \tag{10}$$

where P_d is the distal tubule pressure and R_d is the resistance associated with this pressure drop, assumed constant. In the absence of data on distal tubule hydrostatic pressure, we assume a simple linear proportionality between arterial pressure and P_d:

$$P_d = a_{Pd} P_a, \tag{11}$$

where a_{Pd} is set to 0.02, which gives a value of distal tubule pressure of 2.0–3.6 mmHg over a range of renal perfusion pressure of 100 to 180 mmHg.

Equations (4), (5), (7), and (10), invoking 14 adjustable parameters (see Table 1), are solved for the four unknowns Q_i, Q_e, P_1, and P_2 to provide model predictions of these flows and pressures, as well as functions of input pressure P_a.

Governing equations for nephron

Mass transport in nephrons is represented using a one-dimensionally distributed model accounting for flows and concentrations in a single representative nephron. Thus three-dimensional interactions and the anatomical heterogeneity of loop lengths are not taken into account. Nevertheless, the model is able to effectively match observed pressure-diuresis and pressure-natriuresis relationships. The nephron model, diagramed in Figure 1, simulates flow and sodium concentration in four regions: the descending and ascending limbs of the loop of Henle, the collecting duct, and a combined ascending vasa recta/interstitium region. Fluid flows in these regions are denoted q_d, q_a, q_c, and q_s; sodium concentrations are denoted c_d, c_a, c_c, and c_s, where subscripts 'd', 'a', 'c', and 's' indicate descending limb, ascending limb, collecting duct, and interstitial space. After passing through the proximal tubule, filtrate enters the descending limb at spatial position $x = 0$; the nephron region is defined over the spatial domain $x \in [0, D]$, where $D = 2$ mm is the length of the segments of the nephron.

Fluid transport between the interstitium and the descending limb is assumed to be linearly proportional to the combined mechanical and osmotic pressure driving force, $P_d + \Pi_s - P_s + 2RT(c_d - c_s)$, where P_d is the hydrostatic pressure in the descending limb, Π_s is the osmotic

Table 1 Adjustable parameter values

		Dahl-R	Dahl-S	
		high-salt	low-salt	high-salt
glomerular hydraulic permeability times length	$K_f L$ (ml·min^{-1}·g^{-1}·mmHg^{-1})	0.0886	a	a
resistance associated with distal tubule	R_d (min·g·mmHg·ml^{-1})	7.4959	a	a
afferent arteriole resistance parameter	R_a^0 (ml·min^{-1}·g^{-1}·mmHg^{-1})	37.7673	a	a
minimum afferent arteriole resistance	R_a^{min} (ml·min^{-1}·g^{-1}·mmHg^{-1})	2.8758	4.88	9.84
afferent autoregulation parameter	Q_{i0} (ml·min^{-1}·g^{-1})	5.5796	4.28	b
afferent autoregulation parameter	n_i	9.5614	a	a
maximum efferent arteriole resistance	R_e^{max} (ml·min^{-1}·g^{-1}·mmHg^{-1})	7.4185	13.1	9.10
efferent arteriole resistance parameter	b (ml·min^{-1}·g^{-1}·mmHg^{-1})	37.5995	a	a
efferent arteriole resistance parameter	m (ml·min^{-1}·g^{-1}·mmHg^{-2})	0.5269	0.577	0.54
TGF concentration parameter	C_{TGF} (mM)	25.0	a	a
efferent capillary pressure fitting parameter	P_{e0} (mmHg)	10.4	a	8.32
efferent capillary pressure fitting parameter	P_{e1} (mmHg)	15.1	a	a
efferent capillary pressure fitting parameter	P_{e2} (mmHg)	136.5	a	a
efferent capillary pressure fitting parameter	n_{Pe} (unitless)	5.93	a	a
sodium permeability of the descending limb	H_d (ml·min^{-1}·g^{-1}·mm^{-1})	7.70×10^{-3}	a	a
hydraulic permeability of the descending limb	K_d (ml·min^{-1}·g^{-1}·mmHg^{-1}·mm^{-1})	8.3889×10^{-4}	a	a
hydraulic permeability of the collecting duct	K_c (ml·min^{-1}·g^{-1}·mmHg^{-1}·mm^{-1})	1.8777×10^{-5}	a	a
maximum sodium reabsorption rate in ascending limb	P_{max} (ml·mM·min^{-1}·mm^{-1}·g^{-1})	29.172	a	a
apparent Michaelis-Menten constant for sodium reabsorption	K_m (mM)	50.933	a	a

(a) value same as Dahl-R value.
(b) value same as Dahl-S value.

pressure in the interstitium, P_s is the hydrostatic pressure in the interstitium, and c_d and c_s are the Na$^+$ concentrations in the descending limb and the interstitium. The factor of 2 multiplying the concentration gradient term arises because it is assumed that chloride concentration equals sodium concentration, and sodium plus chloride represent the major contributor to the osmotic gradient. With the hydraulic permeability constant K_d mass conservation yields the equation for q_d, the flow in the descending limb:

$$\frac{dq_d}{dx} = K_d(-\Delta P_d + 2RT(c_d - c_s)), x \in [0, D] \qquad (12)$$

where $\Delta P_d = P_d + \Pi_s - P_s$, and interstitial osmotic and hydrostatic pressures are set to $\Pi_s = 17$ mmHg and $P_s = 3$ mmHg.

The ascending limb is assumed impermeable to water, and thus flow in the ascending limb, q_a, is constant:

$$\frac{dq_a}{dx} = 0. \qquad (13)$$

The governing equation for q_c, the flow in the collecting duct is analogous to the equation for q_d.

$$\frac{dq_c}{dx} = K_c(-\Delta P_c + 2RT(c_c - c_s)), \qquad (14)$$

where $\Delta P_c = P_c + \Pi_s - P_s$ and K_c is the hydraulic permeability in the collecting duct. The hydrostatic pressure in the collecting duct is assumed to be 1 mmHg lower than that in the distal tubule: $P_c = P_d - 1$ mmHg.

Since total volume is conserved

$$\frac{dq_s}{dx} = -\frac{d}{dx}(q_d + q_a + q_c). \qquad (15)$$

Sodium transport is assumed to be governed by passive permeation in the descending limb and collecting duct and by active transport in the ascending limb. The governing equations for Na$^+$ flux in descending limb is given by

$$\frac{d(q_d c_d)}{dx} = H_d(c_s - c_d), \qquad (16)$$

where H_d is the descending limb permeability. The transport rate in the ascending limb is given by

$$\frac{d(q_a c_a)}{dx} = -P(c_a) = -\frac{P_{max}c_a}{c_a + K_m} \cdot \frac{(C_{a,max})^5}{(c_a)^5 + (C_{a,max})^5}, \qquad (17)$$

where the factor

$$\frac{P_{max}c_a}{c_a + K_m}$$

models a saturable process, with P_{max} and K_m adjustable parameters. The factor

$$\frac{(C_{a,max})^5}{(c_a)^5 + (C_{a,max})^5}$$

is applied so that the transport rate goes to zero when concentrations in the nephron exceed an upper limit. Without this factor, concentrations become unbounded when the flow in the collecting duct approaches zero. Physically, this is because the predicted concentration gradient increases as flow through the loop of Henle decreases. Without this factor the solution becomes mathematically unbounded when pressure drops low enough that all of the filtrate is reabsorbed because in this limit q_a and dq_a/dx both approach zero, and the only way for $d(q_a c_a)/dx$ to approach a constant value would be for c_a and/or its gradient to become unbounded. Since the concentration gradient drives fluid loss from the descending limb and the collecting duct, increases in the concentration gradient lead to further decreases in flow. The Hill coefficient of 5 in this multiplying factor is also arbitrarily assigned so that transport rapidly approaches zero when c_a exceeds $C_{a,max}$. The value of the fixed parameter $C_{a,max}$ set to 500 mM, so that the maximal Na$^+$ concentration achieved at low flows is approximately 800 mM, associated with an approximately 5-fold magnification of the input concentration of $c_d(0) = 150$ mM. (See below.) For pressures and flows that result in urine flows that are approximately equal to and greater than the baseline values, c_a remains well below $C_{a,max}$ and the behavior of the model is not sensitive to the values of these fixed parameters.

Sodium reabsorption in the collecting duct is not explicitly accounted for in the model and the equation for Na$^+$ flux in the collecting duct is

$$\frac{d(q_c c_c)}{dx} = 0. \qquad (18)$$

This simplifying assumption is discussed below. Salt transport in the interstitial space combines active transport and passive permeation processes:

$$\frac{d(q_s c_s)}{dx} = +P(c_a) - H_d(c_s - c_d) - H_c(c_s - c_c). \qquad (19)$$

Equation (19) assumes that the combined interstitial and vasa recta space gathers the sum of the fluxes from the other structures. Thus, as expressed by Keener and Sneyd,

$$\frac{d(q_s c_s)}{dx} = -\frac{d}{dx}(q_d c_d + q_a c_a + q_c c_c). \qquad (20)$$

The boundary conditions for input into the descending limb assume that input concentration is equivalent to plasma sodium concentration of 150 mM and input flow is proportional to Q_f, the glomerular filtration rate:

$$\begin{aligned} q_d(0) &= \beta Q_f, \\ c_d(0) &= 150 \, \text{mM}, \end{aligned} \qquad (21)$$

where $Q_f = Q_i - Q_e$ is determined as a function of arterial pressure by the renal blood flow and filtration model component and $\beta = 0.33$ is a fixed constant accounting for reabsorption by the proximal tubule. Thus, the model assumes constant glomerulotubular balance and isotonic reabsorption of water and sodium from the proximal tubule [41].

The boundary conditions for the ascending limb are obtained from the assumption of continuity of concentration and flow at the turn of the loop of Henle:

$$
\begin{aligned}
q_a(D) &= -q_d(D), \\
c_a(D) &= c_d(D).
\end{aligned}
\tag{22}
$$

Similarly, the ascending limb feeds into the collecting duct

$$
\begin{aligned}
q_c(0) &= -q_a(0), \\
c_c(0) &= c_a(0).
\end{aligned}
\tag{23}
$$

The interstitial flow boundary condition is [15]

$$
\begin{aligned}
q_s(D) &= 0 \\
q_d(0) + q_s(0) &= q_c(D).
\end{aligned}
\tag{24}
$$

Equations (20), (21), (22), and (23) provide eight boundary conditions for the eight first-order differential equations described above. The eighth condition comes from conservation of total fluid flow [15], requiring that flow into the system at $x = 0$ equal flow out of the system at $x = D$.

Numerical discretization of the nephron model is described in the Appendix.

Since sodium reabsorption occurs in the model only in the ascending limb and the outflow of the ascending limb feeds directly into the collecting duct, the model does not explicitly account for sodium reabsorption in the distal tubule or the collecting duct. Thus all sodium reabsorption processes are represented by the ascending limb sodium transport rate $P(C_a)$. This simplifying approximation is justified by the fact that during formation of either concentrated or dilute urine, the majority of sodium reabsorption occurs via the ascending limb. Lumping all reabsorption processes into Equation (17) helps keep the model tractable and identifiable. Adding additional processes would add additional uncertainty in parameter values that would not be justified given the available data or yield any additional insight into the operation of the integrated model.

Results

Model identification

Predictions of the renal flow and filtration model component are compared in Figure 2 to data on blood flow, filtration rate, glomerular pressure, and efferent pressure, as functions of arterial pressure in the SS (high-salt and low-salt) and SR (high-salt) rats. Predictions of urine output ($Q_u = Q_c(x = D)$) and sodium excretion ($Q_c(x = D)$.

$C_c(x = D)$) are compared in Figure 3 to data from SS (high-salt and low-salt) and SR (high-salt) rats as functions of arterial pressure. Data plotted in both Figures 2 and 3 used for model identification are obtained from Roman [12]. Additional independent data on urine output and sodium excretion in the SR rat were obtained from Roman and Kaldunski [13].

The 19 adjustable parameters invoked in this model are not identifiable for a given experimental group based on the six data sets (renal blood flow, filtration, glomerular pressure, efferent pressure, urine output, and sodium excretion as function of renal perfusion pressure) represented in these figures. However, the combined data set of pressures and flows versus arterial pressure for three experimental cases— prehypertensive (low-salt fed) and hypertensive (high-salt) SS rats and salt-resistant (high-salt) SR rats—provides independent data that can be compared to sixteen model-predicted functions of P_a: Q_i, Q_f, P_1, P_e, Q_u, and Q_u. $C_c(x = D)$ under both high- and low-salt conditions for the SS and high-salt conditions for the SR. (Data on P_1 and P_e as functions of P_a for the SS on low salt are not available; data for the SR were used to parameterize Equation (9) to represent $P_e(P_a)$ for the SS on low salt.) If we assume that most model parameters attain the same values for all three groups, it is possible to determine identifiable parameter sets and to determine the minimal set of differences between the two conditions that is able to explain the observed data.

Specifically, if it is assumed that only two afferent arterial flow regulation parameters Q_i^o and R_a^0 and the efferent arterial flow regulation parameters m and R_e^{max} are different between the SR and SS (low-salt) cases and that only the parameters R_a^0, R_e^{max}, m, and P_{e0} are different between the SS low-salt and high-salt cases, then there are a total of 27 adjustable parameters that can be estimated by matching data to the 16 model-predicted functions in Figures 2 and 3. These parameters that are allowed to attain different values between the experimental groups govern how afferent arterial resistances are regulated in the model and do not directly affect glomerular filtration or transport in the nephron. Model simulations associated with the parameter values listed in Table 1 are plotted in Figures 2 and 3. The data on flows and pressures in SS and SR rats shown in Figure 2 are effectively captured by the model, with the exception of glomerular filtration rate in the SR rat. (The apparent mismatch between model prediction and reported data on glomerular filtration rate in the SR rat is discussed below.)

The predicted trends in afferent conductivity shown in Figure 1B may be compared to the measurements of Takenaka et al. [42], who observed that: (1.) afferent arterioles from low-salt SS animals maintain higher diameters at low pressures than those from high-salt animals; and (2.) arterioles from low-salt SS animals show a

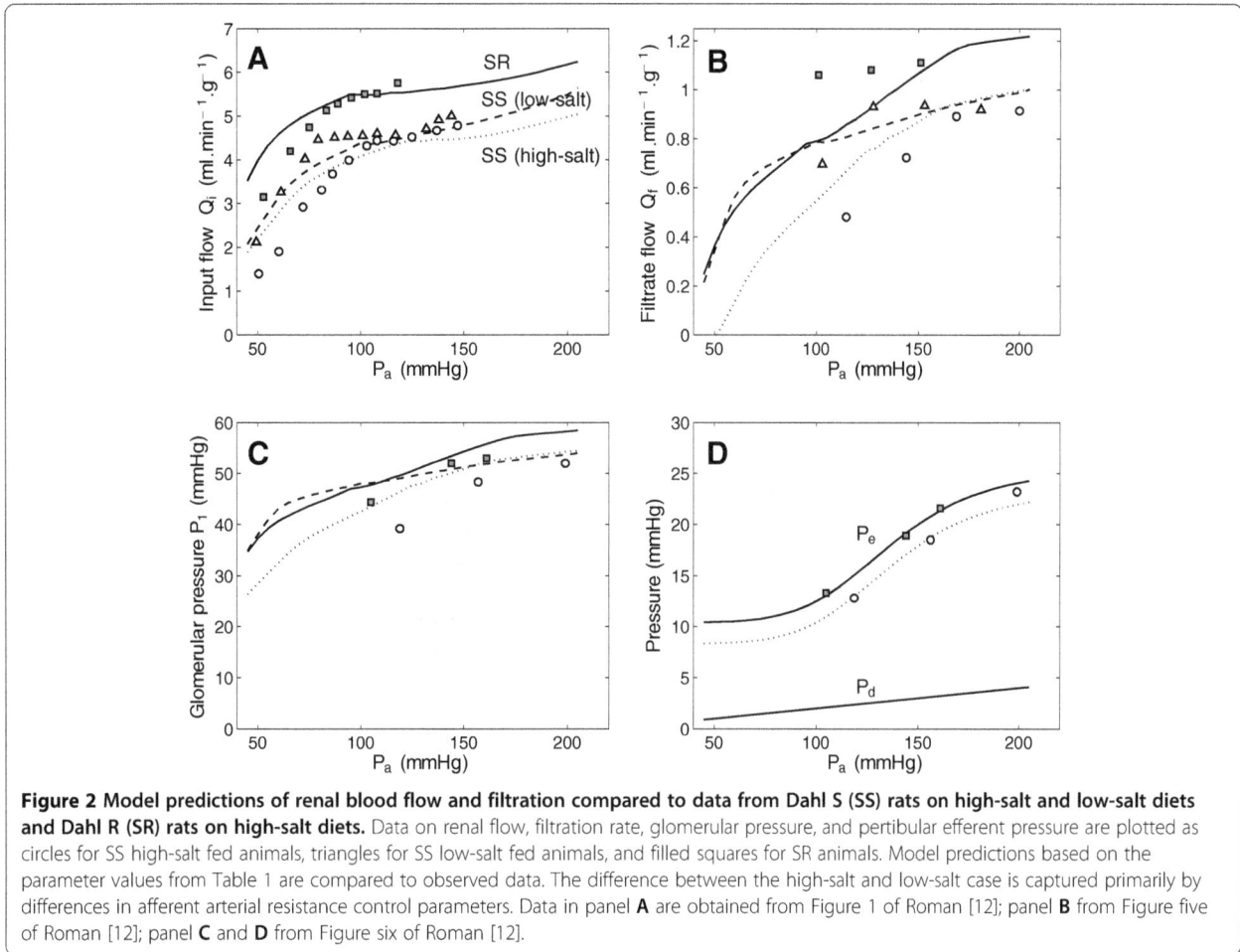

Figure 2 Model predictions of renal blood flow and filtration compared to data from Dahl S (SS) rats on high-salt and low-salt diets and Dahl R (SR) rats on high-salt diets. Data on renal flow, filtration rate, glomerular pressure, and pertibular efferent pressure are plotted as circles for SS high-salt fed animals, triangles for SS low-salt fed animals, and filled squares for SR animals. Model predictions based on the parameter values from Table 1 are compared to observed data. The difference between the high-salt and low-salt case is captured primarily by differences in afferent arterial resistance control parameters. Data in panel **A** are obtained from Figure 1 of Roman [12]; panel **B** from Figure five of Roman [12]; panel **C** and **D** from Figure six of Roman [12].

stronger constriction in response to increasing pressure than those from high-salt animals. These results are consistent with our model predictions. However, the observations of Takenaka et al., which made use of an isolated buffer perfused hydrophonetic kidney preparation, demonstrated total abolishment of the autoregulatory response in afferent arterioles in the high-salt case. An exact match between the model and the in vitro data of Takenaka et al. is not expected because the nature of the experiments of Takenaka et al. altered any sheer-

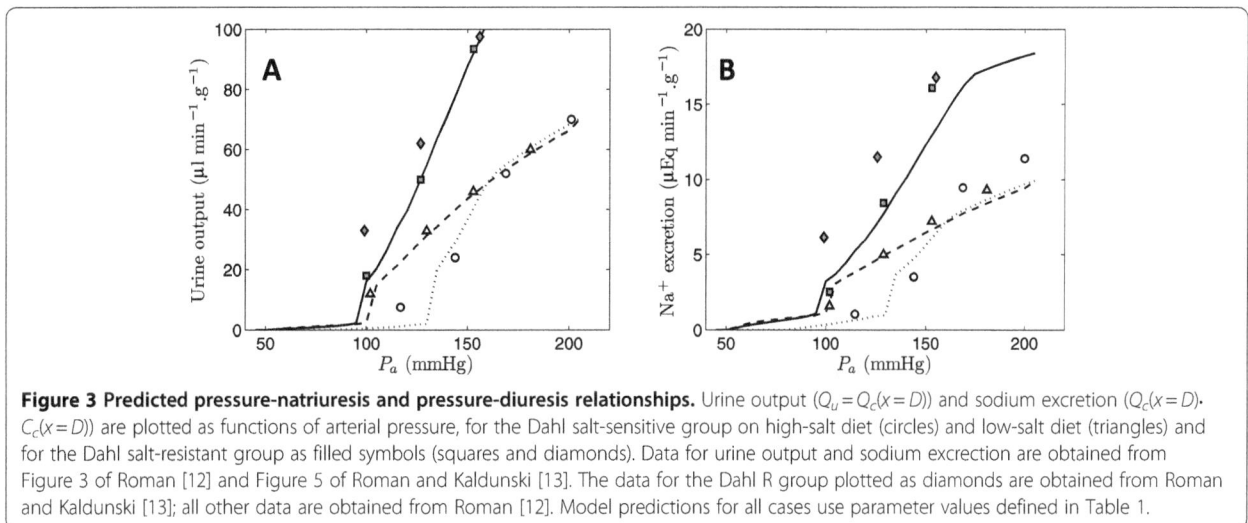

Figure 3 Predicted pressure-natriuresis and pressure-diuresis relationships. Urine output ($Q_u = Q_c(x = D)$) and sodium excretion ($Q_c(x = D) \cdot C_c(x = D)$) are plotted as functions of arterial pressure, for the Dahl salt-sensitive group on high-salt diet (circles) and low-salt diet (triangles) and for the Dahl salt-resistant group as filled symbols (squares and diamonds). Data for urine output and sodium excrection are obtained from Figure 3 of Roman [12] and Figure 5 of Roman and Kaldunski [13]. The data for the Dahl R group plotted as diamonds are obtained from Roman and Kaldunski [13]; all other data are obtained from Roman [12]. Model predictions for all cases use parameter values defined in Table 1.

dependent component of physiological diameter regulation and abolished tubular-glomerular feedback, and because the data of Roman show a clear, if blunted, autoregulation of renal blood flow and filtration in the high-salt animals.

The acute changes in sodium excretion and urine output in response to changes in renal perfusion pressure plotted in Figure 3 are termed the pressure-natriuresis and pressure-diuresis curves. These acute responses should not be confused with long-term relationships between pressure and sodium excretion and urine output, which are influenced by a number of hormonal, neural, and remodeling processes not accounted for here. Here, the acute pressure-natriuresis and diuresis phenomena are effectively reproduced by the model. Since the glomerular filtration and nephron transport parameters are held fixed for all experimental groups, the differences in afferent and efferent arteriole tone are responsible for greatly diminished rates of urine output and increased rate of sodium reabsorption in the SS (on high and low salt) compared to the SR.

Predictions of concentration and flow profiles in the nephron, based on the nephron model, are illustrated in

Figure 4. The upper panel plots model predictions associated with an arterial pressure of 125 mmHg, near the baseline pressure of 126 ± 1 mmHg observed in the (high-salt) SR rats [12]. The lower panel plots model predictions associated with lowering the input pressure to 95 mmHg. Although the differences in input pressure and flow between the upper and lower panels are small, the predicted model behaviors show a major qualitative difference. The slightly lower input flow for the lower pressure simulation results in collecting duct flow that drops to near zero at the outlet at $x = 2$ mm. Also, at lower flow the concentration gradient is greater than at the higher flow. At arterial pressures 95 mmHg and below, the maximal concentrations at $x = 2$ mm are approximately 500 mM, over a three-fold increase of the input concentration of 150 mM.

To summarize the findings of comparing model predictions to data from Roman [12] on high-salt SR and hypertensive (high-salt) and prehypertensive (low-salt) SS rats, the observed differences in renal function may be explained primarily by differences in the control of afferent and efferent resistance and in sodium reabsorption kinetics.

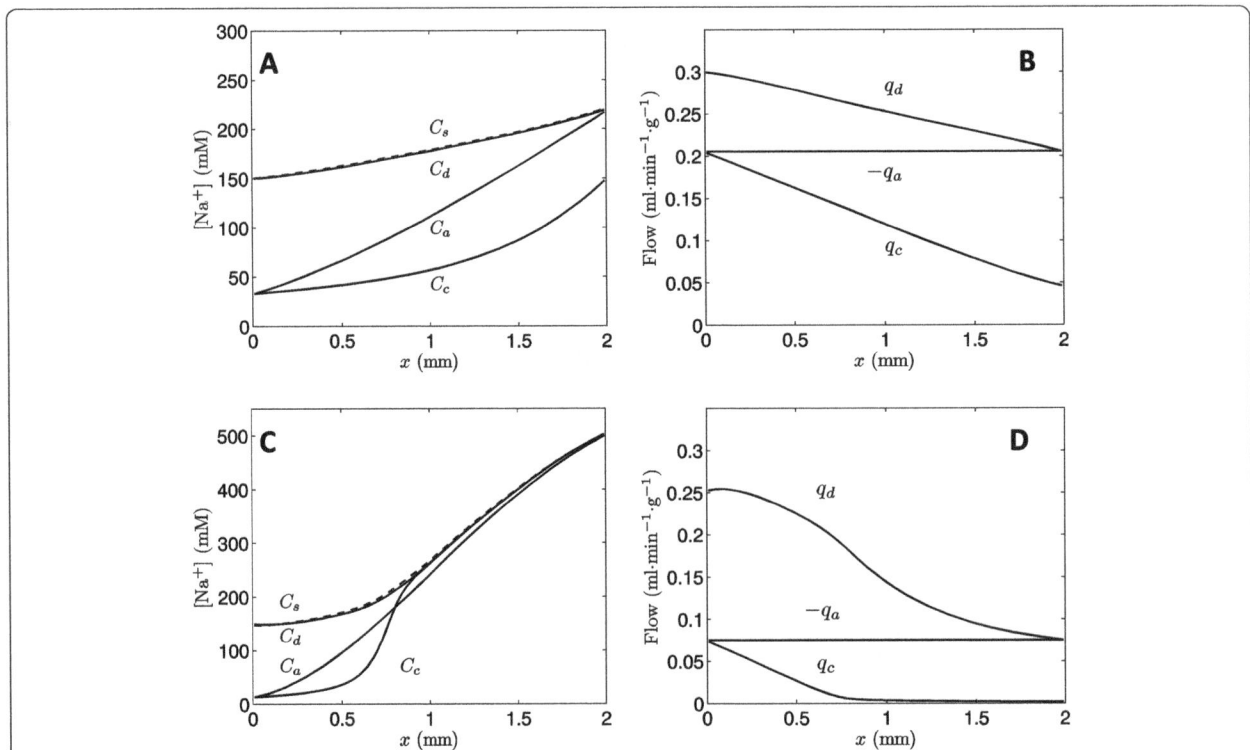

Figure 4 Model-predicted sodium concentration and flow profiles in the nephron model. Simulations are conducted using the parameter values for the Dahl R rat (Table 1). **A**. & **C**. Sodium concentrations as functions of distance along the nephron are plotted for the descending and ascending limb, collecting duct, and interstitium. **B**. & **D**. Flows as functions of distance along the nephron are plotted for the descending and ascending limb and collecting duct. The upper panel (A & B) reports model predictions for the baseline case with $q_d(0) = 0.300$ ml·min^{-1}·g^{-1} and $P_a = 125$ mmHg. The lower panel (**C** & **D**) reports predictions for a lower pressure: $q_d(0) = 0.252$ ml·min^{-1}·g^{-1} and $P_a = 95$ mmHg. At the lower pressure the concentration gradient steepens and output flow drops to near zero.

Discussion

Mechanisms of pressure-natriuresis and pressure-diuresis

Using a simple mathematical model to simulate blood flow regulation, glomerular filtration, and medullary solute transport in the kidney, we have analyzed data from Dahl S and Dahl R rats to investigate the potential mechanistic underpinnings of renal function observed in these animals. While the pressure-natriuresis and pressure-diuresis relationships illustrated in Figure 3 have long been recognized as playing a central role in the long-term control of blood pressure [43], the biophysical mechanisms underlying these phenomena have not been fully resolved. One school of thought maintains that because renal blood flow and glomerular filtration rate do not change over a wide range of arterial pressure, the observed decrease in sodium and water reabsorption associated with an increase in pressure could not be substantially impacted by an increase in the rate of filtrate delivery to nephrons. Observations of reduced sodium-hydrogen exchanger activity in the proximal tubule [44] and increased medullary blood flow [45,46] in response to acute and chronic increases in blood flow point to mechanisms that reduce sodium reabsorption. Another widely held view is that both acute and chronic increases in arterial pressure increase filtration rate and thus directly increase sodium and water excretion through simple mechanical transduction. In a textbook explanation of the pressure-diuresis phenomenon, this primary mechanical response is enhanced by other contributing mechanisms, including the renin-angiotensin system, changes in medullary blood flow, regulation of proximal tubule sodium transport [41].

Our model simulations, as well as the data analyzed here, are consistent with the pressure-natriuresis and pressure-diuresis phenomena emerging from the mechanical relationships between renal pressure, flow, and filtration. Specifically, in the model increasing arterial pressure causes increased glomerular pressure, which causes increasing filtration rate. For the SS rat data sets, an increase in glomerular pressure of 20–30% over the observed pressure range results in an increase in filtration rate of 30% in the low-salt case and almost 90% in the high-salt case. When pressure increases from 100 to 180 mmHg, filtrate flow increases from 700 to over 900 $\mu l \cdot min^{-1} \cdot g^{-1}$ while urine output increases from 10 to 60 $\mu l \cdot min^{-1} \cdot g^{-1}$ in low-salt case. In the high salt case, filtrate flow increases from approximately 480 to 900 $\mu l \cdot min^{-1}$ while urine output increases from 6 to 68 $\mu l \cdot min^{-1} \cdot g^{-1}$ over the pressure range of 120 to 200 mmHg. Thus the slope of filtrate flow (Q_f) versus arterial pressure can be substantially steeper than the slope of urine output (Q_u) versus arterial pressure, even over the pressure range for which blood flow is autoregulated. For these cases the relative change in urine output over the pressure range is much greater than the relative change in filtrate flow because at the lowest pressures nearly all of the filtrate is reabsorbed.

In contrast, the SR data show relatively little increase in filtration over the observed pressure range for the three data points in Figure 2B. For this case, an increase in filtration of approximately 50 $\mu l \cdot min^{-1} \cdot g^{-1}$ is associated with an increase of 65–80 $\mu l \cdot min^{-1} \cdot g^{-1}$ in urine output. For this case the model is not able to capture the nearly constant Q_f as a function of P_a because the glomerular pressure is observed to increase from 44 to 53 mmHg over the same arterial pressure range. Recall that the driving force for filtration is hydrostatic pressure difference minus the oncotic pressure of approximately 28 mmHg. Since the 8 mmHg increase in glomerular pressure over the observed range of arterial pressure represents an approximately 30% increase in driving force for filtration, the model tends to under-represent the slope of P_1 versus P_a while over representing the slope of Q_f versus P_a. It is unclear how to resolve the substantial differences in driving force for filtration with the apparently constant filtration rate observed in the SR rat. The model predicts that Q_f increases roughly 20% over the observed 50 mmHg range of arterial pressure, while measurements in the SS rat and in other rat strains and other species show increases of anywhere from 10% to greater than 20% over the pressure range of autoregulated blood flow [47-49].

The relationship between sodium excretion and glomerular filtrate rate is further explored in Figure 5 by comparing the model predictions of these variables to the data of Thompson and Pitts [14]. Here, model predictions and data are plotted as percent of control since the data are obtained from dog and the model is parameterized for the SR rat. Note that this comparison represents a model prediction where no parameter adjustment has been done to match the data. The non-linear nature of the relationship is effectively captured by the model, where relatively small increases in filtration rate can effect relatively large changes in sodium excretion. Furthermore, the simplified model reveals the extent to which mechanisms not included in the model may be important contributors to the physiological phenomena explored. Specifically, Figure 5 shows that a 20% increase in filtration rate above baseline level elicits a 100% increase in model-predicted urine output rate, for the SR parameter set.

The mechanistic explanation for the pressure-diuresis and pressure-natriuresis phenomena that emerges is illustrated in Figure 6. The upper panel plots conceptualized curves representing glomerular filtration flow and urine flow as functions of arterial pressure. Consistent with the available data, the slopes of glomerular filtration flow and urine flow versus pressure are of the same order of

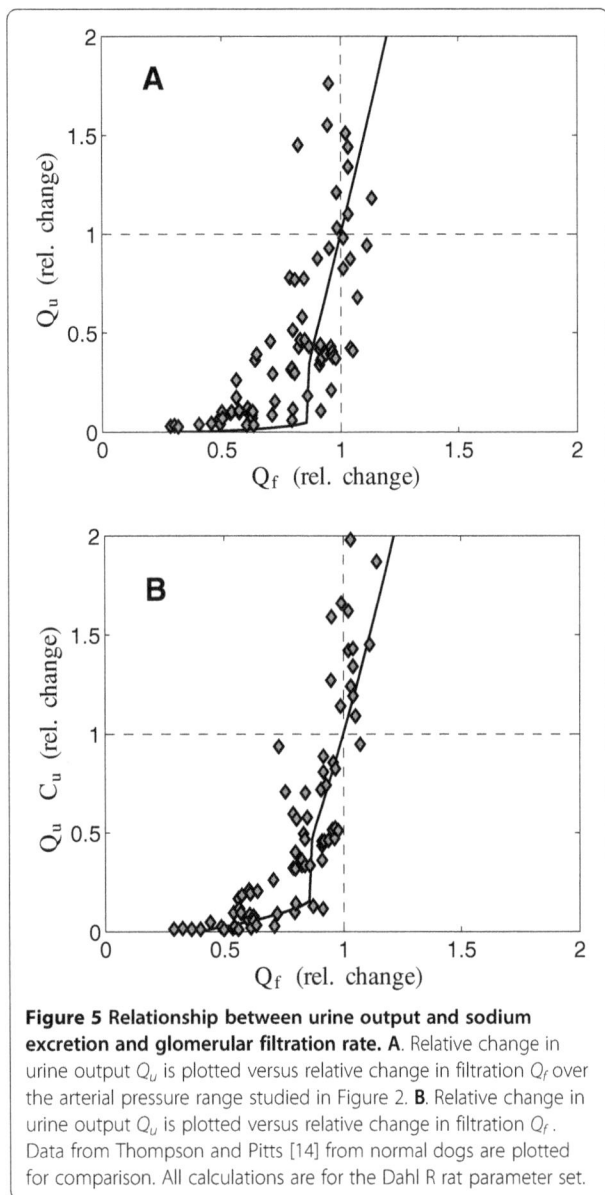

Figure 5 Relationship between urine output and sodium excretion and glomerular filtration rate. A. Relative change in urine output Q_u is plotted versus relative change in filtration Q_f over the arterial pressure range studied in Figure 2. **B**. Relative change in urine output Q_u is plotted versus relative change in filtration Q_f. Data from Thompson and Pitts [14] from normal dogs are plotted for comparison. All calculations are for the Dahl R rat parameter set.

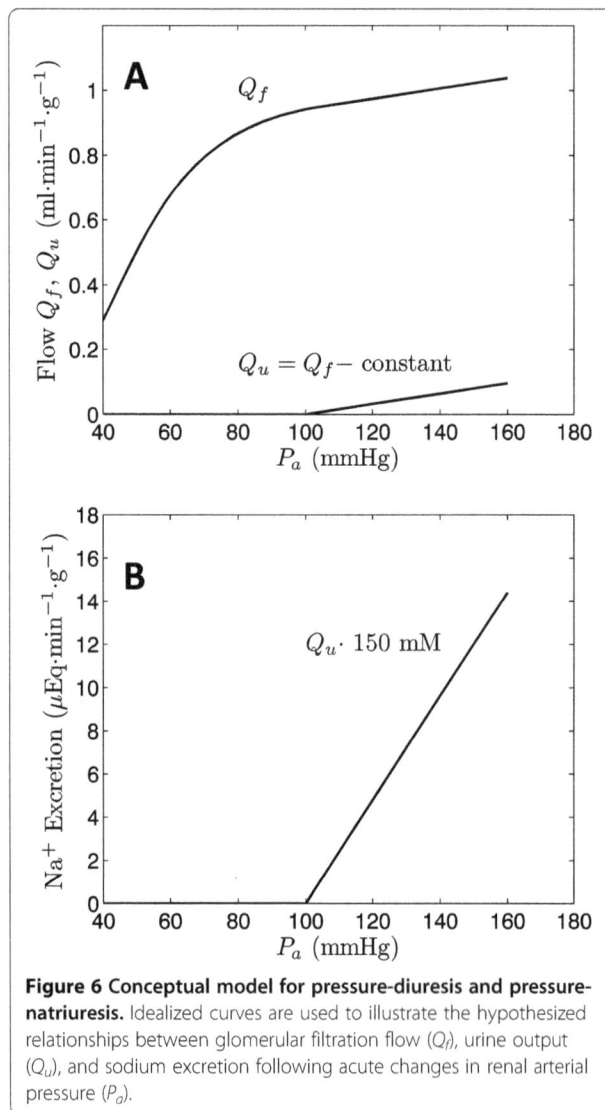

Figure 6 Conceptual model for pressure-diuresis and pressure-natriuresis. Idealized curves are used to illustrate the hypothesized relationships between glomerular filtration flow (Q_f), urine output (Q_u), and sodium excretion following acute changes in renal arterial pressure (P_a).

magnitude over the autoregulated range, here taken to be $P_a = 100$ to 160 mmHg. If the slopes are the same over this pressure range, then Q_u can be approximated as Q_f minus a constant reabsorbed volume. Assuming that sodium concentration remains approximately constant at arterial pressure above the baseline 100 mmHg, the pressure-diuresis relationship of the bottom panel is obtained. While this conceptual model is highly simplified, it does effectively illustrate the basic mechanism that emerges from our mathematical model: since glomerular filtration flow is much larger than urine flow, a relatively small increase in glomerular filtration can cause a relatively large increase in urine output. Thus, this explanation requires that glomerular filtration does increase, albeit slightly, as renal arterial pressure is acutely

increased. If, as has been hypothesized, glomerular filtration remains exactly constant as arterial pressure is acutely increased, then this mechanism cannot explain the observed pressure-diuresis and pressure-natriuresis relationships.

The data from Thompson and Pitts, as well as the data of Roman analyzed in Figures 2 and 3, indicate that the slope of Q_f versus P_a may be lower in normal animals than that captured by the model and that additional secondary mechanisms may be necessary to satisfactorily explain the pressure-diuresis/natriuresis phenomenon. Clearly, mechanical transduction is not the only mechanism at work in vivo. Yet even without a model simulation, it is apparent from the raw data that a given change in pressure can induce a greater change in glomerular filtration than in urine output over the pressure range for which blood flow is autoregulated. The model reveals the extent to which the relationship between acute changes in arterial pressure and glomerular filtration can explain the observed pressure-natriuresis and pressure-diuresis relationships. These findings highlight the direct effects of pressure on influencing urine production by delivering increased filtrate to the proximal tubule. The ability of the model to match observed relationships between arterial pressure and glomerular pressure, urine flow, and sodium excretion depends on the predicted increase in glomerular filtration with pressure that is not apparent in the SR data set. For the model to capture the phenomenon of constant glomerular filtration over the arterial pressure range of 100 to 150 mmHg observed in the SR group would require the introduction of some (unknown) mechanism that reduces glomerular hydraulic permeability in response to acute increases in pressure. Furthermore, since it does not account for hormonal or nervous factors, or changes in medullary blood flow and transporter activities, the model reveals that these factors are not necessary to explain the acute pressure-natriuresis and pressure-diuresis phenomena, at least in the SS rat on low- and high-salt diets.

Physiological differences between SS and SR groups

In addition to revealing insight into how sodium excretion and urine output are influenced by perfusion pressure, model analysis reveals potential mechanistic underpinnings of differences in renal function observed in SR and SS rats when fed on low-salt versus high-salt diets. Our strategy identifies the minimal differences between model parameterizations necessary to explain the data from these groups. Specifically, it was found that differences in five parameters associated with blood flow control (see Table 1) are able to explain a host of differences in renal function observed among the three groups (see Figures 2 and 3).

In developing the model presented here and determining the difference in parameter values necessary to explain the groups, the goal is not to capture all relevant physiological processes impacting renal function and blood pressure regulation in the rat. Indeed several mechanisms important to the renal response to changes in blood pressure, including changes in proximal tubule sodium transport [44] and inner medullary blood flow [45], are not accounted for. In contrast, by focusing on a well-defined set of identifiable physiological processes, we are able to determine a minimal set of processes to explain the data and what differences in those processes are necessary to explain the different experimental cases.

The different parameterizations used to explain the different experimental groups point to increases in afferent resistance and decreases in sodium transport rate as one moves from lower-pressure to higher-pressure animals. The increase in afferent resistance is able to

explain all of the qualitative differences between observed data on renal function—lower flows, filtration rates, and glomerular pressure as well as the shift in the pressure-natriuresis and pressure-diuresis relationships in higher pressure animals. (Since the data analyzed here are obtained from denervated kidneys, the predicted differences in afferent arterial tone cannot be explained based on differences in sympathetic tone, unless chronic differences in sympathetic tone had the effect of chronically altering afferent arterial tone in a way that is reflected in denervated kidneys.)

This observed shift (compared to lower pressure controls) of the pressure-natriuresis relationship to higher pressure necessarily occurs in hypertension. This is because net sodium balance, by definition, must occur at a higher pressure in hypertension than in normotension. The view that the chronic pressure-natriuresis relationship (also called the renal function curve) observed in normal animals is effectively infinitely steep implies that the kidney can maintain blood volume and sodium at nearly constant levels in response to small changes in pressure associated with salt-loading and volume expansion [50]. Furthermore, the steepness of the renal function curve forms the basis of the theory that chronic hypertension in angiotensin- and salt-induced models is caused by renal dysfunction leading to decreased sodium excretion at a given arterial pressure [1-6].

While it is debated whether and/or when renal dysfunction represents the primary cause of chronic hypertension in the SS rat (and other animal models) [51,52], it is clear that the high-salt diet does cause a shift in the acutely measured pressure-natriuresis relationship in the SS rat, as illustrated in Figure 3. These changes are shown here to be underpinned by changes in renal afferent and efferent arterial resistance. If indeed a shift in the pressure-natriuresis relationship is the primary cause of elevated arterial pressure in the Dahl S rat, then alternation in how renal afferent and efferent arterial resistances are regulated represents the primary cause of chronic hypertension in the Dahl S rat.

Assumptions and simplifications of the model

As discussed in the methods section, the developed model for blood flow, glomerular filtration, and sodium transport in the proximal tubule, nephron, and collecting duct developed here is relatively unsophisticated compared to a number of previously developed models of the three-dimensional architecture of the tubules and vasculature [16-19], models of renal flow regulation and tubuloglomerular feedback [20-22], transport in the proximal tubule and cortex [23-25], medulla [17,18,26-35], collecting duct [34,36], and other components [16]. Nor does the model account for different roles for the inner and outer medulla, in terms of tubular function or blood flow, or explicitly for the transport of urea or other solutes. Yet despite the simplifications, the model represents the only available computational model of whole-kidney function that integrates blood flow regulation, glomerular filtration, distributed solute and volume fluxes along a nephron, and tubuloglomerular feedback, to compare whole-kidney pressure-natriuresis and pressure-diuresis phenomena to experimentally observed data.

To a certain degree the level of simplification adopted by the model is justified by the nature of the data analyzed here and the specific questions addressed by the model analysis. The appropriate level of complexity represented by a model is the lowest (most simple) that can capture the biophysical processes underlying the phenomena studied. Based on this standard, the present model may be judged as a reasonable, if imperfect, simplification. The most obvious feature that the model does not capture well is the phenomenon of nearly constant filtration rate observed in the SR group. It is not known what anatomical and physiological features not represented in the current model are critical to improve the behavior of the model in comparison to this observation. While the model makes a number of simplifying assumptions, it is not clear that relaxing any one of those simplifying assumptions would explain the apparent disconnect between driving force for filtration and filtration rate in the SR group. What is clear is that the basic model introduced here represents a useful framework for exploring such questions in a systematic matter.

Conclusions

Analysis of data on renal blood flow, filtration, pressure-diuresis and pressure-natriuresis phenomena in Dahl S and Dahl R rats using a simple mathematical model reveals a hypothetical mechanistic explanation for the observed pressure-diuresis and pressure-natriuresis relationships. Idealized curves plotted in Figure 6 illustrate the hypothesized relationships between glomerular filtration flow (Q_f), urine output (Q_u), and sodium excretion following acute changes in renal arterial pressure (P_a). Increasing pressure is associated with a relatively small increase in glomerular filtration, which increases delivery of filtrate to the nephron, leading to increased urine production. This simplified conceptual model requires that glomerular filtration increases slightly as renal arterial pressure is acutely increased. Furthermore, differences between Dahl salt-sensitive (SS) and salt-resistant (SR) rats in renal filtration and urine production are explained in terms of difference in blood flow regulation.

Appendix: Discretization of nephron equations

Equations (12), (13), and (14) are discretized using finite differences

$$Q_d^{<i>} = Q_d^0 + \Delta x K_d \sum_{j=1}^{i} \left(-\Delta P_d + 2RT \left(C_d^{<j>} - C_s^{<j>} \right) \right)$$

$$Q_a = -Q_d^{<N>}$$

$$Q_c^{<i>} = Q_d^{<N>} + \Delta x K_c \sum_{j=1}^{i} \left(-\Delta P_c + 2RT \left(C_c^{<j>} - C_s^{<j>} \right) \right)$$

$$Q_s^{<i>} = Q_c^{<N>} - \left(Q_d^{<i>} + Q_a^{<i>} + Q_c^{<i>} \right) \tag{25}$$

where $i = 1, 2, \ldots, N$ is the element index and $Q_d^0 = q_d(0)$ is the input flow into the descending limb. The discrete variables $Q_d^{<i>}$, $Q_a^{<i>}$, $Q_c^{<i>}$, and $Q_s^{<i>}$ are numerical approximations for the continuous variables $q_d(x)$, $q_a(x)$, $q_c(x)$, and $q_s(x)$. The equation for $Q_s^{<i>}$ is based on mass conservation and the boundary condition $Q_s^{<N>} = 0$.

The concentrations satisfy numerical approximations of Equations (16) for the descending limb:

$$Q_d^{<i>} C_d^{<i>} - Q_d^0 C_d^0 = \Delta x H_d \left(C_s^{<i>} - C_d^{<i>} \right), i = 1$$
$$Q_d^{<i>} C_d^{<i>} - Q_d^{<i-1>} C_d^{<i-1>}$$
$$\quad = \Delta x H_d \left(C_s^{<i>} - C_d^{<i>} \right), i = 2, 3, \ldots, N \tag{26}$$

Equation (17) for the ascending limb:

$$C_a^{<i>} = C_d^{<N>} + \frac{\Delta x}{Q_a} P \left(C_a^{<i>} \right), i = N$$
$$C_a^{<i>} = C_a^{<i+1>} + \frac{\Delta x}{Q_a} P \left(C_a^{<i>} \right), i = 1, 2, \ldots, N - 1$$
$$\tag{27}$$

Equation (18) or the collecting duct:

$$Q_c^{<i>} C_c^{<i>} - (-Q_a) C_a^{<1>} = \Delta x H_c \left(C_s^{<i>} - C_c^{<i>} \right), i = 1$$
$$Q_c^{<i>} C_c^{<i>} - Q_c^{<i-1>} C_c^{<i-1>}$$
$$\quad = \Delta x H_c \left(C_s^{<i>} - C_c^{<i>} \right), i = 2, 3, \ldots, N \tag{28}$$

and Equation (18) for the interstitium:

$$Q_s^0 = Q_s^{<1>} - \left[Q_d^0 - \left(Q_d^{<1>} + Q_a + Q_c^{<1>} \right) \right]$$
$$Q_s^{<i>} C_s^{<i+1>} - Q_s^0 C_s^{<i>} = \Delta x H_c \left(C_c^{<i>} - C_s^{<i>} \right)$$
$$\quad + \Delta x H_d \left(C_d^{<i>} - C_s^{<i>} \right) + \Delta x P \left(C_a^{<i>} \right), i = 1$$
$$Q_s^{<i>} C_s^{<i+1>} - Q_s^{<i-1>} C_s^{<i>} = \Delta x H_c \left(C_c^{<i>} - C_s^{<i>} \right)$$
$$\quad + \Delta x H_d \left(C_d^{<i>} - C_s^{<i>} \right) + \Delta x P \left(C_a^{<i>} \right), i = 2, 3, \ldots, N - 1$$
$$Q_s^{<i>} C_s^D - Q_s^{<i-1>} C_s^{<i>} = \Delta x H_c \left(C_c^{<i>} - C_s^{<i>} \right)$$
$$\quad + \Delta x H_d \left(C_d^{<i>} - C_s^{<i>} \right) + \Delta x P \left(C_a^{<i>} \right), i = N \tag{29}$$

The input concentration and flow are obtained from the boundary conditions $Q_d^0 = q_d(0)$ and $C_d^0 = c_d(0)$. $Qs^{<N>}$ and C_s^D are the input vasa recta flow and concentration (at $x = D$); $Q_s^{<N>} = q_s(D) = 0$. As long as $Q_s^{<N>} = 0$, the value of C_s^D is arbitrary.

These equations are solved using an iterative method. Computer codes for the model can be obtained by contacting the author.

Authors' contributions
DAB and MM developed the model, carried out the simulation studies, and drafted the manuscript. All authors read and approved the final manuscript.

Acknowledgements
This work was supported by the Virtual Physiological Rat Project funded through NIH grant P50-GM094503.

References
1. Hall JE, Guyton AC, Brands MW: **Pressure-volume regulation in hypertension.** *Kidney Int Suppl* 1996, **55**:S35–S41.
2. Hall JE, Mizelle HL, Hildebrandt DA, Brands MW: **Abnormal pressure natriuresis. A cause or a consequence of hypertension?.** *Hypertension* 1990, **15**(6 Pt 1):547–559.
3. Girardin E, Caverzasio J, Iwai J, Bonjour JP, Muller AF, Grandchamp A: **Pressure natriuresis in isolated kidneys from hypertension-prone and hypertension-resistant rats (Dahl rats).** *Kidney Int* 1980, **18**(1):10–19.
4. Hall JE, Brands MW, Henegar JR: **Angiotensin II and long-term arterial pressure regulation: the overriding dominance of the kidney.** *J Am Soc Nephrol* 1999, **10**(Suppl 12):S258–S265.
5. van der Mark J, Kline RL: **Altered pressure natriuresis in chronic angiotensin II hypertension in rats.** *Am J Physiol* 1994, **266**(3 Pt 2):R739–R748.
6. Hall JE, Granger JP, Hester RL, Coleman TG, Smith MJ Jr, Cross RB: **Mechanisms of escape from sodium retention during angiotensin II hypertension.** *Am J Physiol* 1984, **246**(5 Pt 2):F627–F634.
7. Hall JE, Brands MW, Shek EW: **Central role of the kidney and abnormal fluid volume control in hypertension.** *J Hum Hypertens* 1996, **10**(10):633–639.
8. Hall JE, Guyton AC, Coleman TG, Mizelle HL, Woods LL: **Regulation of arterial pressure: role of pressure natriuresis and diuresis.** *Fed Proc* 1986, **45**(13):2897–2903.
9. Osborn JW, Fink GD, Kuroki MT: **Neural mechanisms of angiotensin II-salt hypertension: implications for therapies targeting neural control of the splanchnic circulation.** *Curr Hypertens Rep* 2011, **13**(3):221–228.
10. Toney GM, Pedrino GR, Fink GD, Osborn JW: **Does enhanced respiratory-sympathetic coupling contribute to peripheral neural mechanisms of angiotensin II-salt hypertension?.** *Exp Physiol* 2010, **95**(5):587–594.
11. Yoshimoto M, Miki K, Fink GD, King A, Osborn JW: **Chronic angiotensin II infusion causes differential responses in regional sympathetic nerve activity in rats.** *Hypertension* 2010, **55**(3):644–651.
12. Roman RJ: **Abnormal renal hemodynamics and pressure-natriuresis relationship in Dahl salt-sensitive rats.** *Am J Physiol* 1986, **251**(1 Pt 2):F57–F65.
13. Roman RJ, Kaldunski M: **Pressure natriuresis and cortical and papillary blood flow in inbred Dahl rats.** *Am J Physiol* 1991, **261**(3 Pt 2):R595–R602.
14. Thompson DD, Pitts RF: **Effects of alterations of renal arterial pressure on sodium and water excretion.** *Am J Physiol* 1952, **168**(2):490–499.
15. Keener JP, Sneyd J: *Mathematical physiology.* New York: Springer; 1998.
16. Thomas SR: **Kidney modeling and systems physiology.** *Wiley Interdiscip Rev Syst Biol Med* 2009, **1**(2):172–190.
17. Wexler AS, Kalaba RE, Marsh DJ: **Three-dimensional anatomy and renal concentrating mechanism. I. Modeling results.** *Am J Physiol* 1991, **260**(3 Pt 2):F368–F383.
18. Layton AT, Pannabecker TL, Dantzler WH, Layton HE: **Two modes for concentrating urine in rat inner medulla.** *Am J Physiol Renal Physiol* 2004, **287**(4):F816–F839.
19. Pannabecker TL, Dantzler WH, Layton HE, Layton AT: **Role of three-dimensional architecture in the urine concentrating mechanism of the rat renal inner medulla.** *Am J Physiol Renal Physiol* 2008, **295**(5):F1271–F1285.
20. Kleinstreuer N, David T, Plank MJ, Endre Z: **Dynamic myogenic autoregulation in the rat kidney: a whole-organ model.** *Am J Physiol Renal Physiol* 2008, **294**(6):F1453–F1464.
21. Holstein-Rathlou NH, Marsh DJ: **Renal blood flow regulation and arterial pressure fluctuations: a case study in nonlinear dynamics.** *Physiol Rev* 1994, **74**(3):637–681.
22. Layton AT, Moore LC, Layton HE: **Multistability in tubuloglomerular feedback and spectral complexity in spontaneously hypertensive rats.** *Am J Physiol Renal Physiol* 2006, **291**(1):F79–F97.
23. Weinstein AM: **Modeling the proximal tubule: complications of the paracellular pathway.** *Am J Physiol* 1988, **254**(3 Pt 2):F297–F305.
24. Weinstein AM: **Glomerulotubular balance in a mathematical model of the proximal nephron.** *Am J Physiol* 1990, **258**(3 Pt 2):F612–F626.
25. Thomas SR, Dagher G: **A kinetic model of rat proximal tubule transport–load-dependent bicarbonate reabsorption along the tubule.** *Bull Math Biol* 1994, **56**(3):431–458.
26. Marsh DJ, Segel LA: **Analysis of countercurrent diffusion exchange in blood vessels of the renal medulla.** *Am J Physiol* 1971, **221**(3):817–828.
27. Kokko JP, Rector FC Jr: **Countercurrent multiplication system without active transport in inner medulla.** *Kidney Int* 1972, **2**(4):214–223.
28. Palatt PJ, Saidel GM: **Countercurrent exchange in the inner renal medulla: vasa recta- descending limb system.** *Bull Math Biol* 1973, **35**(4):431–447.
29. Pallone TL, Morgenthaler TI, Deen WM: **Analysis of microvascular water and solute exchanges in the renal medulla.** *Am J Physiol* 1984, **247**(2 Pt 2):F303–F315.
30. Wexler AS, Kalaba RE, Marsh DJ: **Passive, one-dimensional countercurrent models do not simulate hypertonic urine formation.** *Am J Physiol* 1987, **253**(5 Pt 2):F1020–F1030.
31. Stephenson JL, Jen JF, Wang H, Tewarson RP: **Convective uphill transport of NaCl from ascending thin limb of loop of Henle.** *Am J Physiol* 1995, **268**(4 Pt 2):F680–F692.
32. Weinstein AM: **A mathematical model of the inner medullary collecting duct of the rat: acid/base transport.** *Am J Physiol* 1998, **274**(5 Pt 2):F856–F867.
33. Weinstein AM: **A mathematical model of the inner medullary collecting duct of the rat: pathways for Na and K transport.** *Am J Physiol* 1998, **274**(5 Pt 2):F841–F855.
34. Weinstein AM: **A mathematical model of the outer medullary collecting duct of the rat.** *Am J Physiol Renal Physiol* 2000, **279**(1):F24–F45.
35. Hervy S, Thomas SR: **Inner medullary lactate production and urine-concentrating mechanism: a flat medullary model.** *Am J Physiol Renal Physiol* 2003, **284**(1):F65–F81.
36. Weinstein AM: **A mathematical model of rat collecting duct. I. Flow effects on transport and urinary acidification.** *Am J Physiol Ren Physiol* 2002, **283**(6):F1237–F1251.
37. Ikeda N, Maruo F, Shirataka M: **A model of overall regulation of body fluids.** *Ann Biomed Eng* 1979, **7**:135–166.
38. Karaaslan F, Denizhan Y, Kayserilioglu A, Ozcan Gulcur H: **Long-term mathematical model involving renal sympathetic nerve activity, arterial pressure, and sodium excretion.** *Ann Biomed Eng* 2005, **33**(11):1607–1630.
39. Thomas SR, Baconnier P, Fontecave J, Françoise JP, Guillaud F, Hannaert P, Hernandez A, Le Rolle V, Maziere P, Tahi F, *et al*: **SAPHIR: a physiome core model of body fluid homeostasis and blood pressure regulation.** *Phil Trans Math Phys Eng Sci* 2008, **36**(1878):3175–3197.
40. McLoone VI, Ringwood JV, Van Liet BN: **A multi-component model of the dynamics of salt-induced hypertension in Dahl-S rats.** *BMC Physiol* 2009, **9**:20.
41. Boron WF, Boulpaep EL: *Medical physiology: a cellular and molecular approach.* Updatedthth edition. Philadelphia: Elsevier Saunders; 2005.
42. Takenaka T, Forster H, De Micheli A, Epstein M: **Impaired myogenic responsiveness of renal microvessels in Dahl salt-sensitive rats.** *Circ Res* 1992, **71**(2):471–480.
43. Cowley AW Jr: **Long-term control of arterial blood pressure.** *Physiol Rev* 1992, **72**(1):231–300.
44. McDonough AA, Leong PK, Yang LE: **Mechanisms of pressure natriuresis: how blood pressure regulates renal sodium transport.** *Ann N Y Acad Sci* 2003, **986**:669–677.
45. Cowley AW Jr: **Role of the renal medulla in volume and arterial pressure regulation.** *Am J Physiol* 1997, **273**(1 Pt 2):R1–R15.
46. Pallone TL, Edwards A, Mattson DL: **Renal Medullary Circulation.** *Compr Physiol* 2012, **2**:97–140.

47. Baer PG, Navar LG, Guyton AC: **Renal autoregulation, filtration rate, and electrolyte excretion during vasodilatation.** *Am J Physiol* 1970, **219**(3):619–625.

48. Roman RJ: **Pressure-diuresis in volume-expanded rats. Tubular reabsorption in superficial and deep nephrons.** *Hypertension* 1988, **12**(2):177–183.

49. Roman RJ, Cowley AW Jr: **Abnormal pressure-diuresis-natriuresis response in spontaneously hypertensive rats.** *Am J Physiol* 1985, **248**(2 Pt 2):F199–F205.

50. Guyton AC: **Long-term arterial pressure control: an analysis from animal experiments and computer and graphic models.** *Am J Physiol* 1990, **259**(5 Pt 2):R865–R877.

51. Osborn JW, Averina VA, Fink GD: **Current computational models do not reveal the importance of the nervous system in long-term control of arterial pressure.** *Exp Physiol* 2009, **94**(4):389–396.

52. Montani JP, Van Vliet BN: **Understanding the contribution of Guyton's large circulatory model to long-term control of arterial pressure.** *Exp Physiol* 2009, **94**(4):382–388.

2

Impact of maternal dietary fat supplementation during gestation upon skeletal muscle in neonatal pigs

Hernan P Fainberg[1], Kayleigh L Almond[2,5], Dongfang Li[3], Cyril Rauch[1], Paul Bikker[4,6], Michael E Symonds[2] and Alison Mostyn[1*]

Abstract

Background: Maternal diet during pregnancy can modulate skeletal muscle development of the offspring. Previous studies in pigs have indicated that a fat supplemented diet during pregnancy can improve piglet outcome, however, this is in contrast to human studies suggesting adverse effects of saturated fats during pregnancy. This study aimed to investigate the impact of a fat supplemented (palm oil) "high fat" diet on skeletal muscle development in a porcine model. Histological and metabolic features of the *biceps femoris* muscle obtained from 7-day-old piglets born to sows assigned to either a commercial (C, n = 7) or to an isocaloric fat supplementation diet ("high fat" HF, n = 7) during pregnancy were assessed.

Results: Offspring exposed to a maternal HF diet demonstrated enhanced muscular development, reflected by an increase in fractional growth rate, rise in myofibre cross-sectional area, increased storage of glycogen and reduction in lipid staining of myofibres. Although both groups had similar intramuscular protein and triglyceride concentrations, the offspring born to HF mothers had a higher proportion of arachidonic acid (C20:4n6) and a reduction in α-linolenic acid (C18:3n3) compared to C group offspring. The HF group muscle also exhibited a higher ratio of C20:3n6 to C20:4n6 and total n-6 to n-3 in conjunction with up-regulation of genes associated with free fatty acid uptake and biogenesis.

Conclusion: In conclusion, a HF gestational diet accelerates the maturation of offspring *biceps femoris* muscle, reflected in increased glycolytic metabolism and fibre cross sectional area, differences accompanied with a potential resetting of myofibre nutrient uptake.

Keywords: Nutrition, Muscle, Fetal development, Growth

Background

Despite the success of breeding programs for increasing lean mass, the rate of postnatal death in European "commercial" pig breeds (such as the Large White) has remained high at approximately 10-20% per litter and is therefore a major economic concern to the swine industry [1-3]. The neonatal piglet has body energy reserves of around 270 KJ, mainly in the form of glycogen located in the liver and muscle with little white adipose tissue (~1% body weight comprises adipose tissue) and currently little evidence for brown adipose tissue [4]. Consequently the neonatal pig is reliant on a regular supply of milk to prevent hypoglycaemia, a major cause of neonatal death [3,5,6]. Consequently each dam requires a daily intake of up to 1340 KJ per day to maintain a positive energy balance and support the nutritional requirements of her litter [5,7].

One strategy to reduce neonatal mortality is to add saturated fat to the maternal diet during gestation to promote glycogen and fat deposition in the fetus [8-12] and to promote pre-weaning survival of piglets by improving their energy status [12]. However, there is evidence in both human and animal studies to suggest that consumption of a high-fat diet increases the risk of developing

* Correspondence: alison.mostyn@nottingham.ac.uk
[1]School of Veterinary Medicine and Science, University of Nottingham, Sutton Bonington Campus, Leicestershire LE12 5RD, UK
Full list of author information is available at the end of the article

insulin resistance, sometimes without an increase in fat mass [13-19].

The ability to suckle effectively during the first week of postnatal life is critical to piglet survival, highlighting the importance of physical mobility and therefore appropriate muscular development [3,20]. Formation and contractile differentiation of muscle fibres in the pig, as in most large mammals including humans and sheep, occurs in distinct developmental stages during gestation [21,22] and can be influenced by external factors, including the maternal and postnatal nutritional environments [23,24]. Primary myofibres begin to differentiate at around 35 days gestation, followed by secondary and tertiary fibres and by the first days of postnatal life this process is permanently inhibited [22]. Between 75 days gestation until 8 weeks of postnatal life, each fibre develops its own metabolic phenotype, which is associated with muscular maturation [21,25]. However, during the first 7 days of postnatal life, due to improvements in fatty acid metabolism, there is a rapid maturation in the piglets' skeletal muscle fibre types and growth which requires high levels of protein synthesis [22,26]. Between 7 and 26 days (weaning) protein synthesis declines rapidly [27]. This maturation is characterised by a rise in glycogen storage, leading to an increase in glycolytic metabolism, gene expression plus the activation of enzymes involved in carbohydrate metabolism [28]. These metabolic changes induce fibre hypertrophy and increase muscular strength – both changes are necessary to increase body weight and facilitate mobility and food intake [25,27,28]. Modifications in myofibre development during the first weeks of postnatal life could therefore have important implications for subsequent muscular metabolic capacity. The n-3 (α linolenic acid) and n-6 (linoleic acid) polyunsaturated fatty acids (PUFAs) are considered to be "essential" as they cannot be synthesised by mammalian cells [29], these fatty acids are a crucial component of the phospholipid membrane of skeletal muscle fibres. Whole animal and in vitro studies have highlighted the importance of essential fatty acids in muscle development; improved muscle development, maintenance and function was observed in cattle fed an n-3 PUFA supplemented diet and n-3 PUFA supplementation of L6 skeletal muscle cells also activated differentiation [30,31]. Previous work conducted by our research team, in which we compared the hepatic development of new-born Large White pigs with the slower growing Meishan breed, revealed that these essential fatty acids have a major role in hepatic development during gestation and postnatal growth and metabolism [32]. The ratios of n-6 and n-3 fatty acids within the membrane of skeletal muscle have been implicated in glucose homeostasis [8]. To examine the underlying metabolic and developmental changes during early life, the present study compared two maternal isocaloric gestational diets, a standard commercial diet (control; C) or palmitic acid (a saturated fatty acid) supplemented diet (high fat; HF) upon the *biceps femoris*, a mainly glycolytic muscle, of 7-day-old offspring, when energy requirements are at a peak. Given the impact of fatty acids on muscle development outlined above, we hypothesise that increases in maternal fat intake during gestation would accelerate the *biceps femoris'* maturation from oxidative to glycolytic metabolism; increase energy usage and related parameters of muscular development, including myofibre hypertrophy as well as produce differential fatty acid profiles.

Results

Characteristics of the sows and their offspring

Sow body weight increased throughout gestation, irrespective of diet (P < 0.05, Table 1). Maternal plasma HDL concentrations were raised in the HF group compared to controls, whereas plasma LDL, triglycerides and glucose were unaffected. Sow's milk on day 2 of lactation contained 8% fat, 5% lactose and 6% protein and was unaffected by maternal diet [33]. There was no effect on the length of gestation (C = 117.4 ± 0.3; HF = 116.1 ± 0.7 days (P = 0.19)), mean birth weight (C = 1.22 ± 0.04; HF = 1.25 ± 0.07 kg (P = 0.56)) or litter size (C, 14.9 ± 0.8; FS, 16.4 ± 0.7 piglets/sow (P = 0.07)), but by 7 days of age the offspring born to HF mothers were heavier than controls evidenced by a greater fractional growth rate (Figure 1).

Fibre characteristics and association with body weight

Myofibre cross sectional area (CSA) was higher in the HF group (Figure 2A, B and C), this was positively associated with body weight at 7 days of age as demonstrated in Figure 2D. HF offspring also had reduced myocellular lipids; these were mainly stored on fibres located at the centre of the muscle fascicules (Figure 3A, B and C). Despite the changes in myofibre CSA, there were no differences in CSA of type I fibres (Figure 3D and 3E; C: 232.7 ± 31.3; HF: 317.6 ± 38.9 CSA μm^2 (P = 0.165)).

Gene expression, biochemical and metabolic responses

The gene expression and activities of enzymes involved in muscle metabolism were examined; the activity ratio of LDH (a pro-glycolytic enzyme) and ICDH (an indicator of global mitochondrial oxidation) were higher in the piglets born to mothers fed a HF diet compared to controls (Figure 4A). The ratio of NAD+/NADH, a marker of enhanced cellular oxidative capacity, was significantly lower in the HF group (Figure 4B).

The *biceps femoris* muscle of offspring born to HF fed mothers demonstrated raised expression of the genes ENO3, PGAM2, FAT/CD36 and a reduction in GLUT-1 (Figure 5), but there were no differences in either GLUT-4 (C = 1.0 ± 0.1; HF = 1.5 ± 0.5 (P = 0.12)) or CPT-1

Table 1 Body weight and blood biochemistry of the sows as measured at 0, 40 and 108 days of gestation

Days of gestation	0	40	108	p
Sow weight (Kg)				
C	215.5 ± 13.4	236.6 ± 11.8	287.7 ± 10.5	
HF	209.8 ± 9.2	254.6 ± 8.6	281.8 ± 8.7	
HDL (mmol/l)				
C	0.55 ± 0.05	0.55 ± 0.05*	0.42 ± 0.03[#]	*< 0.05; #< 0.01
HF	0.66 ± 0.05	0.77 ± 0.04*	0.56 ± 0.04[#]	
LDL (mmol/l)				
C	0.68 ± 0.06	0.87 ± 0.05	0.74 ± 0.03	
HF	0.75 ± 0.06	0.98 ± 0.08	0.84 ± 0.08	
Glucose (mmol/l)				
C	3.88 ± 0.57	3.93 ± 0.12	3.93 ± 0.10	
HF	3.58 ± 0.51	4.11 ± 0.08	3.70 ± 0.17	

Values are means ± SEM. C: control (n = 7); HF: high fat (n = 7); HDL: High-density lipoprotein; LDL: Low-density lipoprotein. Superscripts denote significance levels between dietary groups, *< 0.05; #< 0.01.

(C = 1.0 ± 0.1; HF = 1.2 ± 0.1 (0.66)). Consistent with the increases in pro-glycolytic activity, the muscle samples obtained from HF offspring exhibited a higher concentration of glycogen compared to controls (C = 20.3 ± 2.4; HF = 61.8 ± 16.0 mg g tissue^{-1} (P = 0.007)). However, there were no differences between the groups for intramuscular triglyceride (C = 16.7 ± 1.6; HF = 23.8 ± 3.3 mg g tissue^{-1} (P = 0.31) or protein content (C = 39 ± 3; HF = 41 ± 2 mg g tissue^{-1} (P = 0.624)).

Fatty acid content and lipid metabolism

The proportion of n-6 to n-3 phospholipids and linoleic acid (C18:2n6C) to α-linoleic acid (C18:3n3) (p < 0.01), were all higher in the HF offspring than controls (Table 2) as was the percentage of arachidonic acid (C20:4n6) and ratio of C20:4n6 to C20:3n6, a surrogate of 5Δ denaturase activity [34]. In contrast, the amount of C18:3n3 was reduced in offspring born to HF sows (Table 2). The proportions of a majority of non-essential (saturated and

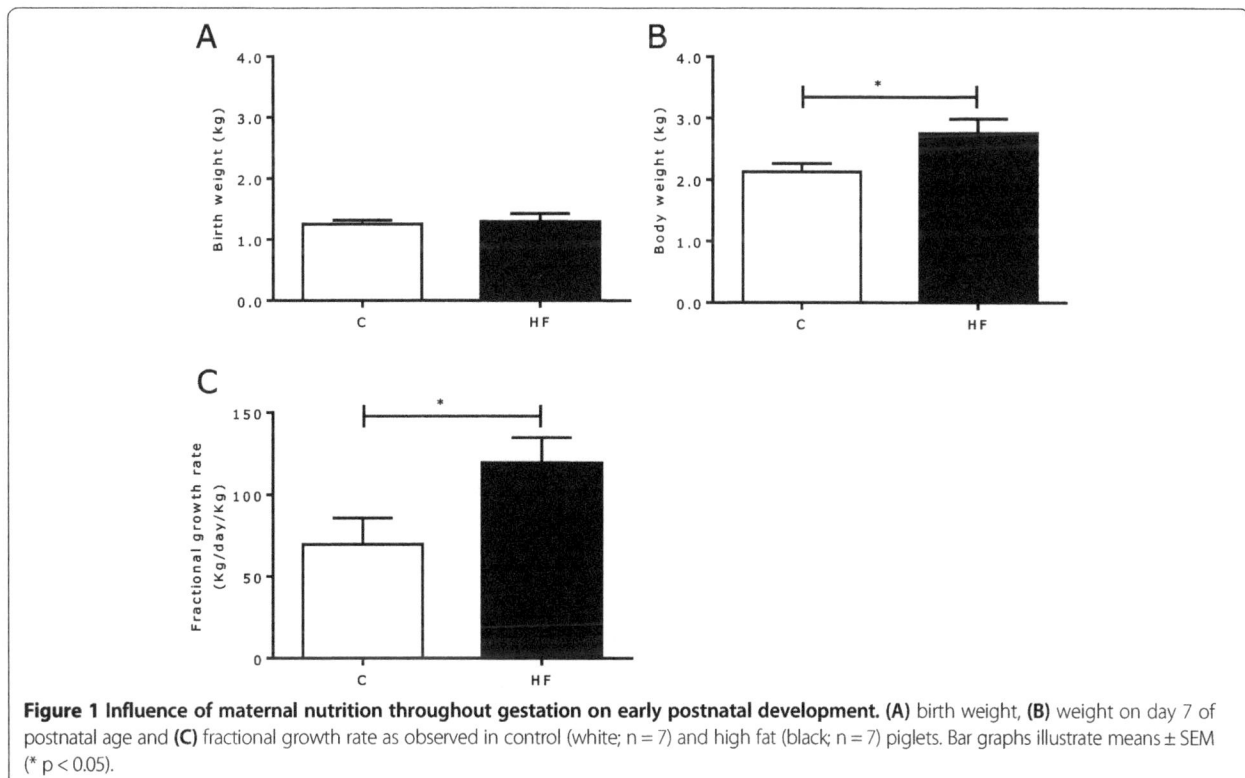

Figure 1 Influence of maternal nutrition throughout gestation on early postnatal development. (A) birth weight, **(B)** weight on day 7 of postnatal age and **(C)** fractional growth rate as observed in control (white; n = 7) and high fat (black; n = 7) piglets. Bar graphs illustrate means ± SEM (* p < 0.05).

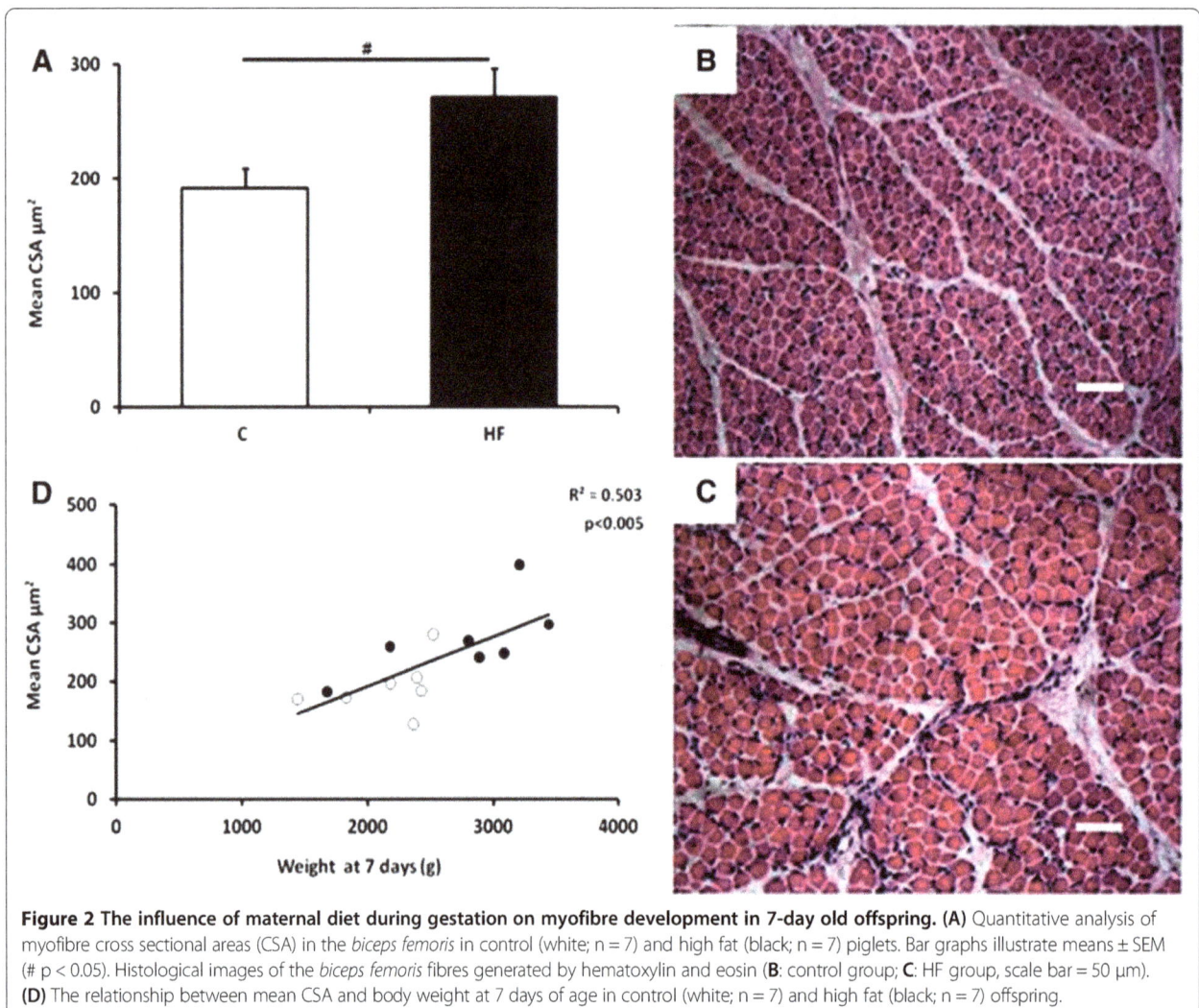

Figure 2 The influence of maternal diet during gestation on myofibre development in 7-day old offspring. (A) Quantitative analysis of myofibre cross sectional areas (CSA) in the *biceps femoris* in control (white; n = 7) and high fat (black; n = 7) piglets. Bar graphs illustrate means ± SEM (# p < 0.05). Histological images of the *biceps femoris* fibres generated by hematoxylin and eosin (**B**: control group; **C**: HF group, scale bar = 50 μm). **(D)** The relationship between mean CSA and body weight at 7 days of age in control (white; n = 7) and high fat (black; n = 7) offspring.

monounsaturated) fatty acids were similar between groups with the exception of arachidic acid (C20:0) in the HF group, which was higher than controls (Table 2).

Discussion

The objective of this study was to explore the potential consequences of fat supplementation of the maternal diet during gestation on skeletal muscle composition in the neonate – a period of intense energy use in the pig. We have demonstrated that the transition from oxidative to glycolytic muscular metabolism was enhanced in offspring born to fat supplemented sows. This was accompanied with changes in muscle phospholipid composition; namely an increase in arachidonic acid and a decrease in α linolenic acid leading to an increase in the n6/n3 ratio and an increased neonatal growth rate in the absence of any effect on offspring birth weight.

We hypothesise that muscle metabolism was reset in utero as a consequence of an increased supply of energy from the mother ultimately leading to improved glycolytic

and lipogenic capacity, thereby promoting myofibre development during early lactation. Although neither individual skeletal muscles nor total muscle mass was assessed due to the limited space and time available during pig sampling within a normal commercial pig unit, we have previously shown that total muscle mass is not influenced by body weight after one week of age [35]. The progeny of fat supplemented sows may have experienced an improvement in the utilization of linoleic acid for conversion to arachidonic acid potentially activating prostaglandin production, an essential pathway for muscular development, although we did not observe differences in expression of cyclo-oxygenase (COX) 1 or 2 in the muscle from offspring [2,36,37]. To date, much of the developmental programming research involving increased fat consumption has investigated the effects of maternal obesity [8,38] but has not examined the effects of macronutrient replacement in an isocaloric manner in a large mammal, such as the pig. Only limited amounts of fatty acids cross the porcine placenta, so their contribution to fetal and muscular

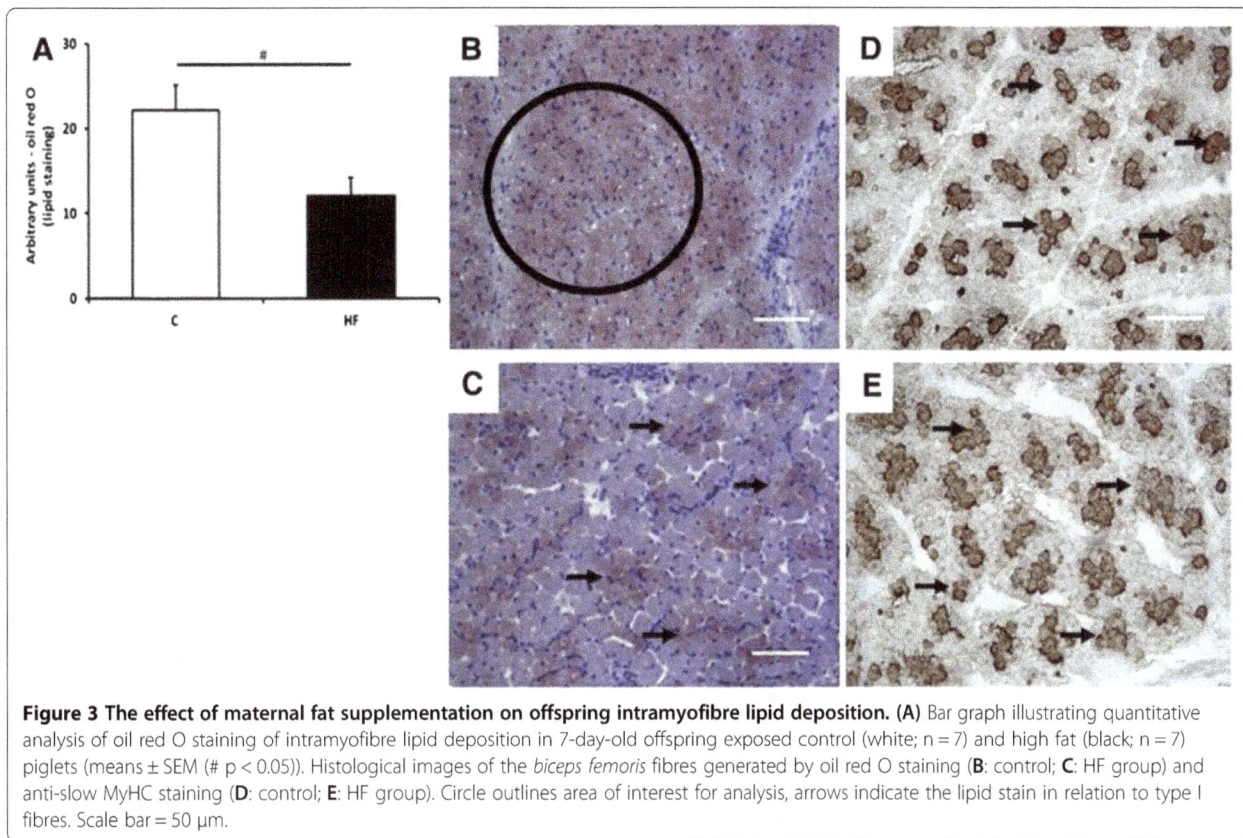

Figure 3 The effect of maternal fat supplementation on offspring intramyofibre lipid deposition. (A) Bar graph illustrating quantitative analysis of oil red O staining of intramyofibre lipid deposition in 7-day-old offspring exposed control (white; n = 7) and high fat (black; n = 7) piglets (means ± SEM (# p < 0.05)). Histological images of the *biceps femoris* fibres generated by oil red O staining (**B**: control; **C**: HF group) and anti-slow MyHC staining (**D**: control; **E**: HF group). Circle outlines area of interest for analysis, arrows indicate the lipid stain in relation to type I fibres. Scale bar = 50 μm.

development is normally minimal [39]. Our dietary manipulation may have promoted a more efficient mobilization of maternal body fat, reflected by the raised maternal HDL which would allow a constant supply of glucose to the growing fetuses [40], for which glucose is a primary substrate for myogenesis [41]. Piglets born to mothers exposed to a fat supplemented diet grew faster up to 7 days and exhibited a proportional expansion of myofibres and a metabolic maturation toward glycolysis, in the *biceps femoris* similar to the findings of Jean and Chiang [42]. Histological analysis, however, failed to indicate which muscle fibre types were affected but decreased lipid staining was found within fibres located in the periphery of the fascicle, in parallel to a substantial increase in muscular glycogen, suggesting more efficient muscle metabolism [43]. Although we cannot exclude reduced carbohydrate having a role in regulating the changes observed, as summarised in a systematic review of animal studies [44] which have adopted fat feeding to mothers, our findings are supportive of the concept that fat is the main nutrient responsible.

Enhanced whole-body growth requires extra nutrition in order to meet the increased metabolic demands, especially within skeletal muscle [45]. An increase in nutrient flux would reset the cellular ratio of NAD^+ to NADH thereby potentially increasing the concentration of NADH, which

in turn, would inhibit activity of ICDH to decrease the influx of glycolytic metabolites through the mitochondria, these findings were observed in the fat supplemented offspring [41,46]. Additionally, the increase in mRNA expression of genes for proteins involved in glycolysis, such as ENO3 and PGAM2, together with greater GLUT-1 (which is independent of insulin) and LDH enzymatic activity are all indicative of greater glucose consumption [47]. Other indicators of muscular development, such as the muscular protein content, total triglyceride content and the mRNA expression of GLUT-4 were unaffected, emphasising that other components of muscle metabolism were unaffected.

Can maternal diet modify the muscular incorporation of essential fatty acids in the neonate?

We also observed differential effects of maternal fat supplementation upon muscle fatty acid composition of the offspring, in particular n-6 and n-3 fatty acids. These essential fatty acids are crucial components of the cellular membrane, affecting structural and regulatory properties that need to adapt to changes in fatty acid supply [48,49]. There is indirect evidence of a different pattern of muscular incorporation of two essential fatty acids, arachidonic acid (C20:4n6) and α-linoleic acid (C18:3n3). Both of these fatty acids are involved in several metabolic pathways

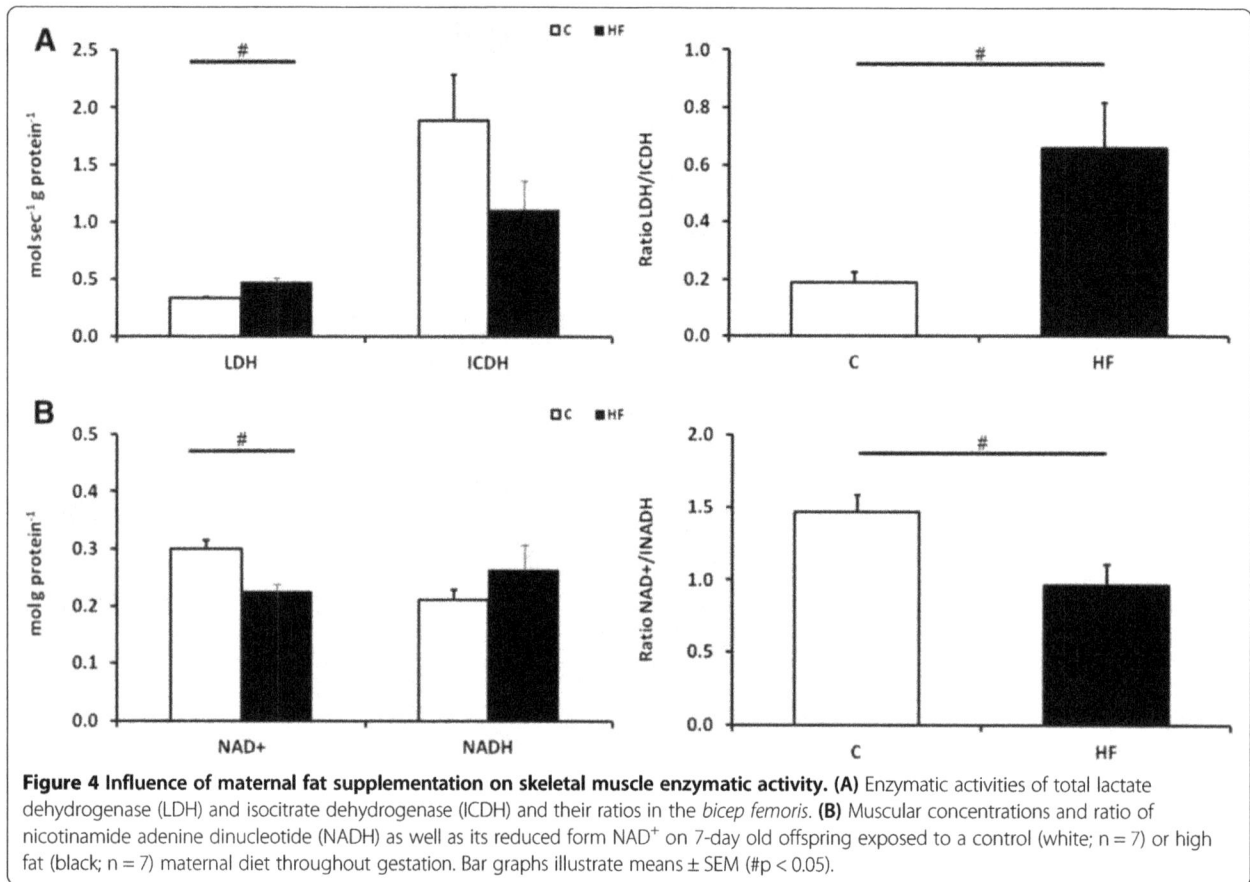

Figure 4 Influence of maternal fat supplementation on skeletal muscle enzymatic activity. (A) Enzymatic activities of total lactate dehydrogenase (LDH) and isocitrate dehydrogenase (ICDH) and their ratios in the *bicep femoris*. **(B)** Muscular concentrations and ratio of nicotinamide adenine dinucleotide (NADH) as well as its reduced form NAD^+ on 7-day old offspring exposed to a control (white; n = 7) or high fat (black; n = 7) maternal diet throughout gestation. Bar graphs illustrate means ± SEM ($\#p < 0.05$).

associated with muscular development and insulin signalling [8]. α-linolenic acid itself can repress the actions of arachidonic acid, it appears likely that reduced α-linolenic acid is responsible for the increased proportion of arachidonic, and may facilitate further muscle growth [50]. The fatty acid composition of skeletal muscle is also influenced by lipid binding proteins such as LPL and CD36/FAT,

which allow circulating triglycerides to be hydrolyzed and free fatty acids to be accumulated [48,51]. Expression of both these genes was increased in fat supplemented offspring, suggesting these processes were enhanced.

Conclusions

Isocaloric replacement of starch with palm oil in the diet of pregnant sows has no effect on birth weight but does promote the ability of offspring to differentiate and develop muscle fibres of the *biceps femoris* by increasing glycolytic capacity [52]. This pattern of growth is sustained by an increase in cellular energy uptake and usage as well as differential activation of elongases and desaturases, that could affect myofibre metabolism [49]. These adaptations, which remain to be quantified in the long-term, may be useful to improve piglet survival.

Methods
Materials and methods
All animal procedures described in this manuscript were approved by the Ethics Committee for Animal Experiments of the Animal Sciences Group of Wageningen Research Centre, and conducted at Schothorst Feed Research in the Netherlands. All laboratory procedures were carried out at The University of Nottingham

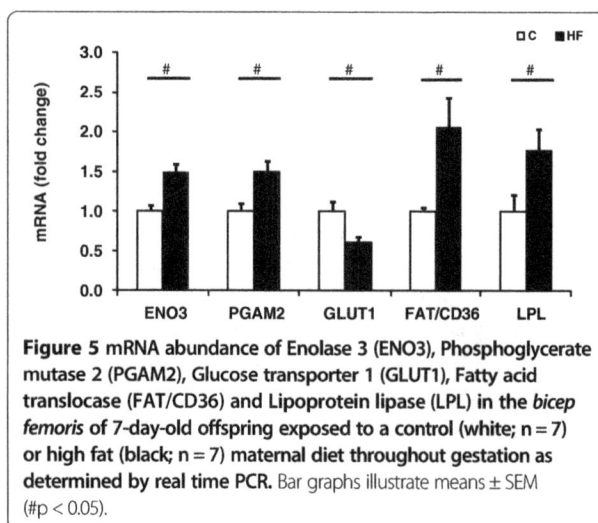

Figure 5 mRNA abundance of Enolase 3 (ENO3), Phosphoglycerate mutase 2 (PGAM2), Glucose transporter 1 (GLUT1), Fatty acid translocase (FAT/CD36) and Lipoprotein lipase (LPL) in the *bicep femoris* of 7-day-old offspring exposed to a control (white; n = 7) or high fat (black; n = 7) maternal diet throughout gestation as determined by real time PCR. Bar graphs illustrate means ± SEM ($\#p < 0.05$).

Table 2 Fatty acid composition of muscular phospholipids as measured in the piglets at 7 days of age after maternal high fat (HF, n = 7) or control (C, n = 7) feeding

Group	C	HF	p
Non-essential fatty acids			
saturated			
Palmitic Acid (C16:0)	21.5 ± 0.7	22.9 ± 0.8	
Stearic Acid (C18:0)	6.50 ± 0.27	6.92 ± 0.15	
Arachidic Acid (C20:0)	0.08 ± 0.02	0.23 ± 0.05	<0.02
C18:0/C16:0 (elongase activity indices)	0.30 ± 0.01	0.30 ± 0.01	
Essential fatty acids n-6			
Linoleic Acid (C18:2n6c)	15.4 ± 0.9	14.9 ± 0.3	
Eicosatrienoic Acid (C20:3n6)	0.32 ± 0.01	0.33 ± 0.02	
Arachidonic Acid (C20:4n6)	2.14 ± 0.17	2.89 ± 0.24	<0.03
SUM n-6	17.9 ± 0.93	18.2 ± 0.47	
C20:4 n6/C20:3 n6 (Δ5 activity indices)	6.68 ± 0.58	8.84 ± 0.58	<0.01
Essential fatty acids n-3			
α-Linolenic Acid (C18:3n3)	1.09 ± 0.12	0.79 ± 0.04	<0.02
Eicosatrienoic Acid (C20:3n3)	0.14 ± 0.03	0.08 ± 0.03	
Eicosapentaenoic Acid (C20:5n3)	0.11 ± 0.04	0.11 ± 0.04	
Docosahexaenoic Acid (C22:6n3)	0.34 ± 0.03	0.42 ± 0.04	
SUM n-3	1.67 ± 0.12	1.40 ± 0.07	
C18:2 6nC/C18:3n3	14.5 ± 1	19.3 ± 1.1	<0.01
Ratio n-6/n-3	10.7 ± 0.34	13.1 ± 0.53	<0.01

Values are means ± SEM. C: control; HF: high fat.

under the United Kingdom code of laboratory practice (COSHH: SI NO 1657, 1988).

Animals and diets

Fourteen Yorkshire X Landrace sows were artificially inseminated, then randomly allocated to one of the two gestational diets, either a commercial control diet (C; n = 7) or a high fat diet generated by supplementing the feed with palm oil ("high fat" HF; n = 7). All sows were between second and sixth parity and equally distributed between dietary groups with a mean parity of 3.8 ± 0.24 and fed to meet their net energy (NE) requirements during pregnancy (*i.e.* from 0 to 70 days of gestation 25.1 MJ NE/day and from 70 to 110 days of gestation 32.6 MJ NE/day). The caloric distribution of macronutrients for each diet was: control 64% starch, 11% fat and 25% protein; high fat 33.8% starch, 40.7% fat and 25.5% protein (Table 3). The feed provided to the HF group contained 50% more linoleic acid (C18:2n6) and 90% more saturated fat in the form of C16:0 and C18:0. In addition, the diets were supplemented to meet adequate essential amino acid, fatty acid, vitamin and mineral needs.

The sows were weighed on 0, 40, 70 and 108 days of gestation prior to feeding. On 0, 40 and 108 days of gestation fasting blood samples were taken from each animal. The plasma was extracted in K⁺EDTA coated tubes,

the samples were immediately separated by centrifugation (3000 g for 10 minutes at 4°C) and stored at –80°C until analysis.

From day 110 of gestation (mean caloric intake ≈ 27.3 MJ/day) and throughout lactation (59 MJ/day) all the sows were fed an identical diet sufficient to meet their energy requirements. Sows gave birth naturally in farrowing crates and all piglets were weighed after birth when litter size plus any still births were recorded. All piglets remained with their mothers and were allowed to suckle *ad libitum*. In all sows, milk was sampled, after milk let down via an intravenous oxytocin injection (10 I.U./mL; Eurovet Animal Health, Bladel, The Netherlands) into the ear on day 2 of lactation. At 7 days after parturition, the median birth weight offspring (C: 6 females, 1 male; HF: 4 females, 3 males) in each litter were weighed, a blood sample collected, the piglet sedated with 10% ketamine and then euthanized with (50 mg/kg) T-61 (Intervet, Boxmeer, Holland) followed by exsanguination.

Laboratory procedures
Plasma and milk analysis
Plasma high-density lipoprotein (HDL), low-density lipoprotein (LDL) and glucose were determined by colorimetric assays and measured using an Imola RX automated apparatus (Randox laboratories Ltd. Co, Antrim, UK). The

Table 3 Composition and quantity of the experimental diets with alterations in macronutrient ratio

a) Maternal dietary composition (%)

Percentage	Gestation diet		Lactation
	Control	Fat substituted	
Tapioca	28.1	3.1	-
Rapeseed meal	10.0	10.0	4.0
Sunflowerseed meal	4.0	4.0	2.0
Soybean hulls	13.0	17.0	2.0
Sugar beet pulp	10.0	10.0	-
Palm oil	-	6.6	3.1
Soybean oil	0.5	0.5	0.97
Maize	-	-	10.0
Sugar beet pulp	-	-	2.0
Soybean meal	-	-	11.7
Wheat	10.0	10.0	26.4
Barley	10.0	10.0	15.0
Wheat middlings	15.0	15.0	15.0
Molasses	4.0	4.0	4.0
Mono calcium phosphate	0.22	0.22	0.48
Salt	-	-	0.37
Limestone	0.50	0.60	1.56
Premix vit. and min.	0.5	0.5	0.5
Lysine (25%)	0.17	0.17	-
Lysine-HCl (L, 79%)	-	-	0.17
Threonine (L, 98%)	-	-	0.02
Phytase	0.5	0.5	0.5
Threonine (15%)	0.01	0.01	-
Sodium bicarbonate	0.6	0.6	0.16
Basic Feed allowance	107.1	92.8	100.0

b) Summary of major dietary components of the maternal diet and net energy. NB these nutrient levels were present in 1.07 Kg of the control diet and 0.92 Kg of the HF diet leading to a 15% reduction in intake in the HF diet. These diets were therefore isocaloric.

	Nutrients	Gestation diet		Lactation
		Control	Fat substituted	
g/Kg	Ash	64	52	61
g/Kg	Crude protein	123	122	161
g/Kg	Crude fat	25	89	63
g/Kg	Crude fibre	120	121	52
MJ/Kg	Net energy	9.3	9.3	9.5

c) Feed quantities provided

	Feed quantity during gestation (Kg/day)		
	Day 0-40	Day 40-70	Day 70-110
Control (n = 8)	2.89	2.89	3.75
Fat substituted (n = 8)	2.51	2.51	3.26

fat, protein and lactose concentrations in fresh milk were determined by infared analysis, using a Fourier Transform InfaRed (FTIR) interferometer (MilkoScan™, Foss Electric, Hillerød, Denmark).

Muscle sampling

The *biceps femoris* is a morphologically and functionally distinct skeletal muscle which forms part of the hamstring muscle group and is located on the posterior thigh. Samples were removed from the centre of each muscle to standardize sampling location and immediately frozen in liquid nitrogen and subsequently stored at −80°C until analysis was performed. All homogenisation carried out during this study was performed using a gentleMACS™ closed homogeniser (Miltenyi Biotec Ltd., Surrey, UK).

Enzymatic kinetics analysis

The lactate dehydrogenase (LDH) and isocitrate dehydrogenase (ICDH) total enzymatic assays were adapted from protocols obtained from SIGMA (http://www.sigmaaldrich.com/life-science/metabolomics/enzyme-explorer/learning-center/assay-library.html). Briefly, the muscular extract used (0.1 g) was homogenised in 4 ml buffer containing 0.25 M sucrose, 0.2 mM EDTA and 0.1 mM Tris (pH7.5). All samples were centrifuged at 6000 g for 15 minutes at 4°C and the supernatant diluted 1:2 with homogenisation buffer for use in subsequent assays. Total LDH enzymatic activity (EC 1.1.1.27) was determined in 1 µl of the muscle homogenate to which 10 µl NADH (0.33 mM) and 290 µl of reaction buffer (2 mM sodium pyruvate, 50 mM TEA, 5 mM EDTA) (Sigma-Aldrich Co LLC, Gillingham, UK) were added. Similarly, total ICDH enzymatic activity (EC 1.1.1.42) was determined in 7.5 µl of the muscle homogenate to which 270 µl of ICDH reaction buffer (38.9 mM Na_2HPO_4, 0.5 mM $MnCl_2$ ($4H_2O$), 0.05% βNADP) and 1 µl of (0.4 M) isocitrate (Sigma-Aldrich Co LLC, Gillingham, UK) were added. Enzymatic activities were measured by changes in absorbance at 340 nm at 28°C on a 96-well spectrophotometer (BIO-TEK Instruments Inc., Vermont, USA). The total LDH and ICDH activity were expressed as oxidised moles of their respective subtracts per second per gram of protein. The kinetic data were analysed by nonlinear regression using a method based on the principles of the Michaelis-Menten equations [53].

Muscle composition

Total protein of the muscle homogenates was determined using a commercial kit (Bio-Rad Laboratories Inc. Hemel Hempstead, UK) based on the Bradford method [54] on. The results were corrected to the dissected muscle weight obtained from each offspring.

Glycogen content was determined using a method developed by Dalrymple and Hamm [55]. The concentration of glucose released from this reaction was determined by a colorimetric commercial assay (Randox Ltd., County Antrim, UK) and the results were expressed as a concentration of milligrams of glycogen per gram of tissue dissected.

NAD+/NADH ratio was determined using a colorimetric commercial kit (Sigma-Aldrich Co LLC, Gillingham, UK) and normalised to the quantity of tissue dissected i.e. moles per gram of protein.

Triglyceride content was assessed using the Folch method [56] followed by colorimetric commercial assay (Randox Ltd., County Antrim, UK) and results expressed in milligrams per gram of tissue dissected.

Phospholipid composition was determined by gas-chromatography in which the chloroform phase was evaporated by applying a nitrogen stream and then 2 ml of hexane was added to each sample. The phospholipids were transmethylated by adding 40 µl of methyl acetate and 40 µl of methylation reagent (30% sodium methoxide, 4.1 ml methanol; Fisher Scientific Ltd. Loughborough, UK) to each reaction and left to react for 10 minutes at room temperature. This was followed by adding 60 µl of termination reagent (0.2 g dried oxalic acid and 6 ml diethyl ether) and methyl ester residues were extracted by adding 200 mg of calcium and followed by short centrifugation. The fatty acid methyl esters were then injected (split ratio 50:1) into a gas chromatograph (GC 6890; Agilent technologies Ltd, Stockport, UK). Separation of fatty acid methyl esters was performed with a Varian CP-88 (Crawford Scientific™ Ltd., Strathaven, UK) capillary column with hydrogen as carrier gas. Oven temperature was programmed from 59°C to 100°C at 8°C per min, then to 170°C at 6°C per minute and held for 10 minutes. The temperature of the injector and detector were set at 255°C and 250°C. The fatty acid methyl esters were identified by comparing the retention times with a fatty acid methyl esters standard (Sigma-Aldrich Co LLC, Gillingham, UK) and the area percentage in moles were used for the statistical analysis.

Histological analysis

Immediately after removing the muscle samples from −80°C storage, approximately 1 cm^3 of frozen tissue was sectioned and left to equilibrate overnight at −20°C. The next day, each sample was embedded on a cryostat metal plate in such a manner as to set the muscle fibres perpendicular to the cutting blade. The mounted samples were cut into 10 µm thickness in a pre-equilibrated at −20°C Leica Cryostat (Leica Microsystems Ltd., Milton Keynes, UK). The slices were then mounted on polysine histological slides (Menzel-Glaser, GmbH &

Co. Braunschweig, Germany) and allowed to equilibrate to room temperature prior to staining.

Haematoxylin and eosin staining was determined on sections placed in filtered 0.1% Harris' haematoxylin for 3 minutes and gently rinsed in cool running water to extract excessive stain. This was followed by further rinsing the sections in acidic alcohol and cool running water before transfer to eosin for 2 minutes. After staining, the slides were dipped in distilled water, dehydrated back through a graded series of alcohol concentrations and placed in xylene for 5 minutes. The stained sections were mounted with a coverslip in resin base medium and finally incubated overnight at room temperature.

Immunostaining of slow myosin (MyHC) was determined using anti-slow myosin pig specific MyHC antibody (Sigma-Aldrich Co. LLC., Gillingham, UK) at 1:4000 dilution. The staining was carried out on the Bond Max histology system using the Bond Polymer Refine Detection System (Vision Biosystems, Mount Waverley, Australia) and Bond software version 3.4A. Briefly, slides were stained as follows: 15 minutes with primary antibody, 8 minutes with secondary antibodies, 10 minutes with 3,3 diaminobenzine and counterstained with hematoxylin. A negative control slide in which the primary antibody stage was excluded was included with each batch.

Oil red O histochemical lipid staining was used to assess the intramyofibre lipid content which detects cellular fat droplets as a light red tint. Briefly, the 10 µm cryosections were placed in a Coplin jar containing 60% isopropanol for 15 minutes. Immediately afterwards, the sections were incubated for 20 minutes in a freshly-prepared solution containing 0.5% w/v oil red-O/isopropanol (Fisher Scientific Ltd. Loughborough, UK) diluted in a 1% w/v solution of dextrin. Thereafter, the stained samples were immersed for 1 minute in 60% isopropanol and then rinsed in cool running water. This was followed by counterstaining of the muscular fibres with Harris' haematoxylin for 3 minutes, followed by a quick rinse in cool running water. In addition, the slides were dipped 3 times in Scott's tap water and fast dried. Finally, a drop of 50% v/v glycerol-water solution was placed over the samples in order to preserve the lipids and the coverslip was sealed by applying an acetone-based nail polish.

Images of the sections were captured using a high performance CCD camera connected to a Leica universal microscope at 20 x magnification (Leica Microsystems Ltd., Milton Keynes, UK). From each image, 10 random pictures were taken for analysis. The mean cross-sectional fibre areas obtained from each image were analysed by dividing them into 12 equal fields and choosing one by random in which at least 150 fibres were measured through the use of image analysis software (Image-pro plus; MediaCybernetics, Bethesda, USA). Irregular-shaped fibres were excluded using a custom-made macro that drew a ring over each myofibre; filtering criteria were applied to reject regions with a CSA $< 50 \ \mu m^2$ or $> 5600 \ \mu m^2$ or regions with circularity (approximation diameter of an ellipse) of <0.3 or >1.0. For type I fibre analysis, a function was incorporated in our custom-made macro to detect the colour intensity of the positive-stained fibres. Finally, for the Oil red O analysis, the colour density threshold was adjusted to distinguish all the fat droplets on a single fibre. Only the droplets with an area $> 0.4 \ \mu m^2$ and $< 1.5 \ \mu m^2$ in those encircled fibres were included in this analysis.

Gene expression

Total RNA was extracted from 100 mg skeletal muscle using a commercially available kit (Qiagen Ltd., Crawley, UK), which included a DNA purification step. The amount and purity of the extracted RNA was determined using a Nanodrop (Thermo Fisher Scientific Ltd. Leicester, UK). 1 µg of total RNA was reverse transcribed using a Thermocycler (Thermo Fisher Scientific Ltd. Leicester, UK). Quantitative PCR (qPCR) was performed using a Roche lightcycler 480 thermocycler and SYBR technology (Roche, Burgess Hill, UK). For quantification of gene expression we applied the comparative C^t method, which was normalised by applying a geometric mean of 3 endogenous housekeeping genes (18 s rRNA, β actin and cyclophillin) [57]. The genomic data is expressed in this study as a ratio to the commercial control animals.

The qPCR primers were designed based on known porcine sequences published on the Genbank using public online software (Primer3) on intra-exonic boundary sequences where possible. A standard curve was included and the samples were run in duplicate as well as having the appropriate positive and negative controls. The primers used were purchased from Eurofins MWG Operon GmbH. (Ebersberg, Germany) and validated as described in previous publications [58]. The following porcine-specific oligonucleotide forward (F) and reverse (R) primers were used:

ENO3: F:GAGCTGGATGGGACAGAAAA–R:GCAA TGTGACGGTAGAGTGG; PGAM2:F:GATCAAGGCA GGCAAGAGAG–R:ACATCCCTTCCAGATGCTTG; FAT/CD36: F:TGAAAGAAGCAGGTGCTGAA–R: AGG ACTGCTCCCAATGACAGC; Primers for cyclophilin, 18S, β-actin, LPL, GLUT-4 and CPT1 have previously been published [58-60].

Statistical analysis

Statistical analysis of the data was performed using SPSS® statistics software (v 16.0 for Windows; IBM, Chicago, USA). The data was tested for normality by applying the Kolmogorov test and controlled by observation of its Gaussian distribution. Depending on the results of the previous tests, the data was analysed by applying Student's unpaired t-test and linear regression analysis with Benjamini & Hochberg False Discovery Rate correction; otherwise the non-parametric Mann Whitney test and Spearman Rank correlation were used. In all cases, the results are given as mean ± SEM, $p < 0.05$ was considered as statistical significant.

Competing interests
The authors declare that they have no competing interests.

Authors' contributions
AM, PB and MES conceived of, designed the study and obtained the funding; AM, PF, KA, DL, CR AM PB and MES conducted the study and analysed the data. AM, PF and MES drafted the manuscript. All authors have read and approved the final manuscript.

Acknowledgements
We are grateful to Prof. Kin-Chow Chang for facilitating the *anti-slow MyHC* monoclonal antibody and Dr. Nigel Kendall for his help with the analysis of serum metabolites. Thanks to Ceri Allen her technical assistance throughout this project. This study was supported by the Biotechnology and Biological Sciences Research Council (BBSRC) (BB/H002650/1) and European Union Sixth Framework Program for Research and Technical Development of the European Community – The Early Nutrition Programming Project (FOOD-CT-2005-007036).

Author details
[1]School of Veterinary Medicine and Science, University of Nottingham, Sutton Bonington Campus, Leicestershire LE12 5RD, UK. [2]Early Life Nutrition Research Unit, Academic Child Health, School of Clinical Sciences, University Hospital, The University of Nottingham, Nottingham NG7 2UH, UK. [3]School of Biosciences, The University of Nottingham, Sutton Bonington Campus, Leicestershire LE12 5RD, UK. [4]Schothorst Feed Research, PO Box 533, 8200 AM Lelystad, The Netherlands. [5]Current address: Primary Diets, Melmerby Industrial state, Melmerby, Ripon, North Yorkshire HG4 5HP, UK. [6]Current address: Wageningen UR Livestock Research, PO Box 338, 6700 AH Wageningen, The Netherlands.

References
1. Leman AD, Knudson C, Rodeffer HE, Mueller AG: Reproductive performance of swine on 76 Illinois farms. *J Am Vet Med Assoc* 1972, 161:1248–1250.
2. Giuffra E, Kijas JMH, Amarger V, Carlborg O, Jeon JT, Andersson L: The origin of the domestic pig: Independent domestication and subsequent introgression. *Genetics* 2000, 154:1785–1791.
3. Mersmann HJ: Metabolic patterns in the neonatal swine. *J Anim Sci* 1974, 38:1022–1030.
4. Le Dividich J, Mormede P, Catheline M, Caritez JC: Body composition and cold resistance of the neonatal pig from European (Large White) and Chinese (Meishan) breeds. *Biol Neonate* 1991, 59:268–277.
5. Elliot JI, Lodge GA: Body composition and glycogen reserves in the neonatal pig during the first 96 h of life. *Canadian J Animal Sci* 1977, 57:141–150.
6. Swiatek KR, Kipnis DM, Mason G, Chao KL, Cornblath M: Starvation hypoglycemia in newborn pigs. *Am J Physiol* 1968, 214:400–405.
7. Le Dividich J, Herpin P, Paul E, Strullu F: Effect of fat content of colostrum on voluntary colostrum intake and fat utilization in newborn pigs. *J Anim Sci* 1997, 75:707–713.
8. Baur LA, O'Connor J, Pan DA, Storlien LH: Relationships between maternal risk of insulin resistance and the child's muscle membrane fatty acid composition. *Diabetes* 1999, 48:112–116.
9. Di Cianni G, Miccoli R, Volpe L, Lencioni C, Ghio A, Giovannitti MG, Cuccuru I, Pellegrini G, Chatzianagnostou K, Boldrini A, Del Prato S: Maternal triglyceride levels and newborn weight in pregnant women with normal glucose tolerance. *Diabet Med* 2005, 22:21–25.
10. Boyd RD, Moser BD, Peo ER Jr, Cunningham PJ: Effect of energy source prior to parturition and during lactation on tissue lipid, liver glycogen

and plasma levels of some metabolites in the newborn pig. *J Anim Sci* 1978, 47:874–882.

11. Newcomb MD, Harmon DL, Nelssen JL, Thulin AJ, Allee GL: **Effect of energy source fed to sows during late gestation on neonatal blood metabolite homeostasis, energy stores and composition.** *J Anim Sci* 1991, 69:230–236.

12. Seerley RW, Pace TA, Foley CW, Scarth RD: **Effect of energy intake prior to parturition on milk lipids and survival rate, thermostability and carcass composition of piglets.** *J Anim Sci* 1974, 38:64–70.

13. Storlien LH, James E, Burleigh KM, Chisholm DJ, Kraegen EW: **Fat feeding causes widespread in vivo insulin resistance, decreased energy expenditure, and obesity in rats.** *Am J Physiol* 1986, 251:E576–E583.

14. Maegawa H, Kobayashi M, Ishibashi I, Takata Y, Shigeta Y: **Effect of diet change on insulin action: difference between muscle and adipocytes.** *Am J Physiol* 1986, 251(5):E616–E623.

15. Storlien LH, Pan D, Kriketos A, Baur LA: **High fat diet-induced insulin resistance.** *Ann N Y Acad Sci* 2006, 683:82–90.

16. Mayer-Davis EJ, Monaco JH, Hoen HM, Carmichael S, Vitolins MZ, Rewers MJ, Haffner SM, Ayad MF, Bergman RN, Karter AJ: **Dietary fat and insulin sensitivity in a triethnic population: the role of obesity. The insulin resistance atherosceloris study (IRIS).** *Am J of Clinical Nutrition* 1997, 65:79–87.

17. Mayer EJ, Newman B, Quesenberry CP, Selby JV: **Usual dietary fat intake and insulin concentrations in healthy women twins.** *Diabetes Care* 1993, 16:1459–1469.

18. Lovejoy JC: **The influence of dietary fat on insulin resistance.** *Current Diabetes Reports* 2002, 2:435–440.

19. Kraegen E, Clark PW, Jenkins AB, Daley EAW, Chisholm DJ, Storlein LH: **Development of muscle insulin resistance after liver insulin resistance in fat fed dams.** *Diabetes* 1991, 40:1397–1403.

20. Goodwin RF: **The relationship between the concentration of blood sugar and some vital body functions in the new-born pig.** *J Physiol* 1957, 136:208–217.

21. Ashmore CR, Addis PB, Doerr L: **Development of muscle fibers in the fetal pig.** *J Anim Sci* 1973, 36:1088–1093.

22. Lefaucheur L, Edom F, Ecolan P, Butler-Browne GS: **Pattern of muscle fiber type formation in the pig.** *Dev Dyn* 1995, 203:27–41.

23. Daniel ZC, Brameld JM, Craigon J, Scollan ND, Buttery PJ: **Effect of maternal dietary restriction during pregnancy on lamb carcass characteristics and muscle fiber composition.** *J Anim Sci* 2007, 85:1565–1576.

24. Wigmore PM, Stickland NC: **Muscle development in large and small pig fetuses.** *J Anat* 1983, 137(Pt 2):235–245.

25. Kovanen V, Suominen H, Peltonen L: **Effects of aging and life-long physical training on collagen in slow and fast skeletal muscle in rats. A morphometric and immuno-histochemical study.** *Cell Tissue Res* 1987, 248:247–255.

26. Kimball SR, Farrell PA, Nguyen HV, Jefferson LS, Davis TA: **Developmental decline in components of signal transduction pathways regulating protein synthesis in pig muscle.** *Am J Physiol Endocrinol Metab* 2002, 282:E585–E592.

27. Davis TA, Burrin DG, Fiorotto ML, Nguyen HV: **Protein synthesis in skeletal muscle and jejunum is more responsive to feeding in 7-than in 26-day-old pigs.** *Am J Physiol Endocrinol Metab* 1996, 270:E802–E809.

28. Lefaucheur L, Ecolan P, Lossec G, Gabillard JC, Butler-Browne GS, Herpin P: **Influence of early postnatal cold exposure on myofiber maturation in pig skeletal muscle.** *J Muscle Res Cell Motil* 2001, 22:439–452.

29. Innis SM: **Essential fatty acids in growth and development.** *Prog Lipid Res* 1991, 30:39–103.

30. Hiller B, Hocquette J-F, Cassar-Malek I, Nuernberg G, Nuernberg K: **Dietary n-3 PUFA affect lipid metabolism and tissue function-related genes in bovine muscle.** *Br J Nutr* 2012, 108:858–863.

31. Briolay A, Jaafar R, Nemoz G, Bessueille L: **Myogenic differentiation and lipid-raft composition of L6 skeletal muscle cells are modulated by PUFAs.** *Biochim Biophys Acta Biomembr* 2013, 1828:602–613.

32. Fainberg HP, Bodley K, Bacardit J, Li D, Wessely F, Mongan NP, Symonds ME, Clarke L, Mostyn A: **Reduced neonatal mortality in meishan piglets: a role for hepatic fatty acids?** *PLoS One* 2012, 7:e49101.

33. Almond K, Fainberg H, Lomax M, Bikker P, Symonds M, Mostyn A: **Impact of maternal palm oil substitution upon offspring survival and hepatic gene expression in the pig.** *Reprod Fertil Dev* 2014. In Press.

34. Andersson A, Sjodin A, Hedman A, Olsson R, Vessby B: **Fatty acid profile of skeletal muscle phospholipids in trained and untrained young men.** *Am J Physiol Endocrinol Metab* 2000, 279:E744–E751.

35. Mostyn A, Litten JC, Perkins KS, Euden PJ, Corson AM, Symonds ME, Clarke L: **Influence of size at birth on the endocrine profiles and expression of uncoupling proteins in subcutaneous adipose tissue, lung, and muscle of neonatal pigs.** *Am J Physiol Regul Integr Comp Physiol* 2005, 288:R1536–R1542.

36. White BR, Lan YH, McKeith FK, Novakofski J, Wheeler MB, McLaren DG: **Growth and body composition of Meishan and Yorkshire barrows and gilts.** *J Anim Sci* 1995, 73:738–749.

37. Wilson ME, Biensen NJ, Youngs CR, Ford SP: **Development of Meishan and Yorkshire littermate conceptuses in either a Meishan or Yorkshire uterine environment to day 90 of gestation and to term.** *Biol Reprod* 1998, 58:905–910.

38. Metzger BE, Lowe LP, Dyer AR, Trimble ER, Chaovarindr U, Coustan DR, Hadden DR, McCance DR, Hod M, McIntyre HD, Oats JJ, Persson B, Rogers MS, Sacks DA: **Hyperglycemia and adverse pregnancy outcomes.** *N Engl J Med* 2008, 358:1991–2002.

39. Thulin AJ, Allee GL, Harmon DL, Davis DL: **Utero-placental transfer of octanoic, palmitic and linoleic acids during late gestation in gilts.** *J Anim Sci* 1989, 67:738–745.

40. Heerwagen MJ, Miller MR, Barbour LA, Friedman JE: **Maternal obesity and fetal metabolic programming: a fertile epigenetic soil.** *Am J Physiol Regul Integr Comp Physiol* 2010, 299(3):R711–R722.

41. Fulco M, Cen Y, Zhao P, Hoffman EP, McBurney MW, Sauve AA, Sartorelli V: **Glucose restriction inhibits skeletal myoblast differentiation by activating SIRT1 through AMPK-mediated regulation of Nampt.** *Dev Cell* 2008, 14:661–673.

42. Jean K-B, Chiang S-H: **Increased survival of neonatal pigs by supplementing medium-chain triglycerides in late-gestating sow diets.** *Anim Feed Sci Technol* 1999, 76:241–250.

43. Halkjaer-Kristensen J, Ingemann-Hansen T: **Microphotometric determination of glycogen in single fibres of human quadriceps muscle.** *Histochem J* 1979, 11:629–638.

44. Ainge H, Thompson C, Ozanne SE, Rooney KB: **A systematic review on animal models of maternal high fat feeding and offspring glycaemic control.** *Int J Obes (Lond)* 2011, 35(3):325–335.

45. Gondret F, Combes S, Lefaucheur L, Lebret B: **Effects of exercise during growth and alternative rearing systems on muscle fibers and collagen properties.** *Reprod Nutr Dev* 2005, 45:69–86.

46. MacDonald MJ, Marshall LK: **Mouse lacking NAD + −linked glycerol phosphate dehydrogenase has normal pancreatic beta cell function but abnormal metabolite pattern in skeletal muscle.** *Arch Biochem Biophys* 2000, 384:143–153.

47. Olson AL, Pessin JE: **Structure, function, and regulation of the mammalian facilitative glucose transporter gene family.** *Annu Rev Nutr* 1996, 16:235–256.

48. Amusquivar E, Sanchez M, Hyde MJ, Laws J, Clarke L, Herrera E: **Influence of fatty acid profile of total parenteral nutrition emulsions on the fatty acid composition of different tissues of piglets.** *Lipids* 2008, 43:713–722.

49. Clandinin MT, Cheema S, Field CJ, Garg ML, Venkatraman J, Clandinin TR: **Dietary fat: exogenous determination of membrane structure and cell function.** *FASEB J* 1991, 5:2761–2769.

50. Garg ML, Thomson AB, Clandinin MT: **Interactions of saturated, n-6 and n-3 polyunsaturated fatty acids to modulate arachidonic acid metabolism.** *J Lipid Res* 1990, 31:271–277.

51. Van Nieuwenhoven FA, Verstijnen CP, Abumrad NA, Willemsen PH, Van Eys GJ, Van der Vusse GJ, Glatz JF: **Putative membrane fatty acid translocase and cytoplasmic fatty acid-binding protein are co-expressed in rat heart and skeletal muscles.** *Biochem Biophys Res Commun* 1995, 207:747–752.

52. Markworth JF, Cameron-Smith D: **Arachidonic acid supplementation enhances in-vitro skeletal muscle cell growth via a COX-2-dependent pathway.** *Am J Physiol - Cell Physiology* 2013, 304(1):C56–C67.

53. Dowd JE, Riggs DS: **A comparison of estimates of Michaelis-Menten kinetic constants from various linear transformations.** *J Biol Chem* 1965, 240:863–869.

54. Bradford MM: **A rapid and sensitive method for the quantitation of microgram quantities of protein utilizing the principle of protein-dye binding.** *Anal Biochem* 1976, 72:248–254.

55. Dalrymple RHR: **A method for the extraction of glycogen and metabolites from a single muscle sample.** *Int J Food Sci Technol* 1972, **8:**439–444.

56. Folch J, Lees M, Sloane Stanley GH: **A simple method for the isolation and purification of total lipides from animal tissues.** *J Biol Chem* 1957, **226:**497–509.

57. Vandesompele J, De Preter K, Pattyn F, Poppe B, Van Roy N, De Paepe A, Speleman F: **Accurate normalization of real-time quantitative RT-PCR data by geometric averaging of multiple internal control genes.** *Genome Biol* 2002, **3:**RESEARCH0034.

58. Sharkey D, Fainberg HP, Wilson V, Harvey E, Gardner DS, Symonds ME, Budge H: **Impact of early onset obesity and hypertension on the unfolded protein response in renal tissues of juvenile sheep.** *Hypertension* 2009, **53:**925–931.

59. Weber TE, Kerr BJ, Spurlock ME: **Regulation of hepatic peroxisome proliferator-activated receptor alpha expression but not adiponectin by dietary protein in finishing pigs.** *J Anim Physiol Anim Nutr (Berl)* 2008, **92:**569–577.

60. Lord E, Ledoux S, Murphy BD, Beaudry D, Palin MF: **Expression of adiponectin and its receptors in swine.** *J Anim Sci* 2005, **83:**565–578.

3

Disease resistance is related to inherent swimming performance in Atlantic salmon

Vicente Castro[1,2,3], Barbara Grisdale-Helland[4,5], Sven M Jørgensen[1], Jan Helgerud[6], Guy Claireaux[7], Anthony P Farrell[8], Aleksei Krasnov[1], Ståle J Helland[2,4,5] and Harald Takle[1,3,5*]

Abstract

Background: Like humans, fish can be classified according to their athletic performance. Sustained exercise training of fish can improve growth and physical capacity, and recent results have documented improved disease resistance in exercised Atlantic salmon. In this study we investigated the effects of inherent swimming performance and exercise training on disease resistance in Atlantic salmon.

Atlantic salmon were first classified as either poor or good according to their swimming performance in a screening test and then exercise trained for 10 weeks using one of two constant-velocity or two interval-velocity training regimes for comparison against control trained fish (low speed continuously). Disease resistance was assessed by a viral disease challenge test (infectious pancreatic necrosis) and gene expression analyses of the host response in selected organs.

Results: An inherently good swimming performance was associated with improved disease resistance, as good swimmers showed significantly better survival compared to poor swimmers in the viral challenge test. Differences in mortalities between poor and good swimmers were correlated with cardiac mRNA expression of virus responsive genes reflecting the infection status. Although not significant, fish trained at constant-velocity showed a trend towards higher survival than fish trained at either short or long intervals. Finally, only constant training at high intensity had a significant positive effect on fish growth compared to control trained fish.

Conclusions: This is the first evidence suggesting that inherent swimming performance is associated with disease resistance in fish.

Background

Diseases represent the main constraint for the success of an expanding aquaculture industry. Atlantic salmon (*Salmo salar*) farmers can experience severe fish losses due to both infectious and non-infectious diseases, usually during the seawater growth stage. Infectious pancreatic necrosis (IPN), pancreas disease (PD), infectious salmon anemia (ISA), as well as the sea lice parasite (*Lepeophtheirus salmonis* K) represent some of the most hazardous diseases [1,2], but losses have also been associated with non-infectious diseases such as cardiac failures [3,4]. Biosecurity countermeasures to control the disease situation include vaccines and pharmaceuticals, as well as improvements of the genetic material, feeds

and husbandry practices. The aim of current and future countermeasures is to strengthen the fish robustness, which is the capability to combine fast growth and normal organ development with improved resistance to both disease and physiological challenges.

Sustained exercise training has been documented to confer higher robustness to cultured fish, including increased somatic and cardiac growth, cardiac performance, aerobic capacity of the muscle, oxygen carrying and extraction capacity and improved bone quality [5-10]. Khovanskiy et al. [11] found that exercised chum salmon (*Oncorhynchus keta*) displayed lower mortality associated with an improved osmoregulatory capacity after seawater transfer when compared to untrained fish. Going further, we have recently demonstrated direct effects of sustained exercise on disease resistance, showing that survival of Atlantic salmon challenged with infectious pancreatic necrosis virus (IPNV) was 13%

* Correspondence: harald.takle@nofima.no
[1] Nofima, Ås, Norway
[3] AVS Chile S.A., Puerto Varas, Chile
Full list of author information is available at the end of the article

higher for fish subjected to a moderate interval-training regime for six weeks prior to smoltification when compared with fish held at a low, constant swimming speed [12]. Thus, sustained exercise in fish can induce a similar robustness effect as in humans, where a moderate aerobic training is also known to decrease the risk of infections and chronic life-style diseases [13,14].

It has been observed that exercised salmonids [12,15] and non-salmonids, (*Plecoglossus altivelis* [16]; *Chalcarburnus chalcoides mento* [17]; *Morone saxatilis* [18]; *Sparus aurata* [19]; *Danio rerio* [20]) exhibit improved growth due to improved feed efficiency, higher feed intake or a mix of both. Several studies have reported on the relationship between improved growth performance and disease resistance in fish (see reviews by Merrifield et al. [21,22]). For example, Gjedrem [23] suggested that a breeding program selecting for growth also induced a positive genetic response for disease resistance, although conflicting results exist [24]. Recently, an association between exercise-induced growth and improved disease resistance was shown in Atlantic salmon [12]. The possibility of a linkage between these two factors, growth and disease resistance, is of obvious importance for the fish farming sector.

Migratory fish such as salmonids have a great inherent capacity for sustained aerobic swimming. Benefits from exercise seem to be maximized at speeds close to the optimal swimming speed (U_{opt}), where energy use is more efficient and the cost of transport is minimized [25]. Exercising fish at speeds other than U_{opt} results in additional energy usage for locomotion, even at low speeds due to behavioral changes (e.g. increased aggression and spontaneous activity). Further, the highest speeds may prove stressful and unsustainable compared with U_{opt} [20]. Because of their natural swimming behavior and high aerobic capacity, salmonids are naturally amenable to long-term continuous exercise training, provided sustainable water velocities are used. This is in contrast to terrestrial animals that more typically require resting periods between bouts of exercise training. In humans, where most exercise training research has been performed, the intensity seems to be a fundamental factor affecting the individual's systemic immunity. While engaging in regular moderate exercise activity seems to enhance immune functions [13], high intensity aerobic training results in acute and chronic states of impaired immunity [26].

On top of training effects, there seems to be an equally large inherent variation in exercise capacity among fish and humans. For example, juvenile rainbow trout (*Oncorhynchus mykiss*) can be classified according to their inherent swimming performance as either poor or good swimmers. Interestingly, such classification was associated with several cardiac and

metabolic capacities after 9 months of common rearing [27].

This study aimed to evaluate if inherent swimming performance in juvenile fish affect disease resistance. Juvenile fish were identified according to their inherent swimming performance by pre-screening them in a swim challenge test. Fish classified as either poor or good swimmers were then trained at four different regimes to investigate if training differentially affected them. After smoltification, a controlled disease challenge with IPNV allowed us to assess differences in disease resistance among and within the two performance groups and four training regimes. This was further examined by analyzing expression levels of sensitive virus responsive genes (VRGs) in head kidney and cardiac tissues. In addition, exercise-induced effects on robustness were evaluated by growth performance and feed efficiency.

Results

Disease resistance is related to inherent swimming performance

Mortality following the IPN challenge started 18 days after the introduction of virus-shedding fish and reached a plateau around day 38 post-challenge. Inherent swimming performance showed a strong association with survival after the IPN challenge test. Fish initially categorized as good swimmers had significantly better survival than poor swimmers (86.1 and 77.6%, respectively; p = 0.02) when analyzed across all groups (Figure 1A). When survival was examined independent of the inherent swimming performance, differences among training regimes showed no significant difference (p = 0.21). The continuous-velocity training regimes tended to improve survival compared to the control trained group (87.1, 84.2 and 82.2% survival for respectively M, H and C), whereas interval-velocity training regimes tended to negatively impact survival (78.2 and 75.3% survival for Sint and Lint, respectively; Figure 1B).

When survival was examined in light of swimming performance, exercise training did not significantly affect disease resistance of poor and good swimmers. Nevertheless, exercise may have had a larger impact on disease resistance of poor swimmers since larger changes in mortality were observed in exercised groups of poor swimmers compared to good swimmers (Figure 2).

Virus responsive gene expression reflects and supports mortality data

To verify mortality data from IPNV, infection level was analyzed in challenged fish at termination of the disease trial. Quantification of IPNV (by real-time qPCR in head-kidney) in surviving fish showed low prevalence of virus-positive fish (33%) and low level of viral transcripts in positive fish. Heart tissue was also tested and found

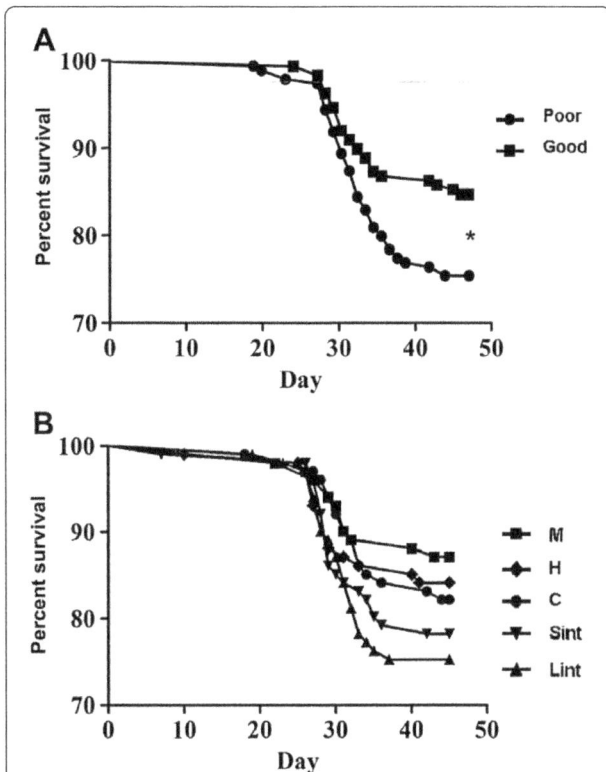

Figure 1 Cumulative survival of swimming performance and exercised groups during IPN challenge. A: The inherent swimming performance of the fish had a significant effect on disease resistance, with the good swimmers showing a higher survival (86.1%) than the poor swimmers (77.6%). **B**: Fish exercised at constant speeds for 10 weeks showed a trend towards higher disease resistance compared to those subjected to interval training regimes (Medium intensity (M) = 87.1%; High intensity (H) = 84.2%; Control (C) = 82.2%; Short interval (Sint) = 78.2% and Long interval (Lint) = 75.3%) (p = 0.21). *indicates significant difference, Mantel-Cox test; p < 0.05.

negative for all fish. Thus, sampled fish were in a late stage of infection with either low levels or no virus replication.

Gene expression analysis was performed to investigate among-groups differences in host immune correlates of disease response. For initial screening of correlates, transcriptome analysis by microarray of poor and good swimmers was assessed, since the strongest contrast in mortality was associated with swimming performance. This resulted in 21 genes with significantly higher transcript abundance in poor compared to good swimmers (t-test, p < 0.05) (Figure 3). By function, all genes were previously identified as virus-responsive genes (VRGs); a group of genes displaying a common activation/transcription to most of the known viruses infecting Atlantic salmon. VRGs are sensitive antiviral markers reflecting the infection status and the level of viral transcripts in cells [28]. Thus, poor swimmers seemed to have higher activation of antiviral immune genes compared to good swimmers at the end of the infection trial.

To further substantiate these results and to evaluate effects of the different training regimes with sufficient biological replication, expression of six VRGs was analyzed in heart ventricle tissue of poor and good swimmers from the C, M and Lint exercise-trained groups using qPCR. Results showed that induced levels of VRGs in poor swimmers were mainly explained by a strong expression in Lint exercised fish (Figure 4A). Control trained (C) and M trained poor swimmers had equal expression level of VRGs. Within the good swimmers, VRG expression levels were higher in M and Lint trained compared to control trained fish.

We further analyzed expression of eight VRGs in head kidney, where IPNV replication was observed. Expression levels within exercised good swimmers showed a similar trend as observed for heart tissue (Figure 4B).

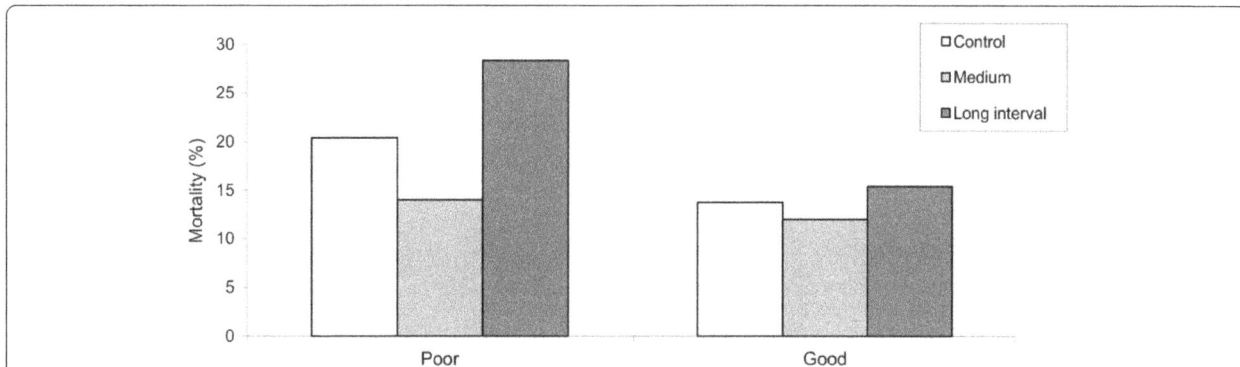

Figure 2 Interaction between inherent swimming performance and exercise training on disease resistance. Only those regimes included in the gene expression analysis are displayed. These reflect the lower (Medium), middle (Control) and higher (Long interval) mortalities found in response to IPN infection. Data is shown within poor (left) and good (right) swimmers. Though not significant, differences in mortalities were larger between poor and good swimmers for the Long interval, smaller for Control and minimum for the Medium intensity regime. Initial number of fish on the challenge ranged from 100 to 112 per regime.

QueryID	Gene Name	Poor	SEM	Good	SEM	Delta ER	ttest
Ssa#S31967511	interferon-induced protein 44	1,06	0,32	-0,05	0,15	1,11	0,01
Omy#S15341095	radical S-adenosyl methionine domain-containing protein 2	2,23	0,34	1,30	0,25	0,94	0,04
Ssa#CL495Contig1	Unknown	0,95	0,34	0,03	0,19	0,92	0,03
Ssa#S50837982	VHSV-inducible protein	1,40	0,36	0,52	0,20	0,88	0,05
Ssa#EG786166	PaTched Related family member	0,46	0,28	-0,31	0,16	0,77	0,03
Ssa#S30269828	interferon-induced protein 44	0,92	0,31	0,16	0,12	0,76	0,03
Ssa#TC112969	fish virus induced TRIM protein	0,62	0,28	-0,13	0,16	0,75	0,03
Ssa#GRASP223648291	poly polymerase 12	0,53	0,20	-0,06	0,10	0,59	0,02
Ssa#KSS1939	IFN-inducible protein Gig1	0,39	0,20	-0,18	0,13	0,57	0,03
Ssa#GRASP209730895	damage-regulated autophagy modulator	0,27	0,17	-0,28	0,12	0,55	0,02
Ssa#S32012561	signal transducer and activator of transcription 3	0,40	0,17	-0,13	0,07	0,53	0,01
Ssa#S31963491	PPAR A-interacting complex 285 kDa protein	0,59	0,18	0,12	0,11	0,48	0,04
Ssa#S35597062	mucin 5, subtype B, tracheobronchial	-0,52	0,16	-0,99	0,13	0,47	0,03
Ssa#DY720543	hect domain and RLD 3	0,56	0,18	0,11	0,07	0,46	0,03
Ssa#DW579399	RING finger protein 135	0,22	0,10	-0,23	0,13	0,46	0,01
Ssa#EG851140	stat1 alpha/beta	0,49	0,18	0,04	0,07	0,45	0,03
Ssa#GRASP223647953	interleukin-10 receptor beta chain precursor	0,33	0,13	-0,11	0,08	0,44	0,01
Ssa#S50837444	nicotinamide phosphoribosyltransferase	0,55	0,14	0,13	0,11	0,42	0,03
Ssa#GRASP223647705	tetraspanin-3	0,43	0,11	0,05	0,08	0,38	0,01
Ssa#S47726724	XIAP-associated factor 1	0,84	0,15	0,46	0,10	0,37	0,05
Ssa#GRASP223647619	CD9 antigen	0,23	0,12	-0,13	0,08	0,36	0,03

Figure 3 Differentially expressed genes in poor versus good swimmers post IPN challenge. Microarray analyses resulted in 21 genes showing higher transcript abundance in cardiac muscle of poor swimmers compared to good swimmers. By function, all of these genes have been previously identified as virus responsive genes (VRGs). Data for Poor and Good swim performance groups is $\log_2$-ER (expression ratio) ± SEM (n = 9).

Within poor swimmers, VRG expression levels were significantly lower in M compared to both control and Lint trained fish (p < 0.05). In contrast to heart tissue, VRG expression levels in head-kidney of control trained good swimmers were significantly lower compared to control trained poor swimmers (p = 0.03). Thus, the increased overall mortality observed for poor swimmers was reflected by stronger expression levels of antiviral immune genes in Lint trained (heart) and control trained (head-kidney) fish as compared to good swimmers. While no evidence for any positive effects of exercise training on mortality and infection status was observed for good swimmers, results implied beneficial effects in terms of reduced infection status (lower VRG expression) from M trained poor swimmers.

Results produced for 8 genes by microarray and qPCR were in close concordance (Pearson r = 0.92; p = 0.001).

Exercise training effects on growth

After six weeks of exercise training, no significant differences in thermal growth coefficient (TGC) were found among training regimes and control trained fish. At the end of the freshwater phase of the experiment (10 weeks of training plus 1 week detraining), TGC was significantly higher (p < 0.05) in the high intensity (H) training regime (1.61) compared with the control (C) trained group (1.50) (Table 1). The other training regimes only

showed a trend towards higher TGC compared to the control trained group (p < 0.1). At the end of exercise training, medium intensity (M) trained fish showed a significantly higher condition factor (CF) than C. Feed intake showed significant differences among training regimes, with the higher values belonging to the H and short interval (Sint) regimes at the end the first six training weeks, while H and long interval (Lint) had the highest feed intake in the second part of the training experiment. After six weeks of training, the only significant differences for feed efficiency ratio (FER) among training groups were H and Sint groups being lower than both C and M (Table 1).

Discussion

In this study we found that the inherent swimming performance of juvenile Atlantic salmon is associated with differences in survival to an infectious disease challenge after seawater transfer, with good swimmers displaying a significantly higher disease resistance than poor swimmers. Exercise training had no significant effect on disease resistance, though a trend towards improved performance was seen for fish being trained at constant compared to interval regimes. Though not significant, results further argue for exercise training affecting poor swimmers more strongly than good swimmers. Mortalities were supported by mRNA expression levels of a

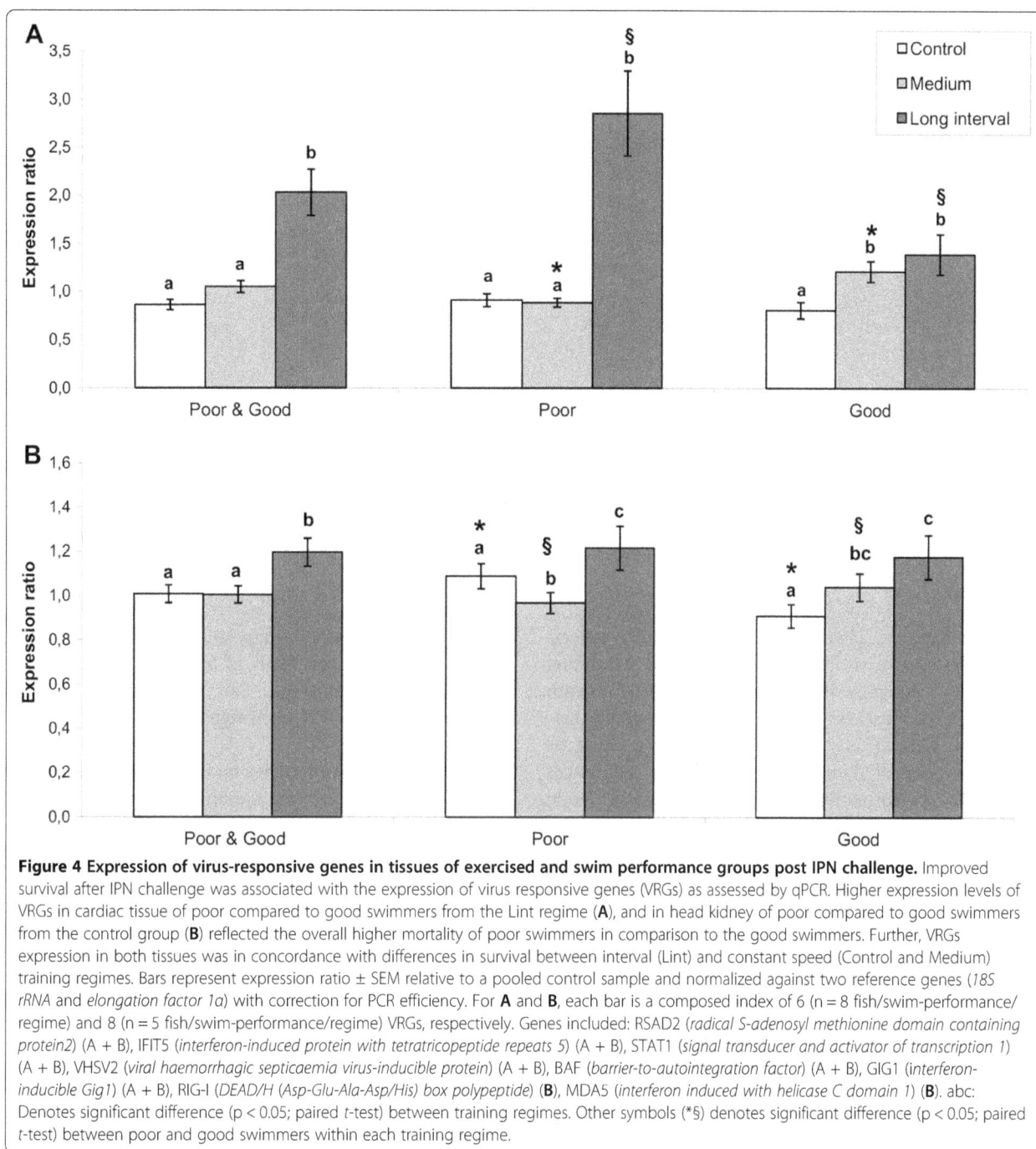

Figure 4 Expression of virus-responsive genes in tissues of exercised and swim performance groups post IPN challenge. Improved survival after IPN challenge was associated with the expression of virus responsive genes (VRGs) as assessed by qPCR. Higher expression levels of VRGs in cardiac tissue of poor compared to good swimmers from the Lint regime (**A**), and in head kidney of poor compared to good swimmers from the control group (**B**) reflected the overall higher mortality of poor swimmers in comparison to the good swimmers. Further, VRGs expression in both tissues was in concordance with differences in survival between interval (Lint) and constant speed (Control and Medium) training regimes. Bars represent expression ratio ± SEM relative to a pooled control sample and normalized against two reference genes (*18S rRNA* and *elongation factor 1a*) with correction for PCR efficiency. For **A** and **B**, each bar is a composed index of 6 (n = 8 fish/swim-performance/ regime) and 8 (n = 5 fish/swim-performance/regime) VRGs, respectively. Genes included: RSAD2 (*radical S-adenosyl methionine domain containing protein2*) (A + B), IFIT5 (*interferon-induced protein with tetratricopeptide repeats 5*) (A + B), STAT1 (*signal transducer and activator of transcription 1*) (A + B), VHSV2 (*viral haemorrhagic septicaemia virus-inducible protein*) (A + B), BAF (*barrier-to-autointegration factor*) (A + B), GIG1 (*interferon-inducible Gig1*) (A + B), RIG-I (*DEAD/H (Asp-Glu-Ala-Asp/His) box polypeptide*) (B), MDA5 (*interferon induced with helicase C domain 1*) (B). abc: Denotes significant difference (p < 0.05; paired *t*-test) between training regimes. Other symbols (*§) denotes significant difference (p < 0.05; paired *t*-test) between poor and good swimmers within each training regime.

subset of VRGs reflecting the antiviral response status. Growth was promoted by exercise training, though only significant for the highest intensity regime (H), while swimming performance did not show an association with growth performance.

The impact of inherent swimming performance on disease resistance

The inherent swimming performance of individual juvenile salmon was positively associated with disease resistance. Fish classified as good swimmers showed 8.5% better survival against IPN virus than poor swimmers when challenged 3 months after the swimming performance classification. Claireaux et al. [27] demonstrated that good swimmers of a cohort of rainbow trout, classified by a similar methodological approach as used in this work, retained this advantage nearly nine months later, despite a common rearing environment and similar growth performance, and displayed a significantly better cardiac capacity and morphology compared

Table 1 Growth parameters and dry matter intake of exercise trained Atlantic salmon

		C	M	H	Sint	Lint
Body weight (BW) (g)	Start	40.9 ± 0.2	40.7 ± 0.2	40.6 ± 0.2	40.2 ± 0.4	41.0 ± 0.4
	W 6	70.5 ± 1.3	70.9 ± 0.7	72.4 ± 2.4	72.3 ± 0.6	71.4 ± 0.4
	W 11	95.4 ± 0.3	99.9 ± 1.1	99.4 ± 2.4	98.2 ± 2.2	100.4 ± 2.2
Length (cm)	Start	15.1 ± 0.03	15.0 ± 0.04	15.0 ± 0.01	15.0 ± 0.05	15.1 ± 0.03
	W 11	20.0 ± 0.04	20.2 ± 0.07	20.2 ± 0.16	20.2 ± 0.14	20.4 ± 0.14
CF	Start	1.18 ± 0.003	1.18 ± 0.002	1.18 ± 0.005	1.18 ± 0.002	1.18 ± 0.001
	W 11	1.18 ± 0.004^b	1.20 ± 0.004^a	1.19 ± 0.004^{ab}	1.18 ± 0.002^b	1.18 ± 0.008^b
TGC	W 1-6	1.56 ± 0.05	1.59 ± 0.04	1.66 ± 0.09	1.68 ± 0.02	1.59 ± 0.01
	W 6-11	1.44 ± 0.08	1.64 ± 0.06	1.53 ± 0.05	1.47 ± 0.12	1.64 ± 0.10
	W 1-11	1.50 ± 0.01^b	1.58 ± 0.03^{ab}	1.61 ± 0.02^a	1.59 ± 0.05^{ab}	1.59 ± 0.03^{ab}
Relative feed intake (% BW d^{-1})	W 1-6	0.87 ± 0.02^c	0.88 ± 0.02^c	0.98 ± 0.03^{ab}	0.99 ± 0.01^a	0.92 ± 0.01^{bc}
	W 6-11	0.65 ± 0.02^c	0.69 ± 0.01^{bc}	0.74 ± 0.01^a	0.70 ± 0.02^{ab}	0.74 ± 0.01^a
FER	W 1-6	1.43 ± 0.04^a	1.42 ± 0.02^a	1.32 ± 0.00^b	1.34 ± 0.00^b	1.37 ± 0.02^{ab}
	W 6-11	1.66 ± 0.08	1.70 ± 0.03	1.52 ± 0.06	1.56 ± 0.11	1.58 ± 0.04

C Control, M medium intensity, H high intensity, Sint short interval, Lint long interval, CF condition factor, TGC thermal growth coefficient, week (W) 6: End of first six weeks of training under a short day light photoperiod. W 11: End of 10 weeks of training and one week of detraining. Means in the same row with different superscripts letters are significantly different based on one-way ANOVA (p < 0.05). Differences between the groups were assessed by the least-squares means procedure. Data are means ± SEM.

to poor swimmers. This and the present study collectively suggest that a simple screening test for swimming performance can efficiently distinguish between fish with low and high robustness, with the latter possessing better cardiac capacity and disease resistance. It must be noted that none of these studies could find differences in growth performance between poor and good swimmers.

In addition to the effects of the inherent swimming performance of fish on robustness, exercise training appeared to have a stronger, though not significant, modulatory effect on the poor swimmer's disease resistance. While the M training regime showed a tendency to improve the survival rate of the poor swimmers, the Lint regime tended to decrease the survival of the poor swimmers. The possible interaction effect between inherent poor swimming performance and training regime on survival was supported by expression analysis of VRGs in surviving fish from the different training regimes and performance groups at the end of the IPN challenge. Results showed that improved survival of good swimmers was associated with lower expression levels of virus responsive genes, probably reflecting an overall lower level of infection pressure, a more rapid or efficient viral clearance and/or a reduced antiviral status to recover and regain homeostasis. Thus, the ability to rapidly clear or reduce virus replication and antiviral immunity at the end of a viral infection might be important for survival. In a previous study, we demonstrated that the improved survival induced by sustained training of juvenile Atlantic salmon, was related to a specific cardiac transcriptome signature, suggesting lower levels of inflammation and higher levels of immune effector molecules, antioxidant enzymes and xenobiotics clearance capacity prior to an IPN challenge [12].

The impact of training regimes on disease resistance
Overall, the three continuous training regimes (including C) displayed a trend, though not significant, towards higher survival compared to the interval training regimes. The continuous 0.65 body lengths (BL)s^{-1} M regime gave the best results, which is in agreement with our previous finding where Atlantic salmon pre-smolts trained at a similar intensity for six weeks (0.8 BLs^{-1} for 16 h and 1 BLs^{-1} for 8 h per day) showed 13% higher survival following an IPN challenge test when compared to control trained fish [12]. Such improvements are very important in an industry context. In contrast to the improvement in disease resistance from utilizing an interval training regime with mild speed changes as in the previously mentioned study, the ~3-fold daily changes in swimming speed applied for the Sint and Lint regimes tended to reduce disease resistance against IPN compared to controls kept continuously at 0.32 BLs^{-1}. Since Sint and Lint trained fish had theoretically swum the same distance as the M trained fish, it could be argued that the relatively strong daily changes in water speed for both interval regimes may be the cause of the apparent negative impact on disease resistance of these fish.

We may speculate that the non-significant trend towards reduced disease resistance of the inherently poor swimmers trained with the Lint regime is due to a lower acclimation capacity of these fish to the relatively strong changes in swimming velocity compared to the good swimmers. It is then plausible to suggest that poor swimmers suffered from higher stress levels when following the Lint compared to the continuous speed regimes, which could potentially cause an impairment of their disease resistance capacities. Inherently good swimmers, however, seem to have sufficient behavioral and/or physiological plasticity as to avoid disease resistance impairment.

The moderate intensity of the M training regime may have promoted an acclimative response in the poor swimmers, boosting their disease resistance to the level of the good swimmers. Thus, if confirmed with new studies, the overall profit of conducting M regime training would be the achievement of a more homogenous population when it comes to disease resistance. This would imply an indisputable benefit for salmon producers.

The impact of training regimes on growth and feed utilization

By definition, a robust fish must possess a good combination of both high growth performance and disease resistance. Jobling et al. [29] and Davison [15] stated that higher growth may be achieved for fish when training intensity lies between 0.75 and 1.5 BLs^{-1}. Our results are in agreement with this; the H training regime (1.31 BLs^{-1}) had significantly higher TGC than the control trained group. Interestingly, the other three regimes (M, Sint and Lint), which had an average water speed of 0.65 BLs^{-1}, showed a tendency towards improved growth compared to control trained fish, suggesting the existence of a correlation between growth and total work load of the swimming-induced exercise. Higher growth given by the H training regime was mainly due to increased feed intake associated with a lower feed efficiency and protein retention. This suggests that fish subjected to that regime required more energy to satisfy the increased demand. Despite a lowered feed efficiency, increases in feed intake were sufficient to overcompensate the needs of simultaneous swimming and growth. It could be argued that training at this intensity stimulated the regulation of neuroendocrine factors involved in controlling feeding, resulting in an anabolic dominant state. It is logical to think though, that growth will be compromised at higher water speeds than those tested here, as has been found in salmonids [30,31] and other species, such as striped bass *Morone saxatilis* [32]. Indeed, routine gut blood flow, which is a basic requirement for effective digestion, is reduced in salmon as they swim progressively faster and can stop with abrupt stresses [33,34].

Another effect that may contribute to exercise-induced growth is the possibility of salmon juveniles changing from active to passive (ram) ventilation. Ram ventilation is the capacity of some fish species to ventilate passively by opening their mouths when swimming or facing high water currents, allowing water to pass through the gills with enough pressure for gas exchange to occur without the need for active branchial pumping [35,36]. The energy sparing effect of ram ventilation ranged from 8.4 to 13.3% in adult rainbow trout, which shifted ventilation mode when swimming above 0.5-1 BLs^{-1} [37]. Nevertheless, we cannot know for certain if this is also the case in this study.

Conclusions

This study provides the first evidence demonstrating that inherent swimming performance in juvenile fish may predetermine disease resistance later in life. Fish classified as good swimmers showed a significantly lower mortality when challenged with IPN than fish classified as poor swimmers. Our results further suggest that the inherently poor swimmers are more sensitive to the intensity and design of the training regimes than good swimmers. Finally, the results confirmed that sustained exercise at high intensity stimulates growth performance of Atlantic salmon, while exercise at lower intensities has less effect.

The great variability in swimming performance within populations of fish opens up novel possibilities for phenotype or marker-assisted selection in breeding programs and as a discrimination tool to sort out poor juvenile fish when it is still cost-effective.

Methods
Experimental fish

Juvenile Atlantic salmon belonging to the Salmobreed strain were produced and reared at Nofima AS, Sunndalsøra, Norway. Freshwater stage procedures took place at the same research station, which is an approved facility under the Norwegian Animal Research Authority (NARA). Stunning and sampling of fish was done in agreement with the Norwegian regulations. As fish were exposed to different sustainable water velocities that did not induce any obvious stressful state, no specific NARA approval was required according to Dr. G. Baeverfjord, member of the NARA board and local NARA officer at Nofima AS.

Swimming performance screening and training experimental setup

A total of 1355 fish were individually tagged (Passive Integrated Transponder (PIT), Glass tag Unique 2.12 × 12 mm, Jojo Automasjon AS, Sola, Norway) and measured (mass ± S.D. = 40.7 ± 0.2 g and fork lengths = 15.0 ± 0.3 cm) before being graded according to their swimming performance. Groups of approximately 100 fish were placed in a pre-conditioned 1.5 m diameter circular tank with an inner ring to reduce the swimming area to a 40 cm radius (Figure 5). The water inlet to the swimming area was tangentially situated on the side of the outer tank so that it generated the maximum water velocity. The inner ring was placed on four pieces of PVC (1 cm high) that allowed the water to drain freely to the center of the tank, while preventing the fish from leaving the swimming area. Maximum water inflow generated water velocities of 42–20 cm s^{-1} nearest the center, 73–58 cm s^{-1} in the middle of the stream and 97–81 cm s^{-1} furthest from the center. A grid (painted metal meshing) was secured downstream of the water inlet to prevent fish from drifting backwards, and a floodlight placed above the grid encouraged fish to remain upstream. Water velocity and height (10–15 cm) were controlled by adjusting the water supply valve and the position of the draining stand pipe. After being introduced into the swimming flume, fish were left undisturbed for 15 min at the lowest speed to acclimatize. Water speed was then increased gradually every 1–2 min until half of a fish group had been removed from the tank. Fish that were unable to swim against the increasing water current typically laid against the back-mesh grid. They were removed with a dip-net, identified (PIT tag reading) and placed back in their rearing tank. During the trial, fish were regularly and gently repositioned to ensure that they would all be exposed to testing conditions and would not evade from the high speed outer portion of the swimming ring. Based on their swimming performance, fish were then allocated to one of two groups. The first 50% that stopped swimming were categorized as "poor swimmers", and the last 50% still swimming were the "good swimmers". Both poor and good swimmers were randomly mixed among 16 cylindro-conical experimental tanks (500 l, 82 cm in diameter, 77–86 fish tank^{-1}) and left undisturbed for one week before the start of the training regimes. The center of each experimental tank was fitted with a plastic pipe (31.5 cm diameter), which reduced the area in the tank with lowest water speed. A frequency-controlled pump (Hanning Elektro Werke, PS 18–300; Oerlinghausen, Germany) directed the water current and a wire mesh fence, attached between the pipe and the edge of the tank, prevented the fish from drifting backwards. The water speeds were calibrated by using the average speed measured at twelve points in the tank (four horizontal locations and three depths at each location (Höntzsch HFA propeller, Waiblingen, Germany with HLOG software)). Five different sustained exercise-training regimes were tested; the control regime in quadruplicate tanks and the other regimes in triplicate tanks. Three of the training regimes were continuous velocity: the control (C; 5.7 cm s^{-1}), medium intensity (M; 11.5 cm s^{-1}) and high intensity (H; 23 cm s^{-1}) regimes. At start of the 10-week training experiment, these speeds were equivalent to 0.38, 0.77 and 1.53 BLs^{-1} for C, M and H, respectively. As fish grew during the trial, average relative water speeds were reduced to 0.32 (C), 0.65 (M) and 1.31 (H) BLs^{-1}. The two remaining training regimes used interval training,

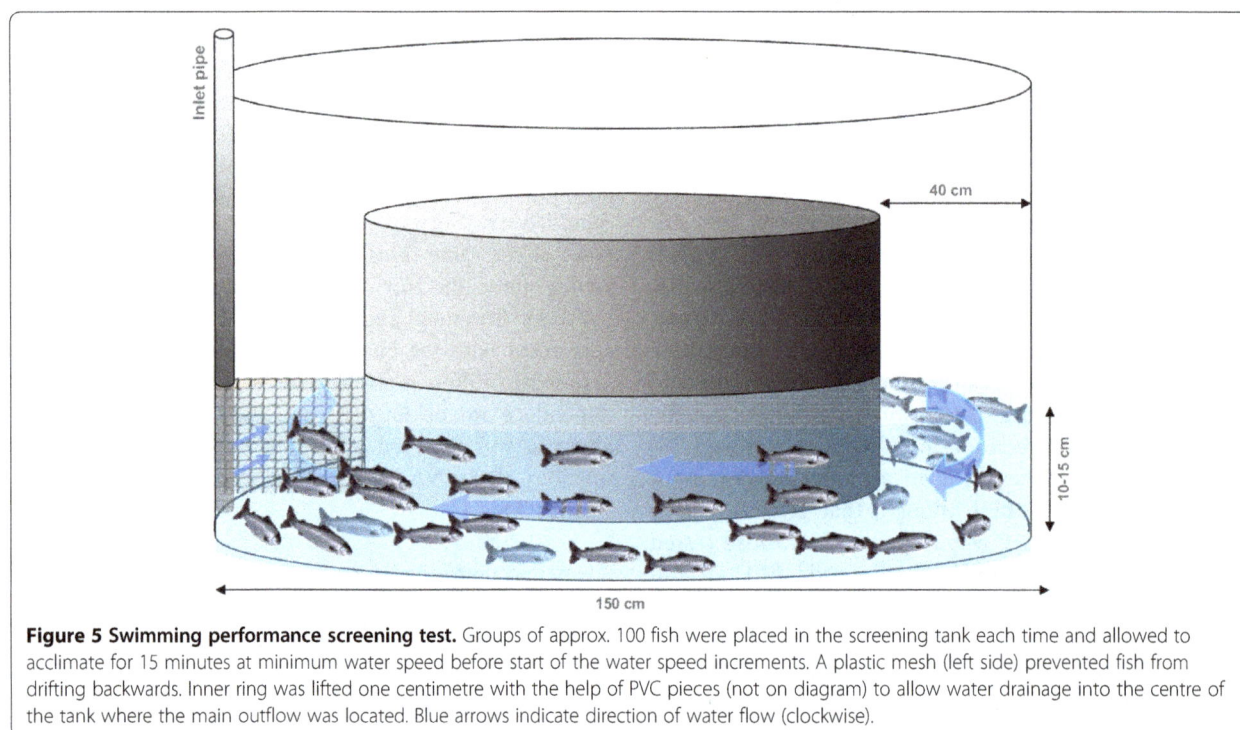

Figure 5 Swimming performance screening test. Groups of approx. 100 fish were placed in the screening tank each time and allowed to acclimate for 15 minutes at minimum water speed before start of the water speed increments. A plastic mesh (left side) prevented fish from drifting backwards. Inner ring was lifted one centimetre with the help of PVC pieces (not on diagram) to allow water drainage into the centre of the tank where the main outflow was located. Blue arrows indicate direction of water flow (clockwise).

with daily increments in the relative water velocity from 0.32 to 1.31 BLs^{-1} for either a single 8 h period (Long interval; Lint) or four 2-h periods for a total high speed training period of 8 h (short interval; Sint). Theoretically, both interval groups swam the same distance as the M group. The 10 weeks of training were followed by a one-week recovery at control speed prior transferring the fish to seawater. To stimulate smoltification during the experiment, fish were exposed to a short daylight regime (12–12 Light–dark) for the first six weeks, followed by continuous light for the remaining five weeks. Measurement of ATPase in gills (n = 10) sampled from each group was conducted in a commercial laboratory, Havbruksinstituttet AS, Bergen, Norway, and confirmed that all fish were sampled within the smolt-window (data not shown). Water temperature was measured daily (10.5 ± 0.8°C) while oxygen saturation was measured weekly and was maintained over 85% with oxygen supplementation. Dead fish were removed with daily inspections and weighed.

Growth and feed intake

During the training experiment, fish were fed to excess an extruded diet based on fish meal, ground wheat and fish oil (produced at Nofima AS, Fyllingsdalen, Bergen, Norway), using automatic feeders. The effluent water of each tank was led into a wire mesh box to enable sieving of waste feed. To minimize feed leaching, the effluent water was directed to two different areas of the wire box using pinch valves on the water pipes, dependent on whether feeding was occurring. The waste feed, expressed as dry matter (DM) content, was used to re-calculate daily feed intake in order to adjust ration level every second day (Helland et al., 1996). After the change in the photoperiod at the sixth week of training, feeding regime was increased from 12 (6.25 min h^{-1}) to 24 (3.12 min h^{-1}) times per day.

Fish were weighed in bulk after six weeks of training and a two-day fast. At the end of the trial, fish were individually re-weighed and re-measured.

Viral challenge test

Following the 1-week detraining period, approx. 110 fish per training regime and training control, including both performance groups, were pooled and transferred to seawater at VESO research station (Vikan, Norway) for an IPN challenge test. An additional nine fish per training regime and training control groups were similarly pooled and transferred to act as infection controls (unchallenged fish). The fish to be challenged as well as those acting as infection controls were acclimatized for one week in a separate 1.5 and 1 m^3 tank (11 ± 0.2°C and

0.5 l kg^{-1} min^{-1}; water volumes were adjusted to achieve similar densities). The IPN challenge test was performed by co-habitation and started when 20% of IPN-infected challenger fish were added to the experimental tank. A similar proportion of uninfected smolts were added to the unchallenged tank, keeping similar densities in both tanks. Challenger fish were previously marked by a fin clip and injected with 5 ml of ~3 × 10^6 TCID$_{50}$/ml of IPNV (strain V-1244 cultured at the Norwegian School of Veterinary Science). Throughout the challenge test, fish were observed and mortalities were recorded daily for 45 days, when the trial was terminated. A representative selection of dead fish was confirmed positive for IPNV and was further bacteriologically examined on 2% NaCl blood agar plates as part of a standard procedure during the challenge at VESO. All trials at VESO were performed according to Norwegian regulations for care and use of fish in research as stated in the Agriculture and Food Department regulation FOR 1996–01–15 Nov. 23.

Gene expression analyzes

Fish used for gene expression analyses were sampled at the end of the IPN challenge test (day 45), when mortality of all groups had leveled off. Challenged fish belonging to both swimming performance categories (poor and good swimmers) were sampled for each of the regimes C, M and Lint, while nine unchallenged control trained (C) fish were used as hybridization controls for microarray analyses. Cardiac ventricle and head kidney tissues were immediately dissected from fish killed by a blow to the head and stored in RNA*later* (Ambion, Austin, TX, USA). Total RNA was extracted using TRIzol and purified with PureLink RNA Mini Kit (Invitrogen, Carlsbad, CA, USA) following manufacturers guidelines. RNA concentration was measured using NanoDrop 1000 spectrophotometer (Thermo Fischer Scientific, Waltham, MA, USA), and RNA integrity was assessed with an Agilent 2100 Bioanalyzer (Agilent Technologies, Waldbronn, Germany). All samples had a RNA Integrity Number (RIN) above 9.

Microarray analyses were performed with the salmonid oligonucleotide microarray (SIQ2.0, NCBI GEO platform GPL10679), consisting of 21 K features printed in duplicate on 4 × 44 K arrays from Agilent Technologies [38]. Eighteen two-color microarray hybridizations were performed. Individual heart ventricle samples of challenged fish from poor and good swimming performers (n = 9 each; 3 from each training regime) were competitively hybridized against a pooled sample consisting of equal amounts of RNA from the infection controls (n = 9) per array. Unless specified otherwise, all reagents and equipment were from Agilent Technologies and used according to manufacturer's protocol. Amplification and labeling of RNA (200 ng) were done using the LowInput-QuickAmp Labeling kit. Cy5 (test) and Cy3 (control) labeled RNA was purified with RNeasy Mini Kit (Qiagen, MD, USA), and the Gene Expression Hybridization Kit was used for RNA fragmentation. Hybridizations were performed for 17 h at 65°C and rotation speed of 10 rpm in a hybridization oven. Arrays were washed twice (Gene Expression wash buffers 1 & 2) and immediately scanned with a GenePix 4100A (Molecular Devices, Sunnyvale, CA, USA) at 5 μm resolution and with manually adjusted laser power to ensure an overall intensity ratio close to unity between Cy3 and Cy5 channels and with minimal saturation of features.

The GenePix Pro 6.1 software was used for spot-grid alignment, feature extraction of fluorescence intensity values and spot quality assessment. Low quality spots were filtered with aid of GenePix flags as well as by the criterion $(I-B)/(S_I-S_B) \geq 0.6$ where I and B are the mean signal and background intensities, respectively, and S_I and S_B are the respective standard deviations. Data were exported into the STARS platform [38] for data transformation and Lowess normalization of $\log_2$-expression ratios (ER). Differentially expressed genes were selected based on spot signal threshold, $\log_2$-ER average $> |0.6|$ in at least two individuals and significant difference between groups (swimming performers) $p < 0.05$, $n = 9$

Table 2 List of primers used for the qPCR reactions

Genes	Short name	Sequence 5' to 3'	Accession
radical S-adenosyl methionine domain-containing protein 2[1]	Rsad2	F-GTACCGCAGATGCACAACAC	AF076620
		R-TTGACACTGCTTGGAGTTGC	
interferon inducible protein Gig1[1]	Gig1	F-GGCAACCTGAATCCAGAAGA	DW569595
		R-GTCTGGACGCAGACTGATGA	
VHSV-inducible protein[1]	Vhsv2	F-GGTGAAGACCTGGACCTGAA	BT072288
		R-TGACCCCTGTTGACCTTCTC	
interferon-induced protein with tetratricopeptide repeats 5[1]	Ifit5	F-CAGAGAGGTGCCAGGCTAAC	BT046021
		R-TGCACATTGACTCTCCTTGG	
interferon induced with helicase C domain 1[1]	Mda5	F-CAGAGGTGGGGTTCAATGAT	NM001195179
		R-AGCTCGCTCCACTTGTTGAT	
DEAD/H (Asp-Glu-Ala-Asp/His) box polypeptide RIG-I[1]	Rig-I	F-GACGGTCAGCAGGGTGTACT	DY714827
		R-CCCGTGTCCTAACGAACAGT	
barrier-to-autointegration factor[1]	Baf	F-ACAGACCCCTCATCATCCTG	BT049316
		R-CGGTGCTTTTGAGAAGTGGT	
signal transducer and activator of transcription 1 isoform alpha[1]	Stat1a	F-CGGTGGAGCCCTACACTAAG	CB513054
		R-GGGATCCTGGGGTAGAGGTA	
interferon-inducible protein Gig2-like[1]	Gig2	F-GATGTTTCATGGCTGCTCAA	BT044026
		R-CTTTTCGGATGTCCCGACTA	
B-type natriuretic peptide[2]	BNP	F-TCGACAAATCCGCAATAAGA	CK883650
		R-TTGAGCCAATTCGGTCTAGC	
putative collagen alpha 1[2]	put_Coll-a1	F-AACCCTGAACCCCTCAGTCT	CA038317
		R-TGGTCCTACCGTCTGGTTTC	
leukocyte elastase inhibitor[2]	LEI	F-TCTCAGATGGCAAAGGCTCT	BT045959
		R-GTTGGCCAGTTTCAGGATGT	
elongation factor 1a[3]	EF1α	F-CACCACGGGCCATCTGATCTACAA	BT072490
		R-TCAGCAGCCTCCTTCTCGAACTTC	
18S rRNA[3]	18S	F-GCCCTATCAACTTTCGATGGTAC	AJ427629
		R-TTTGGATGTGGTAGCCGTTTCTC	
infectious pancreatic necrosis virus_polyprotein[4]	IPNV	F-CCGACCGAGAACAT	AJ877117
		R-TGACAGCTTGACCCTGGTGAT	

[1] Virus-responsive genes (Figure 4).
[2] Genes used for microarray validation.
[3] Reference genes used for normalization.
[4] IPNV gene used for relative virus quantification (described in Results section).

(Student's *t*-test). Recording of microarray experiment metadata was in compliance with the Minimum Information About a Microarray Experiment (MIAME) guidelines (Brazma et al., 2001). Microarray results were submitted to GEO (GSE38603).

Expression of single genes (VRGs) was assessed by quantitative real-time RT-PCR (qPCR) on heart ventricle and head kidney samples from swim performers of the three groups C, M and Lint at day 45 post-challenge. Expression levels were calculated relative to expression levels of the same nine infection control samples used for microarrays. A total of six and eight VRGs were analyzed for heart (n = 16 per regime; 8 good and 8 poor swimmers) and head kidney (n = 10 per regime; 5 good and 5 poor swimmers), respectively. The same samples from both tissues were further scanned for viral presence by using a set of specific IPNV primers (Table 2). Confirmation of array results by qPCR was based on eight genes (4 up- and 4 down-regulated) in the same individual samples as used for microarrays.

All qPCR primers were designed using the ePrimer3 from the EMBOSS online package [39], except for the IPNV primers [40] and synthesized by Invitrogen (Table 2). Synthesis of cDNA was performed on 0.5 μg of DNAse treated (DNA-free; Ambion) RNA samples using TaqMan@ Reverse Transcription reagents (Applied Biosystems, Foster City, CA, USA) and primed with an equal mix of oligo dT and random hexamers. PCR reactions were prepared manually and run in duplicates in 96-well optical plates on a LightCycler® 480 (Roche Diagnostics, Mainheim, Germany) using 2X SYBR Green Master mix (Roche), 5 μl of cDNA samples and a primer concentration of 0.42 μM each in a final volume of 12 μl. For all genes, cDNA was previously diluted 1:10 (1:1000 for 18S). qPCR thermal cycling was as follows: 5 min pre-incubation at 95°C, followed by 45 amplification cycles consisting of 95°C for 10 s, 60°C for 15 s and 72°C for 15 s, followed by a melting curve protocol (95°C for 5 s, continuous increase from 65°C to 97°C) to assess specificity of the amplicon. Fluorescence was measured at the end of every extension step and throughout the melting curve step. Cycle threshold (C_T) values were calculated using the second derivative method. Duplicate reactions differing more than 0.5 C_T values were discarded, and values were averaged for relative quantification. PCR efficiency was assessed by six 10-fold serial dilutions of pooled sample templates for each primer pair. Relative expression ratios were calculated by the Pfaffl method [41] with normalization against two reference genes (*18S* and *Elongation factor 1α*). An index value of VRG expression was calculated for each group (training regime or swimming performance) by averaging the relative expression ratio of the single genes.

Calculation and statistics

Relative feed intake: 100 × (dry feed intake/mean body mass (BM)/days fed).

TGC: $1000 \times [(BM_1^{0.33} - BM_0^{0.33})/\sum \text{day-degrees}]$, where BM_1 and BM_0 are final and initial body masses, respectively.

FER: (Wet fish gain + dead fish mass)/dry feed intake.

CF: $100 \times BM (g) \times \text{fork length (cm)}^{-3}$.

For growth and CF analyses, the individual fish data were analyzed by analysis of variance in a hierarchical model including the fixed effect of training regime and the random effect of tank within regime. The mean data for each tank were tested by variance analysis (means compared using the least-squares means procedure) (SAS software, version 9.1, SAS Institute, Inc., Cary, NC, USA). Percentage data were transformed (arcsine square root) before being subjected to analysis. Differences between training regimes were considered significant at the p < 0.05 level, and are presented as mean ± SEM.

Differences in survival during the IPN challenge test were evaluated using the Mantel-Cox test in GraphPad Prism (version 5.01, GraphPad Software, Inc., San Diego, CA, USA). For the microarray analyses, expression differences between the groups where assessed by Student's *t*-test; p < 0.05, and data are presented as $\log_2 ER \pm SEM$. Difference in expression levels for the indexed values of pooled VRGs, was assessed by paired Student's *t*-test, p < 0.05; between target and control groups in qPCR. Correlation between microarray and qPCR results for selected genes was assessed by Pearsons' *r*.

Competing interests
The authors declare that they have no competing interests.

Authors' contributions
VC carried out the molecular studies, participated in samplings, data interpretation and drafted the manuscript. BG performed the growth and nutrition studies analyses. SMJ interpreted the microarray data and drafted the corresponding section. JH participated in the design of the study and revised the manuscript. GC designed the screening test facilities, performed the classification of fish according to swimming capacities, and revised the manuscript. APF participated in designing the study and critically revised the manuscript. AK analyzed the microarray data and revised the manuscript. SJH designed the fish training facilities and performed and participated in growth analyzes. HT obtained the funding, conceived and designed the study, coordinated and participated in samplings, data interpretation and drafting of the manuscript. All authors have read and approved the final manuscript.

Acknowledgements
We would like to thank the technical staff at Nofima for feed production, caring of the fish and laboratory analyses. This study was funded by The Fishery and Aquaculture Industry Research Fund (FHF) and The Research Council of Norway (Grant number: 190067).

Author details
[1]Nofima, Ås, Norway. [2]Institute of Animal Sciences, Norwegian University of Life Sciences (UMB), Ås, Norway. [3]AVS Chile S.A., Puerto Varas, Chile. [4]Aquaculture Protein Centre, CoE, Ås, Norway. [5]Nofima, Ås, Norway. [6]Norwegian University of Science and Technology, Faculty of Medicine, Trondheim, Norway. [7]Université de Bretagne Occidentale, LEMAR, Unité de Physiologie Fonctionnelle des Organismes Marins, Ifremer, Plouzané, France.

[8]Faculty of Land and Food Systems, & Department of Zoology, University of British Columbia, Vancouver, BC, Canada.

References

1. Johnson SC, Treasurer JW, Bravo S, Nagasawa K, Kabata Z: A review of the impact of parasitic copepods on marine aquaculture. *Zool Stud* 2004, 43:229–243.

2. Robertsen B: Can we get the upper hand on viral diseases in aquaculture of Atlantic salmon? *Aquac Res* 2011, 42:125–131.

3. Poppe TT, Taksdal T: Ventricular hypoplasia in farmed Atlantic salmon *Salmo salar. Dis Aquat Organ* 2000, 42:35–40.

4. Brocklebank J, Raverty S: Sudden mortality caused by cardiac deformities following seining of preharvest farmed Atlantic salmon (*Salmo salar*) and by cardiomyopathy of postintraperitoneally vaccinated Atlantic salmon parr in British Columbia. *Can Vet J* 2002, 43:129–130.

5. Hochachka PW: The effects of physical training on oxygen debt and glycogen reserves in trout. *Can J Zool* 1961, 39:767–776.

6. Davie PS, Wells RMG, Tetens V: Effects of sustained swimming on rainbow-trout muscle structure, blood-oxygen transport, and lactate-dehydrogenase isozymes - evidence for increased aerobic capacity of white muscle. *J Exp Zool* 1986, 237:159–171.

7. Farrell AP, Johansen JA, Steffensen JF, Moyes CD, West TG, Suarez RK: Effects of exercise training and coronary ablation on swimming performance, heart size, and cardiac enzymes in Rainbow-Trout, Oncorhynchus-Mykiss. *Can J Zool* 1990, 68:1174–1179.

8. Gallaugher PE, Thorarensen H, Kiessling A, Farrell AP: Effects of high intensity exercise training on cardiovascular function, oxygen uptake, internal oxygen transport and osmotic balance in chinook salmon (Oncorhynchus tshawytscha) during critical speed swimming. *J Exp Biol* 2001, 204:2861–2872.

9. Anttila K, Jaevilehto M, Manttari S: The swimming performance of brown trout and whitefish: the effects of exercise on Ca^{2+} handling and oxidative capacity of swimming muscles. *J Comp Physiol B* 2008, 178:465–475.

10. Totland GK, Fjelldal PG, Kryvi H, Lokka G, Wargelius A, Sagstad A, Hansen T, Grotmol S: Sustained swimming increases the mineral content and osteocyte density of salmon vertebral bone. *J Anat* 2011, 219:490–501.

11. Khovanskiy IY, Natochin YV, Shakhmatova YI: Effect of physical exercise on osmoregulatory capability in hatchery-reared juvenile chum salmon, Oncorhynchus keta. *J Ichthyol* 1993, 33:36–43.

12. Castro V, Grisdale-Helland B, Helland SJ, Kristensen T, Jorgensen SM, Helgerud J, Claireaux G, Farrell AP, Krasnov A, Takle H: Aerobic training stimulates growth and promotes disease resistance in Atlantic salmon (*Salmo salar*). *Comp Biochem Phys A* 2011, 160:278–290.

13. Gleeson M: Immune function in sport and exercise. *J Appl Physiol* 2007, 103:693–699.

14. Mathur N, Pedersen BK: Exercise as a mean to control low-grade systemic inflammation. *Mediat Inflamm* 2008, doi:10.1155/2008/109502.

15. Davison W: The effects of exercise training on teleost fish, a review of recent literature. *Comp Biochem Physiol A* 1997, 117:67–75.

16. Nakagawa H, Nishino H, Nematipour GR, Ohya S, Shimizu T, Horikawa Y, Yamamoto S: Effects of water velocities on lipid reserves in Ayu. *Nippon Suisan Gakk* 1991, 57:1737–1741.

17. Hinterleitner S, Huber M, Lackner R, Wieser W: Systemic and enzymatic responses to endurance training in 2 Cyprinid species with different life-styles (Teleostei, Cyprinidae). *Can J Fish Aquat Sci* 1992, 49:110–115.

18. Young PS, Cech JJ: Improved growth, swimming performance, and muscular development in exercise-conditioned young-of-the-year striped bass (*Morone saxatilis*). *Can J Fish Aquat Sci* 1993, 50:703–707.

19. Ibarz A, Felip O, Fernandez-Borras J, Martin-Perez M, Blasco J, Torrella JR: Sustained swimming improves muscle growth and cellularity in gilthead sea bream. *J Comp Physiol B* 2011, 181:209–217.

20. Palstra AP, Tudorache C, Rovira M, Brittijn SA, Burgerhout E, van den Thillart GEEJ, Spaink HP, Planas JV: Establishing zebrafish as a novel exercise model: swimming economy, swimming-enhanced growth and muscle growth marker gene expression. *PLoS One* 2010, 5. doi:10.1371/journal.pone.0014483.

21. Merrifield DL, Dimitroglou A, Foey A, Davies SJ, Baker RTM, Bogwald J, Castex M, Ringo E: The current status and future focus of probiotic and prebiotic applications for salmonids. *Aquaculture* 2010, 302:1–18.

22. Sweetman JW, Torrecillas S, Dimitroglou A, Rider S, Davies SJ, Izquierdo MS: Enhancing the natural defences and barrier protection of aquaculture species. *Aquac Res* 2010, 41:345–355.

23. Gjedrem T: Genetic improvement of cold-water fish species. *Aquac Res* 2000, 31:25–33.

24. Overturf K, LaPatra S, Towner R, Campbell N, Narum S: Relationships between growth and disease resistance in rainbow trout, Oncorhynchus mykiss (Walbaum). *J Fish Dis* 2010, 33:321–329.

25. Tucker VA: Energetic cost of locomotion in animals. *Comp Biochem Physiol* 1970, 34:841–846.

26. Nieman DC: Exercise effects on systemic immunity. *Immunol Cell Biol* 2000, 78:496–501.

27. Claireaux G, McKenzie DJ, Genge AG, Chatelier A, Aubin J, Farrell AP: Linking swimming performance, cardiac pumping ability and cardiac anatomy in rainbow trout. *J Exp Biol* 2005, 208:1775–1784.

28. Krasnov A, Timmerhaus G, Schiotz BL, Torgersen J, Alanasyev S, Iliev D, Jorgensen J, Takle H, Jorgensen SM: Genomic survey of early responses to viruses in Atlantic salmon, *Salmo salar* L. *Mol Immunol* 2011, 49:163–174.

29. Jobling M, Baardvik BM, Christiansen JS, Jorgensen EH: The effects of prolonged exercise training on growth performance and production parameters in fish. *Aquacult Int* 1993, 1:95–111.

30. Greer Walker M, Emerson L: Sustained swimming speeds and myotomal muscle function in trout, Salmo gairdneri. *J Fish Biol* 1978, 13:475–481.

31. East P, Magnan P: The effect of locomotor-activity on the growth of brook charr, Salvelinus fontinalis Mitchill. *Can J Zool* 1987, 65:843–846.

32. Young PS, Cech JJ: Optimum exercise conditioning velocity for growth, muscular development, and swimming performance in young-of-the-year striped bass (*Morone saxatilis*). *Can J Fish Aquat Sci* 1994, 51:1519–1527.

33. Thorarensen H, Gallaugher PE, Kiessling AK, Farrell AP: Intestinal blood-flow in swimming chinook salmon Oncorhynchus tshawytscha and the effects of hematocrit on blood-flow distribution. *J Exp Biol* 1993, 179:115–129.

34. Farrell AP, Thorarensen H, Axelsson M, Crocker CE, Gamperl AK, Cech JJ: Gut blood flow in fish during exercise and severe hypercapnia. *Comp Biochem Physiol A* 2001, 128:551–563.

35. Muir BS, Kendall JI: Structural modifications in gills of tunas and some other oceanic fishes. *Copeia* 1968, 2:388–398.

36. Farrell AP, Steffensen JF: An analysis of the energetic cost of the branchial and cardiac pumps during sustained swimming in trout. *Fish Physiol Biochem* 1987, 4:73–79.

37. Steffensen JF: The transition between branchial pumping and ram ventilation in fishes - energetic consequences and dependence on water oxygen-tension. *J Exp Biol* 1985, 114:141–150.

38. Krasnov A, Timmerhaus G, Afanasyev S, Jørgensen SM: Development and assessment of oligonucleotide microarrays for Atlantic salmon (*Salmo salar* L.). *Comp Biochem Phys D* 2011, 6:31–38.

39. Rice P, Longden I, Bleasby A: EMBOSS: The European molecular biology open software suite. *Trends Genet* 2000, 16:276–277.

40. Skjesol A, Skjæveland I, Elnæs M, Timmerhaus G, Fredriksen BN, Jørgensen SM, Krasnov A, Jørgensen JB: IPNV with high and low virulence: host immune responses and viral mutations during infection. *Virol J* 2011, 8:396.

41. Pfaffl MW, Horgan GW, Dempfle L: Relative expression software tool (REST©) for group-wise comparison and statistical analysis of relative expression results in real-time PCR. *Nucleic Acids Res* 2002, 30:e36. doi:10.1093/nar/30.9.e36.

4

Estrogen-related receptor β deficiency alters body composition and response to restraint stress

Mardi S Byerly[1,2,5*], Roy D Swanson[2], G William Wong[1,5] and Seth Blackshaw[2,3,4,6,7]

Abstract

Background: Estrogen-related receptors (ERRs) are orphan nuclear hormone receptors expressed in metabolically active tissues and modulate numerous homeostatic processes. ERRs do not bind the ligand estrogen, but they are able to bind the estrogen response element (ERE) embedded within the ERR response elements (ERREs) to regulate transcription of genes. Previous work has demonstrated that adult mice lacking *Errβ* have altered metabolism and meal patterns. To further understand the biological role of *Errβ*, we characterized the stress response of mice deficient for one or both alleles of *Errβ*.

Results: *Sox2-Cre:Errβ* mice lack *Errβ* expression in all tissues of the developing embryo. *Sox2-Cre:Errβ^{+/lox}* heterozygotes were obese, had increased *Npy* and *Agrp* gene expression in the arcuate nucleus of the hypothalamus, and secreted more corticosterone in response to stress. In contrast, *Sox2-Cre:Errβ^{lox/lox}* homozygotes were lean and, despite increased *Npy* and *Agrp* gene expression, did not secrete more corticosterone in response to stress. *Sox2-Cre:Errβ^{+/lox}* and *Sox2-Cre:Errβ^{lox/lox}* mice treated with the Errβ and Errγ agonist DY131 demonstrated increased corticotropin-releasing hormone (*Crh*) expression in the paraventricular nucleus of the hypothalamus, although corticosterone levels were not affected. *Nes-Cre:Errβ^{lox/lox}* mice, which selectively lack Errβ expression in the nervous system, also demonstrated elevated stress response during an acoustic startle response test and decreased expression of both *Crh* and corticotropin-releasing hormone receptor 2 (*Crhr2*).

Conclusions: Loss of *Errβ* affects body composition, neuropeptide levels, stress hormones, and centrally-modulated startle responses of mice. These results indicate that *Errβ* alters the function of the hypothalamic-pituitary-adrenocortical axis and indicates a role for Errβ in regulating stress response.

Background

ERRs are nuclear hormone receptors that regulate multiple homeostatic processes throughout life [1]. ERRs were initially identified on the basis of sequence homology to estrogen receptors (ERs) [2]. The homology between Errs and Ers is 36% in the ligand binding domain and 68% in the DNA binding domain. ERRs bind both ERR response elements (ERREs) and the closely related estrogen response elements (EREs) embedded within an ERRE sequence on DNA to modulate transcription of target genes [3-8]. Errs activate gene transcription by binding to DNA, either as a monomer, homodimer, or a heterodimer complex, which includes two different Err isoforms [1,6,7,9,10]. While their

binding sites are similar to those of Ers, Errs do not bind estradiol and instead activate transcription in a ligand-independent manner, leading to their classification as orphan nuclear receptors. The three different *Err* genes, α, β and γ, have highly conserved ligand and DNA binding domains and thus may regulate homeostatic processes in a compensatory manner [11].

In mice, *Errβ* and *Errγ* are selectively expressed in the brain and multiple peripheral tissues [2,12-14] and share the highest degree of sequence homology [11], suggesting that they may share overlapping functions. Since Errs recognize the same response elements, they are likely to regulate overlapping subsets of target genes [11].

We have previously reported that whole-body or central nervous system-specific deletion of *Errβ* increases expression of *Errγ* and ultimately alters body composition, metabolism, meal patterns, and energy expenditure of mice [11]. Further, inhibition of *Errβ* or *Errγ* alter

* Correspondence: mardibyerly@gmail.com
[1]Department of Physiology, Johns Hopkins University School of Medicine, Baltimore, MD, USA
[2]Department of Neuroscience, Johns Hopkins University School of Medicine, Baltimore, MD, USA
Full list of author information is available at the end of the article

metabolic parameters, whole-body energy balance (e.g. body composition, food intake and neuropeptide expression), while deletion of *Errβ* reciprocally modulates expression of *Errγ* (and vice versa) suggesting that balanced expression of *Errβ* and *Errγ* is important for control of energy balance and food intake [14-18].

Alterations in glucocorticoid signaling and whole-body energy balance positively correlate with one another, with increased glucocorticoid levels resulting in increased body weight [19-21]. Errβ suppresses glucocorticoid receptor activity in neuroblastoma and kidney cells in a dose-dependent manner, suggesting that it may also regulate metabolism at least in part through modulation of the hypothalamic-pituitary-adrenal (HPA) axis [22]. The HPA axis is regulated by corticotrophin-releasing hormone (Crh) released from neurosecretory cells of the hypothalamic paraventricular nucleus. Crh stimulates release of adrenocorticotropic hormone (ACTH) from the anterior pituitary, and ACTH, in turn, triggers glucocorticoid secretion from the adrenal gland. Negative feedback from ACTH and glucocorticoid secretion ultimately modulates *Crh* expression in the paraventricular nucleus via glucocorticoid receptors [23]. Disrupting glucocorticoid feedback loops can alter whole-body energy balance (e.g. body weight). Glucocorticoid excess (Cushing's disease) increases central fat deposition, whereas decreased body weight is associated with glucocorticoid insufficiency (Addison's disease) [19-21]. In addition to these effects on metabolism, alterations in the HPA axis can also influence anxiety and stress, which increase Neuropeptide Y (Npy) secretion. Npy further augments obesity susceptibility by inducing food intake and contributing to leptin resistance [23-25].

Consequently, we propose that *Errβ* modulates stress responses. Since Errβ suppresses glucocorticoid receptor activity [22], we hypothesized that the HPA axis may be altered in mice that carry heterozygous or homozygous loss of function mutations of *Errβ* in all somatic tissues [14,26,27]. The effects of *Errβ* deficiency on body weight, body composition, neuropeptide levels, stress hormones, and stress responses were examined in *Sox2-Cre:Errβ^{+/lox}* and *Sox2-Cre:Errβ^{lox/lox}* mice, in which *Errβ* expression is disrupted in all somatic tissues. These results indicate that *Errβ* modulates stress responses, at least in part through central mechanisms.

Results

Errβ gene dosage alters body weight and body composition

Sox2-Cre:Errβ^{+/lox} heterozygous mice express one allele of *Errβ*, resulting in higher levels of *Errβ* expression relative to *Sox2-Cre:Errβ^{lox/lox}* homozygous mice. Alterations in energy balance are observed in mice deficient for *Errβ* in all embryonic tissues (*Sox2-Cre:Errβ^{lox/lox}*) [14]. Because

Errβ is proposed to modulate energy balance in a dose-dependent manner, we characterized *Sox2-Cre:Errβ^{lox/lox}* and *Sox2-Cre:Errβ^{+/lox}* mice to determine whether gene dosage altered development of body weight and body composition. We previously showed that *Sox2-Cre:Errβ^{lox/lox}* mice have decreased body weight and fat mass by nine months of age [8]. Body weight and body composition (fat mass and lean mass) were measured in *Sox2-Cre:Errβ^{lox/lox}*, *Sox2-Cre:Errβ^{+/lox}*, and WT mice at three weeks and at nine months of age (Table 1). By three weeks, body composition differences began to emerge between the genotypes: *Sox2-Cre: Errβ^{+/lox}* mice significantly increased fat mass (fat mass: $F_{1,8} = 9.32$, $P = 0.05$), while *Sox2-Cre:Errβ^{lox/lox}* mice trended toward decreased fat mass (fat mass: $F_{1,10} = 4.95$, $P = 0.05$) compared to WT mice. There was no difference in body weight among the genotypes at three weeks, implying that alterations in body composition arise prior to weight changes in *Errβ*-deficient mice.

At nine months of age, *Sox2-Cre:Errβ^{+/lox}* mice had increased fat mass and no change in lean mass relative to WT mice (fat mass: $F_{1,9} = 35.90$, $P = 0.002$). However, *Sox2-Cre:Errβ^{lox/lox}* mice demonstrated the opposite trend in body composition, with decreases in both fat and lean mass (fat free mass) relative to WT mice (fat mass: $F_{1,10} = 46.53$, $P < =0.0001$; lean mass: $F_{1,10} = 6.21$, $P = 0.03$). Accordingly, body weight increased in *Sox2-Cre:Errβ^{+/lox}* mice ($F_{1,9} = 32.31$, $P = < 0.000001$) and decreased in *Sox2-Cre:Errβ^{lox/lox}* mice ($F_{1,10} = 32.57$, $P = 0.0004$) relative to WT mice. Given these differences, the *Sox2-Cre:Errβ^{+/lox}* mice surprisingly had a similar macrostructure of food intake as the *Sox2-Cre:Errβ^{lox/lox}* [14], relative to WT mice. Specifically, after consuming a meal, the duration of time that the mouse was satiated was decreased (satiety ratio), the total number of pellets consumed was increased, and the duration of time between meals (intermeal interval, IMI) was not changed for *Sox2-Cre:Errβ^{+/lox}* mice, but IMI was decreased for *Sox2-Cre:Errβ^{lox/lox}* mice (Table 1). The difference in IMI between the genotypes may be a compensatory change due to peripheral signals modulated by the increases in both body weight and fat mass observed in the *Sox2-Cre:Errβ^{+/lox}* mice.

Hypothalamic neuropeptide expression in *Errβ* mutant mice

In the brain, *Errβ* is primarily expressed in the hindbrain, whereas *Errγ* is expressed in both the hindbrain and hypothalamus [14,28,29]. Nuclei of the hindbrain send primary projections to the hypothalamus (e.g., nucleus tractus solitarius to the paraventricular nucleus) and the amygdala, and activity in these nuclei can modulate hypothalamic gene expression [30-32]. Furthermore, in the absence of *Errβ*, Errγ can modulate food intake [14]. Since *Sox2-Cre:Errβ^{+/lox}* and *Sox2-Cre:Errβ^{lox/lox}* mice demonstrated alterations in body weight and body composition relative to WT mice, we sought to determine if

Table 1 Body weight and body composition, physical activity and meal patterns of wild type (WT), Sox2-Cre:Errβ$^{+/lox}$, and Sox2-Cre:Errβ$^{lox/lox}$ mice

Genotype	Age	Body composition				Meal patterns		
		Body weight (grams)	Fat mass (grams)	Lean mass (grams)	Activity (beam breaks)	Pellets (number)	Satiety ratio (IMI/meal size)	IMI (minutes)
WT	3 weeks	13.1 ± 0.5	2.09 ± 0.09	10.06 ± 0.41				
Sox2-Cre:Errβ$^{+/lox}$	3 weeks	14.0 ± 0.7	2.58 ± 0.16*	10.56 ± 0.62*				
Sox2-Cre:Errβ$^{lox/lox}$	3 weeks	12.9 ± 0.8	1.64 ± 0.17	10.51 ± 0.61				
WT	9 months	36.5 ± 0.9	12.19 ± 0.65	23.09 ± 0.46	67207 ± 8601	128 ± 15	8.3 ± 0.9	107 ± 17
Sox2-Cre:Errβ$^{+/lox}$	9 months	46.1 ± 3.0*	21.43 ± 1.84*	24.00 ± 0.63	93599 ± 9879	238 ± 35* 5.6 ± 0.7$^{\#}$	102 ± 10	
Sox2-Cre:Errβ$^{lox/lox}$	9 months	28.4 ± 1.3*	5.69 ± 0.74*	21.64 ± 0.40*	133741 ± 20533*	260 ± 57*	4.1 ± 0.7*	67 ± 11*

*$P < 0.05$ relative to WT.
$^{\#}P = 0.05$ relative to WT.
Activity is a measurement for the number of beam break, which represents horizontal physical activity that is parallel to the ground.
Meal patterns for Sox2-Cre:Errβ$^{lox/lox}$ mice are adapted from [14].

hypothalamic neuropeptides known to modulate energy balance, Npy and Agrp, were differentially expressed in the brains of these mutants. Brain tissue sections of three-week-old WT, Sox2-Cre:Errβ$^{+/lox}$, and Sox2-Cre:Errβ$^{lox/lox}$ mice were hybridized with cRNA probes specific to Npy and Agrp mRNA. Npy (Figure 1a) and Agrp (Figure 1b) staining were least intense in the hypothalamus of WT brain tissues, more intense in Sox2-Cre:Errβ$^{+/lox}$ brain tissues, and most intense in Sox2-Cre:Errβ$^{lox/lox}$ brain tissues. Expression of Npy and Agrp, as determined by hypothalamic ISH staining, appears to correlate inversely with Errβ expression. Increased staining expression of Npy and Agrp may contribute to the increased fat mass of three-week-old Sox2-Cre:Errβ$^{+/lox}$ mice; conversely, the high levels of Npy and Agrp in Sox2-Cre:Errβ$^{lox/lox}$ mice may be a downstream response to decreased fat mass.

Sox2-Cre:Errβ$^{lox/lox}$ mice show elevated activity levels due to defects in vestibular system development [14,26], which likely contribute to the body weight and body composition differences observed at nine months of age. However, three-week-old Sox2-Cre:Errβ$^{+/lox}$ mice are not hyperactive, suggesting that activity alone does not control hypothalamic neuropeptide levels (Table 1: Sox2-Cre:Errβ$^{lox/lox}$ vs. WT - $F_{1,9} = 16.43$, $P = 0.004$).

Errβ gene dosage alters expression of HPA axis components

Errβ interacts with glucocorticoid receptors in neuroblastoma and kidney cells [22,33] and may also interact in the hindbrain where Errβ is expressed [14]. Since increased Npy expression is often associated with elevated levels of glucocorticoid release, which can influence adiposity [23-25], we hypothesized that Errβ deficiency may alter stress responsiveness via glucocorticoid secretion. Therefore, stress responses of WT, Sox2-Cre:Errβ$^{+/lox}$, and Sox2-Cre:Errβ$^{lox/lox}$ mice were measured by detecting alterations in HPA axis components, Crh expression and corticosterone.

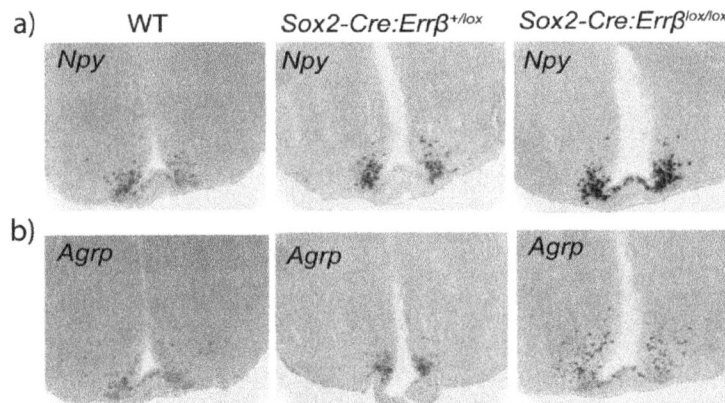

Figure 1 Hypothalamic neuropeptide expression in wild-type (WT), Sox2-Cre:Errβ$^{+/lox}$, and Sox2-Cre:Errβ$^{lox/lox}$ mouse brains. Brain tissues were harvested from three-week-old WT, Sox2-Cre:Errβ$^{+/lox}$, and Sox2-Cre:Errβ$^{lox/lox}$ mice; frozen tissue sections were hybridized in situ with cRNA probes to **a)** Npy and **b)** Agrp (n = 3/genotype).

To investigate the ability of Errγ to compensate for Errβ deficiency, stress responses were investigated in the presence of synthetic agonists of Errγ. Atlhough agonists specific to individual Err isoforms are not commercially available, we were able to perform these studies using DY131, a selective agonist of both Errβ and Errγ [34]. It has been previously determined that DY131 is able to readily penetrate the blood–brain barrier, as it is both hydrophobic and has a topological surface area (TPSA) less than 70 [14]. In $Sox2\text{-}Cre\text{: }Err\beta^{lox/lox}$ null mice, DY131 would exclusively activate Errγ and that this would result in alterations in HPA axis function (e.g. *Crh* expression or corticosterone levels). We utilized a restraint stress paradigm to measure corticosterone serum levels during baseline, stress, and recovery phases. WT mice demonstrated increased stress-induced corticosterone levels, which returned to baseline after one hour of recovery (Figure 2a) (baseline vs. stress: $F_{1,8} = 7.82$, $P = 0.03$). Similar results were measured in WT mice administered DY131 (DY131 WT, baseline vs stress: $F_{1,8} = 6.46$, $P = 0.03$; control WT; DY131 WT, stress vs recovery: $F_{1,11} = 8.54$, $P = 0.01$). $Sox2\text{-}Cre\text{:}Err\beta^{+/lox}$ mice exhibited markedly elevated corticosterone levels during stress, which may arise from altered negative feedback mechanisms that modulate corticosterone secretion (e.g. enhanced Crh secretion from the brain). $Sox2\text{-}Cre\text{:}Err\beta^{+/lox}$ mice exhibit normal recovery to baseline one hour after the stress test (Figure 2b – control $Sox2\text{-}Cre\text{:}Err\beta^{+/lox}$, baseline vs stress: $F_{1,14} = 8.62$, $P = 0.01$). Administration of DY131 yielded similar results (DY131 $Sox2\text{-}Cre\text{:}Err\beta^{+/lox}$, baseline vs stress: $F_{1,14} = 7.02$, $P = 0.02$; control $Sox2\text{-}Cre\text{:}Err\beta^{+/lox}$, stress vs recovery: $F_{1,14} = 7.14$, $P = 0.02$; DY131 $Sox2\text{-}Cre\text{:}Err\beta^{+/lox}$, stress vs recovery: $F_{1,14} = 8.83$, $P = 0.01$).

In contrast, $Sox2\text{-}Cre\text{:}Err\beta^{lox/lox}$ mice had elevated baseline corticosterone levels but exhibited no increase with stress (Figure 2c – control $Sox2\text{-}Cre\text{:}Err\beta^{lox/lox}$, baseline vs stress: $F_{1,8} = 10.86$, $P = 0.02$; DY131 $Sox2\text{-}Cre\text{:}Err\beta^{lox/lox}$, baseline vs stress: $F_{1,8} = 15.14$, $P = 0.01$; control $Sox2\text{-}Cre\text{: }Err\beta^{lox/lox}$; DY131 $Sox2\text{-}Cre\text{:}Err\beta^{lox/lox}$, baseline vs recovery: $F_{1,8} = 21.81$, $P = 0.01$), suggesting that $Err\beta\text{:}Sox2\text{-}Cre^{lox/lox}$ mice are unable to increase corticosterone levels in response to restraint stress. In fact, expression of *Crh*, as determined by ISH staining, was increased in the $Sox2\text{-}Cre\text{:}Err\beta^{lox/lox}$ mice under baseline conditions, a modest increase in ISH staining was also seen in the $Sox2\text{-}Cre\text{: }Err\beta^{+/lox}$ mice, with DY131 further increasing the ISH staining for *Crh*. This data suggests that Errγ may modulate expression of *Crh* in a manner dependent on the level of $Err\beta$ expression (Figure 3).

Neural progenitor-specific deletion of *Errβ* alters acoustic startle response

$Sox2\text{-}Cre\text{:}Err\beta^{+/lox}$ and $Sox2\text{-}Cre\text{:}Err\beta^{lox/lox}$ mice demonstrate differences in HPA activation, which may arise from central and/or peripheral mechanisms. In the central nervous system, $Err\beta$ expression is restricted to the hindbrain. $Nes\text{-}Cre\text{:}Err\beta^{lox/lox}$ mice lack $Err\beta$ in neural progenitor cells, effectively resulting in selective loss of Errβ expression in the hindbrain [14]. Therefore, we investigated the central role of $Err\beta$ in modulating stress responses in $Nes\text{-}Cre\text{:}Err\beta^{lox/lox}$ and WT mice using an acoustic startle test. The neuroanatomical and neurochemical basis of the acoustic startle response has been well mapped and involves neurons found in the amygdala, dorsomedial hypothalamus, and brainstem [35-39]. The amygdala elicits behavioral stress responses associated with the acoustic

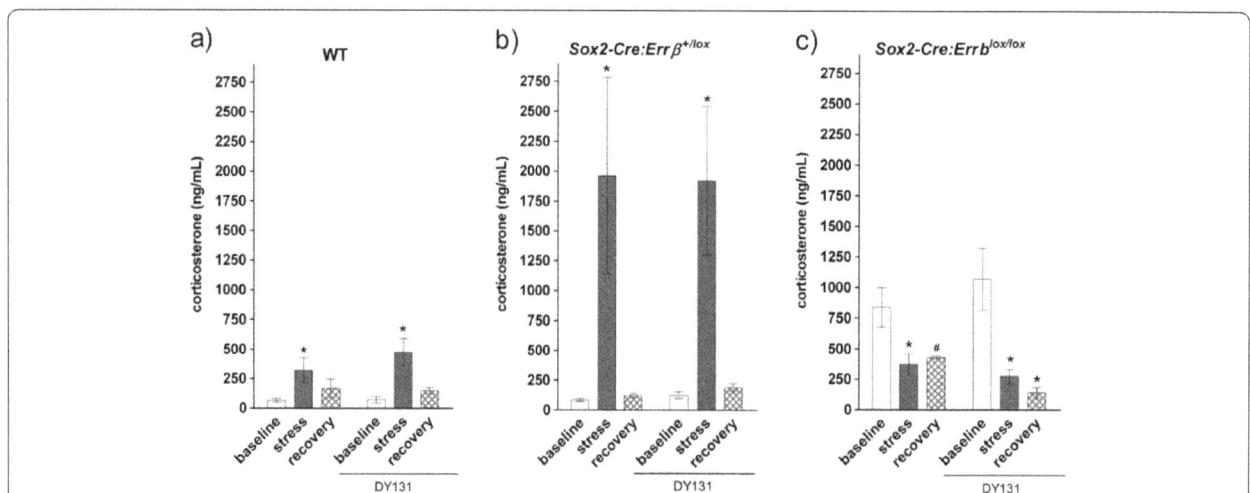

Figure 2 Glucocorticoid levels of wild-type (WT), *Sox2-Cre:Errβ⁺/lox*, and *Sox2-Cre:Errβlox/lox* mice after restraint stress. a) Baseline, stress, and recovery glucocorticoid levels were measured in serum of WT mice and after treatment with Errβ/Errγ agonist DY131 using a corticosterone radioimmunoassay. **b)** Baseline, stress, and recovery glucocorticoid levels were measured in serum of *Sox2-Cre:Errβ⁺/lox* mice and after treatment with Errβ/Errγ agonist DY131 using a corticosterone radioimmunoassay. **c)** Baseline, stress, and recovery glucocorticoid levels were measured in serum of *Sox2-Cre:Errβlox/lox* mice and after treatment with Errβ/Errγ agonist DY131 using a corticosterone radioimmunoassay. *$P < 0.05$.

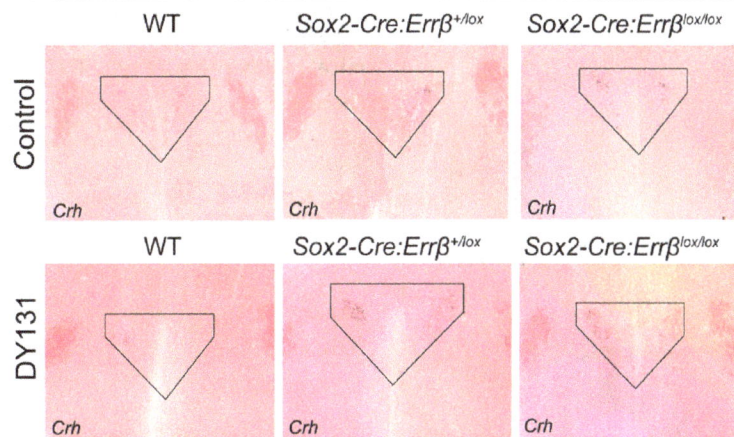

Figure 3 *Crh* **expression of wild-type (WT),** *Sox2-Cre:Errβ*[+/lox], **and** *Sox2-Cre:Errβ*[lox/lox] **mice.** Brain tissue of WT, *Sox2-Cre:Errβ*[+/lox], and *Sox2-Cre:Errβ*[lox/lox] mice injected with saline (top) or Errβ/Erry agonist DY131 (bottom) were stained for *Crh* by ISH (n = 2/genotype).

startle response and expresses the neuromodulators Crh and Npy [36,40]. *Nes-Cre:Errβ*[lox/lox] mice have decreased *Npy* expression in the hindbrain [14], which may modify neural circuitry activated by physical and psychological stress and, more specifically, the acoustic startle response.

We measured PPI and the acoustic startle response to determine if *Nes-Cre:Errβ*[lox/lox] mice had alterations in stress responses that arise from dysfunction of the inhibitory hindbrain circuit associated with PPI or the excitatory circuit associated with the acoustic startle response [41]. The acoustic startle response was measured after delivery of a prepulse intensity signal (0, 74, 78, 82, 86, or 90 dB) followed by the lead interval to a strong auditory stimulus. We observed a greater startle response in *Nes-Cre:Errβ*[lox/lox] mice (n = 8, db120; 1081.5 ±150) compared to WT mice (n = 12, db120; 475.8 ± 27) (Figure 4a, 0db - $F_{1,20} = 0.05$, $P = 0.81$; 0-120db - $F_{1,20} = 9.25$, $P = 0.006$; 74-120db - $F_{1,20} = 15.13$, $P = 0.001$; 78-120db - $F_{1,20} = 15.63$, $P = 0.0009$; 82-120db - $F_{1,20} = 14.04$, $P = 0.001$; 86-120db - $F_{1,10} = 14.17$, $P = 0.001$; 90-120db - $F_{1,8} = 14.98$, $P = 0.001$). However, the amplitude of the startle response decreased in *Nes-Cre:Errβ*[lox/lox] mice when the intensity of the prepulse tone increased. *Crh* expression was measured in the hindbrain of *Nes-Cre:Errβ*[lox/lox] mice and WT mice. Indeed, *Nes-Cre:Errβ*[lox/lox] mice have decreased expression of *Crh* and *Crhr2* relative to WT (Figure 4b, $F_{1,10} = 6.54$, $P = 0.03$ and Figure 4c, $F_{1,10} = 6.23$, $P = 0.03$). These results indicate alterations in the excitatory pathway that generates a startle response, but not the inhibitory pathway arising from the pedunculopontine tegmental nucleus associated with PPI [41-43]. The increased acoustic startle response in *Nes-Cre:Errβ*[lox/lox] mice may thus arise from altered activity of the excitatory pathway involving *Crh* and *Crhr2* expression and the pontine reticular nucleus, bed nucleus of the stria terminalis, amygdala, and hypothalamus [37-39,43-48]. The hindbrain excitatory pathways, which include

catecholaminergic projections to the paraventricular nucleus of the hypothalamus, increase *Crh* expression in the hypothalamus, suggesting that hindbrain signaling may alter the HPA-axis feedback loop [49].

Discussion

ERRs are involved with energy balance and metabolism [14-18]. Using mice globally deficient for *Errβ*, we have shown that *Errβ* modulates body composition, stress signaling, and hypothalamic neuropeptide expression (Table 2). *Errβ* gene dosage affected body composition and stress response with increased fat mass and corticosterone levels in *Sox2-Cre:Errβ*[+/lox] mice and decreased fat mass and corticosterone levels in *Sox2-Cre:Errβ*[lox/lox] mice (Table 1 and Figure 2). Additionally, central nervous system-specific *Errβ* deletion alters stress associated with the acoustic startle response pathways (Figure 4).

Hypothalamic expression of *Npy* and *Agrp*, orexigenic factors that increase fat mass and food intake [50-52], increased in both *Sox2-Cre:Errβ*[+/lox] and *Sox2-Cre:Errβ*[lox/lox] mice (Figure 1). These results suggest that increased anabolic neuropeptide expression may be due to central or peripheral mechanisms that are activated following global deletion of *Errβ*. Increased *Npy* and *Agrp* expression may be due to differences in leptin levels from adipose mass. Increased fat mass and lean mass were measured in *Sox2-Cre:Errβ*[+/lox] mice, although decreased fat mass and lean mass were measured in highly-active *Sox2-Cre:Errβ*[lox/lox] mice at nine months of age (Table 1). Expression of *Npy* and *leptin* are coordinately regulated, as Npy blunts the effects of leptin and increased leptin levels decrease *Npy* expression [23,53-55]. Thus, *Sox2-Cre:Errβ*[+/lox] mice may consume more food and increase *Npy* expression and fat mass due to leptin resistance; *Sox2-Cre:Errβ*[lox/lox] mice may increase *Npy* expression to compensate for decreased fat mass arising from increased physical activity

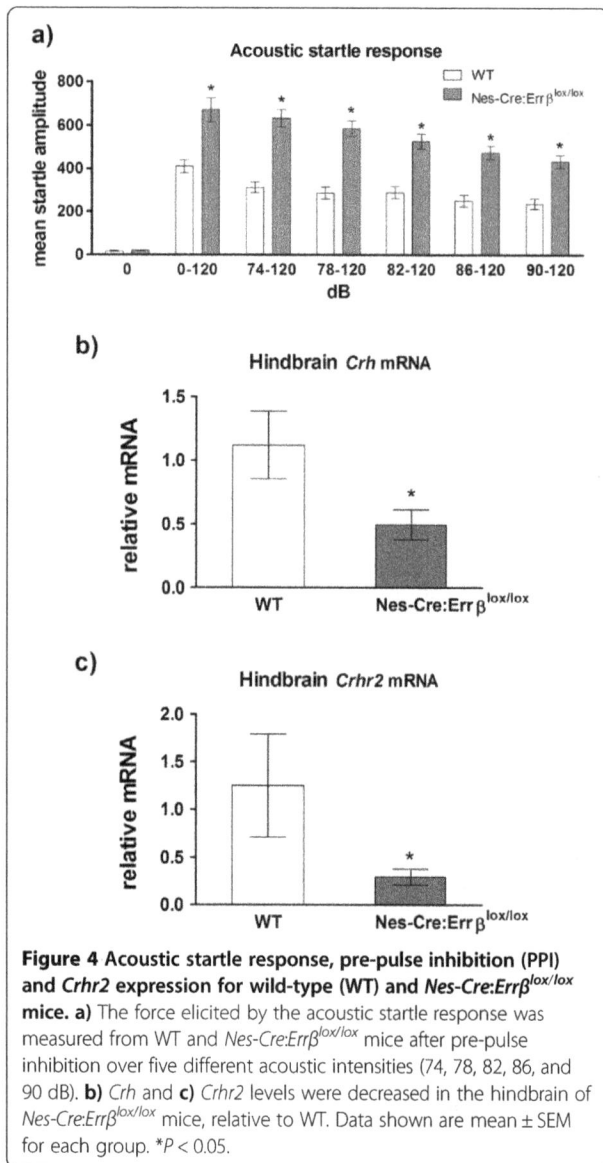

Figure 4 Acoustic startle response, pre-pulse inhibition (PPI) and *Crhr2* expression for wild-type (WT) and *Nes-Cre:Errβ^{lox/lox}* mice. a) The force elicited by the acoustic startle response was measured from WT and *Nes-Cre:Errβ^{lox/lox}* mice after pre-pulse inhibition over five different acoustic intensities (74, 78, 82, 86, and 90 dB). **b)** *Crh* and **c)** *Crhr2* levels were decreased in the hindbrain of *Nes-Cre:Errβ^{lox/lox}* mice, relative to WT. Data shown are mean ± SEM for each group. *$P < 0.05$.

Table 2 Summary of phenotype difference between *Sox2-Cre:Errβ^{+/lox}*, *Sox2-Cre:Errβ^{lox/lox}* and *Nes2-Cre:Errβ^{lox/lox}* mice, relative to wild type (WT)

Phenotype	Sox2-Cre: Errβ^{+/lox}	Sox2-Cre: Errβ^{lox/lox}	Nes2-Cre: Errβ^{lox/lox}
Body Composition			
Body weight	↑,	↓,	↑
Fat mass	↑,	↓,	NC
Lean mass	↓,	↓,	↑
Hormone and Neuropeptides			
Corticosterone	↑,	↓,	NA
Corticosterone (DY131)	↑,	↓,	NA
Crh expression	↑,	↑,	↓
Crh expression (DY131)	↑↑,	↑↑,	NA
Npy expression	↑,	↑,	↓
Agrp expression	↑,	↑,	NA
Stress Behavior			
Acoustic startle response	NA,	NA,	↑
Meal patterns			
Total pellets consumed	↑,	↑,	NC
Inter Meal interval (IMI)	NC,	↓,	↓
Satiety Ratio	↓^#,	↓,	↓

↑ – increase, ↓ – decrease, NC – no change, ↑↑ – increase relative to levels with no DY131 treatment, NA – not available, ^#$P = 0.05$ relative to WT; *Nes2-Cre:Errβ^{lox/lox}* data adapted from [14].

(Figure 1 and Table 1). In support of this, *Nes-Cre:Errβ^{lox/lox}* mice have increased lean mass, no change in physical activity and have decreased *Npy* expression in the hindbrain [14]. Changes in body composition emerged prior to changes in body weight, suggesting that both peripheral and central signals may be altered to regulate the development of increased fat mass (Table 1).

The opposite phenotypes that are seen in the *Sox2-Cre:Errβ^{+/lox}* and *Sox2-Cre:Errβ^{lox/lox}* mice may arise from the ability of Errβ or Errγ to regulate gene transcription as both homodimers and Errβ/Errγ heterodimers [1,6,7,9,10]. Errβ/Errγ heterodimers have been predicted to exist, but to our knowledge it has not been directly detected *in vivo* [1]. RIP140 is a nuclear receptor corepressor that regulates cellular metabolism [56-58]. RIP140 enhanced transcriptional activity for all three mouse *Err* genes [59]. Mice

lacking RIP140 are lean, with increased metabolic rate and insulin sensitivity [58]. Similarly, *Sox2-Cre:Errβ^{lox/lox}* mice are lean with increased metabolic rate (Table 1 and [14]), and *Nes-Cre:Errβ^{lox/lox}* have increased lean mass, increased metabolic rate and insulin sensitivity [14]. Since deletion of both *Errβ* and *RIP140* exhibit similar phenotypes, this suggests that increased lean mass relative to fat mass, metabolic rate and insulin sensitivity may arise from both the RIP140 corepressor and Errβ [59].

ChIP-seq analysis derived from embryonic stem cells revealed that Errβ binds the regulatory element of two genes associated with Crh activity — Corticotropin releasing hormone binding protein (*Crhbp*) and Corticotropin releasing hormone receptor 2 (*Crhr2*) — as well as one gene associated with whole-body energy balance and stress responses, Cholecystokinin B receptor (*Cckbr*) [60]. We hypothesize that *Errβ*, *Crhbp* and *Crhr2* may modulate stress signaling by altering the biological activity of Crh in extrahypothalamic sites and/or corticosterone feedback or secretion [32,39,48,61-64]. Disruption of Errβ-dependent regulation of expression of *Cckbr* and/or *Crhr2* may at least partially explain the abnormal meal patterns and stress behaviors (e.g. acoustic startle response, *Crh* expression or corticosterone levels) observed in *Sox2-Cre:Errβ^{lox/lox}*, *Sox2-Cre:Errβ^{+/lox}*, and *Nes-Cre:Errβ^{lox/lox}* mice [14].

Crh is expressed in the paraventricular nucleus of the hypothalamus and initiates ACTH release from the pituitary [40,65]. Crh has since been found to be synthesized in extra-hypothalamic sites, where it also acts to modulate stress response and food intake [40,65-67]. ERR family members also modulate stress responses by regulating glucocorticoid receptor activity in muscle and neuroblastoma cell lines [22,33]. Further, *Errβ* and *Crh* are expressed in similar regions of the hindbrain [29]. Here we demonstrate that *Errβ* deletion modulates corticosterone levels after exposure to restraint stress, with increased levels in *Sox2-Cre:Errβ*$^{+/lox}$ mice and decreased levels in *Sox2-Cre:Errβ*$^{lox/lox}$ mice relative to WT (Figure 2). Neural connections projecting to the hypothalamus from extra-hypothalamic sites, such as the hindbrain, may also regulate hypothalamic Crh release and *Crh* expression [30,49,68-70].

Biological activity of Crh is inhibited by Crhbp, and Errβ binds to the promoter region of the *Crhbp* gene [60,71], which contains three ERE half sites [72]. Mice that overexpress Crhbp have increased *Crh* expression, potentially resulting from a compensatory response aimed at ameliorating disruptions in stress response [73]. Similarly, increased *Crh* expression was observed when *Errβ* was reduced (*Sox2-Cre:Errβ*$^{+/lox}$) or eliminated (*Sox2-Cre:Errβ*$^{+/lox}$) in somatic tissue, and Erry was activated using DY131 (Figure 3). Therefore, we propose that partial or complete deletion of *Errβ* may alter *Crh* expression by modulating transcription of *Crhbp* or *Crhr2*, resulting in altered corticosterone secretion. Furthermore, *Sox2:Errβ*$^{lox/lox}$ mice lack corticosterone secretion after restraint stress (Figure 2), which may result from altered *Crhr2* expression (Figure 4c) and changes in negative feedback. Therefore, brain regions that express *Crhr2* may show reduced Crh signaling (Figure 4b and 4c), as in the hindbrain [64].

Errβ binds to *cis*-regulatory regions of the *Cckbr* gene [60], which is expressed in the hindbrain [29,74] and the corresponding gene maps to a genomic locus of the genome associated with obesity [75]. *Cckbr* deficient mice (*Cckbr*$^{-/-}$) display a similar phenotype to *Sox2-Cre:Errβ*$^{+/lox}$ mice, and have increased body weight and food intake, which may arise from changes in Cholecystokinin (Cck) signaling (e.g. satiety), and increased metabolism [74,76]. However, *Cckbr*$^{-/-}$ mice also have blunted stress responses associated with anxiety-like behavior [77] and increased *Npy* expression [78], which resembles the phenotype of *Sox2-Cre:Errβ*$^{lox/lox}$ mice (Figure 1 and Table 1). Therefore, heterodimers of Errβ alone, or Errβ in combination with ERRγ, may regulate *Cckbr* transcription, thereby partially accounting for the differences in the phenotypes seen in *Sox2-Cre:Errβ*$^{+/lox}$ and *Sox2-Cre:Errβ*$^{lox/lox}$ mice (Table 2). Differences in developmental compensation arising from Errβ and/or Erry may

also contribute to the phenotype differences in *Sox2-Cre:Errβ*$^{+/lox}$ and *Sox2-Cre:Errβ*$^{lox/lox}$ mice.

Nes-Cre:Errβ$^{lox/lox}$ mice show increased *Erry* expression relative to WT animals [14], while mice deficient for *Erry* show increased *Errβ* expression [17]. This suggests that homozygous mice have reciprocal patterns of *Errβ* and *Erry* expression, potentially arising from developmental compensation and heterozygous mice may partially lack this compensation, contributing to phenotype differences. The Errβ/Erry agonist (DY131) increased *Crh* expression more when *Errβ* expression was reduced (*Sox2:Errβ*$^{+/lox}$ mice) than when *Errβ* expression was absent (*Sox2:Errβ*$^{lox/lox}$ mice) (Figure 3). These results suggest that the ratio of Errβ to Erry signaling may contribute to the observed difference in *Crh* expression, *Crhr2* expression and corticosterone secretion in the two genotypes examined.

Sox2-Cre:Errβ$^{lox/lox}$ and *Sox2-Cre:Errβ*$^{+/lox}$ mice have alterations in the HPA axis (Figures 2 and 3). *Npy*, which modulates corticosterone levels [79], is altered in *Sox2-Cre:Errβ*$^{+/lox}$ and *Sox2-Cre:Errβ*$^{lox/lox}$ (Figures 1 and 2). Both Crh and Npy have been implicated in modulating the acoustic startle response [32,36,40,80], which is altered in *Nes-Cre:Errβ*$^{lox/lox}$ mice (Figure 4 and [14]). Given the results reported here, the phenotype differences between *Sox2-Cre:Errβ*$^{+/lox}$ and *Sox2-Cre:Errβ*$^{lox/lox}$ mice may specifically arise from altered *Crh* expression and corticosterone levels as a result of changes in Errβ-dependent regulation of *Crhbp* or *Crhr2* transcription, as well as through interactions of Errβ with Erry. However, since little is known about Errβ/Erry heterodimers or how different Err family homo and heterodimers may potentially regulate *Crhbp* or *Crhr2* transcription deserves further investigation.

Our data suggest that central *Errβ* modulates stress responses, food intake and body weight, although it remains to be determined whether peripheral *Errβ* also modulates components of the HPA axis and acoustic startle response. *Nes-Cre:Errβ*$^{lox/lox}$ mice lack *Errβ* in the hindbrain and have decreased expression of *Crh*, *Crhr2* and *Npy* [14], suggesting that neuromodulators involved with the acoustic startle response reside in the hindbrain to modulate stress and anxiety. However, other changes in neural circuitry (e.g. altered *Cckbr* expression) regulating the acoustic startle response in *Nes-Cre:Errβ*$^{lox/lox}$ mice are likely to exist and remain to be identified.

Conclusions

Mice heterozygous for *Errβ* deletion have increased fat mass and stress hormone secretion after restraint stress, while those homozygous for *Errβ* deletion have decreased fat mass and secrete higher baseline levels of stress hormones. These effects may be modulated by components of the HPA axis, such as *Crh*, *Crhbp*, *Crhr2*, *Npy* or *Cckrb*. Central Errβ signaling influences stress associated behavior (e.g. the acoustic startle response), possibly through regulation of *Npy*, *Crh* and *Crhr2* expression in the hindbrain or hypothalamic projections to the amygdala [32,62,63,80]. Since the neural circuitry controlling the acoustic startle response is well-conserved between rodents and humans [36,81], these data suggest that ERRβ or ERRγ may be promising candidates for pharmacological treatment of excessive anxiety or stress levels in humans.

Methods

Animals, housing, food intake, and physical activity measurement

Sox2-Cre:Errβ^{lox/lox}, *Sox2-Cre:Errβ^{+/lox}*, and wild-type (WT) (*Errβ^{lox/lox}*) mice were generated as previously described [26]. Briefly, Errβ mice have a conditional allele, with loxP sites flanking exon 2 of the *Errβ* gene that encodes the DNA binding domain (exon 2) [26]. Expression of cre recombinase will excise the loxP-flanked exon 2 from the *Errβ* gene. Sox2-Cre deletes *Errβ* from all embryonic tissues and Nestin-Cre deletes *Errβ* from developing neural tissue. *Sox2-Cre:Errβ^{lox/lox}* mice completely lack functional *Errβ* because both alleles have been removed. *Sox2-Cre:Errβ^{+/lox}* have one wild-type allele of the *Errβ* gene, since the other allele has been excised by the loxP sites. These two mouse lines enable us to address possible phenotypic differences due to differences in gene dosage. Wild-type (WT) mice used for these studies were homozygous for the floxed Errβ allele. Mice were maintained on a 12:12 hour light–dark cycle in a temperature- and humidity-regulated vivarium and had *ad libitum* access to standard laboratory chow (2018, Harlan-Teklad, Harlan Laboratories, Frederick, MD, USA) and water at all times. Different cohorts of mice were analyzed at three weeks and nine months of age. Food intake data and physical activity levels were collected as previously described [14]. Physical activity levels were measured by detecting and counting horizontal beam breaks in a 40 cm × 40 cm × 30 cm plexiglass chamber (Digiscan, Accuscan Instruments, Columbus, OH). All experimental procedures were performed in accordance with the Johns Hopkins University School of Medicine Institutional Animal Care and Use Committee and the National Institutes of Health *Guide for the Care and Use of Laboratory Animals*.

In situ *hybridization assay (ISH) and quantitative real-time PCR*

ISH was performed as previously described [14,82]. Briefly, digoxigenin cRNA probes to *Npy* and *agouti-related protein* (*Agrp*) were synthesized using the Brain Molecular Anatomy Project (BMAP) library containing sequence-verified expressed sequence tags. BMAP clones were purified using a PureLink plasmid miniprep kit per manufacturer's protocol (Invitrogen, Carlsbad, CA, USA) and synthesized using a T3 or T7 RNA polymerase (Roche, Indianapolis, IN, USA). The riboprobe was purified using an RNA extraction kit per manufacturer's protocol (RNeasy, Qiagen, Valencia, CA, USA). Brains were collected from mice, fresh frozen in OCT compound (Tissue Tek, Fisher Scientific, Pittsburgh, PA, USA), and cut using a cryostat into 25-μm sections onto Superfrost Plus slides (Fisher Scientific, Pittsburgh, PA, USA). Hindbrain dissection, mRNA extraction and quantitative real-time PCR was conducted as previously described [14,83]. Briefly, RNA was extracted (RNeasy, Qiagen, Valencia, CA, USA) and cDNA was synthesized using 1 μg of mRNA using Superscript II reverse transcriptase (Invitrogen) and random primers (Invitrogen). Quantitative PCR primer sequences were obtained from PrimerBank and conducted for *Crh*: fwd – 5' CCTCAGC CGGTTCTGATCC 3' and rev – 5' GCGGAAAAAGTTA GCCGCAG 3', *Crhr2*: fwd – 5' CATCCACCACGTCCGA GAC 3' and rev – 5' CTCGCCAGGATTGACAAAGAA 3' and *18S* fwd – 5' GCAATTATTCCCCATGAACG 3' and rev- 5' GGCCTCACTAAACCATCCAA 3'. The Ct value generated was normalized to *18S* in order to obtain a ΔCt value, followed by generating the $2^{-\Delta\Delta Ct}$ value by normalizing the data to control animals as previously described [84].

Restraint stress test, corticosterone radioimmunoassay, and DY131 injections

Baseline blood glucocorticoid levels were measured and mice were placed into a restraining tube (one mouse/tube) for one hour. Upon removal from the restraining tube, blood samples were collected again. Animals were then returned to their housing and blood samples were collected after a one-hour recovery period. Blood was collected in heparin-coated tubes and centrifuged at 3800 rpm for 20 min at 4°C. Corticosterone assays were performed with a radioimmunoassay kit for corticosterone per manufacturer's directions (MP Biomedicals, Solon, OH, USA). DY131 (Tocris, Bristol, BS11, United Kingdom) at a dose of 10 μM/g body weight was injected, and data for meal patterns collected as previously described [14].

Prepulse inhibition (PPI) of acoustic startle response

Startle reactivity and PPI were measured using two startle chambers located inside a sound-attenuating chamber (San Diego Instruments, San Diego, CA, USA). Mice were placed in a Plexiglass tube within the soundproof PPI box for a five-minute acclimation period, which provides exposure to a continuous background noise (70 dB) to elicit an increase in startle amplitude [43]. Mice were then exposed for five minutes without any startle stimulus. The PPI session then began and mice were randomly exposed to the following trials: pulse alone (120 dB), no stimulus, or five prepulse combinations (a 20 ms non-startling prepulse at 74, 78, 82, 86, or 90 dB, followed by an 80 ms startle stimulus at 120 dB). The force from the startle reaction was recorded by an accelerometer with SR-LAB software (San Diego Instruments). Results were analyzed by PPI percentage, which was calculated as:

$$(\text{mean startle amplitude on pulse alone}) -$$
$$(\text{mean startle amplitude on prepulse}) /$$
$$(\text{mean startle amplitude on pulse alone}).$$

Statistical analysis

All value comparisons were made using one-way ANOVA to identify individual differences between groups, and $P < 0.05$ was considered significant (Statistica v.8.0, Tulsa, OK, USA).

Abbreviations

ACTH: Adrenocorticotropic hormone; Agrp: Agouti-related protein; Crh: Corticotropin-releasing hormone; Crhbp: Corticotropin releasing hormone binding protein; Crhr2: Corticotropin releasing hormone receptor 2; ERR: Estrogen-related receptor; ERRE: Estrogen-related receptor response element; HPA: Hypothalamic-pituitary-adrenal axis; IMI: Inter meal interval; ISH: In situ hybridization; Npy: Neuropeptide Y; PPI: Prepulse inhibition; WT: Wild-type.

Competing interests

The authors declare that they have no competing interests.

Authors' contributions

MSB, GWW, and SB; MSB conducted all research; RDS provided technical support for measuring corticosterone levels; MSB analyzed data; MSB drafted the manuscript and MSB, GWW, and SB edited the final version. All authors read and approved the final manuscript.

Acknowledgements

MSB is supported by the National Institute of Diabetes and Digestive and Kidney Diseases training fellowship (T32DK007751), GWW by the National Institutes of Health (DK084171) and the American Heart Association (SDG2260721), and SB by a WM Keck Distinguished Young Scholar Award in Medical Research.

Author details

[1]Department of Physiology, Johns Hopkins University School of Medicine, Baltimore, MD, USA. [2]Department of Neuroscience, Johns Hopkins University School of Medicine, Baltimore, MD, USA. [3]Department of Neurology, Johns Hopkins University School of Medicine, Baltimore, MD, USA. [4]Department of Ophthalmology, Johns Hopkins University School of Medicine, Baltimore, MD, USA. [5]Center for Metabolism and Obesity Research, Johns Hopkins University School of Medicine, Baltimore, MD, USA. [6]Center for High-Throughput Biology, Johns Hopkins University School of Medicine, Baltimore, MD, USA. [7]Institute for Cell Engineering, Johns Hopkins University School of Medicine, Baltimore, MD, USA.

References

1. Giguere V: Transcriptional control of energy homeostasis by the estrogen-related receptors. Endocr Rev 2008, 29:677–696.
2. Giguere V, Yang N, Segui P, Evans RM: Identification of a new class of steroid hormone receptors. Nature 1988, 331:91–94.
3. Pettersson K, Svensson K, Mattsson R, Carlsson B, Ohlsson R, Berkenstam A: Expression of a novel member of estrogen response element-binding nuclear receptors is restricted to the early stages of chorion formation during mouse embryogenesis. Mech Dev 1996, 54:211–223.
4. Lu D, Kiriyama Y, Lee KY, Giguere V: Transcriptional regulation of the estrogen-inducible pS2 breast cancer marker gene by the ERR family of orphan nuclear receptors. Cancer Res 2001, 61:6755–6761.
5. Johnston SD, Liu X, Zuo F, Eisenbraun TL, Wiley SR, Kraus RJ, Mertz JE: Estrogen-related receptor alpha 1 functionally binds as a monomer to extended half-site sequences including ones contained within estrogen-response elements. Mol Endocrinol 1997, 11:342–352.
6. Vanacker JM, Pettersson K, Gustafsson JA, Laudet V: Transcriptional targets shared by estrogen receptor- related receptors (ERRs) and estrogen receptor (ER) alpha, but not by ERbeta. Embo J 1999, 18:4270–4279.
7. Vanacker JM, Bonnelye E, Chopin-Delannoy S, Delmarre C, Cavailles V, Laudet V: Transcriptional activities of the orphan nuclear receptor ERR alpha (estrogen receptor-related receptor-alpha). Mol Endocrinol 1999, 13:764–773.
8. Deblois G, Hall JA, Perry MC, Laganiere J, Ghahremani M, Park M, Hallett M, Giguere V: Genome-wide identification of direct target genes implicates estrogen-related receptor alpha as a determinant of breast cancer heterogeneity. Cancer Res 2009, 69:6149–6157.
9. Huppunen J, Aarnisalo P: Dimerization modulates the activity of the orphan nuclear receptor ERRgamma. Biochem Biophys Res Commun 2004, 314:964–970.
10. Gearhart MD, Holmbeck SM, Evans RM, Dyson HJ, Wright PE: Monomeric complex of human orphan estrogen related receptor-2 with DNA: a pseudo-dimer interface mediates extended half-site recognition. J Mol Biol 2003, 327:819–832.
11. Giguere V: To ERR in the estrogen pathway. Trends Endocrinol Metab 2002, 13:220–225.
12. Chen F, Zhang Q, McDonald T, Davidoff MJ, Bailey W, Bai C, Liu Q, Caskey CT: Identification of two hERR2-related novel nuclear receptors utilizing bioinformatics and inverse PCR. Gene 1999, 228:101–109.
13. Eudy JD, Yao S, Weston MD, Ma-Edmonds M, Talmadge CB, Cheng JJ, Kimberling WJ, Sumegi J: Isolation of a gene encoding a novel member of the nuclear receptor superfamily from the critical region of Usher syndrome type IIa at 1q41. Genomics 1998, 50:382–384.
14. Byerly MS, Al Salayta M, Swanson RD, Kwon K, Peterson JM, Wei Z, Aja S, Moran TH, Blackshaw S, Wong GW: Estrogen-related receptor beta deletion modulates whole-body energy balance via estrogen-related receptor gamma and attenuates neuropeptide Y gene expression. Eur J Neurosci 2013, 37:1033–1047.
15. Herzog B, Cardenas J, Hall RK, Villena JA, Budge PJ, Giguere V, Granner DK, Kralli A: Estrogen-related receptor alpha is a repressor of phosphoenolpyruvate carboxykinase gene transcription. J Biol Chem 2006, 281:99–106.
16. Luo J, Sladek R, Bader JA, Matthyssen A, Rossant J, Giguere V: Placental abnormalities in mouse embryos lacking the orphan nuclear receptor ERR-beta. Nature 1997, 388:778–782.
17. Dufour CR, Wilson BJ, Huss JM, Kelly DP, Alaynick WA, Downes M, Evans RM, Blanchette M, Giguere V: Genome-wide orchestration of cardiac functions by the orphan nuclear receptors ERRalpha and gamma. Cell Metab 2007, 5:345–356.
18. Alaynick WA, Kondo RP, Xie W, He W, Dufour CR, Downes M, Jonker JW, Giles W, Naviaux RK, Giguere V, et al: ERRgamma directs and maintains the transition to oxidative metabolism in the postnatal heart. Cell Metab 2007, 6:13–24.
19. Miller DB, O'Callaghan JP: Neuroendocrine aspects of the response to stress. Metabolism 2002, 51:5–10.
20. Mitchell AL, Pearce SH: Autoimmune Addison disease: pathophysiology and genetic complexity. Nat Rev Endocrinol 2012, 8:306–316.
21. Napier C, Pearce SH: Autoimmune Addison's disease. Presse Med 2012, 41:e626–e635.
22. Trapp T, Holsboer F: Nuclear orphan receptor as a repressor of glucocorticoid receptor transcriptional activity. J Biol Chem 1996, 271:9879–9882.
23. Bjorntorp P: Do stress reactions cause abdominal obesity and comorbidities? Obes Rev 2001, 2:73–86.
24. Erickson JC, Ahima RS, Hollopeter G, Flier JS, Palmiter RD: Endocrine function of neuropeptide Y knockout mice. Regul Pept 1997, 70:199–202.
25. Frankish HM, Dryden S, Hopkins D, Wang Q, Williams G: Neuropeptide Y, the hypothalamus, and diabetes: insights into the central control of metabolism. Peptides 1995, 16:757–771.
26. Chen J, Nathans J: Estrogen-related receptor beta/NR3B2 controls epithelial cell fate and endolymph production by the stria vascularis. Dev Cell 2007, 13:325–337.
27. Onishi A, Peng GH, Poth EM, Lee DA, Chen J, Alexis U, de Melo J, Chen S, Blackshaw S: The orphan nuclear hormone receptor ERRbeta controls rod photoreceptor survival. Proc Natl Acad Sci U S A 2010, 107:11579–11584.

28. Gofflot F, Chartoire N, Vasseur L, Heikkinen S, Dembele D, Le Merrer J, Auwerx J: Systematic gene expression mapping clusters nuclear receptors according to their function in the brain. *Cell* 2007, **131**:405–418.

29. Lein ES, Hawrylycz MJ, Ao N, Ayres M, Bensinger A, Bernard A, Boe AF, Boguski MS, Brockway KS, Byrnes EJ, *et al*: Genome-wide atlas of gene expression in the adult mouse brain. *Nature* 2007, **445**:168–176.

30. Grill HJ, Hayes MR: Hindbrain neurons as an essential hub in the neuroanatomically distributed control of energy balance. *Cell Metab* 2012, **16**:296–309.

31. Gray TS, Cassell MD, Kiss JZ: Distribution of pro-opiomelanocortin-derived peptides and enkephalins in the rat central nucleus of the amygdala. *Brain Res* 1984, **306**:354–358.

32. Yang FC, Connor J, Patel A, Doat MM, Romero MT: Neural transplants. effects On startle responses in neonatally MSG-treated rats. *Physiol Behav* 2000, **69**:333–344.

33. Wang SC, Myers S, Dooms C, Capon R, Muscat GE: An ERRbeta/gamma agonist modulates GRalpha expression, and glucocorticoid responsive gene expression in skeletal muscle cells. *Mol Cell Endocrinol* 2010, **315**:146–152.

34. Yu DD, Forman BM: Identification of an agonist ligand for estrogen-related receptors ERRbeta/gamma. *Bioorg Med Chem Lett* 2005, **15**:1311–1313.

35. Plappert CF, Pilz PK: The acoustic startle response as an effective model for elucidating the effect of genes on the neural mechanism of behavior in mice. *Behav Brain Res* 2001, **125**:183–188.

36. Koch M: The neurobiology of startle. *Prog Neurobiol* 1999, **59**:107–128.

37. Lee Y, Lopez DE, Meloni EG, Davis M: A primary acoustic startle pathway: obligatory role of cochlear root neurons and the nucleus reticularis pontis caudalis. *J Neurosci* 1996, **16**:3775–3789.

38. Davis M, Falls WA, Campeau S, Kim M: Fear-potentiated startle: a neural and pharmacological analysis. *Behav Brain Res* 1993, **58**:175–198.

39. Inglefield JR, Schwarzkopf SB, Kellogg CK: Alterations in behavioral responses to stressors following excitotoxin lesions of dorsomedial hypothalamic regions. *Brain Res* 1994, **633**:151–161.

40. Liang KC, Melia KR, Campeau S, Falls WA, Miserendino MJ, Davis M: Lesions of the central nucleus of the amygdala, but not the paraventricular nucleus of the hypothalamus, block the excitatory effects of corticotropin-releasing factor on the acoustic startle reflex. *J Neurosci* 1992, **12**:2313–2320.

41. Plappert CF, Pilz PK, Schnitzler HU: Factors governing prepulse inhibition and prepulse facilitation of the acoustic startle response in mice. *Behav Brain Res* 2004, **152**:403–412.

42. Hoffman HS, Ison JR: Reflex modification in the domain of startle: I. Some empirical findings and their implications for how the nervous system processes sensory input. *Psychol Rev* 1980, **87**:175–189.

43. Leumann L, Sterchi D, Vollenweider F, Ludewig K, Fruh H: A neural network approach to the acoustic startle reflex and prepulse inhibition. *Brain Res Bull* 2001, **56**:101–110.

44. Yeomans JS, Frankland PW: The acoustic startle reflex: neurons and connections. *Brain Res Brain Res Rev* 1995, **21**:301–314.

45. Heilig M, Koob GF, Ekman R, Britton KT: Corticotropin-releasing factor and neuropeptide Y: role in emotional integration. *Trends Neurosci* 1994, **17**:80–85.

46. Fendt M, Koch M, Schnitzler HU: NMDA receptors in the pontine brainstem are necessary for fear potentiation of the startle response. *Eur J Pharmacol* 1996, **318**:1–6.

47. Alon T, Zhou L, Perez CA, Garfield AS, Friedman JM, Heisler LK: Transgenic mice expressing green fluorescent protein under the control of the corticotropin-releasing hormone promoter. *Endocrinology* 2009, **150**:5626–5632.

48. Meloni EG, Gerety LP, Knoll AT, Cohen BM, Carlezon WA Jr: Behavioral and anatomical interactions between dopamine and corticotropin-releasing factor in the rat. *J Neurosci* 2006, **26**:3855–3863.

49. Khan AM, Kaminski KL, Sanchez-Watts G, Ponzio TA, Kuzmiski JB, Bains JS, Watts AG: MAP kinases couple hindbrain-derived catecholamine signals to hypothalamic adrenocortical control mechanisms during glycemia-related challenges. *J Neurosci* 2011, **31**:18479–18491.

50. Patel HR, Qi Y, Hawkins EJ, Hileman SM, Elmquist JK, Imai Y, Ahima RS: Neuropeptide Y deficiency attenuates responses to fasting and high-fat diet in obesity-prone mice. *Diabetes* 2006, **55**:3091–3098.

51. Segal-Lieberman G, Trombly DJ, Juthani V, Wang X, Maratos-Flier E: NPY ablation in C57BL/6 mice leads to mild obesity and to an impaired refeeding response to fasting. *Am J Physiol Endocrinol Metab* 2003, **284**:E1131–E1139.

52. Wortley KE, Anderson KD, Yasenchak J, Murphy A, Valenzuela D, Diano S, Yancopoulos GD, Wiegand SJ, Sleeman MW: Agouti-related protein-deficient mice display an age-related lean phenotype. *Cell Metab* 2005, **2**:421–427.

53. Sainsbury A, Cusin I, Doyle P, Rohner-Jeanrenaud F, Jeanrenaud B: Intracerebroventricular administration of neuropeptide Y to normal rats increases obese gene expression in white adipose tissue. *Diabetologia* 1996, **39**:353–356.

54. Schwartz MW, Baskin DG, Bukowski TR, Kuijper JL, Foster D, Lasser G, Prunkard DE, Porte D Jr, Woods SC, Seeley RJ, *et al*: Specificity of leptin action on elevated blood glucose levels and hypothalamic neuropeptide Y gene expression in ob/ob mice. *Diabetes* 1996, **45**:531–535.

55. Schwartz MW, Seeley RJ, Campfield LA, Burn P, Baskin DG: Identification of targets of leptin action in rat hypothalamus. *J Clin Invest* 1996, **98**:1101–1106.

56. Christian M, White R, Parker MG: Metabolic regulation by the nuclear receptor corepressor RIP140. *Trends Endocrinol Metab* 2006, **17**:243–250.

57. Rosell M, Jones MC, Parker MG: Role of nuclear receptor corepressor RIP140 in metabolic syndrome. *Biochim Biophys Acta* 2011, **1812**:919–928.

58. Leonardsson G, Steel JH, Christian M, Pocock V, Milligan S, Bell J, So PW, Medina-Gomez G, Vidal-Puig A, White R, *et al*: Nuclear receptor corepressor RIP140 regulates fat accumulation. *Proc Natl Acad Sci USA* 2004, **101**:8437–8442.

59. Castet A, Herledan A, Bonnet S, Jalaguier S, Vanacker JM, Cavailles V: Receptor-interacting protein 140 differentially regulates estrogen receptor-related receptor transactivation depending on target genes. *Mol Endocrinol* 2006, **20**:1035–1047.

60. Chen X, Xu H, Yuan P, Fang F, Huss M, Vega VB, Wong E, Orlov YL, Zhang W, Jiang J, *et al*: Integration of external signaling pathways with the core transcriptional network in embryonic stem cells. *Cell* 2008, **133**:1106–1117.

61. Meloni EG, Reedy CL, Cohen BM, Carlezon WA Jr: Activation of raphe efferents to the medial prefrontal cortex by corticotropin-releasing factor: correlation with anxiety-like behavior. *Biol Psychiatry* 2008, **63**:832–839.

62. Lyons AM, Thiele TE: Neuropeptide Y conjugated to saporin alters anxiety-like behavior when injected into the central nucleus of the amygdala or basomedial hypothalamus in BALB/cJ mice. *Peptides* 2010, **31**:2193–2199.

63. Deo GS, Dandekar MP, Upadhya MA, Kokare DM, Subhedar NK: Neuropeptide Y Y1 receptors in the central nucleus of amygdala mediate the anxiolytic-like effect of allopregnanolone in mice: Behavioral and immunocytochemical evidences. *Brain Res* 2010, **1318**:77–86.

64. Chalmers DT, Lovenberg TW, De Souza EB: Localization of novel corticotropin-releasing factor receptor (CRF2) mRNA expression to specific subcortical nuclei in rat brain: comparison with CRF1 receptor mRNA expression. *J Neurosci* 1995, **15**:6340–6350.

65. Grill HJ, Markison S, Ginsberg A, Kaplan JM: Long-term effects on feeding and body weight after stimulation of forebrain or hindbrain CRH receptors with urocortin. *Brain Res* 2000, **867**:19–28.

66. Bledsoe AC, Oliver KM, Scholl JL, Forster GL: Anxiety states induced by post-weaning social isolation are mediated by CRF receptors in the dorsal raphe nucleus. *Brain Res Bull* 2011, **85**:117–122.

67. Hammack SE, Pepin JL, DesMarteau JS, Watkins LR, Maier SF: Low doses of corticotropin-releasing hormone injected into the dorsal raphe nucleus block the behavioral consequences of uncontrollable stress. *Behav Brain Res* 2003, **147**:55–64.

68. Grill HJ, Kaplan JM: The neuroanatomical axis for control of energy balance. *Front Neuroendocrinol* 2002, **23**:2–40.

69. Grill HJ: Distributed neural control of energy balance: contributions from hindbrain and hypothalamus. *Obesity (Silver Spring)* 2006, **14**(Suppl 5):216S–221S.

70. Sawchenko PE, Swanson LW: Central noradrenergic pathways for the integration of hypothalamic neuroendocrine and autonomic responses. *Science* 1981, **214**:685–687.

71. Potter E, Behan DP, Linton EA, Lowry PJ, Sawchenko PE, Vale WW: The central distribution of a corticotropin-releasing factor (CRF)-binding protein predicts multiple sites and modes of interaction with CRF. *Proc Natl Acad Sci U S A* 1992, **89**:4192–4196.

72. Behan DP, Potter E, Lewis KA, Jenkins NA, Copeland N, Lowry PJ, Vale WW: Cloning and structure of the human corticotrophin releasing factor-binding protein gene (CRHBP). *Genomics* 1993, **16**:63–68.

73. Burrows HL, Nakajima M, Lesh JS, Goosens KA, Samuelson LC, Inui A, Camper SA, Seasholtz AF: Excess corticotropin releasing hormone-binding protein in the hypothalamic-pituitary-adrenal axis in transgenic mice. *J Clin Invest* 1998, **101**:1439–1447.

74. Clerc P, Coll Constans MG, Lulka H, Broussaud S, Guigne C, Leung-Theung -Long S, Perrin C, Knauf C, Carpene C, Penicaud L, *et al*: **Involvement of cholecystokinin 2 receptor in food intake regulation: hyperphagia and increased fat deposition in cholecystokinin 2 receptor-deficient mice.** *Endocrinology* 2007, **148**:1039–1049.

75. Samuelson LC, Isakoff MS, Lacourse KA: **Localization of the murine cholecystokinin A and B receptor genes.** *Mamm Genome* 1995, **6**:242–246.

76. Miyasaka K, Ichikawa M, Ohta M, Kanai S, Yoshida Y, Masuda M, Nagata A, Matsui T, Noda T, Takiguchi S, *et al*: **Energy metabolism and turnover are increased in mice lacking the cholecystokinin-B receptor.** *J Nutr* 2002, **132**:739–741.

77. Horinouchi Y, Akiyoshi J, Nagata A, Matsushita H, Tsutsumi T, Isogawa K, Noda T, Nagayama H: **Reduced anxious behavior in mice lacking the CCK2 receptor gene.** *Eur Neuropsychopharmacol* 2004, **14**:157–161.

78. Chen H, Kent S, Morris MJ: **Is the CCK2 receptor essential for normal regulation of body weight and adiposity?** *Eur J Neurosci* 2006, **24**:1427–1433.

79. Leibowitz SF, Sladek C, Spencer L, Tempel D: **Neuropeptide Y, epinephrine and norepinephrine in the paraventricular nucleus: stimulation of feeding and the release of corticosterone, vasopressin and glucose.** *Brain Res Bull* 1988, **21**:905–912.

80. Gutman AR, Yang Y, Ressler KJ, Davis M: **The role of neuropeptide Y in the expression and extinction of fear-potentiated startle.** *J Neurosci* 2008, **28**:12682–12690.

81. CaH Landis WA: *The Startle Pattern.* New York: Farrar and Rinehart; 1939.

82. Blackshaw S, Snyder SH: **Developmental expression pattern of phototransduction components in mammalian pineal implies a light-sensing function.** *J Neurosci* 1997, **17**:8074–8082.

83. Byerly MS, Simon J, Lebihan-Duval E, Duclos MJ, Cogburn LA, Porter TE: **Effects of BDNF, T3, and corticosterone on expression of the hypothalamic obesity gene network in vivo and in vitro.** *Am J Physiol Regul Integr Comp Physiol* 2009, **296**:R1180–R1189.

84. Livak KJ, Schmittgen TD: **Analysis of relative gene expression data using real-time quantitative PCR and the 2(–Delta Delta C(T)) Method.** *Methods* 2001, **25**:402–408.

5

Matrix metalloproteinases 2 and 9 increase permeability of sheep pleura in vitro

Eleni Apostolidou[1*], Efrosyni Paraskeva[1], Konstantinos Gourgoulianis[2], Paschalis-Adam Molyvdas[1] and Chrissi Hatzoglou[1,2]

Abstract

Background: Matrix metalloproteinases (MMPs) 2 and 9 are two gelatinase members which have been found elevated in exudative pleural effusions. In endothelial cells these MMPs increase paracellular permeability via the disruption of tight junction (TJ) proteins occludin and claudin. In the present study it was investigated if MMP2 and MMP9 alter permeability properties of the pleura tissue by degradation of TJ proteins in pleural mesothelium.

Results: In the present study the transmesothelial resistance (R_{TM}) of sheep pleura tissue was recorded in Ussing chambers after the addition of MMP2 or MMP9. Both enzymes reduced RTM of the pleura, implying an increase in pleural permeability. The localization and expression of TJ proteins, occludin and claudin-1, were assessed after incubation with MMPs by indirect immunofluorescence and western blot analysis. Our results revealed that incubation with MMPs did not alter neither proteins localization at cell periphery nor their expression.

Conclusions: MMP2 and MMP9 increase the permeability of sheep pleura and this finding suggests a role for MMPs in pleural fluid formation. Tight junction proteins remain intact after incubation with MMPs, contrary to previous studies which have shown TJ degradation by MMPs. Probably MMP2 and MMP9 augment pleural permeability via other mechanisms.

Background

Matrix metalloproteinases (MMPs) 2 and 9 are two gelatinase members which have been measured and found to be elevated in pleural exudates of different origin (parapneumonic, malignant, tuberculous). MMPs consist a family of proteolytic enzymes that break down virtually all the protein components of the extracellular matrix. The balance between matrix deposition and degradation is tightly regulated in human tissues and a disruption of this balance has been implicated in several pathological conditions such as cancer, cardiovascular diseases and arthritis [1,2]. MMP2 and MMP9 are thought to be involved in pleural fluid accumulation in the pleural cavity. The disruption of the integrity of the mesothelial layer or the underlying basement membrane, and therefore the facilitation of fluid influx into the pleural space has been proposed as a possible mechanism [3], although no study has been so far conducted.

MMPs have been correlated with the induction of increased capillary permeability in several inflammatory conditions, such as brain and myocardium ischemia injury and diabetic retinopathy [4-6]. In in vitro studies of endothelial cells, MMPs increase paracellular permeability by disrupting tight junction barrier [5,7,8]. Tight junctions (TJs) are a specific type of cell-cell contacts that obstruct paracellular pathway for solute diffusion and they regulate the paracellular passage of small molecules such as water and ions [9]. The two major constituent proteins of TJs are occludin and claudin and the disruption of these proteins in several culture systems has been correlated with increased water and solute flux [9].

This study was designed in order to investigate if MMP2 and MMP9 increase the permeability of sheep pleura and thus contribute to the pathogenesis of pleural effusion formation. The effect of MMP2 and MMP9 on TJ proteins occludin and claudin-1 was examined in order to investigate if MMPs alter paracellular permeability of the mesothelial layer.

---

* Correspondence: elaposto@med.uth.gr
[1]Department of Physiology, University of Thessaly Medical School, Larissa, Biopolis 41110, Greece
Full list of author information is available at the end of the article

Results

MMP2 and MMP9 decrease the transmesothelial resistance of parietal and visceral sheep pleura

We treated parietal and visceral sheep pleura specimens with increasing doses of MMP2 and MMP9 (0.1, 1, 10 and 20 ng/ml) and the R_{TM} was measured over a 40-min period. The R_{TM} decreased in all concentrations studied and this decrease occurred at both parietal and visceral pleura and on both the apical and basolateral side. The decline in R_{TM} suggests for an increase in the permeability of the tissue. As control R_{TM}, we regarded the R_{TM} of the tissue before MMP was added. The mean R_{TM} of parietal pleura was calculated to be 15 ± 3 Ωcm^2 and that of visceral pleura 17 ± 4 Ωcm^2. Sheets of pleura specimens, at which no MMPs where applied, showed a stable value of R_{TM} at least for a period of 40 min (Figures 1 and 2, control experiments).

A time-dependent response occurred both apically and basolaterally for all four concentrations studied. After the addition of MMPs, the R_{TM} decreased significantly and declined progressively thereafter up to the 40 min of incubation when the experiment was terminated (Figures 1 and 2). A significant drop in resistance occurred within 5-15 min for both concentrations 0.1 (Figure 1) and 20 ng/ml (Figure 2). However a delayed response was observed when 0.1 ng/ml MMP2 was incubated with the apical side of the visceral membrane (Figure 2b). The effect of 0.1 ng/ml MMP2 on the apical side of the parietal pleura was not significant (Figure 1a). The changes in R_{TM} for concentrations 1 and 10 ng/ml were comparable to these for 0.1 and 20 ng/ml (data not shown).

A dose-dependent response was observed for both MMPs studied (Figure 3): for MMP2 the decrease in R_{TM} was greatest on the apical side of parietal pleura at concentration 20 ng/ml ($45 \pm 12\%$ of the control value). For MMP9 the greatest effect was observed on the basolateral side of the parietal pleura at the low concentration of 0.1 ng/ml ($59 \pm 17\%$ of the control value).

TIMP2 partially prevented the decrease in R_{TM} induced by MMPs

Next, the MMP inhibitor TIMP2 (200 ng/ml) was applied to the pleura either alone or simultaneously

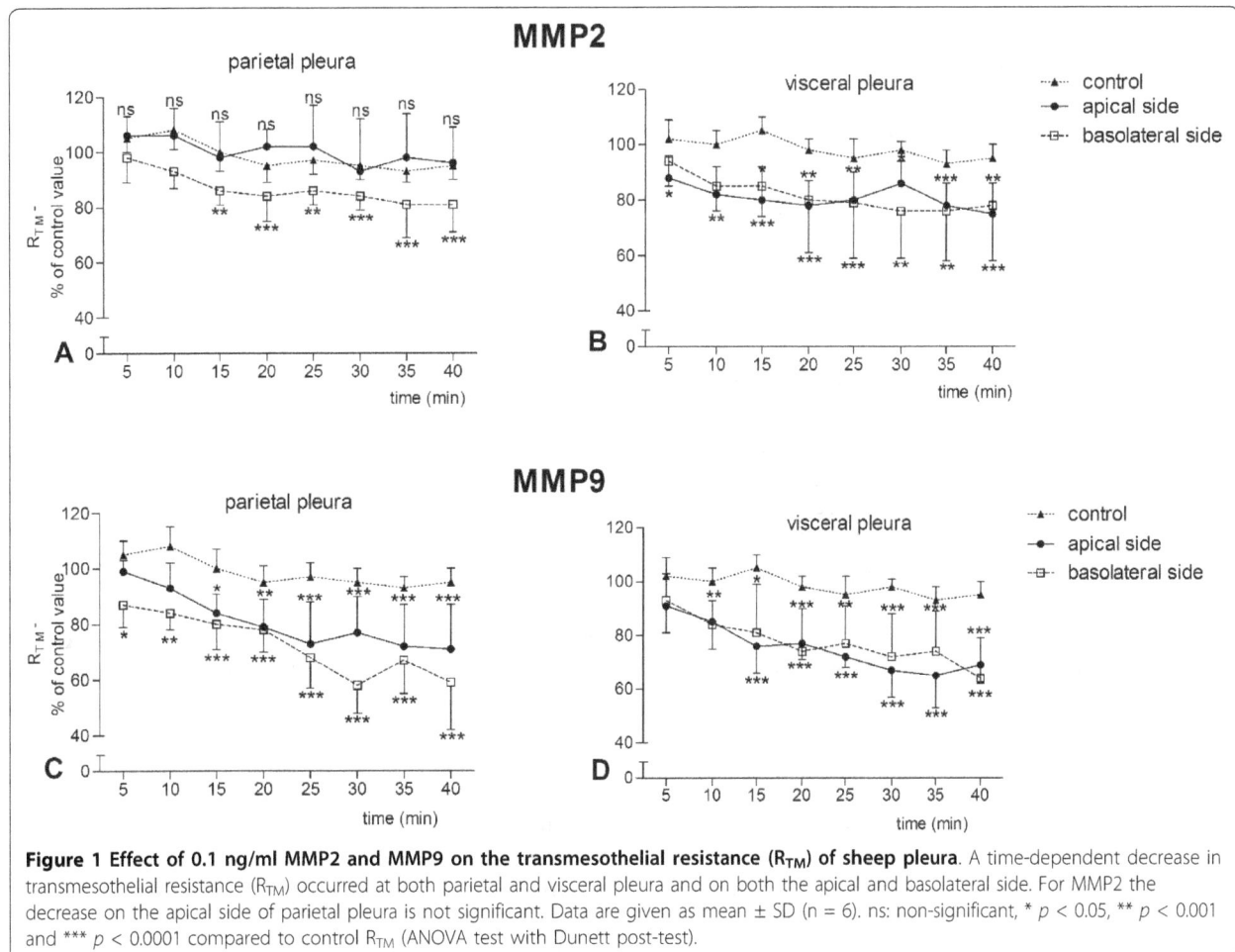

Figure 1 Effect of 0.1 ng/ml MMP2 and MMP9 on the transmesothelial resistance (R_{TM}) of sheep pleura. A time-dependent decrease in transmesothelial resistance (R_{TM}) occurred at both parietal and visceral pleura and on both the apical and basolateral side. For MMP2 the decrease on the apical side of parietal pleura is not significant. Data are given as mean $\pm$ SD (n = 6). ns: non-significant, * $p < 0.05$, ** $p < 0.001$ and *** $p < 0.0001$ compared to control R_{TM} (ANOVA test with Dunett post-test).

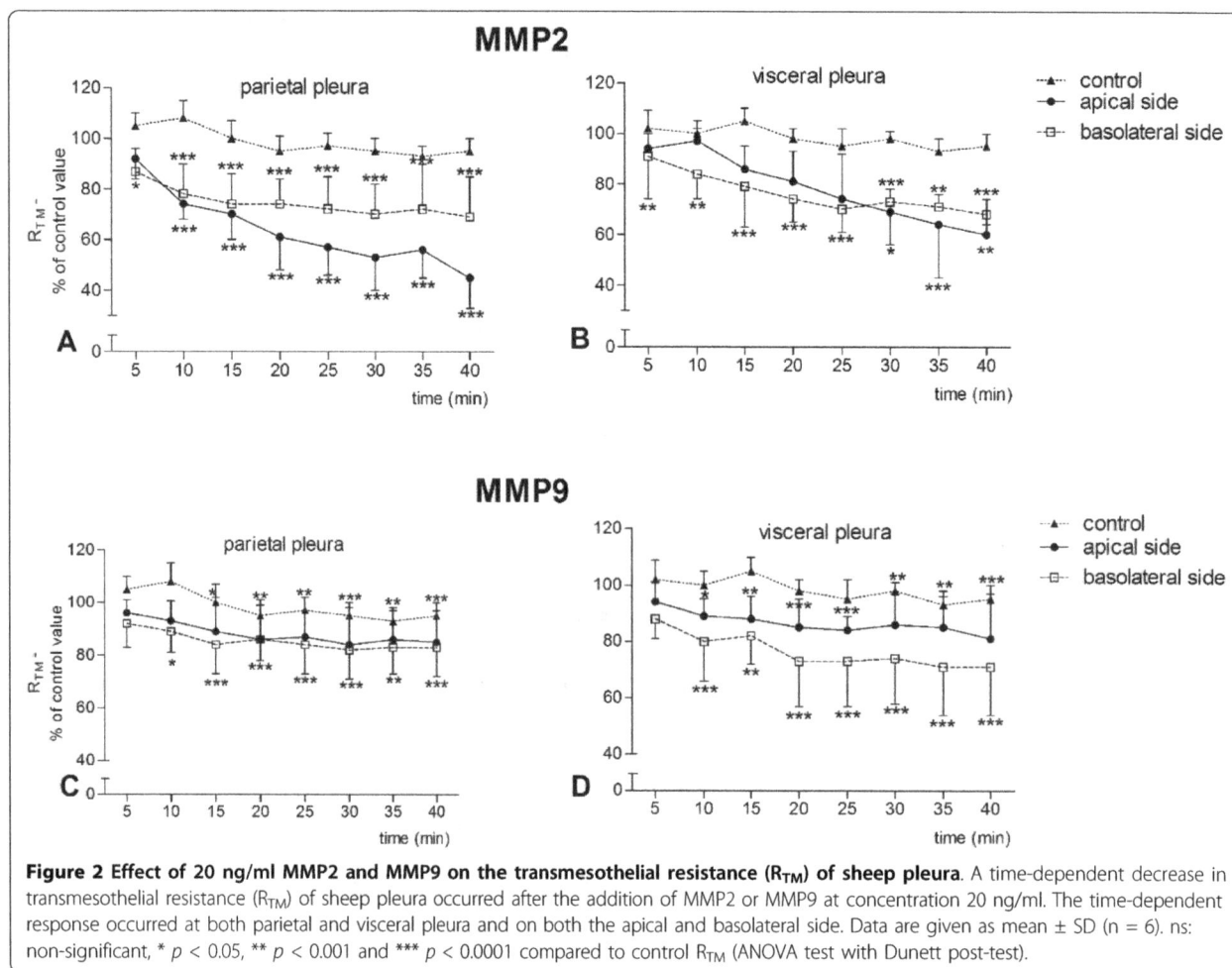

Figure 2 Effect of 20 ng/ml MMP2 and MMP9 on the transmesothelial resistance (R_{TM}) of sheep pleura. A time-dependent decrease in transmesothelial resistance (R_{TM}) of sheep pleura occurred after the addition of MMP2 or MMP9 at concentration 20 ng/ml. The time-dependent response occurred at both parietal and visceral pleura and on both the apical and basolateral side. Data are given as mean ± SD (n = 6). ns: non-significant, * $p < 0.05$, ** $p < 0.001$ and *** $p < 0.0001$ compared to control R_{TM} (ANOVA test with Dunett post-test).

with MMP2 at concentration 20 ng/ml or MMP9 at concentration 0.1 ng/ml. These concentrations of MMPs were chosen because of their maximum effect on R_{TM}. TIMP2 was shown to partially prevent the MMP2 (Figure 4) and MMP9-induced (Figure 5) fall in R_{TM}. This effect was obvious on both the parietal and visceral pleura. Moreover, the application of TIMP2 by itself tended to increase pleural permeability, particularly at visceral pleura and at its basolateral side, as the R_{TM} was 50 ± 5% of control value on the 40th min (Figure 5d).

MMP2 or MMP9 do not alter occludin and claudin-1 immunostaining at cell cultures

We next investigated if the increase in transmesothelial permeability, as occurred by Ussing chamber experiments, is accompanied by loss of tight junction proteins by indirect immunofluorescence. The mesothelial cells in control experiments showed a clear membrane pattern for occludin (Figure 6) and claudin-1 staining (Figure 7). The staining was continuous and decorated the cell periphery. Because cells were well grown to

confluency and occludin and claudin-1 are located at sites of lateral membrane with cell-cell contact, a continuous line resembling to "honeycomb" pattern was obvious. Non-specific staining of the nucleus occurred. The incubation of mesothelial cells with MMPs had no effect on occludin and claudin-1 immunostaining (Figures 6 and 7, respectively), implying that MMPs do not alter occludin and claudin-1 localization at tight junctions.

MMP2 or MMP9 do not alter occludin and claudin-1 expression at mesothelial cells

Western blotting of mesothelial cell extracts showed no alteration for occludin and claudin-1 staining (Figure 8). Occludin migrated as two main bands with apparent molecular weights from 60 to 65 KDa. An additional band at about 85 KDa was also detected (Figure 8a). Claudin-1 was detected as a 28 kDa band (Figure 6b). Neither loss of band intensity nor the appearance of new protein fragments was observed. These findings imply that MMP2 and MMP9 do not degrade TJ proteins.

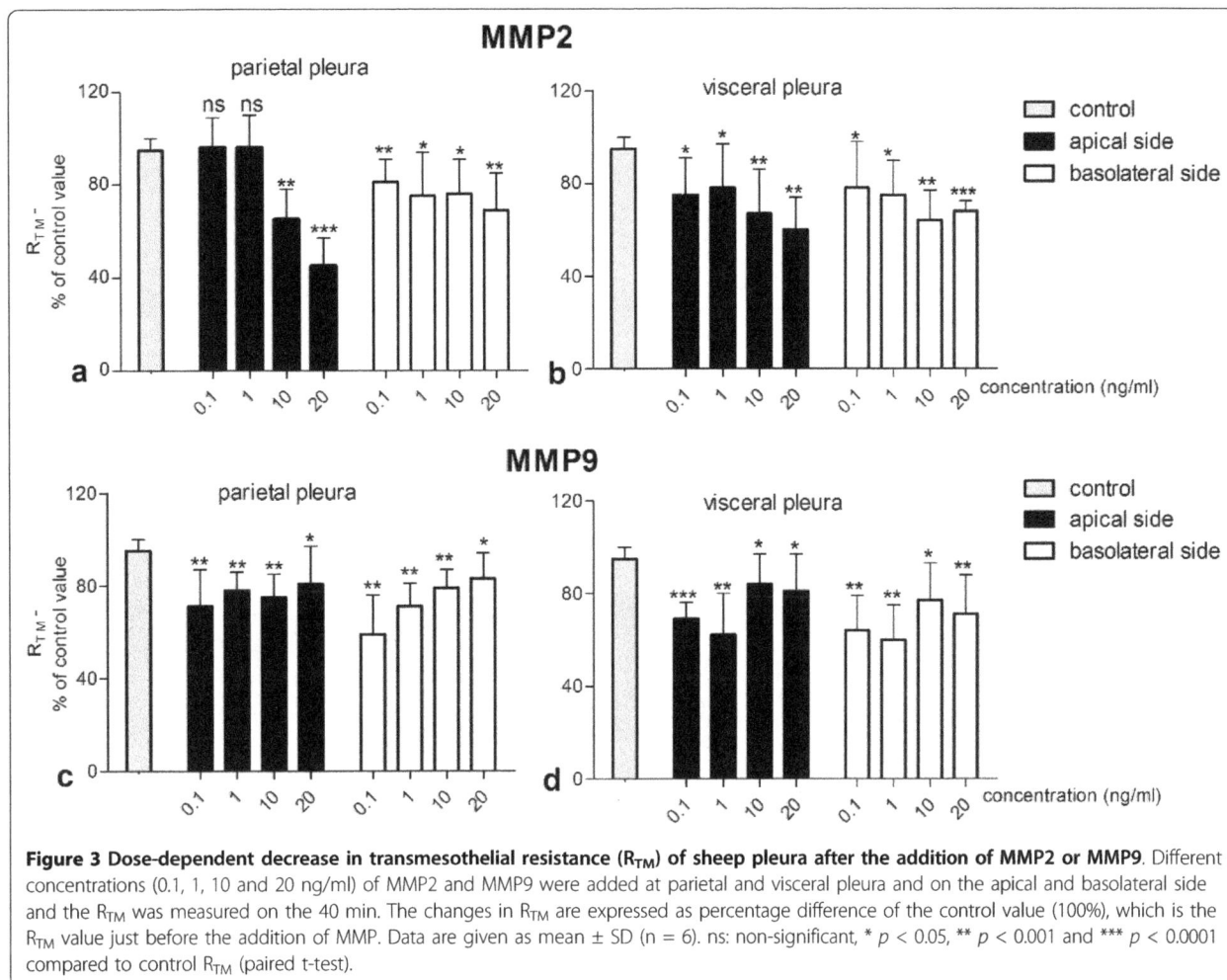

Figure 3 Dose-dependent decrease in transmesothelial resistance (R_{TM}) of sheep pleura after the addition of MMP2 or MMP9. Different concentrations (0.1, 1, 10 and 20 ng/ml) of MMP2 and MMP9 were added at parietal and visceral pleura and on the apical and basolateral side and the R_{TM} was measured on the 40 min. The changes in R_{TM} are expressed as percentage difference of the control value (100%), which is the R_{TM} value just before the addition of MMP. Data are given as mean ± SD (n = 6). ns: non-significant, * $p < 0.05$, ** $p < 0.001$ and *** $p < 0.0001$ compared to control R_{TM} (paired t-test).

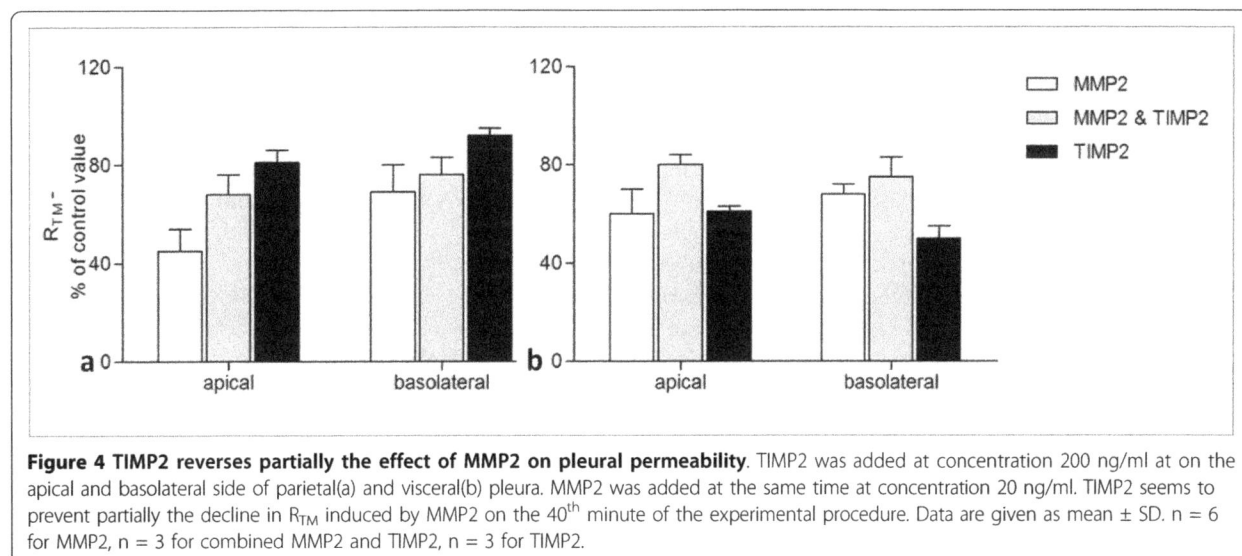

Figure 4 TIMP2 reverses partially the effect of MMP2 on pleural permeability. TIMP2 was added at concentration 200 ng/ml at on the apical and basolateral side of parietal(a) and visceral(b) pleura. MMP2 was added at the same time at concentration 20 ng/ml. TIMP2 seems to prevent partially the decline in R_{TM} induced by MMP2 on the 40th minute of the experimental procedure. Data are given as mean ± SD. n = 6 for MMP2, n = 3 for combined MMP2 and TIMP2, n = 3 for TIMP2.

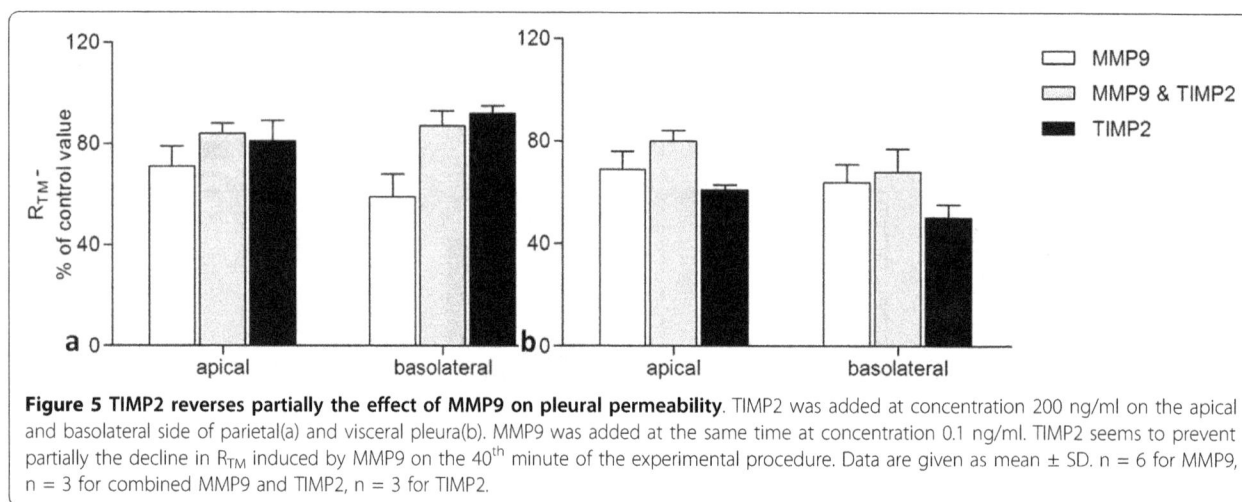

Figure 5 TIMP2 reverses partially the effect of MMP9 on pleural permeability. TIMP2 was added at concentration 200 ng/ml on the apical and basolateral side of parietal(a) and visceral pleura(b). MMP9 was added at the same time at concentration 0.1 ng/ml. TIMP2 seems to prevent partially the decline in R_{TM} induced by MMP9 on the 40th minute of the experimental procedure. Data are given as mean ± SD. n = 6 for MMP9, n = 3 for combined MMP9 and TIMP2, n = 3 for TIMP2.

Discussion and Conclusions

In the present study MMP2 and MMP9 decreased the transmesothelial resistance of parietal and visceral sheep pleura in in vitro experiments. This decrease supports that MMPs augment pleural mesothelial permeability. The paracellular pathway, through which mesothelial permeability may increase, was studied. After incubation of primary mesothelial cells with MMP2 or MMP9, mesothelial monolayer integrity was not disrupted and the expression of TJ proteins occludin and claudin-1 in the cytoplasmic membrane remained intact.

MMP2 and MMP9 were selected for our study because they have been found elevated in exudative pleural effusions of different origin [3,10,11]. MMP2 is expressed and secreted constitutively in the pleural cavity by mesothelial cells [12]. In exudates high levels of MMP2 may be due to increased expression as a result of stimulation of mesothelial cells by cytokines or other cells, such as mononuclear cells, might collaborate in MMP2 release [10]. MMPs can degrade almost all components of the extracellular matrix (ECM) and to date it is widely known that MMPs can cleave not only ECM components, such as collagen and elastin, but also non-ECM protein substrates, such as cell surface molecules, ECM-bound growth factors and cytokines released on the ECM [13,14].

In the present study the decrease in transmesothelial electrical resistance of sheep pleura that occurs after incubation with MMP2 or MMP9 suggests for an increase in the permeability of the pleura. As expected for an enzyme, the decrease in resistance of the pleura was time-dependent with the maximum decline in resistance occurring on the 40 min. Regarding the dose-dependent effect, a remarkable difference between MMP2 and MMP9 occurred: for MMP2 the greatest increase in permeability occurred at the highest concentration studied, which is 20 ng/ml. On the contrary, for MMP9 the greatest increase in permeability occurred at the lowest concentration studied, which is 0.1 ng/ml. The reason for this discrepancy is not elucidated but we should take into account differences between enzyme kinetics and substrate specificity.

TIMP2 is a tissue inhibitor of metalloproteinases and inhibits MMPs activity by binding noncovalently to their active site [15]. TIMP2 is found in exudates whereas in transudates its levels are usually no detectable [3]. The application of TIMP2 on the pleura inhibited the decrease in R_{TM} which was induced by MMPs on both the parietal and visceral pleura. This finding enhances our previous finding and suggests that the decline in R_{TM} is an effect caused by MMPs and not a non-pecific result. TIMP2 was selected at the present study because it is 2-9 times more effective than TIMP1 for the inhibition of MMP2 and MMP9 activity [16]. Moreover, TIMP2 tended to increase pleural permeability particularly at visceral pleura and at its basolateral side, when it was applied alone at the pleura. This finding can be interpreted considering the growth-promoting-activity that has been attributed to TIMP2 [17]. A wide range of human, bovine and mouse cells proliferate when incubated with TIMP2. Indeed, receptors of TIMP2 have been identified at the surface of the above cells [18]. One possible explanation is that TIMP2 acts on mesothelial cells via receptor-binding and influences mesothelial permeability, as is the case for numerous growth factors.

We next looked for a possible mechanism explaining the impact of MMPs on the transmesothelial resistance and asked whether TJ proteins, occludin and claudin-1, may be hydrolyzed by MMPs. TJs are a specific type of cell-cell contact which are located in the most apical region of the lateral plasma membrane. The paracellular passage of small molecules, such as water and solutes, is highly regulated by the TJ proteins, including occludin

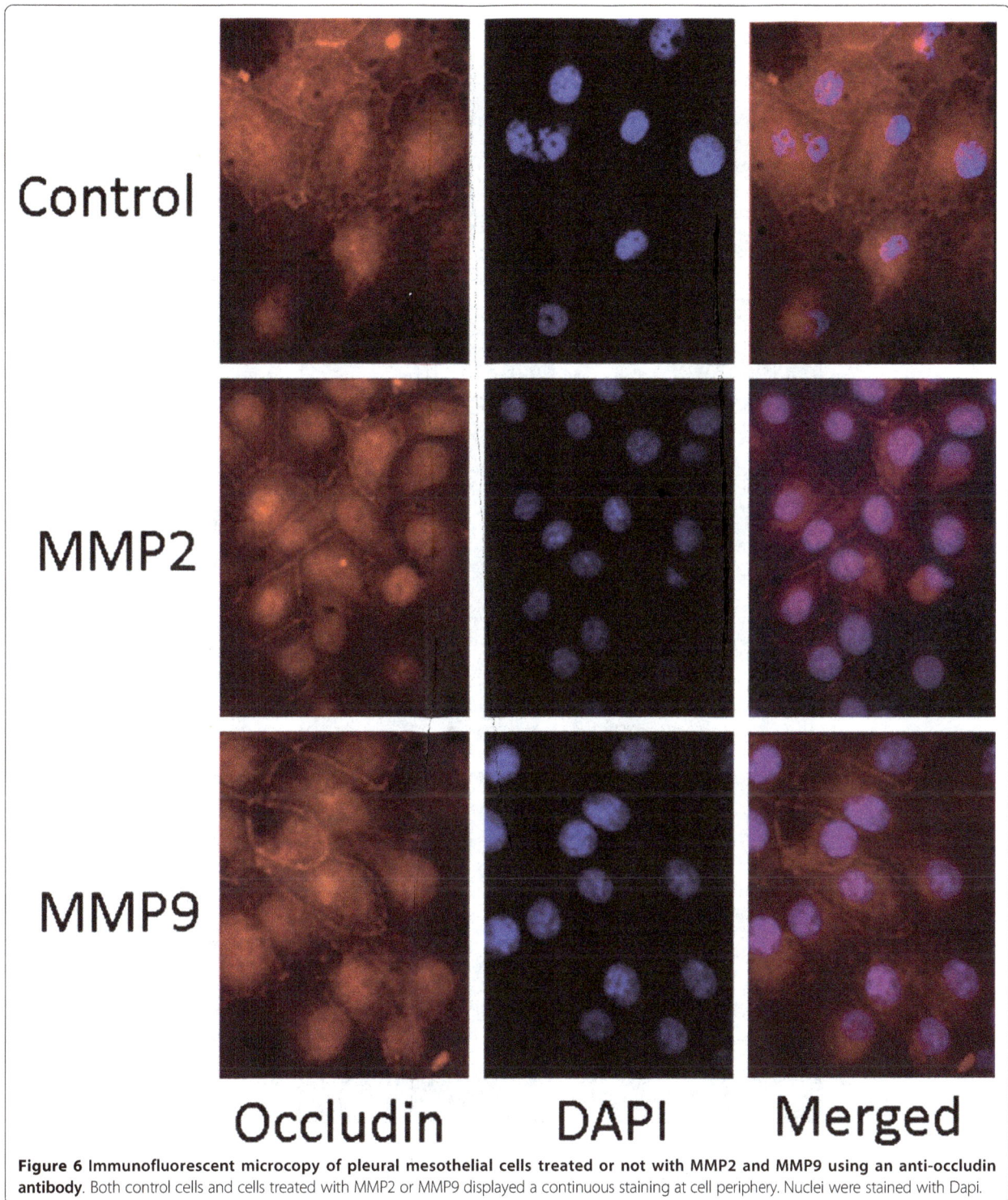

Figure 6 Immunofluorescent microcopy of pleural mesothelial cells treated or not with MMP2 and MMP9 using an anti-occludin antibody. Both control cells and cells treated with MMP2 or MMP9 displayed a continuous staining at cell periphery. Nuclei were stained with Dapi.

and claudin-1 [9]. Indirect immunofluorescence experiments for occludin and claudin-1 showed a continuous staining at cell periphery which was not weakened and remained at the cell borders after incubation with MMPs. Similarly, western blot revealed that these proteins are expressed at pleural mesothelium under normal conditions and are not proteolytically disrupted by MMPs. More specifically for occludin, western blot analysis revealed three distinct bands: at 60 KDa, 85 KDa and a broad band at about > 60 KDa. These bands may be due to occurrence of splice variants or post-transational modification, i.e phosphorylation. Previous

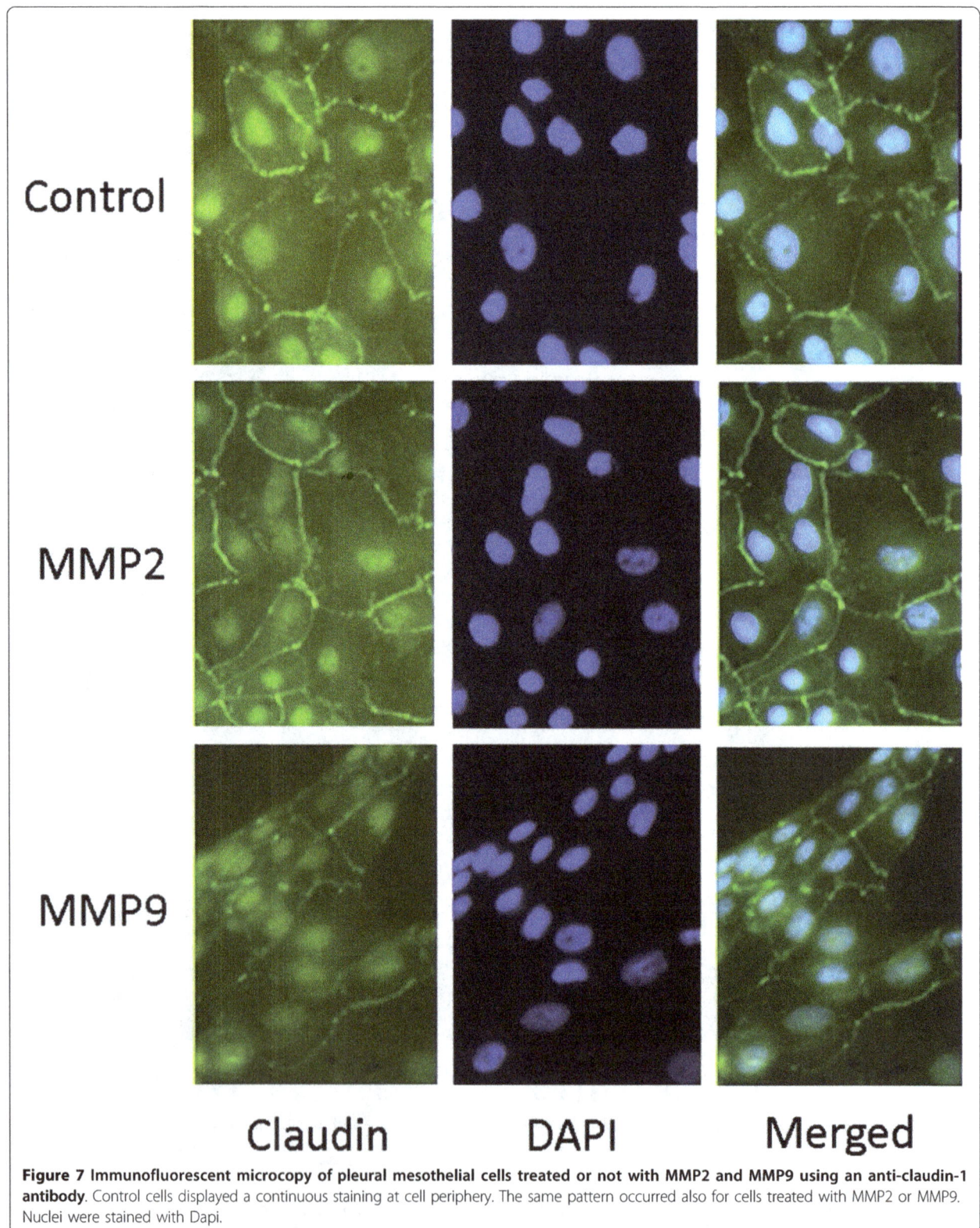

Figure 7 Immunofluorescent microcopy of pleural mesothelial cells treated or not with MMP2 and MMP9 using an anti-claudin-1 antibody. Control cells displayed a continuous staining at cell periphery. The same pattern occurred also for cells treated with MMP2 or MMP9. Nuclei were stained with Dapi.

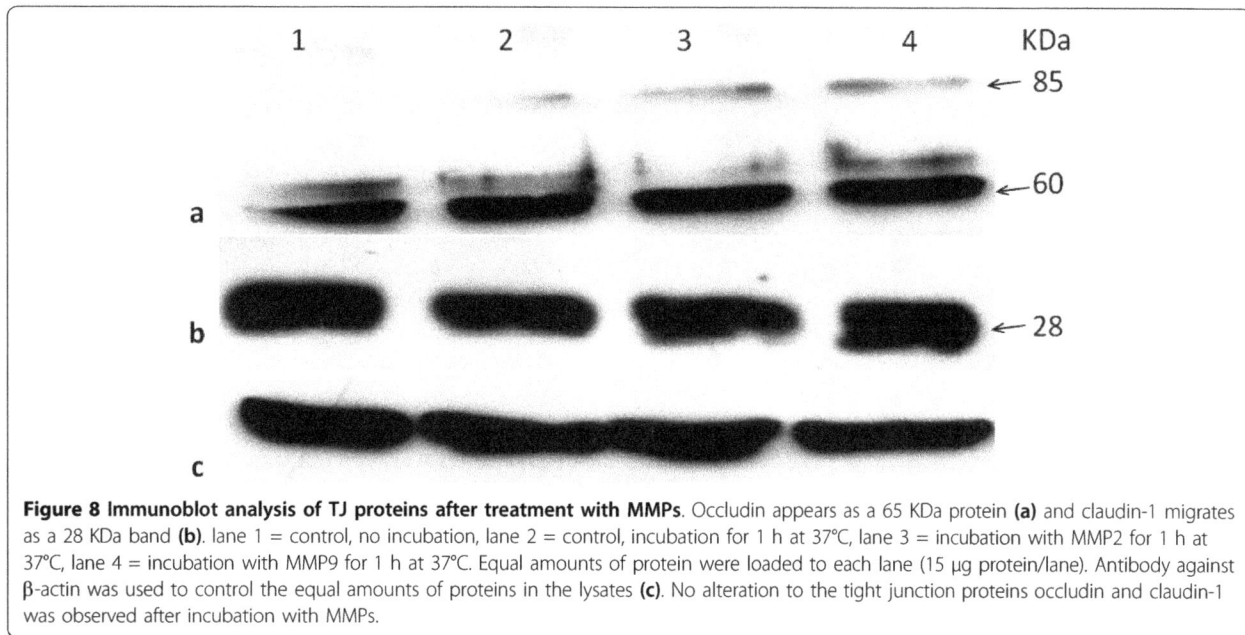

Figure 8 Immunoblot analysis of TJ proteins after treatment with MMPs. Occludin appears as a 65 KDa protein **(a)** and claudin-1 migrates as a 28 KDa band **(b)**. lane 1 = control, no incubation, lane 2 = control, incubation for 1 h at 37°C, lane 3 = incubation with MMP2 for 1 h at 37°C, lane 4 = incubation with MMP9 for 1 h at 37°C. Equal amounts of protein were loaded to each lane (15 μg protein/lane). Antibody against β-actin was used to control the equal amounts of proteins in the lysates **(c)**. No alteration to the tight junction proteins occludin and claudin-1 was observed after incubation with MMPs.

studies have shown that occludin is widely phosphorylated on serine and threonine resides and modulation of occludin phosphorylation regulates cellular localization and paracellular permeability [19,20]. Some degree of phosphorylation may also be the case in the present study. As far as the 80 KDa band is concerned, we cannot rule out the possibility that this band corresponds to a protein complex between occludin and claudin (MWs 60 and 28 KDa respectively). Occludin and claudin do not interact directly to each other, but they crosslink by integral TJ proteins, such as ZO-1, ZO-2 and ZO-3 [9]. The intensity of the above band increased after MMPs incubation, implying that MMPs interfere with occludin and claudin interactions. Because the 80 KDa band appeared enhanced to all three western blot experiments that were performed, it is less likely to represent an artifact. The mesothelial cells used for immunofluorescence and western blotting derived from upper-, middle- and lower-heighted visceral pleura and no difference between them occurred.

Our data is contradictory to previous results which have revealed MMPs as major contributors to the control of paracellular permeability by proteolytic degradation of TJ proteins. More specifically, MMPs have been correlated with an increase in capillary permeability that follows ischemia-reperfusion injury in brain [8], in myocardium [4], in lung [21] and in kidney [22]. These studies attributed to MMPs an elementary role in the inflammatory process and the breakdown of the paracellular capillary permeability during inflammation. In some studies a selective cleavage of TJ proteins occurred [7,23] but the results of our study clearly showed that TJ

integrity is not disrupted at mesothelial cells by MMPs. It is possible that other substrates, different from occludin and claudin-1, are a molecular target for MMPs at pleural mesothelium. For example, MMPs have been found to disrupt or reorganize the basement membrane of endothelial cells and thus result to increased permeability [24,25]. Moreover, adherent junctions are also degraded by MMPs and their hydrolysis leads to TJ disassembly and to increased permeability [22,26].

The limitations of the present study are the followings: Firstly, the Ussing chamber technique investigates permeability alterations provoked on mesothelial membrane, which consists a confluent membrane between the apical and basolateral compartment of a chamber. However, under in vivo conditions it is possible that MMPs act not only on mesothelial cells but also on vascular capillaries lying beneath the basement membrane. Secondly, the precise role of the mesothelial layer at pleural fluid turnover is not fully established. Although we used to believe that mesothelial cells are leaky and display no resistance at pleural fluid passage, more recent investigations indicate that the permeability to solutes of mesothelium is of the same order of magnitude as that of the capillary endothelium [27,28]. This means that pleural fluid is a filtrate of pleural capillaries and mesothelium too. Moreover, damage of pleural mesothelial monolayer by lipopolysaccharide (LPS), thrombin and bacteria increase pleural permeability to proteins and demonstrate to play a central role in the formation of effusions [29,30]. Finally, sheep pleura resembles to human pleura as far as morphology and function is concerned. On both pleurae the blood supply comes from the systemic circulation and microscopically two different types of mesothelial cells are found: the cyboidal cells with less developed TJs and flattened cells with more TJs [31]. However, further studies should be performed at human pleura in order to confirm the results of the present study.

Our findings imply an important role for MMPs in the pathogenesis of pleural effusions. Under normal conditions, MMPs and especially MMP2 are found only in small amounts in the pleural fluid. The balance of MMPs in pleural fluid may serve the degradation and turnover of ECM that underlies mesothelial cells and which normally occurs in low rates. However in pleural exudates MMP2 and MMP9 levels increase, as shown from previous studies, and a role for MMP2 and MMP9 in pleural fluid formation is proposed by our study. Tight junctions do not apparently loosen in mesothelial cells after the addition of MMPs. It is possible that other mechanisms exist through which MMPs increase mesothelial permeability. The revelation of the mechanims by which MMPs compromise the mesothelial barrier will provide a better understanding of the pathogenesis of pleural fluid formation.

Methods

Specimen collection and preparation of sheep pleura

Intact sheets of visceral and parietal sheep pleura were obtained from adult female sheep. The samples were collected from the slaughterhouse immediately after the death of the animals (time of warm ischemia close to 0 minutes). Pieces of parietal pleura were carefully stripped from the chest wall whereas those of visceral pleura were carefully stripped from the underlying lung. Parietal and visceral pleura were examined for evidence of holes or adherent tissue and were discarded if they were not intact. Immediately after removal, the pleural tissue from the animals was placed in oxygenated Krebs-Ringer bicarbonate (KRB) solution at 4°C and transferred to the laboratory within 30 minutes. The KRB solution was balanced at pH 7.4 and bubbled with 95%O_2-5%CO_2. The solution contained (in mM) 117.5 NaCl, 1.15 NaH_2PO_4, 24.99 $NaHCO_3$, 5.65 KCl, 1.18$MgSO_4$, 2.52 $CaCl_2$, and 5.55 glucose.

Electrophysiological transmesothelial measurements

The effect of MMPs on pleural permeability was studied by conducting Ussing experiments under open circuit conditions. The pleura was mounted carefully in Ussing chambers (K Mussler Scientific Instruments, Aachen, Germany) with an opening surface area of 1 cm^2. Tissues were bathed with 4 ml KRB solution on each side of the membrane and were continuously oxygenated with 95%O_2-5%CO_2. Two pairs of Ag/AgCl electrodes monitored the transmesothelial potential difference (Pd,

in mV) and the transmesothelial resistance (R_{TM}, in Ωullet cm^2) under open circuit conditions.

Transmesothelial electrical parameters were measured before and after the addition of active MMP2 or MMP9 (Calbiochem, San Diego, California, USA) at four different concentrations 0.1, 1, 10 and 20 ng/ml. In some experiments TIMP2, a tissue inhibitor of metalloproteinases, was added at concentration 200 ng/ml. MMPs and TIMP2 were added both apically and basolaterally and the electrical parameters were monitored over a period of 40 minutes (at minutes 5, 10, 15, 20, 25, 30, 35, 40). After the addition of the above substances, alterations in the R_{TM} were expressed as the change from the starting value. Activity of matrix metalloproteinases is temperature-dependent, therefore measurements of transmesothelial electrical parameters were conducted at 37°C. The mesothelial cell membrane facing the fluid side is here called the apical membrane, and that facing the blood side is called the basolateral membrane. The voltage response to applied current pulses of 50 μA amplitude and 200 msec duration was measured. The transmesothelial resistance was calculated deducting automatically the resistance of the solution.

Cell cultures

Primary cultures of sheep pleural mesothelial cells were prepared (modified from Stylianou et al [32]). Briefly, specimens of intact visceral sheep pleura were obtained from the slaughterhouse immediately after the death of the animal. The procedure was performed under sterile conditions and pieces of approximately 6 cm^2 were placed in M199 media (Invitrogen, Carlsbad, USA) supplemented with 10% fetal bovine serum (FBS), 100 U/ml penicillin and 100 μg/ml streptomycin. The specimen was transferred on ice to the laboratory, washed with PBS and subjected to enzymatic disaggregation. The specimen was in this incubated for twenty minutes at 37°C in disaggregation solution that contained 0.125% trypsin, 0.01% EDTA and 0.1% glucose in PBS solution. After incubation the pleura membrane was discarded and the suspension was centrifuged at 100 × g for five minutes at 4°C. The resultant supernatant was discarded and the cell pellet was suspended in 10 ml prewarmed M199 media supplemented with 10% fetal bovine serum (FBS), 100 U/ml penicillin, 100 μg/ml streptomycin, 0.4 μg/ml hydrocortisone, 10 mg/ml insulin, 50 mg/ml transferin and 200 mM L-glutamine and subjected to recentrifugation at 100 × g for five minutes at 4°C. Finally the supernatant was discarded, the cell pellet was resuspended in 5 ml of the same medium and seeded in 25 cm^2 tissue culture flasks. The medium was changed every third or fourth day. Cultures contaminated with spindle-like cells, representing probably fibroblasts, were discarded. Confluency of the cells was regarded as a prerequisite for their experimental use. Passages 1 and 2 were used for immunofluorescence experiments and western blot.

Indirect immunofluorescence

For immunofluorescence experiments, mesothelial cells were grown on fibronectin-coated glass coveslips and confluency was reached about 7 days later. After two subsequent washes with PBS, cells were incubated in serum-free media with MMP2 or MMP9 at concentration 10 µg/ml for one hour at 37°C and then were fixed with 3% formaldehyde for 5 minutes at room temperature. Control cells received no MMP treatment and were incubated with serum-free media. After washing, the cells were permeabilized with 1% Triton X-100 in PBS for 15 minutes at 4°C. Samples were washed with PBS and soaked in blocking solution, which consisted of 3% BSA and 0.1% Tween-20 in PBS for 16 hours. Coverslips were incubated with polyclonal anti-occludin (dilution 1:50; Zymed Laboratory, San Fransisco, USA) or polyclinal anti-claudin-1 antibody (dilution 1:50; Zymed Laboratory, San Fransisco, USA) in PBS containing 1% BSA/0.1% Tween-20 for 1 hour at room temperature. Cells were rinsed three times in 1% BSA/0.1% Tween-20/PBS and incubated with a FITC- or CY3-conjugated anti-rabbit IgG secondary antibody (dilution 1:50), for occludin and claudin repectively, for 30 minutes at room temperature. Finally coverslips were washed and mounted with Vectashield containing Dapi. Images were collected with a Leica DFC480 camera (LAS software version V2.3.1R1) on an Axioscope 40 Zeiss microscope.

Western blot

Mesothelial cells were grown in culture dishes and cellular extract was obtained as described previously by Giebel et al [5]. Briefly, mesothelial cells were washed with cold PBS and cellular extract was obtained after scraping the culture dish with 200 µl lysis buffer (0.1% Triton X-100 in 100 Mm PO_4 buffer). The cellular extract was incubated for 30 min on ice and then was subjected to centrifugation at $100 \times g$ for 30 min at 4°C. The pellet was discarded and the supernatant was divided into four equal aliquots each of which had a volume 20 µl. The protein concentration was measured by Bradford method (Bio rad) and each aliquot contained 15 µg proteins. Two aliquots were used as controls and one of them was incubated at 37°C for one hour. Additional aliquots received either MMP2 or MMP9 at concentration 5 µg/ml and were incubated at 37°C for one hour. At the end of incubation period, SDS sample buffer was added to all aliquots and incubation at 95°C for 3 min followed. Samples were loaded on 10% polyacrylamide gel for

electrophoresis and then proteins were transferred to a nitrocellulose membrane. The quality of the transfer was controlled by Ponceau staining of the membrane. The membrane was blocked in 5% milk in PBS-Tween-20 for 30 min at room temperature and then incubated with primary antibodies (polyclonal anti-occludin and anti-claudin-1 at dilution 1:250) for 16 hours at 4°C. After 3 washes with PBS-Tween-20, the membrane was incubated for 1 hour at room temperature with HRP-secondary antibody (anti-rabbit IgG at dilution 1:3000) and the immunoreactive bands were detected with enhanced chemiluminescence (Roche).

Statistical analysis

Statistical analysis for quantative experiments was performed using GraphPad Prism 5. For permeability experiments, comparisons between control and MMP-treated tissues were made using one way ANOVA test with Dunnett post-test. For short-circuit experiments, the comparison between control experiments and experiments with application of MMPs was performed with unpaired t-test. Values of $p < 0.05$ were regarded as significant.

Abbreviations
MMPs: Matrix metalloproteinases; TJs: Tight junctions; R_{TM}: Transmesothelial resistance; SD: Standard deviation; TIMP2: Tissue inhibitor of metalloproteinases 2; ECM: Extracellular matrix; FBS: Fetal bovine serum.

Author details
[1]Department of Physiology, University of Thessaly Medical School, Larissa, Biopolis 41110, Greece. [2]Department of Respiratory Medicine, University of Thessaly Medical School, University Hospital of Larissa, Larissa, Biopolis 41110, Greece.

Authors' contributions
EA wrote this manuscript. EP contributed to the performance of indirect immunofluorescence and western blotting. CH, KG and PAM conceived the study and participated in the design of the experiments. All authors read and approved the final manuscript.

References
1. Kerrigan JJ, Kerrigan JJ, Mansell JP, Sandy JR: Matrix turnover. *J Orthod* 2000, **27**:227-233.
2. Nagase H, Visse R, Murphy G: Structure and function of matrix metalloproteinases and timps. *Cardiovasc Res* 2006, **69**:562-573.
3. Eickelberg O, Sommerfeld CO, Wyser C, Tamm M, Reichenberger F, Bardin PG, Soler M, Roth M, Perruchoud AP: MMP and TIMP expression pattern in pleural effusions of different origins. *Am J Respir Crit Care Med* 1997, **156**:1987-1992.
4. Danielsen CC, Wiggers H, Andersen HR: Increased amounts of collagenase and gelatinase in porcine myocardium following ischemia and reperfusion. *J Mol Cell Cardiol* 1998, **30**:1431-1442.
5. Giebel SJ, Menicucci G, McGuire PG, Das A: Matrix metalloproteinases in early diabetic retinopathy and their role in alteration of the blood-retinal barrier. *Lab Invest* 2005, **85**:597-607.
6. Rosenberg GA, Estrada EY, Dencoff JE: Matrix metalloproteinases and TIMPs are associated with blood-brain barrier opening after reperfusion in rat brain. *Stroke* 1998, **29**:2189-2195.

7. Lohmann C, Krischke M, Wegener J, Galla HJ: **Tyrosine phosphatase inhibition induces loss of blood-brain barrier integrity by matrix metalloproteinase-dependent and -independent pathways.** *Brain Res* 2004, **995**:184-196.

8. Yang Y, Estrada EY, Thompson JF, Liu W, Rosenberg GA: **Matrix metalloproteinase-mediated disruption of tight junction proteins in cerebral vessels is reversed by synthetic matrix metalloproteinase inhibitor in focal ischemia in rat.** *J Cereb Blood Flow Metab* 2007, **27**:697-709.

9. Schneeberger EE, Lynch RD: **The tight junction: a multifunctional complex.** *Am J Physiol Cell Physiol* 2004, **286**:C1213-C1228.

10. Iglesias D, Alegre J, Aleman C, Ruiz E, Soriano T, Armadans LI, Segura RM, Angles A, Monasterio J, de Sevilla TF: **Metalloproteinases and tissue inhibitors of metalloproteinases in exudative pleural effusions.** *Eur Respir J* 2005, **25**:104-109.

11. Vatansever S, Gelisgen R, Uzun H, Yurt S, Kosar F: **Potential role of matrix metalloproteinase-2,-9 and tissue inhibitors of metalloproteinase-1,-2 in exudative pleural effusions.** *Clin Invest Med* 2009, **32**:E293-E300.

12. Marshall BC, Santana A, Xu QP, Petersen MJ, Campbell EJ, Hoidal JR, Welgus HG: **Metalloproteinases and tissue inhibitor of metalloproteinases in mesothelial cells. Cellular differentiation influences expression.** *J Clin Invest* 1993, **91**:1792-1799.

13. Arribas J, Coodly L, Vollmer P, Kishimoto TK, Rose-John S, Massague J: **Diverse cell surface protein ectodomains are shed by a system sensitive to metalloprotease inhibitors.** *J Biol Chem* 1996, **271**:11376-11382.

14. McQuibban GA, Gong JH, Tam EM, McCulloch CA, Clark-Lewis I, Overall CM: **Inflammation dampened by gelatinase A cleavage of monocyte chemoattractant protein-3.** *Science* 2000, **289**:1202-1206.

15. Woessner F Jr: **Matrix metalloproteinases and their inhibitors in connective tissue remodeling.** *Faseb* 1991, **5**:2145-2154.

16. Kahari VM, Saarialho-Kere U: **Matrix metalloproteinases and their inhibitorsin tumour growth and invasion.** *Ann Med* 1999, **31**:34-45.

17. Hayakawa T: **Tissue inhibitors of metalloproteinases and their cell growth- promoting activity.** *Cell Struct Funct* 1994, **19**:109-114.

18. Hayakawa T, Yamashita K, Ohuchi E, Shinagawa A: **Cell growth-promoting activity of tissue inhibitor of metalloproteinases-2 (TIMP-2).** *J Cell Sci* 1994, **107**:2373-2379.

19. Sakakibara A, Furuse M, Saitou M, Ando-Akatsuka Y, Tsukita S: **Possible involvement of phosphorylation of occludin in tight junction formation.** *J Cell Biol* 1997, **137**:1393-1401.

20. Harhaj NS, Antonetti DA: **Regulation of tight junctions and loss of barrier function in pathophysiology.** *Int J Biochem Cell Biol* 2004, **36**:1206-1237.

21. Yano M, Omoto Y, Yamakawa Y, Nakashima Y, Kiriyama M, Saito Y, Fujii Y: **Increased matrix metalloproteinase 9 activity and mRNA expression in lung ischemia-reperfusion injury.** *J Heart Lung Transplant* 2001, **20**:679-686.

22. Covington MD, Burghardt RC, Parrish AR: **Ischemia-induced cleavage of cadherins in NRK cells requires MT1-MMP (MMP-14).** *Am J Physiol Renal Physiol* 2006, **290**:F43-F51.

23. Chen F, Ohashi N, Li W, Eckman C, Nguyen JH: **Disruptions of occludin and claudin-5 in brain endothelial cells in vitro and in brains of mice with acute liver failure.** *Hepatology* 2009, **50**:1914-1923.

24. Fukuda S, Fini CA, Mabuchi T, Koziol JA, Eggleston LL Jr, del Zoppo GJ: **Focal cerebral ischemia reduces active proteases that degrade microvascular matrix.** *Stroke* 2004, **35**:998-1004.

25. Lacherade JC, Van De Louw A, Planus E, Escudier E, D' Ortho MP, Lafuma C, Harf A, Delclaux C: **Evaluation of basement membrane degradation during TNF-alpha-induced increase in epithelial permeability.** *Am J Physiol Lung Cell Mol Physiol* 2001, **281**:L134-L143.

26. Navaratna D, McGuire PG, Menicucci G, Das A: **Proteolytic degradation of VE-cadherin alters the blood-retinal barrier in diabetes.** *Diabetes* 2007, **56**:2380-2387.

27. Bodega F, Zocchi L, Agostoni E: **Macromolecule transfer through mesothelium and connective tissue.** *J Appl Physiol* 2000, **89**:2165-2173.

28. Agostoni E, Bodega F, Zocchi L: **Equivalent radius of paracellular "pores" of the mesothelium.** *J Appl Physiol* 1999, **87**:538-544.

29. Kroegel C, Antony VB: **Immunobiology of pleural inflammation: potentialimplications for pathogenesis, diagnosis and therapy.** *Eur Respir J* 1997, **10**:2411-2418.

30. Antony VB: **Immunological mechanisms in pleural disease.** *Eur Respir J* 2003, **21**:539-544.

31. Wheeldon EB, Mariassy AT, McSporran KD: **The pleura: a combined light microscopic and scanning and transmission electron microscopic study in the sheep. II. Response to injury.** *Exp Lung Res* 1983, **5**:125-140.

32. Stylianou E, Jenner LA, Davies M, Coles GA, Williams JD: **Isolation, culture and characterization of human peritoneal mesothelial cells.** *Kidney Int* 1990, **37**:1563-1570.

6

Linking nutritional regulation of *Angptl4, Gpihbp1, and Lmf1* to lipoprotein lipase activity in rodent adipose tissue

Olessia Kroupa[1], Evelina Vorrsjö[1], Rinke Stienstra[2], Frits Mattijssen[2], Stefan K Nilsson[1,3], Sander Kersten[2], Gunilla Olivecrona[1] and Thomas Olivecrona[1*]

Abstract

Background: Lipoprotein lipase (LPL) hydrolyzes triglycerides in lipoproteins and makes fatty acids available for tissue metabolism. The activity of the enzyme is modulated in a tissue specific manner by interaction with other proteins. We have studied how feeding/fasting and some related perturbations affect the expression, in rat adipose tissue, of three such proteins, LMF1, an ER protein necessary for folding of LPL into its active dimeric form, the endogenous LPL inhibitor ANGPTL4, and GPIHBP1, that transfers LPL across the endothelium.

Results: The system underwent moderate circadian oscillations, for LPL in phase with food intake, for ANGPTL4 and GPIHBP1 in the opposite direction. Studies with cycloheximide showed that whereas LPL protein turns over rapidly, ANGPTL4 protein turns over more slowly. Studies with the transcription blocker Actinomycin D showed that transcripts for ANGPTL4 and GPIHBP1, but not LMF1 or LPL, turn over rapidly. When food was withdrawn the expression of ANGPTL4 and GPIHBP1 increased rapidly, and LPL activity decreased. On re-feeding and after injection of insulin the expression of ANGPTL4 and GPIHBP1 decreased rapidly, and LPL activity increased. In ANGPTL4$^{-/-}$ mice adipose tissue LPL activity did not show these responses. In old, obese rats that showed signs of insulin resistance, the responses of ANGPTL4 and GPIHBP1 mRNA and of LPL activity were severely blunted (at 26 weeks of age) or almost abolished (at 52 weeks of age).

Conclusions: This study demonstrates directly that ANGPTL4 is necessary for rapid modulation of LPL activity in adipose tissue. ANGPTL4 message levels responded very rapidly to changes in the nutritional state. LPL activity always changed in the opposite direction. This did not happen in Angptl4$^{-/-}$ mice. GPIHBP1 message levels also changed rapidly and in the same direction as ANGPTL4, i.e. increased on fasting when LPL activity decreased. This was unexpected because GPIHBP1 is known to stabilize LPL. The plasticity of the LPL system is severely blunted or completely lost in insulin resistant rats.

Keywords: Gene expression, Insulin, Gene inactivation, Cycloheximide, Actinomycin D, Transcription, Translation, Posttranslational

* Correspondence: Thomas Olivecrona@medbio.umu.se
[1]Department of Medical Biosciences/Physiological Chemistry, Umeå University, Umeå SE-90187, Sweden
Full list of author information is available at the end of the article

Background

Lipoprotein lipase (LPL) is produced by parenchymal cells in some tissues (e.g. adipocytes, myocytes), secreted, and transported to the luminal side of capillaries. Here the enzyme hydrolyzes triglycerides in chylomicrons and VLDL and thereby makes fatty acids available for tissue metabolism. LPL activity is rapidly modulated by the nutritional state and plays a major role in distribution of fatty acids between tissues [1,2] .

The rapid daily modulations of LPL activity are mainly post-transcriptional [1-3]. One mechanism involves changes in the proportion of active to inactive species of the enzyme without significant changes in total LPL protein [4]. Down-regulation of adipose tissue LPL activity upon fasting requires that a gene, other than the LPL gene, is switched on [5]. This implies a protein that can transform LPL from an active to an inactive form. The fasting-induced, PPAR-responsive angiopoietin-like protein-4 (ANGPTL4) has emerged as a strong candidate for the role of such an LPL-controlling protein in adipose tissue [6,7]. *In vitro* studies show that ANGPTL4 interacts with LPL and converts active LPL dimers to inactive monomers [8,9]. Inactivation of *Angptl4* in mice is associated with low plasma triglycerides and high postheparin LPL activity [10]. A special case is that *Angptl4*[−/−] mice on a diet with high content of saturated fat develop severe abdominal inflammation due to excessive LPL-mediated lipid uptake in mesenteric lymph nodes [11]. Similarly, a loss of function mutation in ANGPTL4 in humans is associated with low levels of plasma triglycerides [12]. Conversely, overexpression of *Angptl4* in mice results in low LPL activity and high plasma triglycerides [10,13,14]. Taken together these data convincingly show that ANGPTL4 is involved in modulating the activity of LPL and thereby metabolism of plasma triglycerides. It should be noted however that ANGPTL4 also has effects on angiogenesis and several other processes, and that there are additional members in the ANGPTL protein family that have effects on plasma lipid metabolism [15] .

Another protein important for LPL action is the newly discovered glycosylphosphatidylinositol-anchored high density lipoprotein-binding protein 1, GPIHBP1 [16]. This protein, which is expressed only in endothelial cells, is crucial for transfer of LPL to the luminal side of the capillary endothelium [17]. Inactivation of the gene for GPIHBP1 in mice results in gross chylomicronemia. Genetic deficiency in humans produces a clinical phenotype similar to that in LPL deficiency. It is not known if GPIHBP1 has any direct role in the modulation of LPL action. Like *Angptl4* [6] the *Gpihbp1* is PPAR-responsive [18], suggesting that the two genes might be similarly regulated.

A third, newly discovered, protein involved with the lipase system is the lipase maturation factor (LMF1). This is an ER-based chaperone which appears to be necessary for maturation of LPL and the related hepatic lipase and endothelial lipase into their active forms [19,20].

In this paper we have explored how this landscape of LPL controlling proteins behaves in rat adipose tissue under a number of conditions previously shown to be associated with rapid changes of LPL activity. Specifically we have studied (1) if ANGPTL4 is needed for the rapid modulation of LPL activity; (2) if the message levels show circadian oscillations, (3) at what rates the messages for the three LPL-controlling proteins and the proteins themselves are being turned over, (4) how the messages for the LPL controlling proteins change on changes in the nutritional state, known to cause large changes of adipose tissue LPL activity and (5) what happens to the expression of the three proteins when rats become insulin resistant.

Results

Circadian rhythm

The expressions in adipose tissue of many of the genes involved in energy metabolism undergo circadian changes [21]. We followed the changes with time of day of a number of parameters related to LPL activity (Figure 1). Rats eat mainly during the dark period (18:00 h – 6:00 h). Mean food consumption was $0.88 \pm 0.10\%$ of body weight per hour during the night (Figure 1A). During the first hours of the light period (6:00 h – 9:00 h) the rats ate $0.04 \pm 0.01\%$ of body weight per hour. This is less than 5% of what they ate per hour during the night. From 9:00 h –15:00 h food consumption per hour was about one quarter of that during the dark period. During the last hours of the light period, 15:00 h – 18:00 h, food consumption increased to about half of that during the dark period.

The changes in plasma glucose and non-esterified fatty acids (NEFA) over the day were moderate (Figure 1B). Adipose tissue LPL mRNA (Figure 1C) showed its highest value at 22:00 h. This was 2.8 fold higher than the lowest value (at 10:00 h, p=0.028). Changes in GPIHBP1 mRNA (Figure 1C) were modest and the tendency was opposite to that for LPL mRNA, with higher values during the light than during the dark period. The increase in ANGPTL4 mRNA during the light period was more pronounced compared to GPIHBP1, but the levels were down again by 18.00 h. LPL activity (Figure 1D) in adipose tissue showed its highest value at 2:00 h and its lowest value at 10:00 h (p<0.01). The difference was about two-fold. LPL mass (Figure 1D) followed a similar pattern, and the ratio between LPL activity and mass (specific activity) did not change significantly.

Response of the proteins studied and of LPL activity when mRNA or protein synthesis was blocked

To directly study the turnover of the proteins involved, cycloheximide was injected in rats to block synthesis of

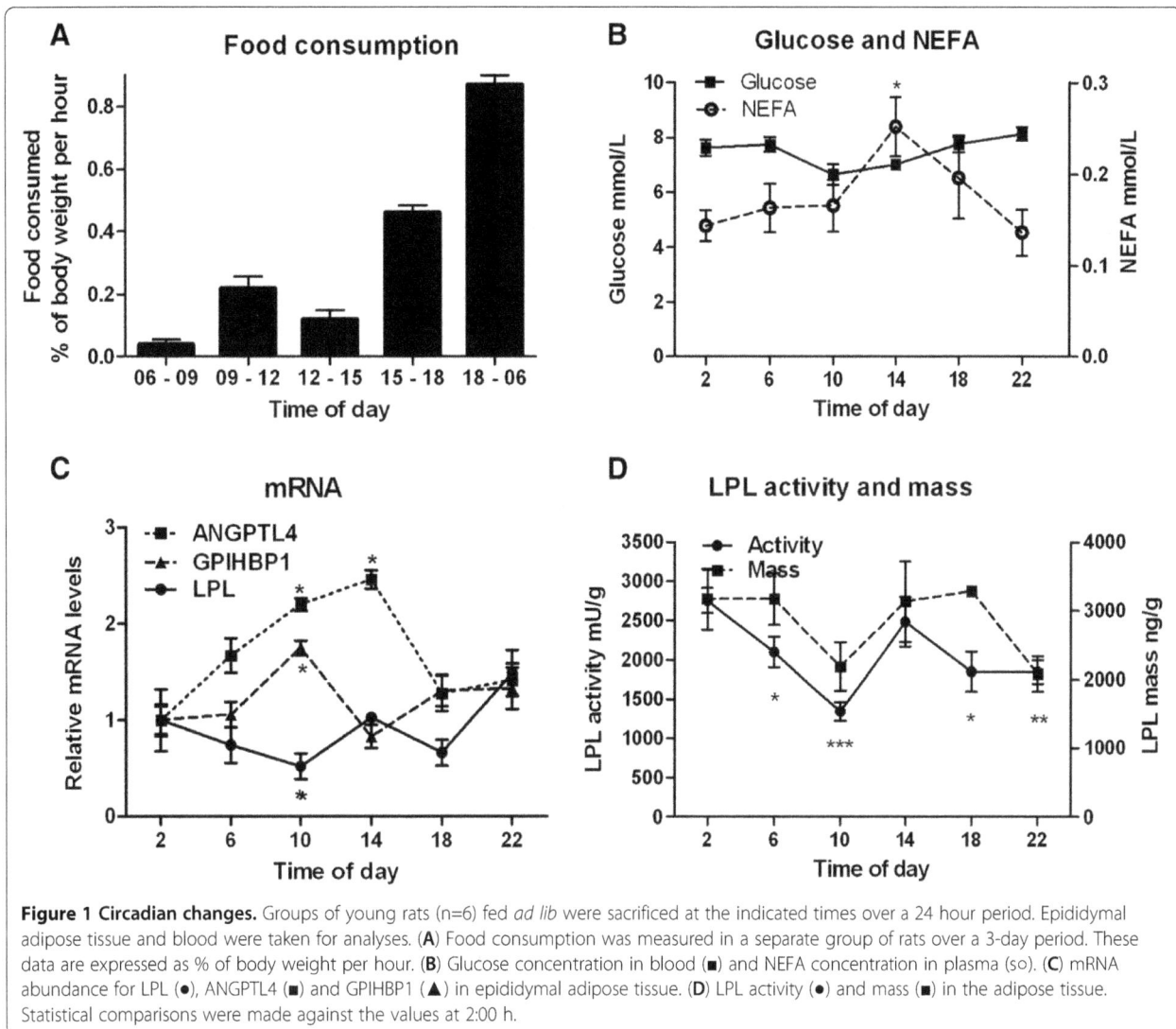

Figure 1 Circadian changes. Groups of young rats (n=6) fed *ad lib* were sacrificed at the indicated times over a 24 hour period. Epididymal adipose tissue and blood were taken for analyses. (**A**) Food consumption was measured in a separate group of rats over a 3-day period. These data are expressed as % of body weight per hour. (**B**) Glucose concentration in blood (■) and NEFA concentration in plasma (so). (**C**) mRNA abundance for LPL (●), ANGPTL4 (■) and GPIHBP1 (▲) in epididymal adipose tissue. (**D**) LPL activity (●) and mass (■) in the adipose tissue. Statistical comparisons were made against the values at 2:00 h.

new proteins (Figure 2). LPL activity decreased by 60% in 3 hours (Figure 2A). LPL mass, measured by ELISA (Figure 2A), and estimated from Western blots (Figure 2D), decreased at a similar rate as the activity. These data are in line with earlier observations that the LPL protein turns over rapidly [22,23]. In contrast, ANGPTL4 protein showed bands of similar intensity on western blots throughout the four hours studied (Figure 2E and F). The pattern was the same when antibodies to the C-terminal (Figure 2E) or N-terminal domain (Figure 2F) of ANGPTL4 were used. Almost all of the protein was full length (here 68 kDa compared to MW standards). With antibodies to the C-terminal domain small amounts of a 45 kDa fragment was seen (Figure 2E), probably representing the fibrinogen-like domain of ANGPTL4. These data show that the ANGPTL4 protein turns over relatively slowly, much slower than the LPL protein. The turnover of the GPIHBP1 and LMF1 proteins could not be studied since suitable antibodies were not available.

To directly study the turnover of the corresponding messages, the transcription blocker actinomycin D (ActD) was injected (Figure 2). Fasted rats were used since the level of ANGPTL4 and GPIHBP1 messages in adipose tissue are several-fold higher in the fasted than in the fed state [6,18]. In concert with earlier studies [5], LPL activity in adipose tissue rose from 340 ± 43 to 1225 ± 112 mU/g in six hours after ActD (Figure 2B). The value for LPL mRNA decreased by 8% by 4 h and by 33% by 6 h (Figure 2C), but these changes did not reach statistical significance. LPL mass as measured by the ELISA increased by 40% (p<0.05) in 6 h. Consistent with these data, Western blots showed that the level of LPL protein was essentially stable over the six h studied (Figure 2G). These data confirm that the LPL transcript is relatively stable.

While LPL activity went up, mRNA levels for ANGPTL4, GPIHBP1 and LMF1 were reduced by 93%, 75% and 29% by six hours after ActD (Figure 2C). These results show that the ANGPTL4 and GPIHBP1 transcripts are turned

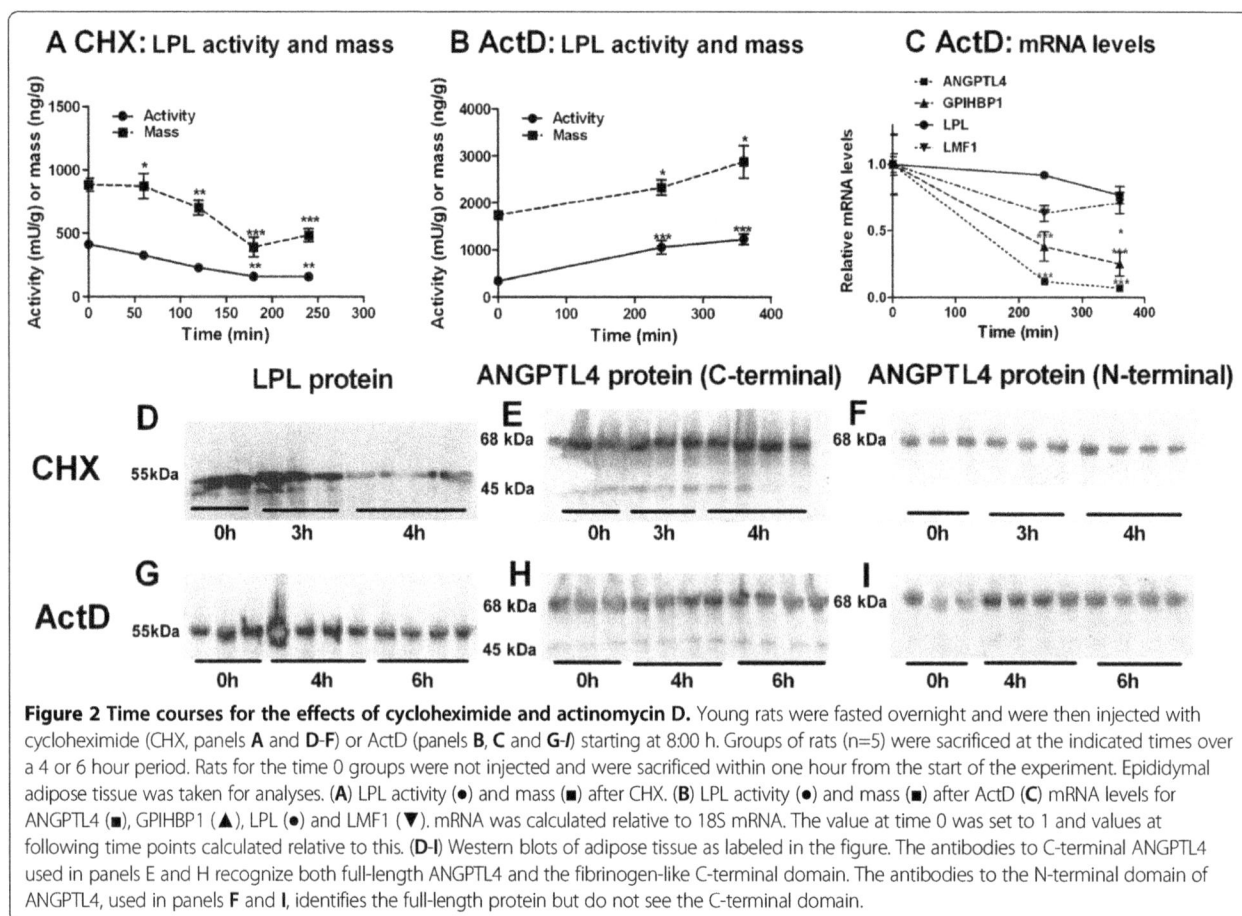

Figure 2 Time courses for the effects of cycloheximide and actinomycin D. Young rats were fasted overnight and were then injected with cycloheximide (CHX, panels **A** and **D-F**) or ActD (panels **B**, **C** and **G-I**) starting at 8:00 h. Groups of rats (n=5) were sacrificed at the indicated times over a 4 or 6 hour period. Rats for the time 0 groups were not injected and were sacrificed within one hour from the start of the experiment. Epididymal adipose tissue was taken for analyses. (**A**) LPL activity (●) and mass (■) after CHX. (**B**) LPL activity (●) and mass (■) after ActD (**C**) mRNA levels for ANGPTL4 (■), GPIHBP1 (▲), LPL (●) and LMF1 (▼). mRNA was calculated relative to 18S mRNA. The value at time 0 was set to 1 and values at following time points calculated relative to this. (**D-I**) Western blots of adipose tissue as labeled in the figure. The antibodies to C-terminal ANGPTL4 used in panels **E** and **H** recognize both full-length ANGPTL4 and the fibrinogen-like C-terminal domain. The antibodies to the N-terminal domain of ANGPTL4, used in panels **F** and **I**, identifies the full-length protein but do not see the C-terminal domain.

over rapidly. On Western blots, the ANGPTL4 protein showed bands of similar intensity throughout the six hours (Figure 2H and I). This pattern was the same when antibodies to the C-terminal or N-terminal domain were used. Almost all of the protein was full length but traces of a 45 kDa fragment were seen with the antibody specific for the C-terminal domain of ANGPTL4. These data again show that the ANGPTL4 protein turns over relatively slowly.

Early response to food withdrawal

To study the early events in adaptation of the LPL system in adipose tissue to fasting, food was withdrawn from rats in the morning. At this time the animals ate rather little (Figure 1A). Their stomachs were about half full and emptied almost completely within two hours after food was removed. Insulin (Figure 3A) and glucose (Figure 3B) decreased whereas NEFA increased (Figure 3B). Triglycerides decreased, presumably because the inflow of chylomicrons from the intestine faded (data not shown). LPL mRNA in adipose tissue did not change significantly, in accordance with earlier observations [24] (data not shown). The level of mRNA for LMF1 also did not change significantly (data not shown).

In contrast, the levels of ANGPTL4 mRNA and GPIHBP1 mRNA increased markedly (about 6-fold and 2-fold, respectively) in adipose tissue over the six hours studied (Figure 3C). LPL activity in adipose tissue had decreased by 40% at four hours and by 53% at six hours (Figure 3D). In contrast there was no significant change of LPL mass (Figure 3D). All of these responses to food withdrawal were similar in a parallel experiment on female rats, but data are shown only for males. These data indicate that short term fasting is associated with reciprocal changes in adipose ANGPTL4 mRNA and LPL activity.

Relation to changes in expression of other genes

To get a perspective on the rapid and large response of *Angptl4* transcript on fasting [8] we carried out an array analysis of the changes of RNA abundances in adipose tissue under the conditions used for our experiments. For this, food was removed from one group of rats in the early morning. Seven h later the rats were sacrificed, epididymal adipose tissue was cut out, RNA prepared and analyzed on Illumina arrays. N = 6 for both the fasted and the *ad lib* group. After filtering the data for P < 0.01 and signal intensity > 50, there remained 22

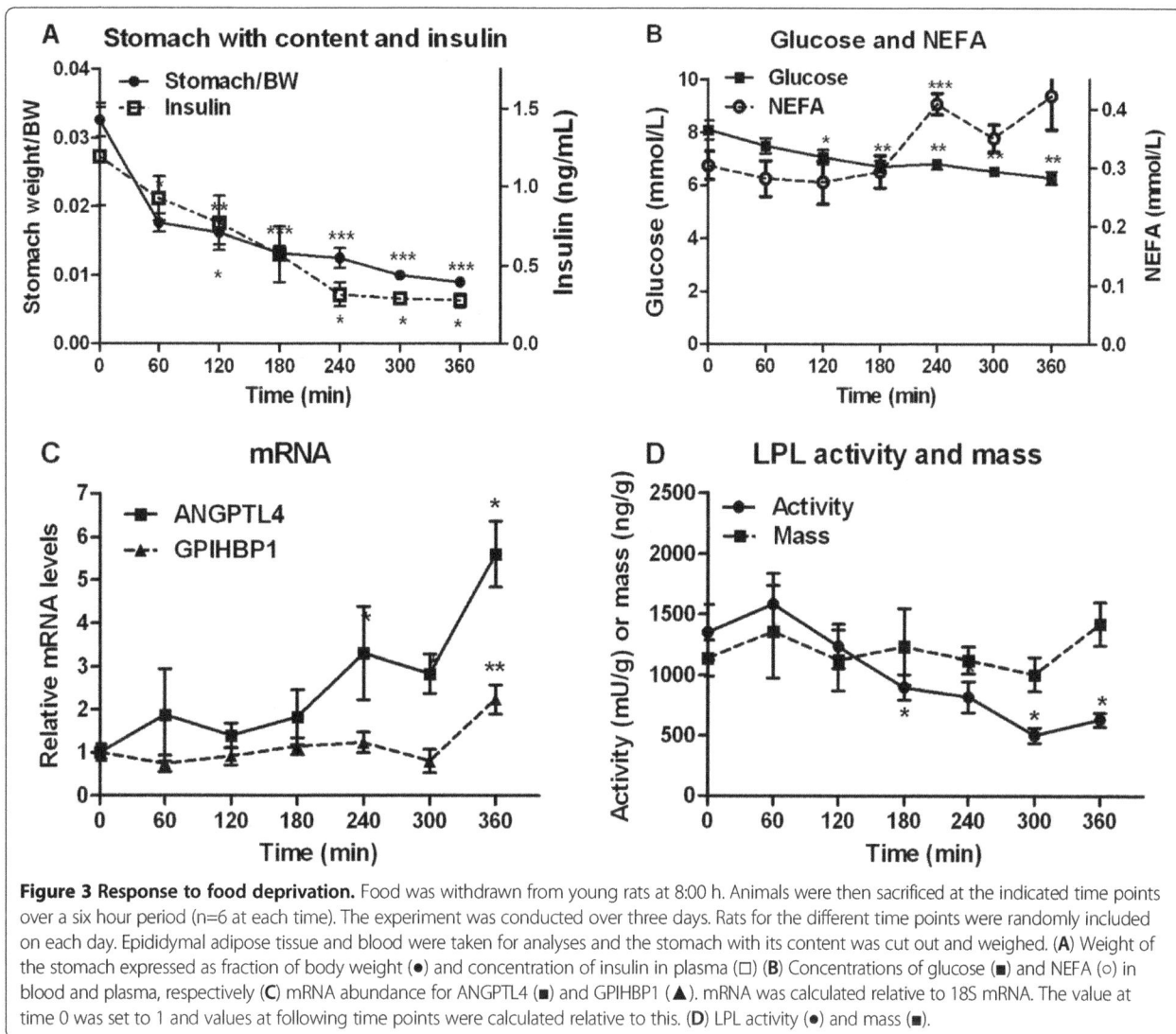

Figure 3 Response to food deprivation. Food was withdrawn from young rats at 8:00 h. Animals were then sacrificed at the indicated time points over a six hour period (n=6 at each time). The experiment was conducted over three days. Rats for the different time points were randomly included on each day. Epididymal adipose tissue and blood were taken for analyses and the stomach with its content was cut out and weighed. (**A**) Weight of the stomach expressed as fraction of body weight (●) and concentration of insulin in plasma (□) (**B**) Concentrations of glucose (■) and NEFA (o) in blood and plasma, respectively (**C**) mRNA abundance for ANGPTL4 (■) and GPIHBP1 (▲). mRNA was calculated relative to 18S mRNA. The value at time 0 was set to 1 and values at following time points were calculated relative to this. (**D**) LPL activity (●) and mass (■).

transcripts that had increased, and 21 that had decreased by a factor of 2.0 or more.

Sorting by foldchange+, *Angptl4* came out as number four from the top (foldchange 3.37, $p < E * 10^{-17}$), preceded only by *Pdk4*, pyruvate dehydrogenase kinase 4, a key regulator of glycolysis/glyceroneogenesis, *Gpr109a*, the ketone body/niacin receptor, a key regulator of lipolysis, and *RGD1565690_*predicted, a gene of unknown function (Table 1). In concert with the results of the experiment in Figure 3 and earlier observations [24], the expression of *LPL* did not change significantly (foldchange 1.02). Neither *Gpihbp1* or *LmfF1* was represented on this chip.

Responses to re-feeding

To study a situation when adipose tissue LPL activity increases rapidly we turned to re-feeding as a physiological model that we had used before [8]. For this, rats were fasted overnight and food was given back in the

Table 1 The eight genes that increased their expression in adipose tissue the most when food was removed

Symbol	Foldchange +	DiffScore
Pdk4	4.97	70.6
Gpr109a	3.86	54.8
RGD1565690_predicted	3.83	55.7
Angptl4	3.58	330.8
Per1	3.25	39.4
Pfkfb3	3.15	12.7
Pck1	2.91	40.9
Net1	2.82	56.3
Lpl	1.02	0.00004

Food was removed from one group of rats in the early morning. Seven h later the rats were sacrificed, epididymal adipose tissue was cut out, RNA prepared and analyzed on Illumina arrays. N = 6 for both the fasted and the *ad lib* group. Full data are deposited at NCBI GEO, accession no GSE 41800.

morning. The animals started to eat within 5 to 10 min. By one hour their stomachs contained 2.0 ± 0.03 g/100 g body weight (Figure 4A), similar to what was found in the stomach of regularly fed rats (Figure 3A). Insulin (Figure 4A) followed a time course similar to that for weight of stomach contents. Glucose increased (Figure 4B), and NEFA decreased (Figure 4B). ANGPTL4 and GPIHBP1 mRNA levels decreased rapidly and after two hours were only 35 and 21% of the initial levels, respectively (Figure 4C). LPL activity and mass increased (Figure 4D). Thus, similar to fasting, fasting-refeeding is associated with reciprocal changes in adipose ANGPTL4 and GPIHBP1 mRNA on the one hand, and LPL activity on the other hand.

Response of the LPL system to fasting and re-feeding in Angptl4 $^{-/-}$ mice

To directly investigate the role of ANGPTL4 in the rapid modulation of LPL activity we turned to studies in mice in

which *Angptl4* had been inactivated [10]. Groups of mice (n=6) were fed *ad lib*, fasted over night, or fasted over night and then re-fed in the morning for 3 h. Plasma lipid levels were in accordance with previous results on *Angptl4* $^{-/-}$ mice [10]. Separation of lipoprotein classes by FPLC high-lighted that the fasted *Angptl4* $^{-/-}$ mice had no TG in the VLDL fraction, while after re-feeding the levels of VLDL TG were similar in *Angpt4* $^{-/-}$ compared to wild-type mice (Figure 5A). The peak of HDL cholesterol was slightly higher in *Angptl4* $^{-/-}$ and was shifted towards larger particles in all three groups of mice compared to wild-type (Figure 5A). The increase in NEFA on fasting was blunted in the *Angptl4* $^{-/-}$ mice (Figure 5B). This is in accordance with a role of ANGPTL4 for intracellular lipolysis [25].

In the wild-type animals, fasting caused a decrease of adipose tissue LPL activity, as expected (Figure 6A). In contrast, fasting caused an increase of adipose tissue LPL activity in the *Angptl4* $^{-/-}$ mice compared to fed or

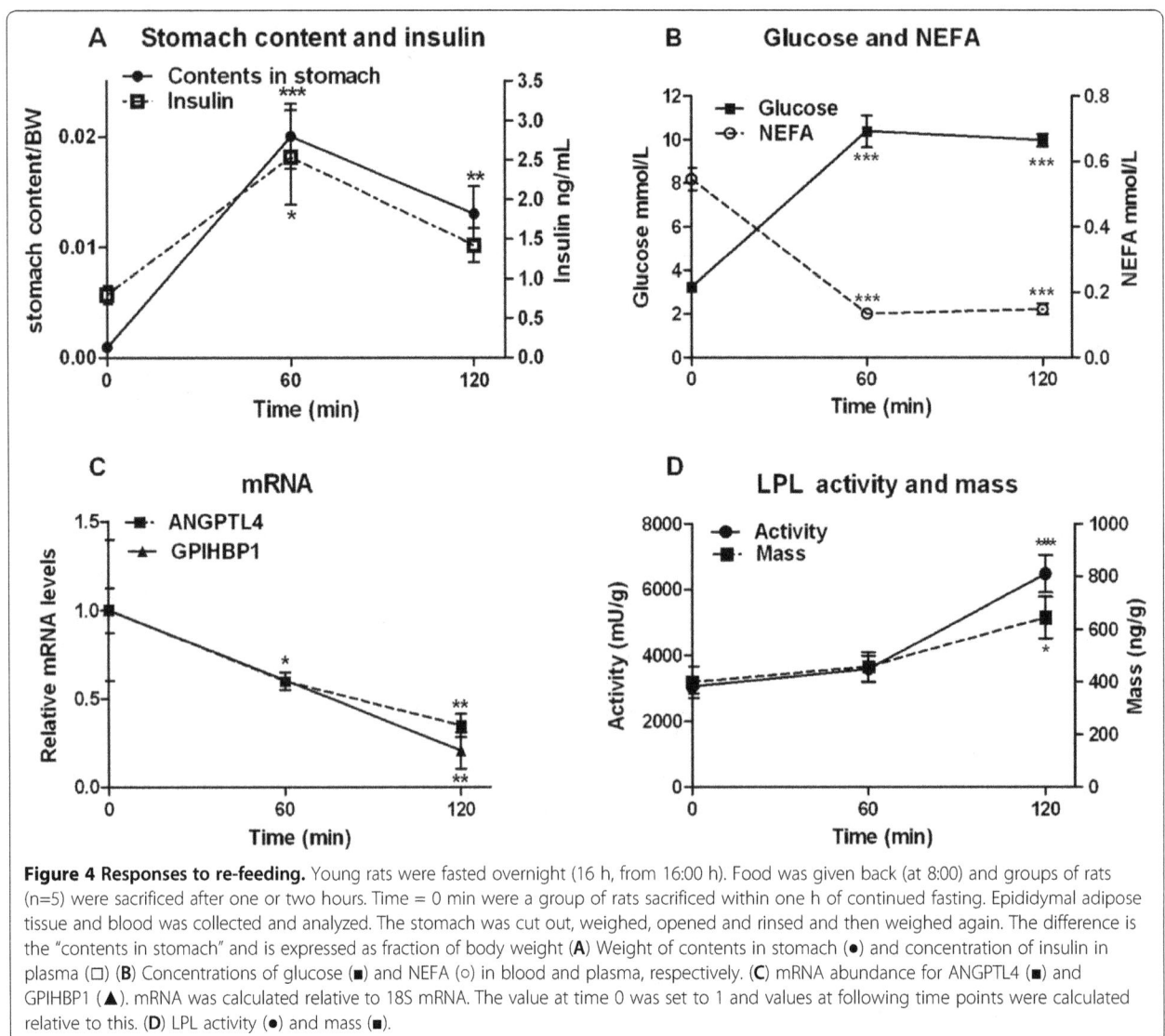

Figure 4 Responses to re-feeding. Young rats were fasted overnight (16 h, from 16:00 h). Food was given back (at 8:00) and groups of rats (n=5) were sacrificed after one or two hours. Time = 0 min were a group of rats sacrificed within one h of continued fasting. Epididymal adipose tissue and blood was collected and analyzed. The stomach was cut out, weighed, opened and rinsed and then weighed again. The difference is the "contents in stomach" and is expressed as fraction of body weight (**A**) Weight of contents in stomach (●) and concentration of insulin in plasma (□) (**B**) Concentrations of glucose (■) and NEFA (○) in blood and plasma, respectively. (**C**) mRNA abundance for ANGPTL4 (■) and GPIHBP1 (▲). mRNA was calculated relative to 18S mRNA. The value at time 0 was set to 1 and values at following time points were calculated relative to this. (**D**) LPL activity (●) and mass (■).

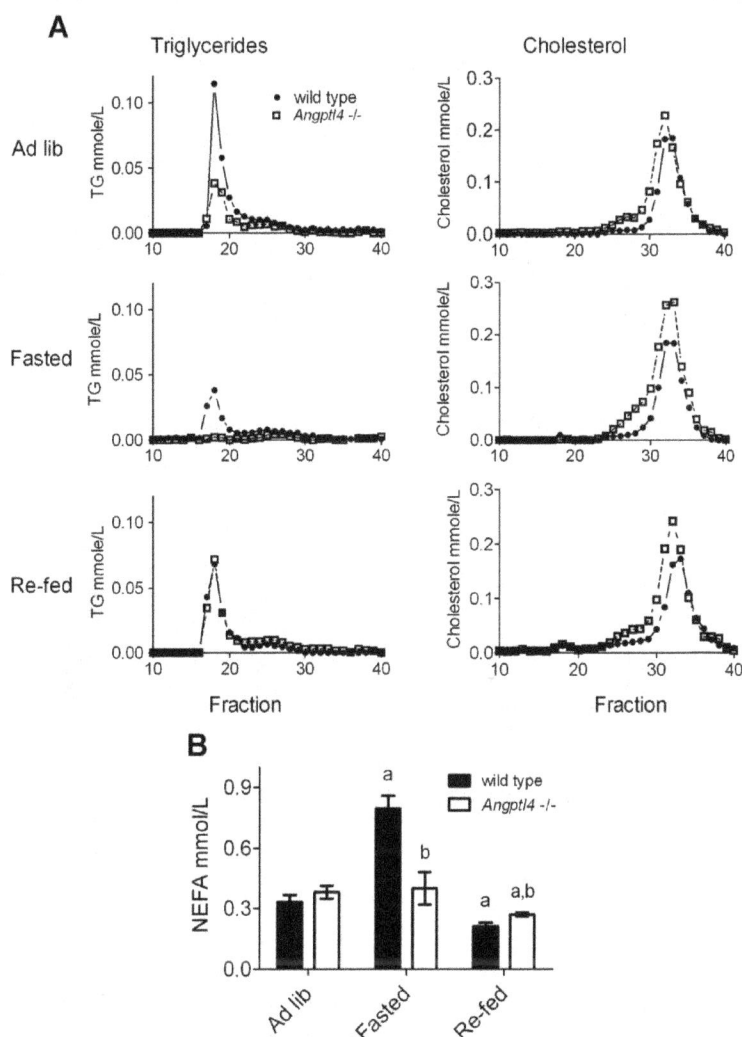

Figure 5 Plasma lipids in Angptl$^{-/-}$ mice. Wild-type and Angptl$^{-/-}$ mice were fasted overnight or fed *ad lib*. Food was given back to groups of fasted mice at 6:00 h (re-fed), while others continued fasting or eating (n=6 per group). All animals were sacrificed between 9:00 h – 10:00 h. (**A**) FPLC analyses of pooled plasma samples representing the 6 different groups. (**B**) Fatty acids (NEFA) in individual plasma samples. Statistically significant (p<0.05) differences are indicated by: a when comparing fasted or re-fed animals to *ad lib* for the same genotype b when comparing the two genotypes for the same nutritional state.

re-fed *Angptl4$^{-/-}$* animals. LPL activity was significantly higher in all three nutritional states in *Angptl4$^{-/-}$* compared to wild-type animals, indicating that ANGPTL4 represses LPL activity to some extent also in fed animals. ANGPTL4 mRNA was about two-fold increased in fasted compared to *ad lib* fed wild-type mice, while, as expected, there was no detectable ANGPTL4 mRNA in the *Angptl4$^{-/-}$* mice (Figure 6C). GPIHBP1 mRNA was also increased about two-fold in fasted wild-type mice compared to the fed groups. Interestingly, this difference was not seen in the *Angptl4$^{-/-}$* mice (Figure 6D). LPL mRNA was not significantly changed in wild-type mice, but was decreased in the fasted *Angptl4$^{-/-}$* mice compared to the fed groups (Figure 6B). Taken together these data demonstrate that the reduction in adipose

LPL activity upon fasting is dependent on increased expression of ANGPTL4.

Response to insulin

To study direct effects of insulin on the LPL system, fasted rats were given an intraperitoneal injection of insulin, 1 U/kg body weight, which is in the range used for insulin tolerance tests in rodents [26]. The injection resulted in levels of insulin in blood that were about five times higher than the mean level in controls at 60 min. Glucose and NEFA both decreased (data not shown). Already one hour after the injection, adipose tissue LPL activity had almost doubled (Figure 7). LPL mass did not change significantly (data not shown). ANGPTL4 and GPIHBP1 mRNA both decreased (Figure 7). One hour

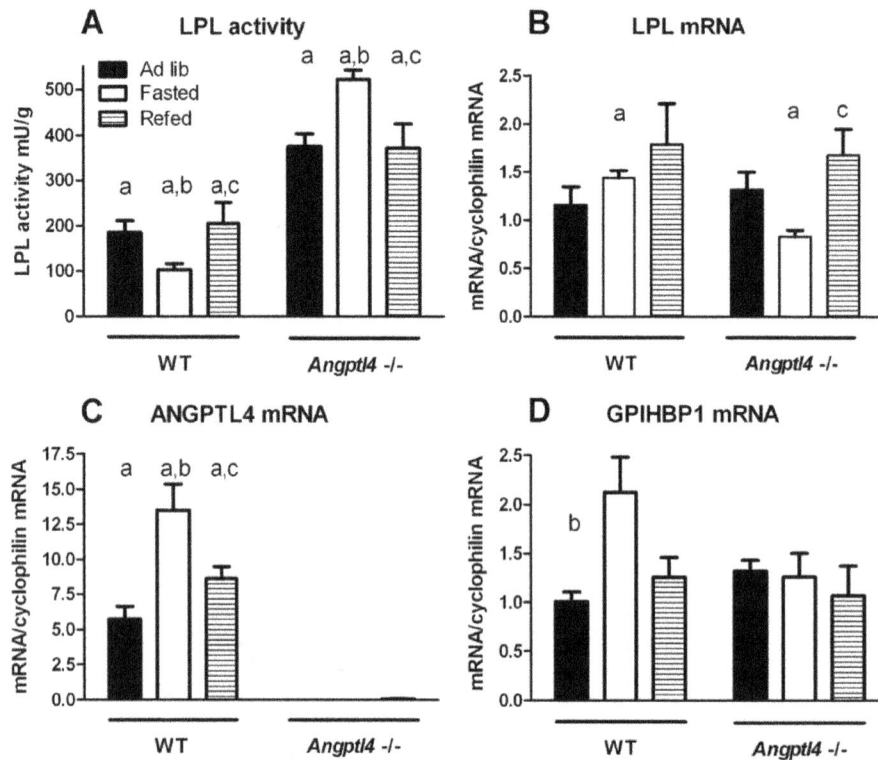

Figure 6 Response of the LPL system to fasting and re-feeding in Angptl4 $^{-/-}$ mice. Epididymal adipose tissue from the same mice as described in Figure 5 was cut out and analyzed for LPL activity and mRNA abundance for LPL, ANGPTL4, and GPIHBP1. The levels of mRNA were calculated relative to cyclophilin mRNA. Statistically significant ($p < 0.05$) differences are indicated by: a when comparing Angptl4 $^{-/-}$ and WT for the same nutritional state b when comparing fasted and *ad lib* for the same genotype c when comparing refed and *ad lib* for the same genotype.

after injection of insulin the levels were 33% and 50% of the initial levels, respectively.

Changes with age and/or weight of the rats

Previous studies have shown that the response of adipose tissue LPL activity to feeding/fasting is blunted in old, obese rats [5,27]. To probe this we studied rats at three different ages, 5 weeks old, lean, body weight 199 ± 20 g; 25 weeks old, moderately obese, body weight 695 ± 66 g; and 52 weeks old, grossly obese, body weight 1006 ± 82 g. One set of rats from each age group was fasted overnight and compared to *ad lib* fed controls.

In the fasted state, the young lean rats had low blood glucose, about 3.3 mmol/L. The intermediate and old rats had much higher blood glucose, about 6.0 mmol/L (Figure 8A). In the fed state the three groups had similar blood glucose levels, around 8 mmol/L. The fed/fasted ratio for glucose was around 2.3 in the young, lean rats, but only 1.3 and 1.2 in the old and intermediate groups, respectively. NEFA levels were similar in all three groups in the fed state (Figure 8B). On fasting, the level increased almost three-fold in the young rats, but did not change significantly in the intermediate or old rats.

Plasma insulin levels (Figure 8C) showed large differences between the groups. The fasting level was below 0.6 ng/ml in the young rats, four times higher in the intermediate group and 12 times higher in the oldest group. The fed/fasted ratio was about 5 in the young lean rats, but only 1.35 in the intermediate group. In the old group insulin levels in plasma did not differ between fed or fasted animals.

In accordance with the observations for food withdrawal (Figure 3) and re-feeding (Figure 4), ANGPTL4 and GPIHBP1 mRNA levels were much higher in the fasted than in the fed state in the young rats (Figure 8D and E). In contrast there were no statistically significant changes with nutritional state in the older rats.

Adipose tissue LPL activity, expressed per gram wet tissue weight, was high in the young rats, about 1600 mU/g. In the intermediate and old rats the activity was less than one-third (Figure 8F). These rats had much larger fat pads than the young lean ones so that the total LPL activity per pad was actually larger in the older groups (2.1-fold and 3.6-fold for the intermediate and old rats, respectively), compared to the young rats. Remarkably, the response to nutritional state was more

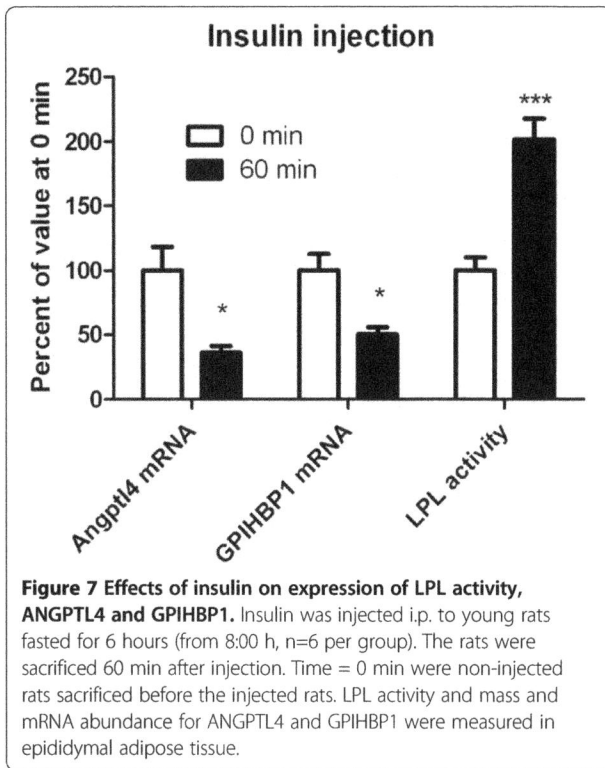

Figure 7 Effects of insulin on expression of LPL activity, ANGPTL4 and GPIHBP1. Insulin was injected i.p. to young rats fasted for 6 hours (from 8:00 h, n=6 per group). The rats were sacrificed 60 min after injection. Time = 0 min were non-injected rats sacrificed before the injected rats. LPL activity and mass and mRNA abundance for ANGPTL4 and GPIHBP1 were measured in epididymal adipose tissue.

pronounced in the young rats with a fed/fasted ratio more than twice as high as that in the two older groups (Figure 8F).

Discussion

The present study reinforces previous observations that rapid modulation of LPL activity (in rodent adipose tissue) is not exerted at the level of LPL gene expression [1,24,27,28]. LPL mRNA levels remained essentially stable under the conditions we tested. Likewise, the mRNA for LMF1, an ER protein needed for proper maturation of LPL into its active form [19,20], did not change significantly, in accordance with an earlier study in Zucker diabetic rats [29]. In contrast, the mRNAs for ANGPTL4 and GPIHBP1, changed much more rapidly than most mRNAs in mammalian cells [30]. These two proteins interact with LPL and we will designate them collectively as 'LPL controlling proteins'. There may well be more, yet undiscovered, proteins that participate in the LPL system. A major mechanism for the modulation of adipose LPL activity is conversion of catalytically active LPL dimers into inactive monomers [4,8]. This process is virtually irreversible [31,32]. The LPL protein, active or inactive, turns over with a half-life of less than two hours [22,23] which is much more rapid than the

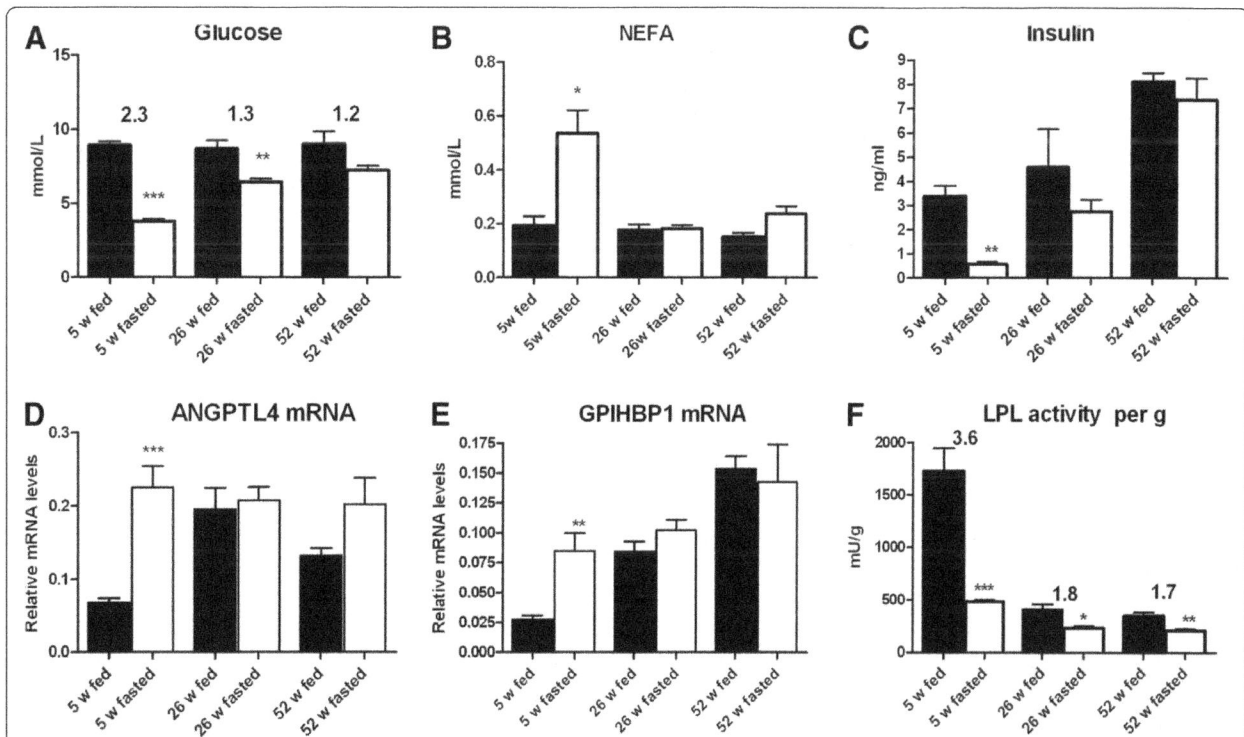

Figure 8 Effects of age and/or obesity. Groups of rats of different ages (5 weeks, 26 weeks and 52 weeks) were either fed *ad lib* (solid bars) or fasted overnight for 16 h (open bars). At 8:00 h groups of fed and fasted rats of the indicated age were sacrificed (n=5 per group). The epididymal fat body was cut out and weighed. Blood was also taken for analyses of (**A**) glucose, (**B**) NEFA and (**C**) Insulin. mRNA levels for ANGPTL4 (**D**) and GPIHBP1 (**E**) and are expressed relative to 18S RNA. (**F**) LPL activity expressed per g wet weight of tissue. Statistical comparisons are made between fed and fasted animals. The numbers above some of the bars represent the relative change from the fasted to the fed state.

turnover of most proteins in mammalian cells [30]. Hence, the overall design of the LPL system appears to be relatively constant production and secretion of short-lived enzyme molecules that either retain or loose their catalytic activity in response to a number of controlling proteins. This design may have evolved to meet the need to modulate the activity of secreted/extracellular LPL molecules.

The expression of many genes involved in energy metabolism undergo profound circadian oscillations in the adipose tissue presumably to adapt the animal to predictable changes in the environment [21], LPL mRNA, mass and activity all shoved higher values in the middle of the dark period. For LPL activity the amplitude was about two-fold, in accordance with previous studies [24,33-37]. ANGPTL4 and GPIHBP1 mRNA showed modest changes opposite in direction to that for LPL. Hence, it appears that the LPL system displays a moderate circadian oscillation in phase with the eating behavior, but can respond rapidly and profoundly whenever food becomes scarce. Of note, the circadian oscillations of adipose tissue LPL are more pronounced in mice, with a more than three-fold higher activity in the middle of the dark period compared to the middle of the light period [38]. A significant circadian variation has also been reported for post-heparin LPL activity in humans [39].

A possible confounding factor for studies of how LPL activity is modulated in adipose tissue is changes in the rate at which proteins are being synthesized in the adipocytes [1]. Parkin et al. found that insulin more than doubled the rate of incorporation of amino acids into proteins in rat fat pads and caused a corresponding increase in LPL activity [40]. Other groups have reported similar observations [1,2]. Kern and his associates have described a more specific mechanism that affects LPL synthesis whereby stimulation of the protein kinase A system leads to formation of a protein complex that binds to the 3'UTR of LPL mRNA and blocks its translation [28]. It seems likely that part of the early responses of LPL activity in our studies, e.g. after injection of a large dose of insulin, reflect decreased/increased rates of LPL translation. This can not, however, fully explain the changes seen. For instance, during food deprivation (Figure 3) LPL activity decreased by more than 50%, while there was no significant change in LPL mass.

The experiment on $Angptl4^{-/-}$ mice clearly demonstrated the important role of ANGPTL4 for suppression of adipose tissue LPL activity in the fasted state. Even though LPL mRNA levels were significantly reduced in adipose tissue of the $Angptl4^{-/-}$ mice, compared to all other groups of mice, LPL activity was the highest in adipose tissue of fasted $Angptl4^{-/-}$ mice. Also in the ad lib fed and the re-fed states, adipose tissue LPL activity was significantly higher in $Angptl4^{-/-}$ mice than in wild-

type mice, indicating that some LPL is depressed by ANGPTL4 even under conditions when LPL activity is at demand. These data are compatible with those of Köster et al. [10], demonstrating 2–3 fold higher LPL activity in post-heparin plasma in $Angptl4^{-/-}$ mice compared to wild-type mice in both fed and fasted animals. Similarly, blocking transcription by ActD led to a decrease in ANGPTL4 mRNA levels in adipose tissue and to a 3-fold increase in LPL activity in fasted rats [8], and to a 3-fold increase in post-heparin plasma LPL activity in ad lib fed rats [41]. In fed animals, most of the LPL activity in post-heparin plasma originates from adipose tissue, while in fasted animals the dominating source is presumably skeletal muscle and heart [38,42]. Taken together the data demonstrate that ANGPTL4 is an important modulator of LPL activity in both fasted and fed animals.

The present data show that ANGPTL4 mRNA turns over rapidly in adipose tissue, in concert with an earlier study [8]. When transcription was blocked by injection of ActD, the mRNA decreased more than 90% in 4 hours. The mRNA level responded rapidly to the perturbations of the nutritional state that we used. It increased more than 200% from 3 to 6 hours after food deprivation. It decreased by about 50% in one hour after injection of insulin and by about 65% within two hours after re-feeding of rats that had fasted overnight. In all of these situations, the expression of $Angptl4$ changed as expected for a gene that negatively controls LPL activity. Whenever the expression of $Angptl4$ increased, LPL activity decreased and conversely when the expression of $Angptl4$ decreased, LPL activity increased. The time courses for the changes were compatible with a major role for ANGPTL4 in modulation of LPL activity, if one takes into account that the general rate of protein synthesis, and hence LPL synthesis, probably changed (see above). In contrast to the rapid changes of ANGPTL4 message levels, the ANGPTL4 protein remained essentially unchanged over several hours, as evaluated by Western blots. This was true whether we used antibodies to the N-terminal or C-terminal domains, and was true both in experiments where syntheses of new protein was blocked by cycloheximide and in experiments where message levels changed several-fold in response to a transcription block or in response to food withdrawal, re-feeding or insulin injection. This suggests compartmentalization, such that only newly synthesized ANGPTL4 protein can inactivate LPL. Within cells the ANGPTL4 protein exists as monomers but they form oligomers when they reach the cell surface [43]. It is only after oligomerization that the ANGPTL4 protein can interact with and inactivate LPL [12,43]. Hence, it is possible that LPL and ANGPTL4 monomers do not interact when they travel through the secretory pathway, but there is a critical event when the proteins emerge at the cell surface that triggers oligomerization of ANGPTL4 and thereby inactivation of LPL. LMF1 may have a role here [20]. Once LPL transfers to the endothelial cells the enzyme may be rescued by interaction with heparan sulfate proteoglycans [44] and/or GPIHBP1 [45].

The message for GPIHBP1 also turned over rapidly. When transcription was blocked by ActD the message decreased by more than 60% within 4 hours. It increased 4-fold from 3 to 6 hours after food deprivation. It decreased by about 50% in one hour after injection of insulin and by about 80% within 2 hours after re-feeding of overnight fasted rats. This is in accordance with the studies of Davis et al. who found that GPIHBP1 message in adipose tissue is higher in 16 h fasted than in fed rats [18]. Comparing the amplitudes of the changes, *Gpihbp1* was at least as responsive as *Angptl4*. This is impressive considering that array analysis showed that *Angptl4* was one of the genes whose expression had increased most seven hours after food withdrawal (Table 1). The changes of GPIHBP1 mRNA were in the same direction as the changes of ANGPTL4 mRNA in all the situations that we studied. This is surprising. According to present hypotheses ANGPTL4 protein suppresses LPL activity. GPIHBP1 on the other hand stabilizes the enzyme and promotes its delivery to the site of action at the vascular endothelium [45]. One should note that the changes presumably take place in different cells in the tissue. *Gpihbp1* is expressed in endothelial cells [16] whereas *Angptl4* is presumably expressed mainly in adipocytes. It is possible that GPIHBP1 not only delivers LPL to the luminal side of the endothelium, but that under certain circumstances, like during fasting, GPIHBP1 may predominantly transport LPL in the opposite direction leading to LPL-inactivation and or degradation within the tissue [46].

Rapid, tissue-specific modulation of LPL activity is important for whole body energy homeostasis by directing lipid uptake to the appropriate tissues and limiting the need for re-transport [1,2]. Earlier studies have shown that the response of adipose tissue LPL activity to feeding-fasting becomes blunted as rats grow older and become obese [5,24]. The present study confirms these observations and links them to the development of insulin resistance. In young, lean rats (5 weeks old) adipose tissue LPL activity decreased by a factor of 3.6 – 3.9 on fasting overnight. In older, obese rats the response was less than half, 1.7 – 1.9-fold. The older rats appeared to be insulin-resistant. Fasting blood glucose and insulin was elevated compared to the young rats and the difference fed versus fasted was less for all parameters studied. It is of interest to note that these rats were not manipulated in any way but housed by normal routines and fed chow *ad lib* [47]. The responses of the LPL controlling genes, *Angptl4* and *Gpihbp1* were blunted. The

large change in GPIHBP1 mRNA (about 3-fold) seen when young rats were fasted was completely abolished in the older rats. For ANGPTL4 mRNA some response remained but it was much less than in the young rats. It is of interest to note that the values seen in either the fed or fasted state in the older rats were similar to those seen in fasted young rats. Hence, it appears that it was the ability to down-regulate the expression in the fed state that caused the loss of metabolic plasticity. In line with this it was recently shown that mRNA of Angptl4 is upregulated in diabetic mice [48] whereas insulin inhibited Angptl4 mRNA expression in 3 T3-L1 adipocytes [49]. Moreover, FFA, which are increased in the insulin-resistant state, were shown to upregulate mRNA expression of Angptl4 in human adipocytes [50]. A study on groups of human subjects (young, lean compared to old, obese with or without diabetes type II) demonstrated a blunting of the response of *Angptl4* to feeding/fasting in both groups of elderly individuals compared to the young, while no effect was in this case seen on *GPIHBP1* expression [42]. Bergö et al. found that blocking transcription by ActD (which relieves the suppression of LPL activity) increased adipose tissue LPL activity severalfold in fasted young rats, but had only a small effect in old, obese rats [5]. These data are compatible with the hypothesis that expressions of *Angptl4* and/or *Gpihbp1* are main determinants for LPL activity in adipose tissue of rats.

Modulation of LPL activity is important for partitioning of lipids between tissues in accordance with changes in the metabolic situation [1,2]. It is becoming evident that that modulation of LPL action occurs by interplay of several factors. The central player, the LPL enzyme, appears to be produced at a relatively constant rate. The activity and the distribution of the enzyme between the endothelial cell surface and other places in the tissue are determined by LMF1, ANGPTLl4 and GPIHBP1 and perhaps other proteins in a context dependent manner. In addition LPL action is modulated by factors pertaining to the lipoprotein substrate [1]. Apolipoprotein CII is a necessary cofactor. Apolipoprotein CIII and other apolipoproteins can suppress lipase action. In this case the action of the enzyme is inhibited but not irreversibly lost.

Conclusions

The main conclusion from this study is that ANGPTL4 is necessary for the rapid modulation of LPL activity in adipose tissue. ANGPTL4 message levels responded very rapidly to changes in the nutritional state. LPL activity always changed in the opposite direction. This did not happen in Angptl4$^{-/-}$ mice. GPIHBP1 message levels also changed rapidly and in the same direction as ANGPTL4, i.e. increased on fasting when LPL activity decreased. This was unexpected because GPIHBP1 is known to stabilize LPL.

In old, obese rats that showed signs of insulin resistance, the responses of ANGPTL4 and GPIHBP1 mRNA and of LPL activity were severely blunted (at 26 weeks of age) or almost abolished (at 52 weeks of age). Hence, the plasticity of the LPL system is severely blunted or completely lost in insulin resistant rats.

Methods
Animal procedures
Inbred male Sprague–Dawley rats weighing 150–210 g were used, except in the exp on the effect of ageing/insulin resistance in Figure 8. The rats were housed with free access to a standard pellet diet and water in a 12-h light cycle (6:00 h – 18:00 h). Experiments were, unless otherwise stated, carried out with rats fed or fasted overnight (food removed at 16:00 h) or fasted for 6 h (food removed at 8:00 h). During fasting the rats were kept in cages with a perforated floor to prevent coprophagia. In experiments with re-feeding, rats were fasted overnight and then food was given back at 8:00 h. The experiment then continued for 2 h. The rats were killed by decapitation. The fat depot studied was the epididymal. Tissues were collected into Eppendorf tubes and immediately frozen in liquid nitrogen. Blood samples to be analyzed for LPL activity and metabolites were collected in EDTA blood collection tubes (Sarstedt). Plasma was obtained by centrifugation of the blood at 4°C and the samples were then stored at –70°C. the bars represent the relative change from the fasted to the fed state

Male pure-bred WT and *Angptl4–/–* mice on a C57Bl/6 background between ages 4–6 months were used [10]. Fasted mice were fasted from 15:00 h and sacrificed the next day between 9:00 h and 10:00 h. Refed mice were fasted from 15:00 h, refed with chow the next day at 6:00 h and sacrificed between 9:00 h and 10:00 h. Mice were anaesthetized with a mixture of isoflurane (1.5%), nitrous oxide (70%) and oxygen (30%). Blood was collected by orbital puncture into EDTA tubes. Mice were killed by cervical dislocation, after which tissues were excised and directly frozen in liquid nitrogen.

All animal procedures were approved by the local animal ethics committees in Umeå (rats) and Wageningen (mice), respectively.

In experiments on rats, insulin (Actrapid, Novo Nordisk A/S, Denmark) was injected intraperitoneally (1U/kg bw) to rats fasted for 6 h. Controls were injected with saline only. Actinomycin D (Sigma Aldrich), dissolved in pure ethanol to a concentration of 2 mg/ml, was injected intraperitoneally (2 mg/kg bw) to rats fasted for 6 h. Controls were injected with ethanol. Cycloheximide (Sigma Aldrich), dissolved in saline to a concentration of 35 mg/ml, was injected intraperitoneally (35 mg/kg bw) to rats fasted for 16 h. Controls were injected with saline.

LPL activity assay
Frozen tissues were homogenized in 9 volumes of buffer at pH 8.2 containing 0.025 M ammonia, 1% Triton X-100, 0.1% SDS and protease inhibitor cocktail tablets (Complete Mini, Roche Diagnosis, Germany) using a Polytron PT 3000 Homogenizer (Kinematica). The homogenates were centrifuged for 15 min at 10,000 rpm, 4°C. Aliquots of the supernatants were used for determination of LPL activity as previously described [5] using a phospholipid-stabilized emulsion of soy bean triacylglycerols and ^{3}H-oleic acid-labeled triolein with the same composition as Intralipid 10% (Fresenius Kabi, Uppsala, Sweden). The incubation was at 25°C for 100 or 120 min. One milliunit of enzyme activity corresponds to 1 nmol of fatty acids released per min. Enzyme activity is expressed per g wet tissue weight. In the exp in Figure 8 LPL activity per whole epididymal fat pad was also calculated. All samples were assayed in triplicates.

LPL mass determination
Mass was measured by an Elisa method previously described [4,5]. Affinity purified immunoglobulins (IgY) from chicken, raised against bovine LPL were used for capture of the antigen during an overnight incubation. Bound LPL was detected with 5D2 monoclonal antibody raised against bovine LPL (a generous gift from Prof. J. Brunzell, University of Washington, Seattle WA), followed by detection with peroxidise-labelled anti-mouse IgG. LPL purified from bovine milk was used as standard.

Quantitative RT-PCR analyses
For determination of the levels of LPL, ANGPTL4, GPIHBP1 and LMF1 mRNA in rat tissues, total RNA was extracted from adipose tissues using TRIzol reagent (Life Technologies) and treated with DNA-free kit (Ambion). cDNA was prepared from 50 ng total RNA using Moloney Murine Leukemia Virus Reverse Transcriptase, RNase H Minus (Fermentas) and pd(N)$_6$ Random Hexamer (Fermentas) in total volume of 20 µl. The expression of the genes of interest were quantified by real time PCR using TaqMan Universal PCR Master Mix and the ABI Prism 7700 Sequence Detection System (Applied Biosystems, Foster City, CA) and normalized to endogenous control (18S rRNA). ANGPTL4, LPL, GPIHBP1 and LMF1 primers and probes were designed from the published sequences for rat ANGPTLl4, LPL, GPIHBP1 and LMF-1 (corresponding GenBank accession numbers are: NM_199115, NM_000237, NM_001130547, and XM_340769. The sequences for primers and probes used were as follows:

5′-Fam-CTTGGAGCCCATGCTGCTGGC-TAMRA (LPL probe)

5'-ACTGGTGGGACAGGATGTGG
(LPL forward primer)
5'-CCGTTCTGCATACTCAAAGTTAGG
(LPL reverse primer)
5'-Fam-TCCCCAAGGCGAGTTCTGGCTG- TAMRA
(ANGPTL4probe)
5'-GACGCCTGAACGGCTCTGT
(ANGPTL4forward primer)
5'-CCCCTGTGATGCTGTGCAT
(ANGPTL4reverse primer)
5'-Fam-TGCCAGCACGAAATTCTCCCCG-TAMRA
(GPIHBP1 probe)
5'-TCAAAGGCTCATTCTCATCTTGA
(GPIHBP1 forward primer)
5'-ACACTCTTGGTTTCCTTCCAACA
(GPIHBP1 reverse primer)
5'-Fam CGCTTTCATTTACTTTGTGGCCTTCTTGG-
TAMRA (LMF1 probe)
5'-CAGCCTGGCTACACACGGGC
(LMF1 forward primer)
5'-CAGCCAGTGCTGCCGTGGAA
(LMF1 reverse primer)

Expression levels were normalized to 18S rRNA using the Eukaryotic18S rRNA Endogenous Control Reagent Set supplied from Applied Biosystems. All calculation was done in accordance with recommendation from Applied Biosystems (User Bulletin #2).

For analyses of mRNAs for LPL, GPIHBP1 and ANGPTL4 in mouse adipose tissue, total RNA was isolated with TRIzol reagent (Invitrogen, Breda, The Netherlands) according to manufacturer's instructions. One μg of total RNA was reverse transcribed using iScript (Bio-Rad, Veenendaal, The Netherlands). cDNA was amplified on a Bio-Rad CFX384 Real Time System using Sensimix (Bioline, GC Biotech, Alphen aan de Rijn, The Netherlands). Cyclophilin was used as housekeeping gene. PCR primer sequences were taken from the PrimerBank and ordered from Eurogentec (Seraing, Belgium). Sequences of the primers used are available upon request.

Gene expression array
Food was removed from one group of rats (n=6) at 1:30 h while another group (n=6) remained fed *ad lib*. The animals were killed starting from 8:15 h and epididymal adipose tissue was collected. Aliquots of total RNA were converted to biotinylated double-stranded cRNA using Illumina Totalprep RNA Amplification Kit according to manufacturer's instructions (Ambion, Austin, TX, USA). The labeled cRNA samples were hybridized to RatRef-12 Expression BeadChip (Illumina, San Diego, CA, USA), incubated with streptavidin-Cy3 and scanned on the Illumina Beadstation GX (Illumina, San Diego, CA, USA). To determine differentially expressed genes microarray

data were analyzed using Illumina Beadstudio software (version 3.3). The data were normalized and significant differential expression was calculated using Beadstudio's cubic spline algorithm. False discovery rate was applied. The gene expression fold change for the fasted group was calculated as the average signal value relative to the average signal value for the *ad lib* fed group. Statistical significance cutoff was set to $P < 0.01$; minimum signal intensity was set at 50 A. Full data are deposited at NCBI GEO, accession no GSE41800.

Western analyses
The same homogenates as prepared for assay of LPL activity and mass were used. Protein was determined by the BDH protein assay (Pierce) and 20 μg of total protein was separated on 4-20% Tris-glycine gradient gels (Lonza), and blotted onto PVDF membranes (Hybone-C, Amersham Biosciences). The membranes were blocked by ECL Advance blocking agent (GE Healthcare). For detection of LPL we used a rabbit polyclonal antibody from Santa Cruz Biotechnology at a dilution of 1:2000. For detection of ANGPTL4 we used a polyclonal goat anti-human antibody against the N-terminal domain (N-15, Santa Cruz Biotechnology), a goat polyclonal anti-mouse against the C-terminal domain (L-17, Santa Cruz Biotechnology) and a rabbit polyclonal antibody against full-length ANGPTL4 from Abcam, Cambridge, UK. All of these antibodies were used at a dilution of 1:3000. For detection we used the ECL detection system (GE Healthcare).

Metabolite assessments and plasma lipid profiles
For rats, NEFA-HR (WAKO Chemicals, Germany) was used for measurements of plasma NEFA. Plasma insulin was measured using coated plates from Mercodia, Sweden. Trig/GB (Roche Diagnostics, Germany) was used for TG measurements. One Touch Ultra (Life Scan, Milpitas, CA) glucose sticks were used for blood glucose determinations on whole blood immediately after collection.

For mice, plasma cholesterol was determined using the Cholesterol PAP SL kit from Elitech (Sopachem, Ochten, Netherlands). Plasma triglycerides were determined using the GPO PAP kit from Instruchemie (Delfzijl, Netherlands). Plasma lipoproteins were separated using fast protein liquid chromatography (FPLC). For this 0.2 ml of pooled plasma was injected into a Superose 6B 10/300 column (GE Healthcare Bio-Sciences AB, Roosendaal, Netherlands) and eluted at a constant flow of 0.5 ml/minute with phosphate buffered saline (pH 7.4). The effluent was collected in 0.5 ml fractions and TG and cholesterol levels were determined.

Statistical analysis
Data are presented as mean ± SEM. Statistical analyses were performed using unpaired *t*-test of variances or

one-way ANOVA, where *= p<0.05, ** = p<0.01 and *** = p<0.001. Unless otherwise stated, comparisons were made to time = 0 min or to matched controls.

Abbreviations
ANGPTL: Angiopoietin-like protein; ActD: ActinomycinD; CHX: Cycloheximide; GPIHBP1: Glycosylphosphatidylinositol-anchored high density lipoprotein-binding protein 1; LPL: Lipoprotein lipase; NEFA: Non-esterified fatty acids also called free fatty acids FFA; PPAR: Peroxisome proliferator activated receptor.

Authors' contributions
OK, GO, and TO did the conception and design of the research and conducted most of the animal experiments. OK performed most of the analytical work. VS, GO, and TO had conducted preliminary experiments on which the study was designed. EV and SKN contributed to mRNA analyses and to design and performance of the gene array study, respectively, together with OK. RS, FM, and SK conducted the experiments on *Angptl–/–* mice and most of the analyses on these animals. All authors contributed to analyses of data and to interpretation of the results. OK, GO and TO prepared the figures. GO and TO drafted the manuscript. All authors contributed to edition and revision of the manuscript. KS, GO, and TO approved the final version.

Acknowledgements
This work was supported by the Research Council Medicine (project 12203), the Swedish Heart and Lung Foundation and the Kempe Research Foundations. We thank Dr. Anja Köster from Eli Lilly & Company, Indianapolis for the gift of Angptl4$^{-/-}$ mice and we thank Solveig Nilsson, Department of Medical Biosciences, Umeå University, for technical assistance and Nina Gennebäck, Department of Public Health and Clinical Medicine, Umeå University, for help with analyses of gene expression arrays.

Author details
[1]Department of Medical Biosciences/Physiological Chemistry, Umeå University, Umeå SE-90187, Sweden. [2]Nutrition, Metabolism and Genomics group, Division of Human Nutrition, Wageningen University, Wageningen 6700EV, The Netherlands. [3]Present address: Department of Medicine, University of Gothenburg, Gothenburg SE-405 30, Sweden.

References
1. Olivecrona T, Olivecrona G: **The ins and outs of adipose tissue**. In *Cellular lipid metabolism*. Edited by Ehnholm C. Heidelberg: Springer; 2009:315–369.
2. Wang H, Eckel RH: **Lipoprotein lipase: from gene to obesity**. *Am J Physiol Endocrinol Metab* 2009, **297**(2):E271–E288.
3. Semb H, Olivecrona T: **Two different mechanisms are involved in nutritional regulation of lipoprotein lipase in guinea-pig adipose tissue**. *Biochem J* 1989, **262**(2):505–511.
4. Bergo M, Olivecrona G, Olivecrona T: **Forms of lipoprotein lipase in rat tissues: in adipose tissue the proportion of inactive lipase increases on fasting**. *Biochem J* 1996, **313**(Pt 3):893–898.
5. Bergo M, Wu G, Ruge T, Olivecrona T: **Down-regulation of adipose tissue lipoprotein lipase during fasting requires that a gene, separate from the lipase gene, is switched on**. *J Biol Chem* 2002, **277**(14):11927–11932.
6. Kersten S, Mandard S, Tan NS, Escher P, Metzger D, Chambon P, Gonzalez FJ, Desvergne B, Wahli W: **Characterization of the fasting-induced adipose factor FIAF, a novel peroxisome proliferator-activated receptor target gene**. *J Biol Chem* 2000, **275**(37):28488–28493.
7. Yoshida K, Shimizugawa T, Ono M, Furukawa H: **Angiopoietin-like protein 4 is a potent hyperlipidemia-inducing factor in mice and inhibitor of lipoprotein lipase**. *J Lipid Res* 2002, **43**(11):1770–1772.
8. Sukonina V, Lookene A, Olivecrona T, Olivecrona G: **Angiopoietin-like protein 4 converts lipoprotein lipase to inactive monomers and modulates lipase activity in adipose tissue**. *Proc Natl Acad Sci USA* 2006, **103**(46):17450–17455.
9. Yau MH, Wang Y, Lam KS, Zhang J, Wu D, Xu A: **A highly conserved motif within the NH2-terminal coiled-coil domain of angiopoietin-like protein 4 confers its inhibitory effects on lipoprotein lipase by disrupting the enzyme dimerization**. *J Biol Chem* 2009, **284**(18):11942–11952.
10. Koster A, Chao YB, Mosior M, Ford A, Gonzalez-DeWhitt PA, Hale JE, Li D, Qiu Y, Fraser CC, Yang DD, *et al*: **Transgenic angiopoietin-like (angptl)4 overexpression and targeted disruption of angptl4 and angptl3: regulation of triglyceride metabolism**. *Endocrinology* 2005, **146**(11):4943–4950.
11. Lichtenstein L, Mattijssen F, de Wit NJ, Georgiadi A, Hooiveld GJ, van der Meer R, He Y, Qi L, Koster A, Tamsma JT, *et al*: **Angptl4 protects against severe proinflammatory effects of saturated fat by inhibiting fatty acid uptake into mesenteric lymph node macrophages**. *Cell Metab* 2010, **12**(6):580–592.
12. Yin W, Romeo S, Chang S, Grishin NV, Hobbs HH, Cohen JC: **Genetic variation in ANGPTL4 provides insights into protein processing and function**. *J Biol Chem* 2009, **284**(19):13213–13222.
13. Mandard S, Zandbergen F, van Straten E, Wahli W, Kuipers F, Muller M, Kersten S: **The fasting-induced adipose factor/angiopoietin-like protein 4 is physically associated with lipoproteins and governs plasma lipid levels and adiposity**. *J Biol Chem* 2006, **281**(2):934–944.
14. Lei X, Shi F, Basu D, Huq A, Routhier S, Day R, Jin W: **Proteolytic processing of angiopoietin-like protein 4 by proprotein convertases modulates its inhibitory effects on lipoprotein lipase activity**. *J Biol Chem* 2011, **286**(18):15747–15756.
15. Hato T, Tabata M, Oike Y: **The role of angiopoietin-like proteins in angiogenesis and metabolism**. *Trends Cardiovasc Med* 2008, **18**(1):6–14.
16. Young SG, Davies BS, Voss CV, Gin P, Weinstein MM, Tontonoz P, Reue K, Bensadoun A, Fong LG, Beigneux AP: **GPIHBP1, an endothelial cell transporter for lipoprotein lipase**. *J Lipid Res* 2011, **52**(11):1869–1884.
17. Davies BS, Beigneux AP, Barnes RH 2nd, Tu Y, Gin P, Weinstein MM, Nobumori C, Nyren R, Goldberg I, Olivecrona G, *et al*: **GPIHBP1 is responsible for the entry of lipoprotein lipase into capillaries**. *Cell Metab* 2010, **12**(1):42–52.
18. Davies BS, Waki H, Beigneux AP, Farber E, Weinstein MM, Wilpitz DC, Tai LJ, Evans RM, Fong LG, Tontonoz P, *et al*: **The expression of GPIHBP1, an endothelial cell binding site for lipoprotein lipase and chylomicrons, is induced by peroxisome proliferator-activated receptor-gamma**. *Mol Endocrinol* 2008, **22**(11):2496–2504.
19. Doolittle MH, Ehrhardt N, Peterfy M: **Lipase maturation factor 1: structure and role in lipase folding and assembly**. *Curr Opin Lipidol* 2010, **21**(3):198–203.
20. Peterfy M: **Lipase maturation factor 1: A lipase chaperone involved in lipid metabolism**. *Biochim Biophys Acta* 2012, **1821**(5):790–794.
21. Gimble JM, Floyd ZE: **Fat circadian biology**. *J Appl Physiol* 2009, **107**(5):1629–1637.
22. Olivecrona T, Chernick SS, Bengtsson-Olivecrona G, Garrison M, Scow RO: **Synthesis and secretion of lipoprotein lipase in 3 T3-L1 adipocytes. Demonstration of inactive forms of lipase in cells**. *J Biol Chem* 1987, **262**(22):10748–10759.
23. Wu G, Olivecrona G, Olivecrona T: **The distribution of lipoprotein lipase in rat adipose tissue. Changes with nutritional state engage the extracellular enzyme**. *J Biol Chem* 2003, **278**(14):11925–11930.
24. Bergo M, Olivecrona G, Olivecrona T: **Diurnal rhythms and effects of fasting and refeeding on rat adipose tissue lipoprotein lipase**. *Am J Physiol* 1996, **271**(6 Pt 1):E1092–E1097.
25. Gray NE, Lam LN, Yang K, Zhou AY, Koliwad S, Wang JC: **Angiopoietin-like 4 (Angptl4) protein is a physiological mediator of intracellular lipolysis in murine adipocytes**. *J Biol Chem* 2012, **287**(11):8444–8456.
26. Harndahl L, Wierup N, Enerback S, Mulder H, Manganiello VC, Sundler F, Degerman E, Ahren B, Holst LS: **Beta-cell-targeted overexpression of phosphodiesterase 3B in mice causes impaired insulin secretion, glucose intolerance, and deranged islet morphology**. *J Biol Chem* 2004, **279**(15):15214–15222.
27. Bergo M, Olivecrona G, Olivecrona T: **Regulation of adipose tissue lipoprotein lipase in young and old rats**. *Int J Obes Relat Metab Disord* 1997, **21**(11):980–986.
28. Ranganathan G, Pokrovskaya I, Ranganathan S, Kern PA: **Role of A kinase anchor proteins in the tissue-specific regulation of lipoprotein lipase**. *Mol Endocrinol* 2005, **19**(10):2527–2534.
29. Forcheron F, Basset A, Del Carmine P, Beylot M: **Lipase maturation factor 1: its expression in Zucker diabetic rats, and effects of metformin and fenofibrate**. *Diabetes Metab* 2009, **35**(6):452–457.
30. Schwanhausser B, Busse D, Li N, Dittmar G, Schuchhardt J, Wolf J, Chen W, Selbach M: **Global quantification of mammalian gene expression control**. *Nature* 2011, **473**(7347):337–342.

31. Zhang L, Lookene A, Wu G, Olivecrona G: **Calcium triggers folding of lipoprotein lipase into active dimers.** *J Biol Chem* 2005, **280**(52):42580–42591.

32. Zhang L, Wu G, Tate CG, Lookene A, Olivecrona G: **Calreticulin promotes folding/dimerization of human lipoprotein lipase expressed in insect cells (sf21).** *J Biol Chem* 2003, **278**(31):29344–29351.

33. De Gasquet P, Griglio S, Pequignot-Planche E, Malewiak MI: **Diurnal changes in plasma and liver lipids and lipoprotein lipase activity in heart and adipose tissue in rats fed a high and low fat diet.** *J Nutr* 1977, **107**(2):199–212.

34. Goubern M, Portet R: **Circadian rhythm and hormonal sensitivity of lipoprotein lipase activity in cold acclimated rats.** *Horm Metab Res* 1981, **13**(2):73–77.

35. Sugden MC, Holness MJ, Howard RM: **Changes in lipoprotein lipase activities in adipose tissue, heart and skeletal muscle during continuous or interrupted feeding.** *Biochem J* 1993, **292**(Pt 1):113–119.

36. Benavides A, Siches M, Llobera M: **Circadian rhythms of lipoprotein lipase and hepatic lipase activities in intermediate metabolism of adult rat.** *Am J Physiol* 1998, **275**(3 Pt 2):R811–R817.

37. Tsutsumi K, Inoue Y, Kondo Y: **The relationship between lipoprotein lipase activity and respiratory quotient of rats in circadian rhythms.** *Biol Pharm Bull* 2002, **25**(10):1360–1363.

38. Ruge T, Bergo M, Hultin M, Olivecrona G, Olivecrona T: **Nutritional regulation of binding sites for lipoprotein lipase in rat heart.** *Am J Physiol Endocrinol Metab* 2000, **278**(2):E211–E218.

39. Arasaradnam MP, Morgan L, Wright J, Gama R: **Diurnal variation in lipoprotein lipase activity.** *Ann Clin Biochem* 2002, **39**(Pt 2):136–139.

40. Parkin SM, Walker K, Ashby P, Robinson DS: **Effects of glucose and insulin on the activation of lipoprotin lipase and on protein-synthesis in rat adipose tissue.** *Biochem J* 1980, **188**(1):193–199.

41. Wu G, Zhang L, Gupta J, Olivecrona G, Olivecrona T: **A transcription-dependent mechanism, akin to that in adipose tissue, modulates lipoprotein lipase activity in rat heart.** *Am J Physiol Endocrinol Metab* 2007, **293**(4):E908–E915.

42. Ruge T, Svensson A, Eriksson JW, Olivecrona T, Olivecrona G: **Food deprivation increases post-heparin lipoprotein lipase activity in humans.** *Eur J Clin Invest* 2001, **31**(12):1040–1047.

43. Makoveichuk E, Sukonina V, Kroupa O, Thulin P, Ehrenborg E, Olivecrona T, Olivecrona G: **Inactivation of lipoprotein lipase occurs on the surface of THP-1 macrophages where oligomers of angiopoietin-like protein 4 are formed.** *Biochem Biophys Res Commun* 2012, **425**(2):138–143.

44. Lookene A, Chevreuil O, Ostergaard P, Olivecrona G: **Interaction of lipoprotein lipase with heparin fragments and with heparan sulfate: stoichiometry, stabilization, and kinetics.** *Biochemistry* 1996, **35**(37):12155–12163.

45. Sonnenburg WK, Yu D, Lee EC, Xiong W, Gololobov G, Key B, Gay J, Wilganowski N, Hu Y, Zhao S, *et al*: **GPIHBP1 stabilizes lipoprotein lipase and prevents its inhibition by angiopoietin-like 3 and angiopoietin-like 4.** *J Lipid Res* 2009, **50**(12):2421–2429.

46. Davies BS, Goulbourne CN, Barnes RH 2nd, Turlo KA, Gin P, Vaughan S, Vaux DJ, Bensadoun A, Beigneux A, Fong LG, Young SG: **Assessing mechanisms of GPIHBP1 and lipoprotein lipase movement across endothelial cells.** *J Lipid Res* 2012, **53**(12):2690–2697.

47. Martin B, Ji S, Maudsley S, Mattson MP: **"Control" laboratory rodents are metabolically morbid: why it matters.** *Proc Natl Acad Sci USA* 2010, **107**(14):6127–6133.

48. Mizutani N, Ozaki N, Seino Y, Fukami A, Sakamoto E, Fukuyama T, Sugimura Y, Nagasaki H, Arima H, Oiso Y: **Reduction of insulin signaling upregulates angiopoietin-like protein 4 through elevated free fatty acids in diabetic mice.** *Exp Clin Endocrinol Diabetes* 2012, **120**(3):139–144.

49. Yamada T, Ozaki N, Kato Y, Miura Y, Oiso Y: **Insulin downregulates angiopoietin-like protein 4 mRNA in 3 T3-L1 adipocytes.** *Biochem Biophys Res Commun* 2006, **347**(4):1138–1144.

50. Gonzalez-Muniesa P, de Oliveira C, de Perez HF, Thompson MP, Trayhurn P: **Fatty acids and hypoxia stimulate the expression and secretion of the adipokine ANGPTL4 (angiopoietin-like protein 4/ fasting-induced adipose factor) by human adipocytes.** *J Nutrigenet Nutrigenomics* 2011, **4**(3):146–153.

7

Identification of novel Kirrel3 gene splice variants in adult human skeletal muscle

Peter Joseph Durcan[1], Johannes D Conradie[1], Mari Van deVyver[2] and Kathryn Helen Myburgh[1*]

Abstract

Background: Multiple cell types including trophoblasts, osteoclasts and myoblasts require somatic cell fusion events as part of their physiological functions. In Drosophila Melanogaster the paralogus type 1 transmembrane receptors and members of the immunoglobulin superfamily Kin of Irre (Kirre) and roughest (Rst) regulate myoblast fusion during embryonic development. Present within the human genome are three homologs to Kirre termed Kin of Irre like (Kirrel) 1, 2 and 3. Currently it is unknown if Kirrel3 is expressed in adult human skeletal muscle.

Results: We investigated (using PCR and Western blot) Kirrel3 in adult human skeletal muscle samples taken at rest and after mild exercise induced muscle damage. Kirrel3 mRNA expression was verified by sequencing and protein presence via blotting with 2 different anti-Kirrel3 protein antibodies. Evidence for three alternatively spliced Kirrel3 mRNA transcripts in adult human skeletal muscle was obtained. Kirrel3 mRNA in adult human skeletal muscle was detected at low or moderate levels, or not at all. This sporadic expression suggests that Kirrel3 is expressed in a pulsatile manner. Several anti Kirrel3 immunoreactive proteins were detected in all adult human skeletal muscle samples analysed and results suggest the presence of different isoforms or posttranslational modification, or both.

Conclusion: The results presented here demonstrate for the first time that there are at least 3 splice variants of Kirrel3 expressed in adult human skeletal muscle, two of which have never previously been identified in human muscle. Importantly, mRNA of all splice variants was not always present, a finding with potential physiological relevance. These initial discoveries highlight the need for more molecular and functional studies to understand the role of Kirrel3 in human skeletal muscle.

Keywords: Kirrel3, Human, Myogenesis, Biopsy, Drosophila

Background

Somatic cell fusion events are critical for development of multicellular eukaryotic organisms. Postnatal growth and repair also frequently rely on somatic cell fusion events, especially in tissues such as skeletal muscle that contain multinucleated cells. However, the genes and molecular mechanisms underpinning this fundamental cellular process in humans are largely unknown. Multiple cell types including trophoblasts, osteoclasts and skeletal muscle require somatic cell fusion events in order to perform their physiological functions [1-3]. The occurrence of cell fusion events in skeletal muscle provides a potential mechanism for the introduction of exogenous DNA to

cure genetic myopathies, while increasing evidence is emerging that fusion of cancer cells and bone marrow derived cells may enable and promote cancer metastasis [4-7]. Therefore, an improved understanding of how somatic cells fuse will likely have diverse clinical benefits.

In humans, a single skeletal muscle fibre can contain thousands of nuclei [8]. Each nucleus present in the muscle fibre arises from asynchronous cell fusion events. Post birth, skeletal muscle is a very adaptable tissue that is capable of repairing itself in response to injury such as that which accrues from damage-inducing exercise bouts [9,10]. The regeneration capacity of skeletal muscle is largely due to the presence of stem cell-like progenitor cells, termed satellite cells, that reside between the basal lamina and plasma membrane [11]. Satellite cells are typically found in an inactive state, however, in response to muscle injury they proliferate and also fuse (either

* Correspondence: khm@sun.ac.za
[1]Department of Physiological Science, Stellenbosch University, Private Bag X1 Matieland, 7602 Stellenbosch, South Africa
Full list of author information is available at the end of the article

together or with damaged fibres) in order to facilitate muscle repair [12-14]. The large amount of fusion events that occur during development, growth and repair of skeletal muscle make it a suitable tissue for studies aiming to identify the genes and mechanisms that underpin the somatic cell fusion process.

Research findings from Drosophila have highlighted that key events in the muscle cell fusion process are cell-cell attraction, adhesion and subsequent actin nucleation at sites of cell-cell adhesion, the latter enabling membrane fusion [15-17]. A wide variety of genes impact on the muscle cell fusion process ranging from actin nucleation factors, such as those found in the actin related protein 2/3 complex [18], to type 1 transmembrane receptors [19,20]. Of particular interest to this research paper has been the discovery of two paralogus type 1 transmembrane receptors and members of the immunoglobulin (Ig) superfamily Kirre [21] and Rst [22]. Loss of both Kirre and Rst from the Drosophila genome results in muscle cell fusion inhibition [19].

Present within the human genome are three Kirre homologs termed Kin of Irre like (Kirrel) 1 ,2 and 3 [23]. This family of genes have also been referred to in the literature as the Neph family, Neph1 (Kirrel1), Neph2 (Kirrel3), and Neph3 (Kirrel2)[23,24]. Kirrel3 has been implicated in diverse functions including pontine nuclei formation in the developing brain [25] male-male aggressive behaviour [26] and inhibition of hematopoietic stem cell differentiation [27]. Notably, no detailed investigation has been performed on any of the Kirrel family members and their presence in human skeletal muscle. Of particular interest to this research paper is the Kirrel3 gene as murine kirrel3 has been reported to be present in the kidney [28], brain [25] and also in cultured stromal cells [27], yet, results from mRNA analysis of murine skeletal muscle suggest that Kirrel3 is absent [27]. However, a different study reported Kirrel3 immunoreactivity in lysates obtained from mouse skeletal muscle [28]. These conflicting reports on Kirrel3 in mammalian skeletal muscle merit further investigation.

Our primary aim was to assess whether Kirrel3 is present in uninjured and regenerating human skeletal muscle following mild damage-inducing exercises such as plyometric jumping and downhill running. Presence of Kirrel3 in the afore mentioned samples would raise questions about its function in skeletal muscle. Currently nothing is known about Kirrel3 in this tissue, or if it is indeed present in adult human skeletal muscle. While its presence alone would not confirm a role in the human muscle cell fusion process, it would provide initial support for further investigation. It is possible that it could mirror the role of Kirre, its Drosophila homolog, in regulating myoblast fusion events in adult human muscle.

Our research findings demonstrate that at least three alternative splice variants of Kirrel3 are present in adult

human skeletal muscle. Two of these splice variants have not been previously reported in the published literature. Detection of Kirrel3 mRNA in adult human skeletal muscle using standard PCR was sporadic with occasional detection in uninjured and regenerating skeletal muscle samples. Semi nested PCR increased the detection rate. Such sporadic detection, using standard PCR assessment, demonstrates that in adult human skeletal muscle Kirrel3 mRNA is present at very low levels. At the protein level, Kirrel3 immunoreactive proteins in uninjured and regenerating adult human skeletal muscle were observed. Further work is now required in order to ascertain the function of all Kirrel3 splice variants in human skeletal muscle and to provide more insight into stimuli promoting its expression and its subsequent post-transcriptional regulation.

Results

Analysis of the National Centre for Biotechnology (NCBI) gene database highlighted the presence of two human Kirrel3 reference sequences NM_032531.3 (hereafter referred to as Kirrel3 A) containing 3777 nucleotides and NM_001161707.1 (hereafter referred to as Kirrel3 B) containing 2534 nucleotides. Aligning Kirrel3 A and B mRNA transcripts to the human genome via DNA sequence present in the genomic contig NT_033899.8, demonstrated that Kirrel3 A has 17 exons while B has 14 exons (see Figure 1A for schematic). Of particular note in both transcripts was the very large first intron which spanned approximately 438 kilo bases (KB). Both transcripts are predicted to start their translation initiation in their first exons. The first 2057 nucleotides of Kirrel3 A and B are identical. This region spans exons 1-14 of Kirrel3 A. Subsequently Kirrel3 A has a splice site that is not present in B thus resulting in exon 14 of Kirrel3 B containing an additional 477 nucleotides. The predicted stop codon (TAA) in Kirrel3 B is 107 nucleotides 3′ to the missed splice site. In comparison to Kirrel3 B, Kirrel3 A has an additional 3 exons totalling 1720 nucleotides 3′ to the missed spliced site. The stop codon (TAA) for Kirrel3 A is located in exon its 17th exon 641 nucleotides 3′ to the missed spliced site in B. The 3′ untranslated regions of Kirrel3 A and B are 1079 and 370 nucleotides respectively.

In silico analysis of Kirrel3 protein domains

Kirrel3 A is the larger of the two Kirrel3 proteins with 778 amino acids (AA) while Kirrel3 B has 600 AA. The first 565 AA of Kirrel3 A and B are identical. Domains predicted within this region (see Figure 1B for schematic) are a signal peptide (AA1-21 http://www.cbs.dtu.dk/services/SignalP/), five extracellular Ig domains (AA 49-146, 152-239, 251-332, 336-417, 420-516 http://scansite.mit.edu/) and a transmembrane domain (AA 536-558 http://www.cbs.dtu.dk/services/TMHMM/). Five putative N-linked

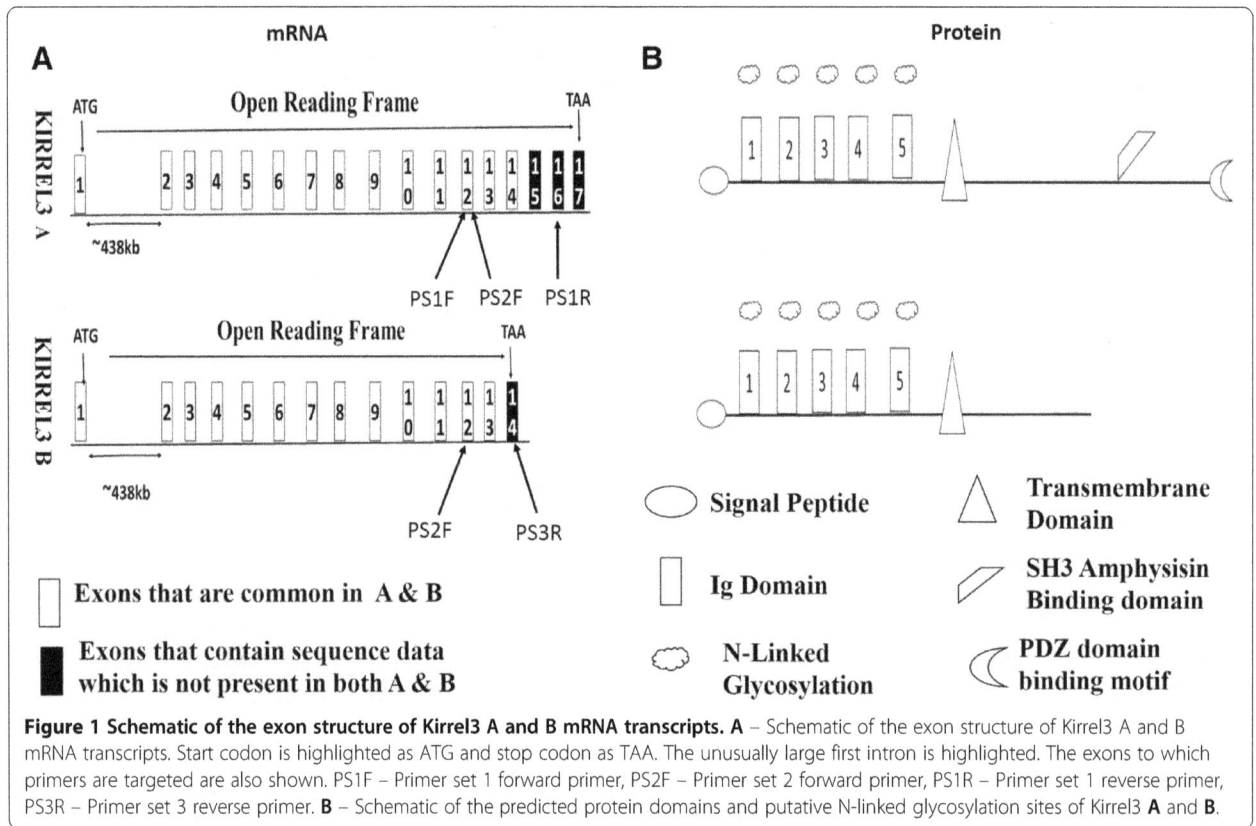

Figure 1 Schematic of the exon structure of Kirrel3 A and B mRNA transcripts. A – Schematic of the exon structure of Kirrel3 A and B mRNA transcripts. Start codon is highlighted as ATG and stop codon as TAA. The unusually large first intron is highlighted. The exons to which primers are targeted are also shown. PS1F – Primer set 1 forward primer, PS2F – Primer set 2 forward primer, PS1R – Primer set 1 reverse primer, PS3R – Primer set 3 reverse primer. **B** – Schematic of the predicted protein domains and putative N-linked glycosylation sites of Kirrel3 **A** and **B**.

glycosylation sites (AA 167, 253, 324, 361 & 498 http://www.cbs.dtu.dk/services/NetNGlyc/) are predicted to be present in the extracellular domain of both Kirrel3 proteins. The intracellular domain of Kirrel3 A is predicted to contain an amphysisin SH3 binding domain (AA 759-773 http://scansite.mit.edu/). Also present at its C-terminal end is a Post Synaptic density protein 95, Drosophila discs Large tumour suppressor, zonula occludens (PDZ) binding domain corresponding to the amino acids THV [29]. Kirrel3 B is not predicted to contain either of the afore mentioned intracellular domains.

Analysis of mRNA

To assess for the presence of Kirrel3 A and B mRNA in adult human skeletal muscle, gene specific primers were designed. We initially investigated Kirrel3 mRNA expression in adult human male skeletal muscle biopsies obtained pre and 4 and 24 hr post a plyometric jumping exercise in order to assess for Kirrel3 in uninjured and mildly injured skeletal muscle. The plyometric jumping protocol used here has previously been demonstrated to induce mild muscle damage [30]. Kirrel3 has previously been reported to be present in the mouse brain [31] and for the current study human astrocytes were used as a positive control for Kirrel3 mRNA expression.

Primer set 1 was specific to Kirrel3 A with a forward primer targeting exon 12 and a reverse primer targeting

exon 16 of Kirrel3 A (see Figure 1A for schematic on primer position). The expected amplicon is 391 nucleotides. Two distinct amplicons migrating at approximately 370 and 400 nucleotides were detected in the biopsy taken from subject 1 at 24 hr post plyometric exercise (Figure 2A). In contrast, only the approximately 370 nucleotide amplicon was detectable in the biopsy sample that was taken at the 4 hr post plyometric exercise time point from the same subject (Figure 2A). No biopsy from Subject 2 presented with either the approximately 370 or 400 nucleotide amplicon. Subject 3 had the approximately 370 nucleotide amplicon present at the baseline time point, but not at 4 hr or 24 hr post plyometric exercise (Figure 2A). The quality of cDNA template in all human skeletal muscle samples (except for subject 1 baseline) was confirmed as satisfactory via assessing for GAPDH mRNA expression (Figure 2A). A semi nested PCR was performed with primer sets 1 and 2 to assess if this approach would yield more consistent Kirrel3 mRNA detection. Primer set 2 contained a forward primer that was targeted towards exon 12 of Kirrel3 A with the reverse primer being the same as in primer set 1 (see Figure 1A for schematic of primer location). Three samples from subject 2 were negative for all amplicons in the first analysis. However, in one of these an amplicon of approximately 370 nucleotides was detected at the 4 hr time point using the semi-nested PCR (Figure 2B). In human astrocytes two amplicons were

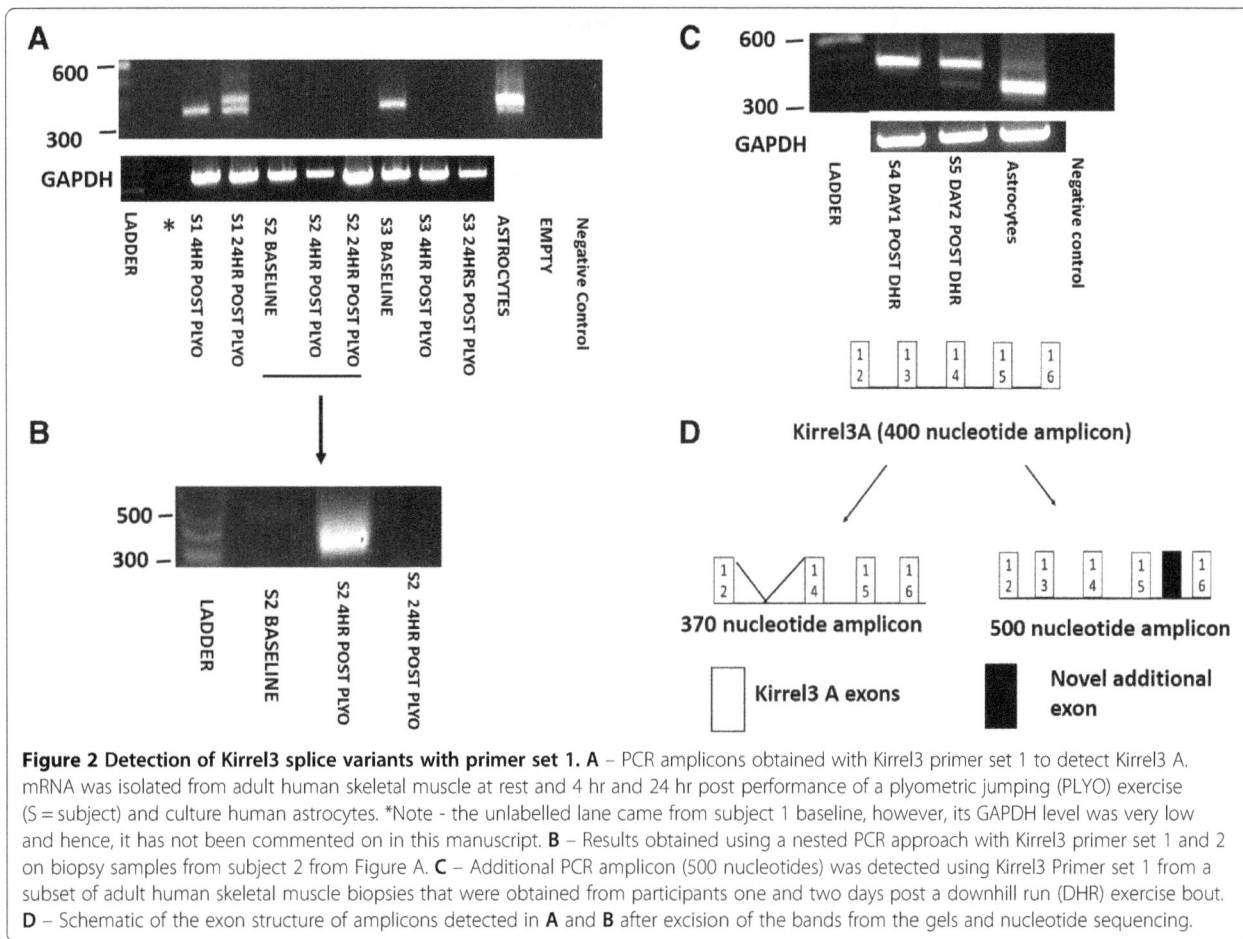

Figure 2 Detection of Kirrel3 splice variants with primer set 1. A – PCR amplicons obtained with Kirrel3 primer set 1 to detect Kirrel3 A. mRNA was isolated from adult human skeletal muscle at rest and 4 hr and 24 hr post performance of a plyometric jumping (PLYO) exercise (S = subject) and culture human astrocytes. *Note - the unlabelled lane came from subject 1 baseline, however, its GAPDH level was very low and hence, it has not been commented on in this manuscript. **B** – Results obtained using a nested PCR approach with Kirrel3 primer set 1 and 2 on biopsy samples from subject 2 from Figure A. **C** – Additional PCR amplicon (500 nucleotides) was detected using Kirrel3 Primer set 1 from a subset of adult human skeletal muscle biopsies that were obtained from participants one and two days post a downhill run (DHR) exercise bout. **D** – Schematic of the exon structure of amplicons detected in **A** and **B** after excision of the bands from the gels and nucleotide sequencing.

observed with primer set 1 at approximately 370 and 400 nucleotides (Figure 2A) thus matching those observed in human skeletal muscle. A much fainter amplicon was also detected in astrocytes at approximately 500 nucleotides (Figure 2A). We also analysed mRNA extracted from biopsies obtained from a previous study by our research group that investigated the effects of downhill running on skeletal muscle [32]. In some of these samples, an amplicon was detected that matched of the approximate 500 nucleotide amplicon observed in astrocytes (Figure 2C).

All three differently sized amplicons detected in adult human skeletal muscle samples were excised from the gel and sequenced. Aligning the sequence data obtained from the approximately 370, 400 and 500 nucleotide sized amplicons to the human genome via the Basic Local Alignment Search Tool (BLAST available at http://blast.ncbi.nlm.nih.gov/Blast.cgi) demonstrated that they were all variants of Kirrel3 (see Figure 2D for schematic of exon structure and Table 1 for raw sequence data). The approximately 400 nucleotide amplicon corresponded to a known sequence present in Kirrel3 A. The 37 nucleotide containing exon 13 of Kirrel3 A was spliced out of the approximately 370 nucleotide amplicon. Analysis of the

approximate 500 nucleotide amplicon sequence highlighted the presence of an additional exon of 93 nucleotides between exon 15 and 16 of Kirrel3A. This novel exon is located approximately 3100 nucleotides 3′ to exon 15 of Kirrel3 A and 355 nucleotides 5′ to exon 16 of Kirrel3 A.

Subsequently it was of interest to ascertain whether Kirrel3 B mRNA was present in adult human skeletal muscle and astrocytes. The same samples as those from the plyometric jumping exercise intervention were assessed for Kirrel3 B mRNA using primer set 3 that contained the same forward primer as primer set 2 and a reverse primer targeted towards a Kirrel3 B specific sequence present in its 14th exon. The predicted amplicon was 607 nucleotides. No amplicon was detectable in adult human skeletal muscle samples from either the plyometric jumping protocol (Figure 3B) or the downhill running samples (Data not shown), however, two amplicons migrating at approximately 610 and 590 nucleotides were detected in astrocytes (Figure 3B). Both amplicons were excised from the gel and sequenced. The amplicon migrating at approximately 610 nucleotide corresponded to Kirrel3 B while the amplicon that migrated at approximately 590 nucleotides lacked the 13th exon of Kirrel3 B which

Table 1 Sequence data obtained from amplicons with Kirrel3 primer set 1

370 amplicon nucleotide sequence	TARRCWACTGCTGGATMCCCCGGTCATCATCAGCTGCTTGATGGTGGAGTGCTCCTCACCCTCCCGACCAGAGGCTGGTT
	CCTTGTGGACAATTTCCACTCGGATATCATTTTTGGCTGACACAACACCTTTGAGATTTCTCTGGGAACGGGCACAGCAG
	AACGCCACGATGGTTGCCATAAGGACGAGGAAGGCCACACCAGCTCCTACGGCCACCCCAATGATGACGGCCATCGGCAC
	AGACTCTTGCTCCTTGAGCCGGATGATCTCAGTGTCGGAGCCGAAGCTGTTCCAGGCCGTGCAGTTGTAGATGGTCTGGA
	AGTCGGCAAA
400 amplicon nucleotide sequence	GTRMGTACTGCTGGATTMCCCCGGTCATCATCAGCTGCTTGATGGTGGAGTGCTCCTCACCCTCCCGACCAGAGGCTGGT
	TCCTTGTGGACAATTTCCACTCGGATATCATTTTTGGCTGACACAACACCTTTGAGATTTCTCTGGGAACGGGCACAGCA
	GAACGCCACGATGGTTGCCATAAGGACGAGGAAGGCCACACCAGCTCCTACGGCCACCCCAATGATGACGGCCATCGGCA
	CAGACTCTGGTTCCWKSCCSGSTCCCAACTTCRTTTCCGAACCTTGCTCCTTGARCCSGATGATCTCRKWGWYGGASYCG
	AAGYTGKYACAGGCCGTGCAGTTGTAGATGGTCTGGAAGTCGGCA
500 nucletotide sequence	GGRARWRGTCKCACGCTTCGGCTCCGACACTGAGATCATCCGGCTCAAGGAGCAAGGTTCGGAAATGAAGTCGGGAGCCG
	GGCTGGAAGCAGAGTCTGTGCCGATGGCCGTCATCATTGGGGTGGCCGTAGGAGCTGGTGTGGCCTTCCTCGTCCTTATG
	GCAACCATCGTGGCGTTCTGCTGTGCCCGTTCCCAGAGAAATCTCAAAGGTGTTGTGTCAGCCAAAAATGATATCCGAGT
	GGAAATTGTCCACAAGGAACCAGCCTCTGGTCGGGAGGGTGAGGAGCACTCCACCATCAAGCAGCTGATGCAGAGCAACT
	GGCCGGCATTTTACAATAAACGTTCAGTCAATGGAATTGAATCAKCCATGGGAGATCTCTGGTGATGCCCTCGCCCACRC
	GAGATGGACCGGGGTGAATTCCAGCAAGACTCASTCCTGAAACARCTGGAGGTCCTCAAAARACACTYCCTTTYYCCCCC
	CCYCCTTTAMCCCCCTTTTCTCCTCTTTTTTTTCTTCTTTT

Amplicons correspond to those shown in Figure 2A and B. These sequences were blasted against the human genome via BLAST available at the NCBI to confirm their identity as Kirrel3 splice variants.

contains 37 nucleotides (see Table 2 for raw sequence data obtained).

Analysis of protein

Based on results obtained from our mRNA analysis we wished to investigate Kirrel3 protein presence in human skeletal muscle samples. A commercially available antibody that was raised against the intracellular AA 596-626 of Kirrel3 A was utilised. Lysates obtained from a previous downhill run (DHR) study by our group [32] were utilised for the analysis. Baseline, 1 and 2 days post DHR were the time points assessed. Multiple immunoreactive proteins were detected in all human skeletal muscle samples ranging in size from approximately 45-110 kDa

(Figure 4A). To assess for Kirrel3 specificity of the antibody, a blocking peptide was incubated with the antibody prior to addition to the membrane. The immunoreactive proteins observed at approximately 50-100 kDa with antibody alone were eliminated (Figure 4B), thus providing support that these immunoreactive proteins may be isoforms of Kirrel3. To confirm the protein presence of Kirrel3 a second commercially available antibody that was raised against a recombinant human Kirrel3 protein (AA33-535 of NP_001288026) was tested on a selection of lysates from the downhill running study. Immunoreactive proteins were detected at approximately 70-75 kDA while no immunoreactive proteins were detected at approximately 50-55 kDA and 110 (Figure 4C), which is in

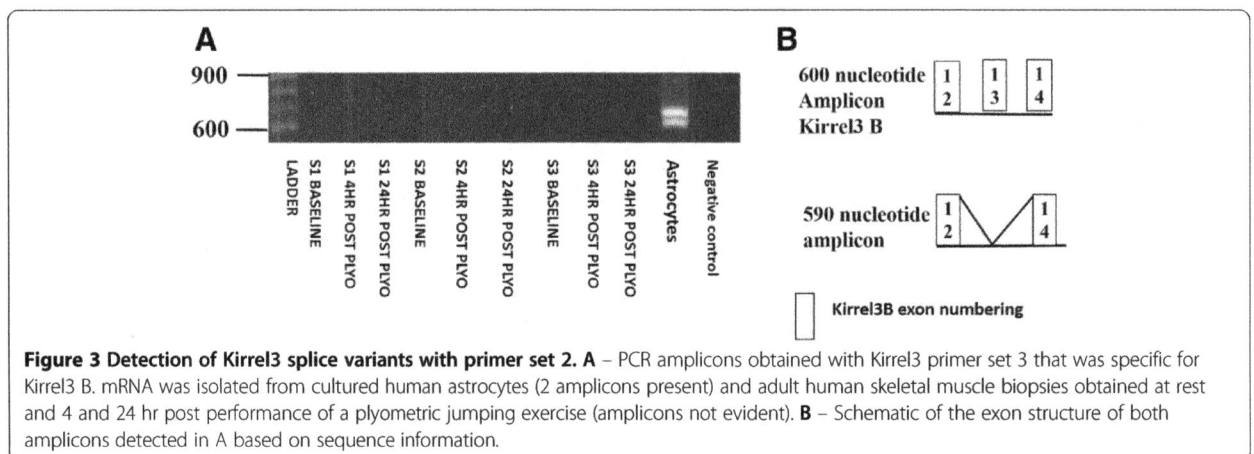

Figure 3 Detection of Kirrel3 splice variants with primer set 2. A – PCR amplicons obtained with Kirrel3 primer set 3 that was specific for Kirrel3 B. mRNA was isolated from cultured human astrocytes (2 amplicons present) and adult human skeletal muscle biopsies obtained at rest and 4 and 24 hr post performance of a plyometric jumping exercise (amplicons not evident). **B** – Schematic of the exon structure of both amplicons detected in A based on sequence information.

Table 2 Sequence data obtained from amplicons with Kirrel3 primer set 2

610 nucleotide sequence	AATARMATTGMGAGAGCTATGTGTTCATCCAAAATGCTGGCTGCCCTGCAGATGAAGTTCAGTCTAGTCCAGGTCAACCT
	CAGCCTAGCGCCCACTCTGCCAGGCGCCATGTTGCCCAGGCTCACATACACCGATGCATCAGACCCACTCCCTGCCCCAG
	GAGCTCACAGCACTGTTAGGACCCCTGTTCATTGCACTCCTGCTTACTTGCTCTCCGGGGCAGCCTAAGCCTGGCCTTTT
	TCTCTGTCCCCCTCCCTGAGATCCCGGATCTCCCTCCCGTACTTCTCTGGGAACGGGCACAGCAGAACGCCACGATGGTT
	GCCATAAGGACGAGGAAGGCCACACCAGCTCCTACGGCCACCCCAATGATGACGGCCATCGGCACAGACTCTKGTTCCWK
	GCSSGSTACGAACTTCRTGTCCGARCCTAGSTCCTTGARSGSCATGATSTCGKWGATGGASTGGAAGYTGKYCCRSGCCA
	TGYWGYTGATGATGGKGTGGAAGATGACCCCCTCSATGKTGCTGATGGTCWCGRYCGAAAAGAGRCCCTCCT
590 nucleotide sequence	CATTCGATCGATTRSCGMKAGAGCWTGTGTTCATCCAAATGCTGGCTGCCCTGCAGATGAAGTTCAGTCTAGTCCAGGTC
	AACCTCAGCCTAGCGCCCACTCTGCCAGGCGCCATGTTGCCCAGGCTCACATACACCGATGCATCAGACCCACTCCCTGC
	CCCAGGAGCTCACAGCACTGTTAGGACCCCTGTTCATTGCACTCCTGCTTACTTGCTCTCCGGGGCAGCCTAAGCCTGGC
	CTTTTTCTCTGTCCCCCTCCCTGAGATCCCGGATCTCCCTCCCGTACTTCTCTGGGAACGGGCACAGCAGAACGCCACGA
	TGGTTGCCATAAGGACGAGGAAGGCCACACCAGCTCCTACGGCCACCCCAATGATGACGGCCATCGGCACAGACTCTTGC
	TCCTTGAGCCGGATGATCTCAGTGTCGGAGCCGAAGCTGTTCCAGGCCGTGCAGTTGTAGATGGTCTGGAAGTCGGCCCG
	CACGATGTTGCTGATGGTCAGGGTGGAGATGACGCCCTCCTCGGTGCTGATGGTCTCCACCGTATAGCGA

Amplicons correspond to those shown in Figure 3A. These sequences were blasted against the human genome via BLAST available at the NCBI to confirm their identity as Kirrel3 splice variants.

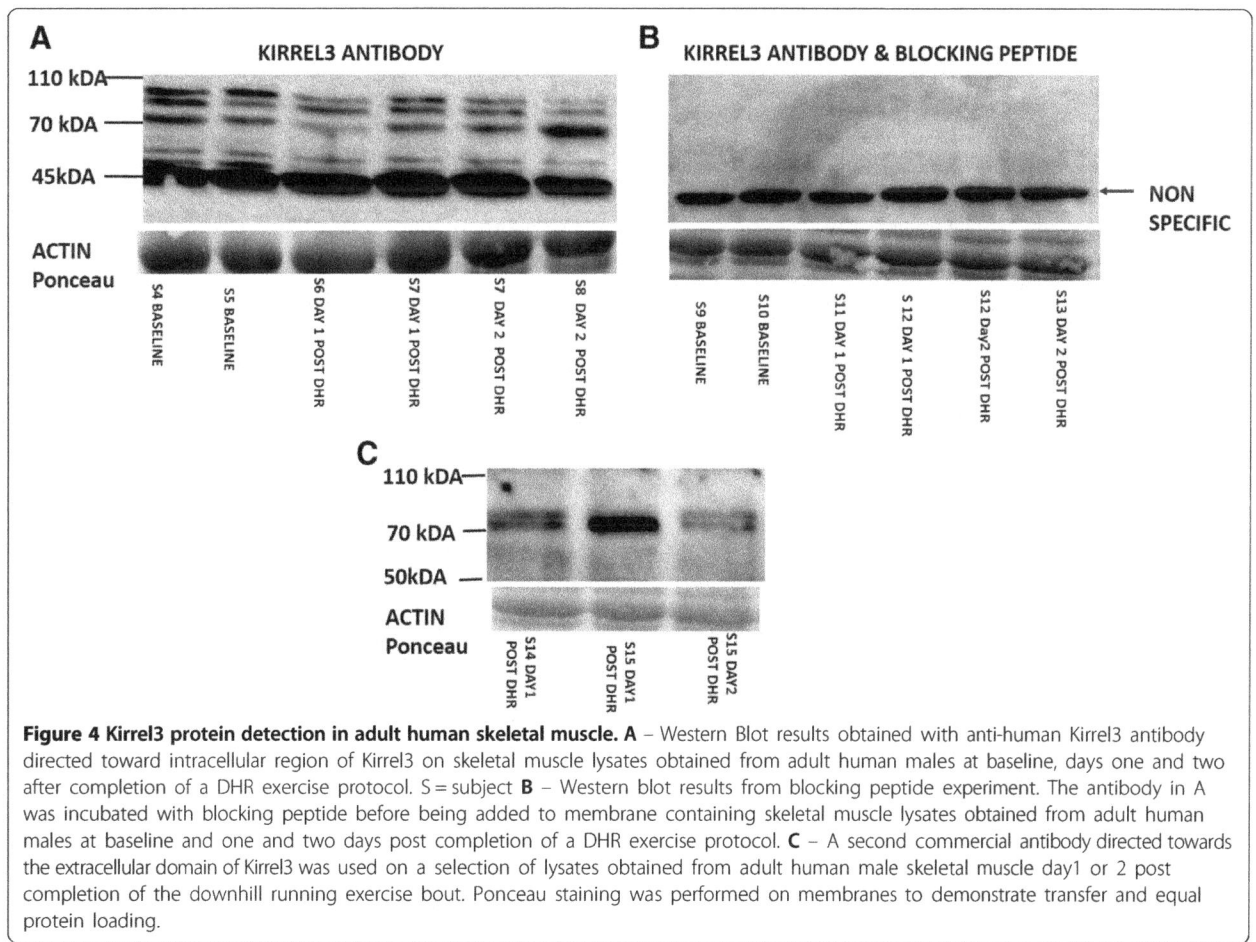

Figure 4 Kirrel3 protein detection in adult human skeletal muscle. A – Western Blot results obtained with anti-human Kirrel3 antibody directed toward intracellular region of Kirrel3 on skeletal muscle lysates obtained from adult human males at baseline, days one and two after completion of a DHR exercise protocol. S = subject **B** – Western blot results from blocking peptide experiment. The antibody in A was incubated with blocking peptide before being added to membrane containing skeletal muscle lysates obtained from adult human males at baseline and one and two days post completion of a DHR exercise protocol. **C** – A second commercial antibody directed towards the extracellular domain of Kirrel3 was used on a selection of lysates obtained from adult human male skeletal muscle day1 or 2 post completion of the downhill running exercise bout. Ponceau staining was performed on membranes to demonstrate transfer and equal protein loading.

contrast to results obtained with the intracellular targeting antibody.

Discussion

Skeletal muscle is made up of multinucleated cells (muscle fibres). The Drosophila homolog of Kirrel3, Kirre is involved in enabling muscle cell fusion events. Hence, Kirrel3 may be a putative muscle cell fusion regulator in humans. There is currently no published data available regarding Kirrel3 in adult human skeletal muscle. Therefore, the primary aim of this research was to assess for the presence of Kirrel3 in adult human skeletal muscle. By using PCR and transcript sequencing, we provide the first evidence that three alternatively spliced Kirrel3 mRNA transcripts are present in adult human skeletal muscle. Results from western blot analysis provide support for the presence of Kirrel3 protein in adult human skeletal muscle.

The mRNA data highlight that in adult human skeletal muscle Kirrel3 mRNA expression levels are very low and that using standard PCR may result in false negatives. A nested PCR approach yielded a higher rate of Kirrel3 detection. It will be of interest for future studies to examine Kirrel3 mRNA expression in a model that is known to include a large amount of myogenesis such as can be seen in some muscle pathologies. Primary human myoblast cell cultures would provide a useful system to further investigate Kirrel3 and ascertain its importance to human muscle cell fusion. Murine proprioceptive neurons have been reported to express Kirrel3 [33], therefore their contribution to Kirrel3 mRNA expression in adult human skeletal muscle should also be investigated.

The physical process of transcribing Kirrel3 can be regarded as a specialised event because, compared to the vast majority of other genes within the human genome, Kirrel3 spans a very large genomic region of approximately 580kB. Such a long genome span is likely to impact on the rate of Kirrel3 mRNA transcript production. RNA polymerase II has been reported to be capable of transcribing large human genes at a rate of approximately 4 kb^{-min} [34]. This rate of transcription suggests that production of Kirrel3 mRNA transcripts would take approximately 145 minutes. Previously produced transcripts are likely to be translated or degraded within the time period required to produce a Kirrel3 mRNA transcript. Such a time frame may result in a pulsatile occurrence of Kirrel3 mRNA in adult human skeletal muscle, unless Kirrel3 is being continually transcribed. Such a scenario may help explain the apparent discrepancy between the mRNA results in relation to Kirrel3 protein that was detectable in all biopsy samples analysed from both pre and post the DHR exercise intervention. Interestingly, our findings in relation to human Kirrel3 are largely in agreement with two different mouse studies focussing specifically on Kirrel3. In the first study, mRNA has been reported to be absent from mouse skeletal muscle [27], while the second study reported strong protein detection of Kirrel3 in mouse skeletal muscle [28].

Results from our western blot experiments varied depending on the commercial antibody being used. Each antibody targeted different epitopes with one being extracellular and the other intracellular. The fact two immunoreactive proteins that migrated at approximately 70 and 75 kDa were detected by both antibodies, appears to support that these are Kirrel 3 proteins rather than breakdown products. However, the predicted molecular weight of Kirrel3A is 85 kDa therefore the Kirrel proteins within the 70 kDa range are likely to be one or two of the other Kirrel3 splice variants present in human skeletal muscle. It is possible that they represent one splice variant with the larger having undergone post-translational modification. Immunoprecipitation and mass spectrometry analysis will be useful in determining the identity of these immunoreactive proteins.

The proteins detected at 50 and 55 kDa were detected only when using the Kirrel3 antibody targeting the intracellular domain. This antibody may be recognising partially degraded Kirrel3 proteins or these could be alternative truncated isoforms.

For analysis of mRNA, our primers were directed towards the 3′ end region of Kirrel3 (intracellular coding region) and we can only speculate on whether or not alternative splicing may occur further downstream towards the 5′ end (extracellular coding region) that would produce even smaller Kirrel3 protein isoforms. If alternative splicing occurs at the 5′ end this could explain why the extracellular targeting antibody did not detect proteins of similar size as those detected by the intracellular targeting antibody. In future, we suggest that 5′ race experiments should be performed to provide useful information in evaluating this possibility.

Our rationale for investigating Kirrel3 in human skeletal muscle was derived from research studies in Drosophila that demonstrated the involvement of two genes, Kirre and Rst, in the muscle cell fusion process during embryonic development [19]. While our research findings do not prove a role for Kirrel3 in the cell fusion process in adult human muscle, they do raise interesting questions regarding the function of Kirrel3 in human myogenesis and even in uninjured human skeletal muscle fibres. Murine Kirrel3 is present in stromal cells [27] and co-culture studies of Kirrel3 expressing stromal with hematopoietic stem cells, demonstrated a role for the extracellular domain of Kirrel3 in inhibiting hematopoietic stem cells' differentiation [27]. Such a finding is particularly notable since adult human skeletal muscle also contains stem cells termed satellite cells [14]. Satellite cells, located within the space between the basal lamina and plasma membrane of skeletal muscle fibres, are kept in an undifferentiated state until activated by events such as muscle damage [11]. It will therefore be of future interest to ascertain whether Kirrel3 may be involved in regulating satellite cell differentiation in human skeletal muscle.

In vitro, the extracellular domain of Kirrel3 is capable of binding to the extracellular domain of nephrin, a type 1 transmembrane protein and member of the immunoglobulin superfamily [28]. Nephrin is the mammalian homolog to the Drosophila gene, sticks and stones, that is essential for the muscle cell fusion process during embryonic fly development [20]. Considering that a significant body of evidence has emerged describing similarities in cellular processes between fly and man [35] it is tempting to hypothesise that interaction of Kirrel3 and nephrin in human skeletal muscle may facilitate the muscle cell fusion process. Indeed, in a small mammal model, nephrin$^{-/-}$ murine myoblasts displayed reduced fusion capabilities during in vitro myogenesis [36].

Kirrel3 is part of the Kirrel gene family that contains another two structurally similar members: Kirrel and Kirrel2 [24]. In Drosophila redundancy is present between Kirre and Rst with regard to the muscle cell fusion process [19] and redundancy may also be present among the Kirrel family members for the muscle cell fusion process in humans. Such redundancy should be considered when attempting to ascertain the possible roles of the Kirrel family members in the human muscle cell fusion process. In vitro primary myoblast culture studies should be fruitful in this regard.

The splice variants, Kirrel3 A and B, that are present in adult human skeletal muscle and/or astrocytes are predicted to contain significantly different cytoplasmic domains. Kirrel3 A, but not Kirrel3 B, is predicted to contain a SH3 amphysisin binding domain and also a PDZ binding domain. Such differences are likely to result in the two isoforms having divergent functions. Amphysisin is a protein whose function is not completely understood, however, it is highly concentrated at nerve terminals [37]. The C-elegans homolog of Kirrel3 (an adhesion molecule named syg-1) is located at synapses [38] and hence, amphysisin binding may regulate Kirrel3 A presence at neural synapses or neuromuscular junctions.

The PDZ binding domain present in Kirrel3 A may confer Kirrel3 with the ability to alter the polarity of the cell in which it is expressed as the PDZ binding domain of human Kirrel3 is capable of binding to the cell polarity protein partitioning defective 3 (PARD3) [39]. Satellite cells require PARD3 function in order to achieve asymmetric cell division [40]. The asymmetric cell division of satellite cells enables diversity that is thought to be important in the maintenance of the satellite cell pool. A subset of satellite cells in injured skeletal muscle are highly proliferative while another subset of cells retains the ability to return to quiescence [40]. It will therefore be of future interest to ascertain whether Kirrel3 is present in satellite cells and if so, whether it regulates asymmetric division via its interaction with PARD3.

Conclusion

In conclusion, the results presented here demonstrate for the first time that there are at least 3 splice variants of Kirrel3 present in adult human skeletal muscle, two of which have never previously been identified in human muscle. Importantly, mRNA of all splice variants was not always present, a finding with potential physiological relevance. These initial discoveries highlight the need for more molecular and functional studies. Full length sequence information should be obtained on all Kirrel3 mRNA transcripts in order to predict the translated Kirrel3 proteins. Physiological studies should be done to confirm involvement in fusion, or not. Production of isoform specific anti Kirrel3 antibodies will enable identification of the cellular localisation of the different Kirrel3 isoforms. Obtaining such information will aid in our understanding of Kirrel3 and its function in human skeletal muscle.

Methods
Ethics statement
Healthy young men aged between 18-28 years of age volunteered to participate in one of two studies aiming to describe molecular and physiological responses to exercise-induced muscle damage. Participants were informed about the purpose and risks of the study in which they were to participate before signing an informed consent document. The experimental protocols were approved by the Committee for Human Research at Stellenbosch University and the studies were conducted according to the ethical guidelines and principles of the International Declaration of Helsinki.

Plyometric jumping protocol
Participants were first taught how to perform the squat jump exercise. Subsequently their maximum squat jump height was measured. For the squat jump exercise intervention participants preformed 100 squat jumps at 90% of their maximum jump height. Jumps were divided into sets of 10 with 1 minute rest interval between each set. Prior to performing the 100 squat jumps participants exercised at a light to moderate intensity for 5 minutes on a treadmill.

Downhill running protocol
The protocol used here was previously described [32]. In brief, participants performed a 60-minute intermittent DHR protocol (12 × 5 min bouts at 85% VO$_2$max, 10% decline) on a motorized treadmill. They were allowed a

2 min standing rest between bouts and all the participants were able to complete all twelve bouts.

Biopsies

Muscle biopsies were obtained from the *vastus lateralis* muscle using a 5 mm trephine biopsy needle with assisted suction. Baseline biopsies were obtained from participants who had not engaged in any strenuous physical activity 7 days prior to the biopsy. Biopsies from participants who had performed the plyometric jumping protocol were obtained 4 and 24 hrs post completion of the protocol. Baseline and 24 hr biopsies were taken from the right leg while the 4 hr biopsy was taken from the left leg. Similarly, biopsies from participants who completed the downhill running protocol were taken at baseline and one and two days post downhill running in a consistent manner. Biopsies were frozen in liquid nitrogen cooled isopentane and stored at -80°C until use.

Cell culture

Human astrocytes (SciencCell research laboratories San Diego CA Catalog #1800) were seeded at a density of 10^5 in 6 well plates (BD Bioscience) in growth media which contained 89% Dulbecco's Modified Eagle Medium, 1% N-2 Supplement 100X, 10% Fetal Bovine serum (all Life Technologies). Once cells had reached 70% confluence they were lysed for RNA and protein isolation. Growth media was removed from wells before 200 ul of Tripure (Roche) was added per well of a 6 well plate and incubated at room temperature for 5 minutes with occasional gentle agitation. For protein isolation 150 ul of protein lysis buffer was added per well and incubated on ice for 5 minutes with occasional gentle agitation.

RNA isolation and RT-PCR

Muscle biopsies were sectioned on a cryostat (Leica Bio systems) at -20°C to obtain approximately 20 mg of tissue. Samples were then homogenised on ice in 1 ml of Tripure (Roche). RNA was isolated according to manufacturer's guidelines and suspended in TE Buffer and stored at -20°C until use. For reverse transcription (RT) 1ug of RNA was DNAse treated according to manufacturers (Roche) guidelines. Subsequently the 1 ug of DNAse treated RNA was reverse transcribed using random hexamers in accordance with manufacturers (Roche – Transcriptor First strand cDNA synthesis kit) guidelines. For PCR a 2 ul aliquot of cDNA corresponding to 50 ng of RNA was used. Each PCR consisted of a total volume of 25 ul. Primers (Sigma Life Science) were used at a 1 uM concentration and remaining components of PCR followed manufacturers (Roche – Faststart PCR Master) recommended protocol. For semi nested PCR a 2 ul volume from the initial PCR was used in the second PCR instead of 2 ul of cDNA. Post PCR the 25 ul volume was mixed with 6 ul of loading buffer (75% v/v glycerol, 0.02% w/V bromophenol blue, 10 mM Tris Base, 1 mM EDTA, 0.2% w/v SDS) and loaded onto a 1% agarose gel which contained sybr safe (Life Technologies) at 1X concentration and electrophoresed alongside a 100 bp ladder (Life Technologies). Gels were visualised on a Chemidoc MP (Biorad) that was supported with Image Lab software (Biorad). Kirrel3 Primer sets used were as follows **Primer set 1 – Forward primer** GCCGACTTCCAGACCATCTA, **Reverse primer –** TTTGAGGACCTCCAGCTGTT, **Primer set 2 - Forward Primer** CGCTATACGGTGGAGACCAT, **Reverse Primer** Same as primer set 1. **Primer set 3 – Forward primer** same as primer set 2, **Reverse Primer –** CGCTTTT CCCCCTATCTTTC. Amplicons were excised from the agarose gel, purified and sequenced at the central analytical facility at Stellenbosch University. For GAPDH primer set used was **Forward primer –** AATCCCATCACCATCTTC CA, **Reverse primer -** TGACAAAGTGGTCGTTGAGG.

Protein isolation and Western blot

Muscle biopsies were sectioned on a cryostat (Leica Biosystems) at 12 μm to obtain ~20 mg of tissue. Samples were homogenised on ice in 700 ul of lysis buffer (50 mM Tris HCL PH 7.5, 150 mM NaCl, 1 mM EDTA, 1% v/v nonidet p40, 0.25% w/v sodium deoxycholate 1 mM NaF, 1 mM Na3V04, 1 mM PMSF, 1 ug/ml leupeptin, 1 ug/ml pepstatin, 1 ug/ml aprotinin). Protein concentration was measured via a Bicinchoninic acid *(*BCA) kit (Thermo Fischer Scientific) using Bovine serum albumin (Roche) as standards. 30 ug of protein lysate was mixed with 5× Lamelli buffer (60 mM Tris HCL PH6.8, 2% SDS, 10% glycerol, 5% B-mercaptoethanol, 0.01% bromophenol blue) to yield 1× and electrophoresed using the Mini Protean Tetra system (Biorad). Post electrophoresis proteins were transferred to a nitrocellulose membrane (Amsheram Hybond ECL Nitrocellulose membranes GE Healthcare) via Trans Blot Turbo (Biorad) and membranes were stained with ponceau S to confirm transfer and equal protein loading. Subsequently membranes were washed 3 times for 5mins with 1× TBST (50 mM Tris, 150 mM NaCl, 0.1% tween 20, pH 8.3) and then blocked for 1 hr at room temp in 1× TBST and 5% semi skimmed milk. The intracellular targeting primary rabbit anti human Kirrel 3 antibody (102960 Abcam Cambridge UK) and the extracellular targeting primary sheep anti Kirrel 3 antibody (AF4910 R and D systems Minneapolis USA) were incubated over night at room temp with gentle agitation in 1× TBST with 5% semi skimmed milk. For blocking peptide experiment intracellular targeting primary anti human Kirrel 3 antibody was incubated with blocking peptide at a ratio of 1:4 for 3 hrs at room temperature with gentle agitation. Post primary antibody incubation or antibody and blocking incubation membranes were washed 3 times for 5 mins and subsequently incubated either with goat anti rabbit secondary (7074 Cell Signalling) at 1:15,000 or donkey anti sheep HRP conjugated secondary (6900 Abcam Cambridge UK) at 1:30,000 for 1 hr at room temp in 1x TBST and 5% milk. Membranes were subsequently washed 6X for 5mins followed by incubation with chemiluminescence detection reagents (Femto, Pierce Thermo Fischer Scientific). Membranes were visualised on a Chemidoc MP (Biorad) which was supported with Image Lab software (Biorad).

Abbreviations

Kirre: Kin of irregular Chiasm; Rst: Roughest; Kirrel: Kin of irregular chiasm like; Ig: Immunoglobulin; KB: Kilobases; NCBI: National center for biotechnology; AA: Amino acids; PDZ: Post Synaptic density protein 95, Drosophila discs Large tumour suppressor, zonula occludens.

Competing interests

The authors declare that they have no competing interests.

Authors' contributions

PJD and KHM designed the study and wrote the manuscript. PJD carried out the molecular studies and in silico analysis. JDC recruited subjects, performed exercise testing for the plyometric jumping exercise group and obtained biopsies. MVDV recruited subjects, performed testing for the downhill run exercise group and obtained biopsies. All authors read and approved the final manuscript.

Acknowledgements

Authors would like to acknowledge Luan Africa for culturing of astrocyte cells, Jeandre Viljoen and Paul Steyn for assistance in recruiting subjects and exercise testing. Funding was provided by the National Research Foundation (NRF) of South Africa. Funders had no role in this study other than to provide the funding.

Author details

[1]Department of Physiological Science, Stellenbosch University, Private Bag X1 Matieland, 7602 Stellenbosch, South Africa. [2]Division of Endocrinology, Department of Medicine, Stellenbosch University, Tygerberg, South Africa.

References

1. Dupressoir A, Vernochet C, Bawa O, Harper F, Pierron G, Opolon P, Heidmann T: **Syncytin-A knockout mice demonstrate the critical role in placentation of a fusogenic, endogenous retrovirus-derived, envelope gene.** *Proc Natl Acad Sci U S A* 2009, **106:**12127–12132.
2. Ishii M, Saeki Y: **Osteoclast cell fusion: mechanisms and molecules.** *Mod Rheumatol* 2008, **18:**220–227.
3. Horsley V, Pavlath GK: **Forming a multinucleated cell: molecules that regulate myoblast fusion.** *Cells Tissues Organs* 2004, **176:**67–78.
4. Lazova R, Laberge GS, Duvall E, Spoelstra N, Klump V, Sznol M, Cooper D, Spritz RA, Chang JT, Pawelek JM: **A melanoma brain metastasis with a donor-patient hybrid genome following bone marrow transplantation: first evidence for fusion in human cancer.** *PLoS One* 2013, **8:**e66731.
5. Chakraborty AK, Funasaka Y, Ichihashi M, Pawelek JM: **Upregulation of alpha and beta integrin subunits in metastatic macrophage-melanoma fusion hybrids.** *Melanoma Res* 2009, **19:**343–349.
6. Pawelek JM, Chakraborty AK: **The cancer cell–leukocyte fusion theory of metastasis.** *Adv Cancer Res* 2008, **101:**397–444.
7. Carter A: **Cell fusion theory: can it explain what triggers metastasis?** *J Natl Cancer Inst* 2008, **100:**1279–1281.
8. Mitchell WK, Williams J, Atherton P, Larvin M, Lund J, Narici M: **Sarcopenia, dynapenia, and the impact of advancing age on human skeletal muscle size and strength; a quantitative review.** *Front Physiol* 2012, **3:**260.
9. Clarkson PM, Tremblay I: **Exercise-induced muscle damage, repair, and adaptation in humans.** *J Appl Physiol (1985)* 1988, **65:**1–6.
10. Warhol MJ, Siegel AJ, Evans WJ, Silverman LM: **Skeletal muscle injury and repair in marathon runners after competition.** *Am J Pathol* 1985, **118:**331–339.
11. Relaix F, Zammit PS: **Satellite cells are essential for skeletal muscle regeneration: the cell on the edge returns centre stage.** *Development* 2012, **139:**2845–2856.
12. Chargé SBP, Rudnicki MA: **Cellular and molecular regulation of muscle regeneration.** *Physiol Rev* 2004, **84:**209–238.
13. Dreyer HC, Blanco CE, Sattler FR, Schroeder ET, Wiswell RA: **Satellite cell numbers in young and older men 24 hours after eccentric exercise.** *Muscle Nerve* 2006, **33:**242–253.
14. Scharner J, Zammit PS: **The muscle satellite cell at 50: the formative years.** *Skelet Muscle* 2011, **1:**28.
15. Abmayr SM, Pavlath GK: **Myoblast fusion: lessons from flies and mice.** *Development* 2012, **139:**641–656.
16. Richardson BE, Nowak SJ, Baylies MK: **Myoblast fusion in fly and vertebrates: new genes, new processes and new perspectives.** *Traffic* 2008, **9:**1050–1059.
17. Sens KL, Zhang S, Jin P, Duan R, Zhang G, Luo F, Parachini L, Chen EH: **An invasive podosome-like structure promotes fusion pore formation during myoblast fusion.** *J Cell Biol* 2010, **191:**1013–1027.
18. Richardson BE, Beckett K, Nowak SJ, Baylies MK: **SCAR/WAVE and Arp2/3 are crucial for cytoskeletal remodeling at the site of myoblast fusion.** *Development* 2007, **134:**4357–4367.
19. Strünkelnberg M, Bonengel B, Moda LM, Hertenstein A, de Couet HG, Ramos RG, Fischbach KF: **rst and its paralogue kirre act redundantly during embryonic muscle development in Drosophila.** *Development* 2001, **128:**4229–4239.
20. Bour BA, Chakravarti M, West JM, Abmayr SM: **Drosophila SNS, a member of the immunoglobulin superfamily that is essential for myoblast fusion.** *Genes Dev* 2000, **14:**1498–1511.
21. Ruiz-Gómez M, Coutts N, Price A, Taylor MV, Bate M: **Drosophila dumbfounded: a myoblast attractant essential for fusion.** *Cell* 2000, **102:**189–198.
22. Ramos RG, Igloi GL, Lichte B, Baumann U, Maier D, Schneider T, Brandstätter JH, Fröhlich A, Fischbach KF: **The irregular chiasm C-roughest locus of Drosophila, which affects axonal projections and programmed cell death, encodes a novel immunoglobulin-like protein.** *Genes Dev* 1993, **7:**2533–2547.
23. Völker LA, Petry M, Abdelsabour-Khalaf M, Schweizer H, Yusuf F, Busch T, Schermer B, Benzing T, Brand-Saberi B, Kretz O, Höhne M, Kispert A: **Comparative analysis of Neph gene expression in mouse and chicken development.** *Histochem Cell Biol* 2012, **137:**355–366.
24. Neumann-Haefelin E, Kramer-Zucker A, Slanchev K, Hartleben B, Noutsou F, Martin K, Wanner N, Ritter A, Gödel M, Pagel P, Fu X, Müller A, Baumeister R, Walz G, Huber TB: **A model organism approach: defining the role of Neph proteins as regulators of neuron and kidney morphogenesis.** *Hum Mol Genet* 2010, **19:**2347–2359.
25. Nishida K, Nakayama K, Yoshimura S, Murakami F: **Role of Neph2 in pontine nuclei formation in the developing hindbrain.** *Mol Cell Neurosci* 2011, **46:**662–670.
26. Prince JEA, Brignall AC, Cutforth T, Shen K, Cloutier J-F: **Kirrel3 is required for the coalescence of vomeronasal sensory neuron axons into glomeruli and for male-male aggression.** *Development* 2013, **140:**2398–2408.
27. Ueno H, Sakita-Ishikawa M, Morikawa Y, Nakano T, Kitamura T, Saito M: **A stromal cell-derived membrane protein that supports hematopoietic stem cells.** *Nat Immunol* 2003, **4:**457–463.
28. Gerke P, Sellin L, Kretz O, Petraschka D, Zentgraf H, Benzing T, Walz G: **NEPH2 is located at the glomerular slit diaphragm, interacts with nephrin and is cleaved from podocytes by metalloproteinases.** *J Am Soc Nephrol* 2005, **16:**1693–1702.
29. Sellin L, Huber TB, Gerke P, Quack I, Pavenstädt H, Walz G: **NEPH1 defines a novel family of podocin interacting proteins.** *FASEB J* 2003, **17:**115–117.
30. Macaluso F, Isaacs AW, Myburgh KH: **Preferential type II muscle fiber damage from plyometric exercise.** *J Athl Train* 2012, **47:**414–420.
31. Tamura S, Morikawa Y, Hisaoka T, Ueno H, Kitamura T, Senba E: **Expression of mKirre, a mammalian homolog of Drosophila kirre, in the developing and adult mouse brain.** *Neuroscience* 2005, **133:**615–624.
32. Van de Vyver M, Myburgh KH: **Variable inflammation and intramuscular STAT3 phosphorylation and myeloperoxidase levels after downhill running.** *Scand J Med Sci Sports* 2014, **24:**e360–e371.
33. Komori T, Gyobu H, Ueno H, Kitamura T, Senba E, Morikawa Y: **Expression of kin of irregular chiasm-like 3/mKirre in proprioceptive neurons of the

dorsal root ganglia and its interaction with nephrin in muscle spindles. *J Comp Neurol* 2008, **511**:92–108.

34. Singh J, Padgett RA: **Rates of in situ transcription and splicing in large human genes.** *Nat Struct Mol Biol* 2009, **16**:1128–1133.

35. Bier E: **Drosophila, the golden bug, emerges as a tool for human genetics.** *Nat Rev Genet* 2005, **6**:9–23.

36. Sohn RL, Huang P, Kawahara G, Mitchell M, Guyon J, Kalluri R, Kunkel LM, Gussoni E: **A role for nephrin, a renal protein, in vertebrate skeletal muscle cell fusion.** *Proc Natl Acad Sci U S A* 2009, **106**:9274–9279.

37. Zhang B, Zelhof AC: **Amphiphysins: raising the BAR for synaptic vesicle recycling and membrane dynamics. Bin-Amphiphysin-Rvsp.** *Traffic* 2002, **3**:452–460.

38. Shen K, Bargmann CI: **The immunoglobulin superfamily protein SYG-1 determines the location of specific synapses in C. elegans.** *Cell* 2003, **112**:619–630.

39. Hartleben B, Schweizer H, Lübben P, Bartram MP, Möller CC, Herr R, Wei C, Neumann-Haefelin E, Schermer B, Zentgraf H, Kerjaschki D, Reiser J, Walz G, Benzing T, Huber TB: **Neph-Nephrin proteins bind the Par3-Par6-atypical protein kinase C (aPKC) complex to regulate podocyte cell polarity.** *J Biol Chem* 2008, **283**:23033–23038.

40. Troy A, Cadwallader AB, Fedorov Y, Tyner K, Tanaka KK, Olwin BB: **Coordination of satellite cell activation and self-renewal by Par-complex-dependent asymmetric activation of p38α/β MAPK.** *Cell Stem Cell* 2012, **11**:541–553.

8

*Kcnq*1-5 (Kv7.1-5) potassium channel expression in the adult zebrafish

Calvin Wu[1,2,3], Kanishk Sharma[1], Kyle Laster[1], Mohamed Hersi[1], Christina Torres[1], Thomas J Lukas[1] and Ernest J Moore[1,3*]

Abstract

Background: *KCNQx* genes encode slowly activating-inactivating K^+ channels, are linked to physiological signal transduction pathways, and mutations in them underlie diseases such as long QT syndrome (*KCNQ*1), epilepsy in adults (*KCNQ*2/3), benign familial neonatal convulsions in children (*KCNQ*3), and hearing loss or tinnitus in humans (*KCNQ*4, but not *KCNQ*5). Identification of *kcnqx* potassium channel transcripts in zebrafish (Danio rerio) remains to be fully characterized although some genes have been mapped to the genome. Using zebrafish genome resources as the source of putative *kcnq* sequences, we investigated the expression of *kcnq1-5* in heart, brain and ear tissues.

Results: Overall expression of the *kcnqx* channel transcripts is similar to that found in mammals. We found that *kcnq1* expression was highest in the heart, and also present in the ear and brain. *kcnq2* was lowest in the heart, while *kcnq3* was highly expressed in the brain, heart and ear. *kcnq5* expression was highest in the ear. We analyzed zebrafish genomic clones containing putative *kcnq4* sequences to identify transcripts and protein for this highly conserved member of the Kcnq channel family. The zebrafish appears to have two *kcnq4* genes that produce distinct mRNA species in brain, ear, and heart tissues.

Conclusions: We conclude that the zebrafish is an attractive model for the study of the KCNQ (Kv7) superfamily of genes, and are important to processes involved in neuronal excitability, cardiac anomalies, epileptic seizures, and hearing loss or tinnitus.

Keywords: Zebrafish (Danio rerio), *kcnq1-5*, RNA transcripts, Kcnq protein, Zebrafish genome, qRTPCR, Tinnitus

Background

Potassium channels are well-established biological targets for diseases including neuropathic pain, epilepsy, cardiac arrhythmia, hearing loss, deafness, or tinnitus [1]. In particular, mutations in the *KCNQ4* potassium gene and perhaps *KCNQ3* are associated with progressive high frequency hearing loss [2,3]. Of the several ion channels used by the sensory hair cell, the K^+ channel KCNQ4 is thought to modulate the membrane potential of hair cells to adjust the sensitivity of hearing in a variety of mammals [1,4,5]. Similarly, KCNQ4 and KCNQ5 are key modulators of L-type Ca^{2+} channel activity in cardiovascular cells [6]. Variants of *KCNQ5* are not

associated with sensory hearing loss in humans, but there is high abundance in the larval zebrafish ear [7,8], and thus, may be related to yet to be defined developmental factors related to hearing [9].

A recent study characterized the expression of *kcnq2*, *kcnq3*, and *kcnq5* in whole larval zebrafish (*Danio rerio*) [7], but we know little about the expression of the complement of *kcnq* genes and the K^+ ion channels that they encode in various organs of the adult zebrafish. Since certain drugs and metal ions affect the function of Kcnq channels [10-12] in a dose-dependent manner, these agents can be used to alter ion permeability across the membrane of zebrafish hair cells and thus create a fish model of sensory cell dysfunction. KCNQ2-5 channels are also regulated by intracellular signal transduction effectors such as phospholipids [13], phosphorylation [14], and calmodulin [15]. However, little is known about how these signaling systems impact the *kcnq* channels in zebrafish sensory pathways. Thus, the zebrafish offers a

---

* Correspondence: ernest.moore@unt.edu
[1]Department of Molecular Pharmacology & Biological Chemistry, Northwestern University, Chicago, IL 60611, USA
[3]Department of Speech & Hearing Sciences, University of North Texas, Denton, TX 76203, USA
Full list of author information is available at the end of the article

unique opportunity to study Kcnq channel modulation, function and dysfunction.

The zebrafish has served as an especially attractive model for the study of the development and function of the vertebrate inner ear [8,16]. It has three methods of sensing sound within its environment. The first involves the lateral line system, which is comprised of a set of neuromasts containing hair cells arrayed along each side of the body. Neuromasts contain bundles of sensory hair cells beneath a cupula, which are responsible for sensing the displacement of water molecules [17]. The second means of sensing sound are structures of the inner ear composed of the utricle, saccule, lagena and pars neglecta. Each of these anatomical structures house patches of sensory hair cells and supporting cells that are embedded in the epithelial lining of the macula [18]. The hair cells found in these structures are similar to those found in mammals, and contain voltage gated and ligand gated ion channels presumably linked to several signal transduction pathways. Third, there are sets of motion detectors or neuromasts arrayed around the head, particularly the orbital regions. In this report, we have studied Kcnq channel expression and localization in several tissues of the zebrafish. Using the deduced mRNA sequences in the available databases, we probed for the presence of Kcnq channel mRNA transcripts in the ear, brain and heart, and partially characterized the amino acid sequence of one channel protein. The zebrafish genome has two different *kcnq4* genes, one of which has been localized to chromosome 19. The mRNA from this gene is also expressed in zebrafish brain and ear. We prepared a specific antibody to zebrafish Kcnq4, quantified its levels using qRT-PCR, and further verified its expression using Western blots of brain and ear tissues.

Results

Detection of Kcnq Expression in Zebrafish

Amplicons representing *kcnq1-5* were detected by RT-PCR analyses and observed under UV illumination. Table 1 shows the primers, amplicon size, and primer sequences used for all PCR reactions. Primers and nested primers were designed to cross several exons of the specific PCR template sequence.

Several of the *kcnq* RNA transcripts were expressed in the zebrafish brain (Figure 1A) consistent with observations in other species [19]. *Kcnq1* and *kcnq5* were absent in the gel (Figure 1A), but were detected in the quantitative data (Figure 2, top), at the same approximate levels. The PCR data for *kcnq5* were done with *kcnq5b* primers while the quantitative PCR was done with *kcnq5a* primers. *Kcnq4* was probed by three different sets of primers (KCNQ4-a, KCNQ4-b, KCNQ4-c) for downstream cDNA sequencing. Bands for *kcnq4* for the three

Table 1 Summary of primers designed to amplify *kcnq* 1-5 and β-actin mRNAs

Primer	Nucleotide sequence	Expected size (bp)
KCNQ1 fwd	5'- TCC AGT CGC TCA TGT GTC TC -3'	203
KCNQ1 rev	5'- TTT CAT CCC ACC TTC TTT GC -3'	
KCNQ2 fwd	5'- GAG CCA GTG CAG GAG AAA AG -3'	344
KCNQ2 rev	5'- TGA GGT AGA AGG CCG ACA CT -3'	
KCNQ3 fwd	5'- GAG AAG GAT TCG GCT CAC TG -3'	443
KCNQ3 rev	5'- GCG TCT GCA TAG GTG TCA AA -3'	
KCNQ4 (a) fwd	5'-TAT GCA GAC TCC CTC TGG TG-3'	175
KCNQ4 (a) rev	5'-CCT GCA CTT TCA GAG CAA AG-3'	
KCNQ4 (b) fwd	5'-GGG CCG CAG GGT TTC TTT AAA CTT-3'	400
KCNQ4 (b) rev	5'-ATG ACA GTA TGC TGC CGT CCT TCA-3'	
KCNQ4 (c) fwd	5'-CGG CCG CAG GGT TTC TTT AAA CTT-3'	400
KCNQ4 (c) rev	5'-TCC TTC AGT GGG AAG ATG GGC TTT-3'	
KCNQ4 ch19(a) fwd	5'-TGC CTG TAC AAT GTG CTG GAG AGA-3'	265
KCNQ4 ch19(a) rev	5'-AAG GCT TTC TGG CAA AGC GTA GTC-3'	
KCNQ4 ch19(b) fwd	5'-ATC AGC CAA TGA TGA CAG ACG GGT-3'	458
KCNQ4 ch19(b) rev	5'-AAG GCT TTC TGG CAA AGC GTA GTC-3'	
KCNQ5b fwd	5'- TGC CTG GTA TAT TGG GTT CC -3'	261
KCNQ5b rev	5'- TGA ACC TTC AAG GCA AAA CC -3'	
β-actin fwd	5'- TCC CCT TGT TCA CAA TAA CC- 3'	350
β-actin rev	5'- TCT GTG GCT TTG GGA TTC A-3'	

sets of primers were readily detected. *Kcnq2* and *kcnq3* showed the strongest signal, while *kcnq3* displayed two almost overlapping bands. A negative control (PCR reaction without RNA, or "No RNA") is shown in the last lane. The expression strength of the mRNA transcript was compared to the intensity of the *β*-actin control.

The inner ear tissue of zebrafish included the sensory epithelium (culled from 6 fish, both ears), consisting also portions of the utricle, saccule and lagena tissues, but not semicircular canals. Figure 1B shows mRNA expression of *kcnq1-5* in the zebrafish ear - all *kcnq* transcripts were detected. However, *kcnq1* was somewhat weak, while *kcnq5b* provided a much stronger signal. Figure 1C shows the expression pattern in zebrafish heart. Except for *kcnq5b*, transcripts for *kcnq1-4* were detected.

As mentioned in the Introduction, the partial sequence of a *kcnq4* gene has also been mapped to chromosome 19. We detected expression of transcripts based upon this gene in brain and ear (Figure 3A) and the heart (Figure 3B). The sequence is located at the 5' end (519 bp) of the

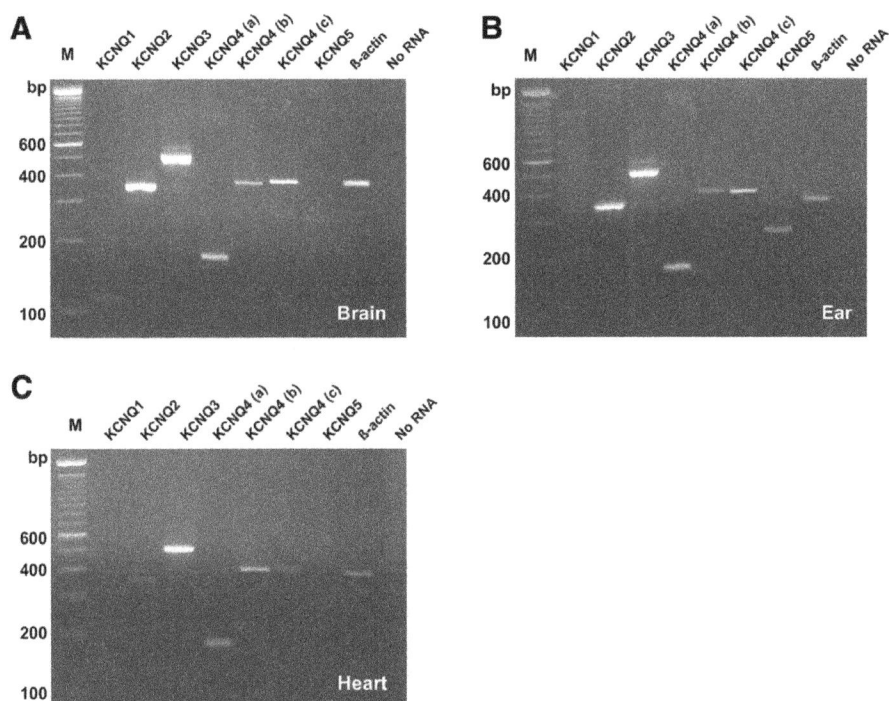

Figure 1 Expression of *kcnq* in zebrafish brain (A), ear (B) and heart (C). Lanes labeled M are the 100 bp ladder molecular standards. Lane 9 and 10, respectively, is a positive control with β-actin, and a negative control without RNA.

transcript encoding a 173 amino acid sequence, homologous to *KCNQ4* from human as well as other species (See Figure 4). Using various combinations of primers in the RT-PCR experiments, all attempts to link sequences of the chromosome 19 transcripts to the more 3′ *kcnq4* sequences in our mRNA, which is not yet mapped to a chromosome, failed to show up in our data (not shown). Therefore, we conclude from these observations that there are two separate *kcnq4* genes expressed in the zebrafish.

qRTPCR of kcnq1-5 expression in brain, ear, or heart

End point PCR is not applicable to quantitative measures of expression, and detection of bands can be variable using electrophoretic separation. Therefore, we performed qRTPCR using reverse-transcribed mRNA templates from each tissue. Different primers were designed to produce amplicons (100-200 bp) suitable for SYBR green-based real time quantitative analysis (Table 2). As shown in Figure 2, the brain has very high expression of *kcnq2* and *kcnq3* compared to other tissues. *Kcnq2-5* transcripts are lower than *kcnq1* in the heart, while *kcnq5*a is particularly elevated in the ear, when compared to the brain.

Kcnq4 *protein expression using Western Blots*

To further verify the presence of Kcnq4 protein, we probed Western blots of ear (Figure 5, lane A) and brain (Figure 5, lane B) tissue with rabbit polyclonal antipeptide

antisera. A major band at ~80 kDa corresponding to the size of Kcnq4 in mammalian species was readily detected in ear, and brain tissue extracts. The band was absent (Figure 5, lane C) when the immunizing peptide was present along with the primary antibody. Pre-immune sera from the rabbit showed no reactivity to proteins in zebrafish brain or ear tissue extracts (not shown). Using appropriately designed primers, we also performed DNA sequencing on the *kcnq4* PCR products that are summarized in Table 2. The sequenced data maps to various zebrafish genomic clones, and the translation of the mRNA provide amino acid sequences consistent with KCNQ4 (Figure 4), indicating that the clones represent active transcripts of a Kcnq4 protein.

Genetic and comparative analysis of Kcnq4 *Proteins (channels)*

We checked the putative *kcnq4* cDNA sequence against the zebrafish genome assembly and clones by BLAST searching. We retrieved the sequences of two genomic clones that contained *kcnq4* sequences (Figure 6A). Using two exon prediction programs, Net2Gene [20] and HMM [21], we generated a mRNA sequence comparable to the GenBank sequence, except that the 300 bp of 5′ end and the 200 bp of 3′ end sequence were not found. In the genomic clones, NW_001881069 contains three exons, while the scaffold Zv9_NA546:9, 520-23,017 contains 4 exons. We originally analyzed an earlier sequence deposited in GenBank (NW_00188744)

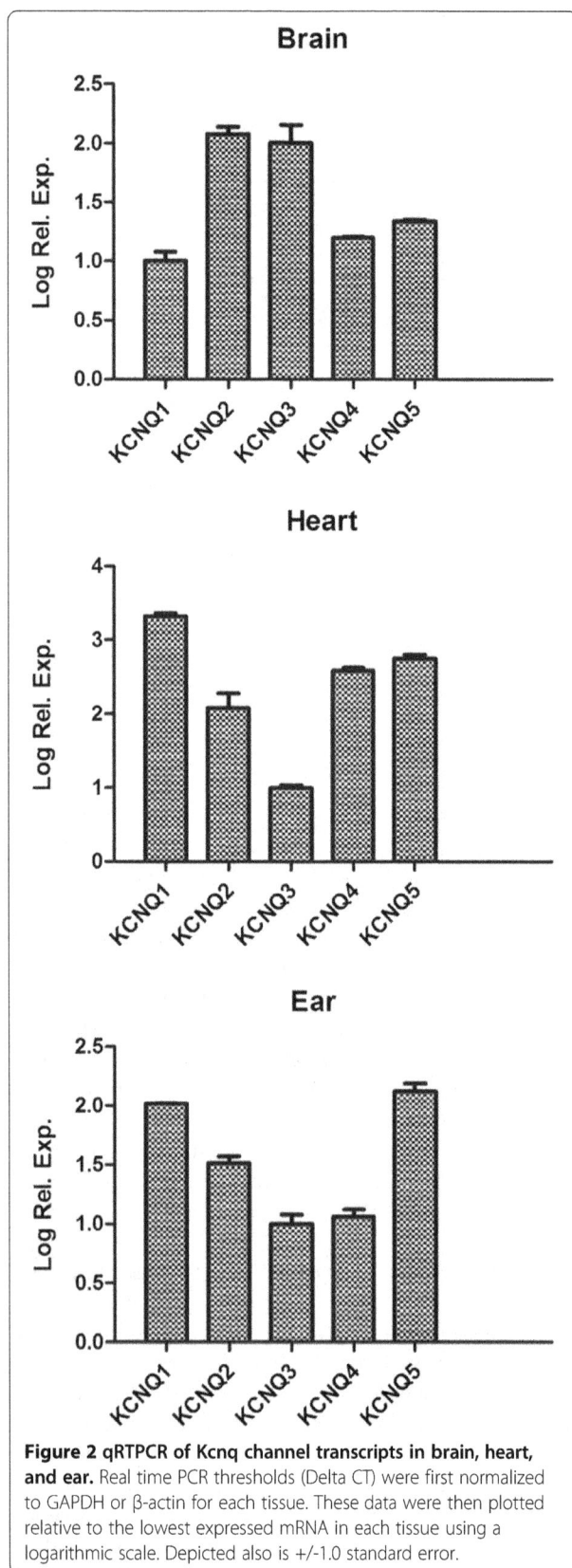

Figure 2 qRTPCR of Kcnq channel transcripts in brain, heart, and ear. Real time PCR thresholds (Delta CT) were first normalized to GAPDH or β-actin for each tissue. These data were then plotted relative to the lowest expressed mRNA in each tissue using a logarithmic scale. Depicted also is +/-1.0 standard error.

that contains the same exons as the scaffold Zv9_NA546: 9,520-23,017. Two cryptic exons in NW_00188074 detected by the exon predictions programs are not used in the zebrafish Kcnq4. Moreover, ORFs within these two cryptic exons do not contain amino acid sequences related to the Kcnq family of channels. For comparison, the exon structure of the partial *kcnq4* gene from chromosome 19 is shown in Figure 6B. Our PCR data confirmed that the transcript contains a sequence from the three exons in this partial gene.

The derived coding sequence from the 7 exons of NW_001881069 + Zv9_NA546: 9, 520-23,017 matches very well to other Kcnq4 amino acid sequences from chimpanzee, frog, and humans (Figure 4A). Similarly, the translation of the 5′ mRNA from chromosome 19 KCNQ4 is also very well conserved in the same species (Figure 4B). Table 3 summarizes all of the known Kcnq genes in zebrafish as of January 2013. *Ensembl* IDs are used for the gene, mRNA, and translated protein sequences, as these are referenced directly in the ZFIN database. Cross-references to entries in GenBank and Uniprot are also tabulated. *Kcnq1* on chromosome 7 has three potential splice products of differing lengths that have not been fully characterized. *Kcnq1* also has another gene identified on chromosome 25, but no transcripts have yet to be reported. *Kcnq2* has two genes, one on chromosome 6 that we also detected in this work, and another on chromosome 8 that was detected in zebrafish larvae [7]. *Kcnq5* has also two genes, and in this paper, we focused mostly on transcripts derived from chromosome 13 (*kcnq5a*). The chromosome 1 derived *kcnq5b* has also been detected in zebrafish larvae [7].

Discussion

In this study, we characterized Kcnq-type proteins/channel expression in brain, heart, and ear tissues of the zebrafish. We show that members of the Kcnq (Kv7.x) family of mRNAs are present in these tissues. Further, we demonstrated mRNA as well as the protein for Kcnq4 in ear and brain extracts from adult zebrafish. Although signals for *kcnq1* and *kcnq5* were weak using end-point PCR, the transcripts were readily detected in all tissues using qRTPCR. These data are consistent with previous reports of the Kcnq1 channel expressed during development [22].

As previously found in mammals [1,3-5,23-25], *kcnq2* was expressed in zebrafish brain, heart and ear. Similarly, in mammals, *kcnq3* is usually found co-expressed in the same tissues. Kcnq4 was detected in ear and brain tissue using a Kcnq4 selective antibody. KCNQ4 is found in auditory hair cells in mammals and we suggest that it may be present in homologous cells in the zebrafish.

The amino acid sequences of zebrafish Kcnq4, as well as other members of the KCNQ channel family, are

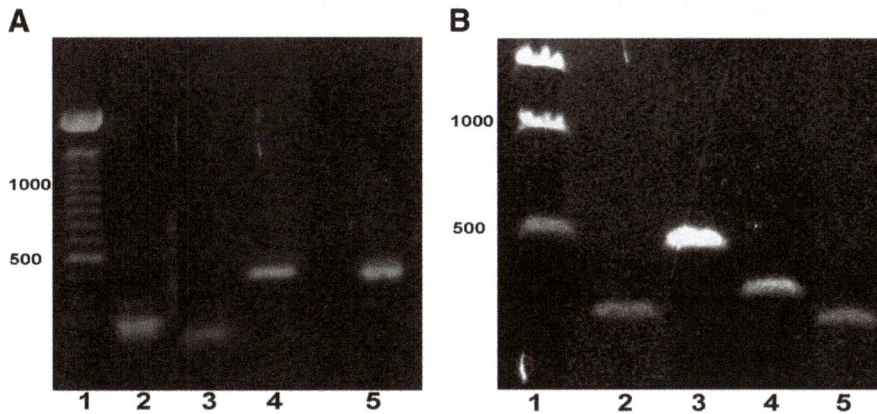

Figure 3 Expression of *kcnq4* transcripts from chromosome 19. A. PCR products from reverse transcriptase PCR reactions using primers (Table 1) for *kcnq*4. Lanes 2 and 5 are brain mRNA products, while lanes 3 and 4 are zebrafish ear mRNA-derived products. Lane 1 is a 100 bp ladder standard. **B**. PCR products from reverse-transcriptase PCR reactions using primers (Table 1) for Chr 19 (Lanes 2 and 3) and the Zv9_NA546 scaffold *kcnq*4 (lanes 4 and 5) of mRNA from zebrafish heart. Lane 1 is a 500 bp ladder standard.

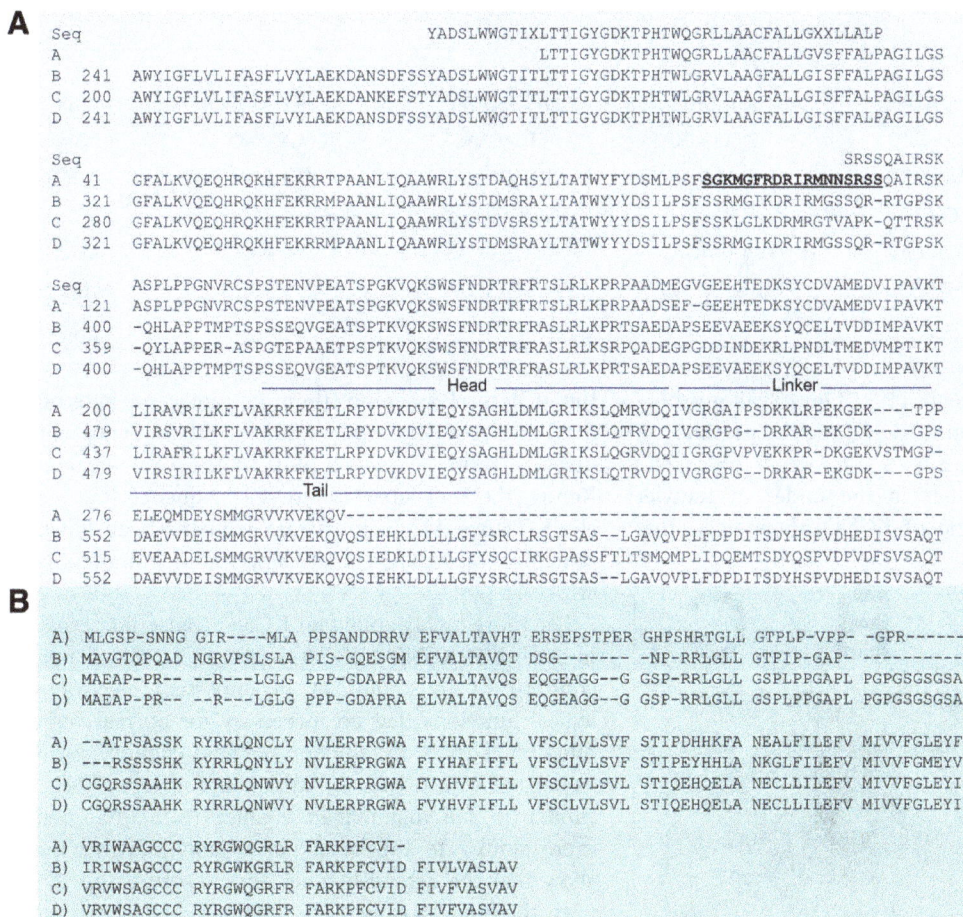

Figure 4 A. Alignment of the partial zebrafish *kcqn4* sequence (A), with KCNQ4 sequences from chimpanzee (B), frog (C) and human (D). The sequences on top of the KCNQ4 groups are the translation of the sequences that we obtained from the sequencing of PCR products (Table 2). The carboxyl region that contains the sequences implicated in the assembly of homo- vs. hetero-tetramers is indicated with bars, with the Head-Linker-Tail designations. **B**. Alignment of the translation of the Chr 19 sequence of zebrafish Kcnq4 (A) with the amino termini of Frog (B), Chimpanzee (C) and Human (D).

Table 2 Partial sequences of KCNQ4 obtained from PCR products

KCNQ4 (a) primers

5'-

NNNNNNNNNN	CGGGCAGGGC	AAGAAGNNCT	CCCAGAAGGG	CAAAACAAGC	TGCTAAAAGA
CGACCTTGCC	AGGTGTGTGG	AGTCTTGTCA	CCGTAGCCGA	TCGTAGTCAG	GGTTATCGTC
CCCCACCAGA	GGGAGTCTGC	ATAA			

-3' (144 bp)

KCNQ4 (b) primers

5'-

NNNNNNTNNG	ATGATATTCT	CGCTCCTCTC	AGGCCATCCG	GAGCAAGGCT	TCTCCTTTA
CTCCAGGTAA	CGTGCGGTGT	TCACCCAGCA	CTGAGAACGT	CCCAGAAGCC	ACCAGCCCTG
GGAAAGTGCA	GAAAAGCTGG	AGCTTCAATG	ACCGGACACG	TTTTCGCACA	TCTCTGCGCC
TCAAACCACG	ACCCGCTGCA	GACATGGAGG	GAGTCGGAGA	AGAGCACACT	GAGGACAAAT
CTTACTGTGA	CGTGGCCATG	GAGGATGTGA	TTCCCGCAGT	GAAGACCCTG	ATTCGAGCGG
TTCGGATCCT	GAAGTTCCTG	GTGGCCAAGA	GGAAGTTTAA	AGANCCCCTT	GCCGGCCGAA
NNG					

-3'(363 bp)

KCNQ4 (c) primers

5'-

CNNNNNNTNG	GATGATNTTC	TCGCTCCTCT	CAGGCCATCC	GGAGCAAGGC	TTCTCCTTTA
CCTCCAGGTA	ACGTGCGGTG	TTCACCCAGC	ACTGAGAACG	TCCCAGAAGC	CACCAGCCCT
GGGAAAGTGC	AGAAAAGCTG	GAGCTTCAAT	GACCGGACAC	GTTTTCGCAC	ATCTCTGCGC
CTCAAACCAC	GACCCGCTGC	AGACATGGAG	GGAGTCGGAG	AAGAGCACAC	TGAGGACAAA
TCTTACTGTG	ACGTGGCCAT	GGAGGATGTG	ATTCCCGCAG	TGAAGACCCT	GATTCGAGCG
GTTCGGATCC	TGAAGTTCCT	GGTGGCCAAG	AGGAAGTTTA	AAGAAACCCT	GCGGCCGA

-3' (358 bp)

conserved across phylogeny [19]. One distinguishing characteristic of KCNQ2 and KCNQ3 is the presence of a clustering domain that allows interaction of KCNQ channels with Na+ channels in the nodes of Ranvier [26]. Another characteristic of KCNQ channels is that

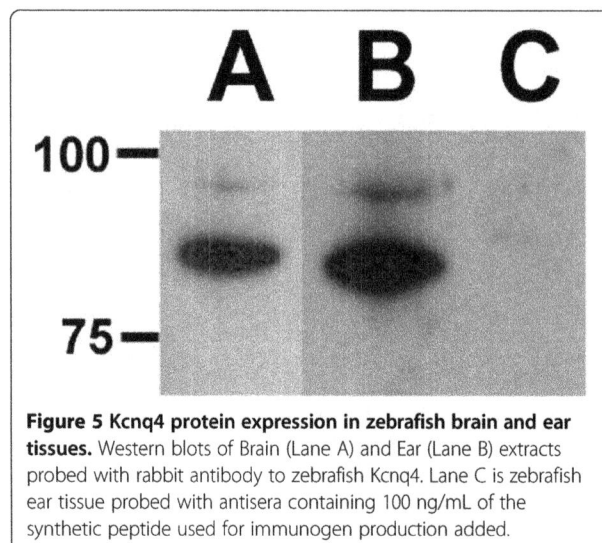

Figure 5 Kcnq4 protein expression in zebrafish brain and ear tissues. Western blots of Brain (Lane A) and Ear (Lane B) extracts probed with rabbit antibody to zebrafish Kcnq4. Lane C is zebrafish ear tissue probed with antisera containing 100 ng/mL of the synthetic peptide used for immunogen production added.

the structural assembly (homotetramer vs. heterotetramer) is dependent upon amino acid sequences in the carboxyl-terminal region [23]. In the case of zebrafish Kcnq4, the translated amino acid sequence that we derived (Figure 4A) is consistent with the head-linker-tail structure of KCNQ4 that supports a homotetrameric structure [23].

The more highly abundant KCNQ transcripts expressed in the brain (KCNQ2, KCNQ3, and KCNQ5) are possible contributors to a number of important electrophysiological functions that are necessary for normal cognitive function. That is, dysfunction of these channels has been associated with dementia, stroke, and epilepsy [24]. Very similar to the mammalian cochlea [4,25], but perhaps more similar to the vestibular system [27], our results show that the zebrafish inner ear sensory tissues do express the *kcnq2-5* genes. The inhibition of KCNQ4 activity in the mammalian cochlea [28] or knockout mouse [29] causes sensory cell degeneration followed by deafness. However, unlike mammals, the zebrafish hair cells are capable of regeneration after acoustic or chemical insult [30,31], and selected transcription factors among other putative molecules are key mediators of the regeneration

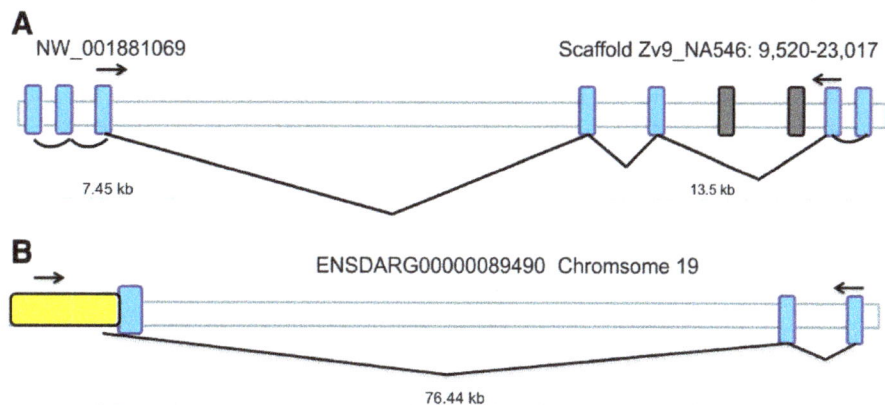

Figure 6 Analysis of *kcnq4* genomic structures. A. Schematic representation of zebrafish genomic clone containing *kcnq4*-related sequences - these have not at the time of the publication of this work been mapped to a chromosome. **B**. Partial structure of the Chr 19 Kcnq4 genomic clone. Only the first three exons have been identified. Blue boxes indicate active exons, while white boxes indicate silent exons. A yellow box shows the 5′ untranslated region of Kcnq4 from chromosome 19. Arrows indicate the location of primers used for mRNA detection across the largest number of exons.

[32,33]. No variants of *KCNQ5* are associated with sensory hearing loss in humans so perhaps its high abundance in the zebrafish ear is associated with regenerative capabilities.

Studies of the effects of exogenous regulators of zebrafish hair cell regeneration are at various stages of investigation [34]. Our identification of Kcnq channels in zebrafish may offer a new *in vivo* model system for screening KCNQ channel modulators/drugs and their effects on regeneration. Certain classes of drugs are being designed to modulate the activity of specific KCNQ-type channels [35-37], and our work suggests that screening this class of chemotherapeutic agents for functional [38-40], as well as for adverse effects (such as behavioral

abnormalities) in the zebrafish is promising. Further, expression of the channels cloned from the zebrafish in heterologous systems [15,41,42] provides an attractive platform for electrophysiological studies since dissociated hair cells from the inner ear of the zebrafish are extremely difficult to patch (Moore, unpublished observations, 2010; however, see [43]).

Conclusions

Recent advances in sequencing the zebrafish genome have provided further insight into modeling human diseases [44,45]. Nevertheless, the chromosomal localizations and/or complete sequencing of the *kcnq4* gene

Table 3 Summary of *kcnq* genes in zebrafish (2013)

Name	Chr.	Gene	mRNA	Protein	RefSeq	UniProt
kcnq1	25	ENSDARG 00000088397				
kcnq1	7	ENSDARG 00000059798	ENSDART 00000125483	ENSDARP 00000106445		A1L1U6
	7	ENSDARG 00000059798	ENSDART 00000083516	ENSDARP 00000077951		F1QG65
	7	ENSDARG 00000059798	ENSDART 00000083516	ENSDARP 00000077949	NP_001116714 NM_001123242	B0R0K2
kcnq2a	8	ENSDARG 00000075307	ENSDART 00000131736	ENSDARP 00000122368		B8JIR6
kcnq2	6	ENSDARG 00000091130	ENSDART 00000130440	ENSDARP 00000107870	XM_003198845 XP_00319889	E7F4W4
kcnq3	2	ENSDARG00000060085	ENSDART00000084303	ENSDARP 00000078738	XM_003197933 XP_003197981	F1RE25
kcnq4	Zv9 NA546	ENSDARG00000089559	ENSDART 00000125605	ENSDARP 00000108227		
kcnq4'	19	ENSDARG00000089490	ENSDART 00000129915	ENSDARP 00000108792		
kcnq5a	13	ENSDARG 00000069954	ENSDART 00000139904	ENSDARP 00000118905	XM_679763 XP_684855	B8JHS5, F1Q5A8
kcnq5b	1	ENSDARG 00000069953	ENSDART 0000085370	ENSDARP 00000079805	XP_697081 XM_691989	F1RB62

remain to be completed. Western blots demonstrated that the Kcnq4 protein is expressed in the brain as well as the ear. Thus, using the zebrafish with its rapid developmental period as a laboratory specimen may accelerate genetic screening for more specific KCNQ channel mutants, and perhaps foster drug discovery strategies for chemotherapeutic intervention in diseases associated with mutations in the Kv (x) family of genes, e.g., conditions manifested in humans such as hearing loss, and tinnitus.

Methods
Animals
Animal procedures were approved by the NU-ACUC (Approval number 2006 - 1034) and were performed in accordance with regulations for the care and use of laboratory animals. Adult zebrafish (initial stock was a kind gift from Dr. Jacek Topczewski, Ann Lurie Children's Research Medical Center, Northwestern University, Chicago, IL) were kept in an aquarium that was maintained at 25°C, filtrated, pH balanced, with frequent removal of excess nitrate, nitrite, ammonia, chloramines, and chloride. Exchange of conditioned tap water occurred at regular intervals. Two bottom feeder fish (Bristle nose catfish, *Ancistrus temmincki*) were kept in the aquarium to reduce the accumulation of waste. Animals were fed twice daily using a combination of flake or morsels that had been sterilized (UV illumination overnight) before usage. Wild type embryos were collected from natural matings in our lab, or ordered from ZIRC (University of Oregon, Eugene, OR), and were kept in 12-well clusters (~n = 6 each well) at 28.5°C in an air-only incubator. Stages were referred to in hours post-fertilization (hpf) or days post-fertilization (dpf) [9]. After 24-hpf, some larvae were maintained in 0.03% phenylthiourea to prevent melanin pigment formation [46] to ease the identification of a normally developed lateral line.

Tissue extraction
Zebrafish were sacrificed using a combination of Tricaine Methylsulphonate (MS-222) and ice, and the various tissues were rapidly removed. Zebrafish brain, heart, and ear were dissected, used immediately for experimentation, or pooled separately in 1.5 ml Cryovials and placed in liquid nitrogen until use. Total RNA was extracted from the tissues using TRIzol reagent (Invitrogen, Carlsbad, CA). Ear tissues were placed in 6.0 ml of low calcium saline (LCS, 10 mM HEPES, 100 µM CaCl2, 110 mM NaCl, 2.0 mM KCl, 2.0 mM MgCl2, 3.0 mM D-glucose, pH 7.3). EDTA and $MgCl_2$ (12 µl) were added to the ear tissues and incubated for 15 min to prevent calcium carbonate leakage from the inner ear otolithic structures.

RT-PCR and PCR
Primers for *kcnq1-5* and controls were designed based on zebrafish DNA sequences found in publically available databases such as the NCBI (GenBank), and Ensembl. The nucleotide sequence was searched using BLASTN to determine the number and location of different exons. Primers were designed using PrimerQuest (IDT, Coralville, IA). Nested primers were designed to cross exon boundaries and selected to amplify a 200 – 600 bp fragment of the desired *kcnq* mRNA. Primers were selected for optimum base content and annealing properties to the desired mRNA. Searching the zebrafish genome and expressed mRNAs was conducted using the BLAST suite of programs [47].

Total RNA pellets were washed with 75% ethanol, dried, suspended in RNAse free water and stored at a temperature of 4°C. The RNA concentration and purity was quantified by spectrophotometry (Beckman DU-7500, Fullerton, CA) using the absorbance ratio of A260/A280. Individual PCR reactions contained forward and reverse primers for the desired target, and control reactions contained primers for β-actin. The one-step RT-PCR system (Invitrogen, Carlsbad, CA) was used for amplification of target mRNAs. For each reaction, 200 - 400 ng of total RNA was used for the RT-PCR.

Reactions were performed in a thermocycler for 30 cycles (Techne, TC-312, Minneapolis, MN) with recommended denaturation (94°C, 2 min), annealing (55°C, 30 s), extension (72°C, 2 min), and hold (72°C, forever). The PCR products were separated using 1.0 – 2.0% agarose gel electrophoresis with gels containing ethidium bromide. Gel photographs were taken (Kodak, DC 290, Rochester, NY), transferred and stored to a microcomputer (Dell Dimension 8200). The molecular ladder (M) of the gels was separated by 100 bp bands with the first band at the bottom being 100 bp; the brightest band near the top of the ladder is at 600 bp.

Sequencing of kcnq4 PCR products
Gel bands were excised and purified using purification columns (Catalog #K2100, Invitrogen, Carlsbad, CA) designed for agarose gel extracts. The purified DNA products were sequenced at Sequetech (Mountain View, CA). The 5′ PCR primers for each product were used as sequencing primers (see Table 1).

Quantitative RTPCR (qRTPCR)
qRTPCR was conducted using a Biorad MyIQ detection system. Second strand synthesis was conducted using the IScript cDNA synthesis kit (Biorad, Grand Island, NY) starting with 0.45 to 0.74 µg of mRNA from the target tissues (brain, ear, or heart). An aliquot of the cDNA (5-10 ng) was then subjected to quantitative PCR in 96 well plates in the BioRAD Icycler using IQ supermix

(Biorad, Grand Island, NY) and primers (100 nM each) selected to generate 100-200 bp amplicons for *kcnq1-5*. GAPDH was used as an internal control (Table 4). After initial denaturation, samples were subjected to 40 cycles of PCR (95°: 15 s, 60°: 60 s) with SYBR green dye fluorescence read at the end of each cycle. Melting curves were obtained at the end of the runs to verify that single melting point species were generated in each reaction. Well factors were collected to compensate for differences in responses across the plate. Cycle times were calculated, and data were transferred to a spreadsheet for calculation of deltaCTs. Dilutions of the mRNA (1:2, 1:10, 1:50, and 1:250) of the mixed cDNA were used to determine amplification efficiency, as reported previously [48].

Antibody preparation

A synthetic peptide CSGKMGFRDRIRMNNSRSS based upon the reported partial cDNA, and putative amino acid sequences for zebrafish *Kcnq4* was prepared and conjugated to Kehoe Limpet hemocyanin (KLH) for immunization. Two rabbits were used for antibody production by Bio-Synthesis (Lewisberg, TX). Antisera were obtained 6 -10 weeks after immunization and characterized for immunoreactivity against zebrafish tissue extracts.

Table 4 Sequences of primers used for qRTPCR

Primer ID	Sequence 5' – 3'	Sequence source
KCNQ1 FOR	TTC ACA GGG CCA TCT CAA CCT CAT	NM_001123242
KCNQ1 REV	TCA AGC GCT CTG AAC TTG TCT GGA	
KCNQ2 FOR	TCA GCG GAT TCA GCA TCT CAC AGT	XM_003198845
KCNQ2 REV	TGT CCG ATT CAC CCT CTG CAA TGT	
KCNQ3 FOR	AAC TCC ATT TCC GTA CCC ATC CCA	XM003197933
KCNQ3 REV	TGT CTC TCC ACC CGC ACA AAT CTA	
KCNQ4 FOR	TTT CGC ACA TCT CTG CGC CTC AAA	ENSDART00000125606
KCNQ4 REV	TCC ATG GCC ACG TCA CAG TAA GAT	
KCNQ5aFOR	ACA ACC AAC CTT CCA GTC CAG ACA	XM_679763.4
KCNQ5a REV	TAA CTC ACT AAA CCG CTG GTG GCT	
GAPDH FOR	TTG CCG TTC ATC CAT CTT TGA CGC	NM_001115114
GAPDH REV	TCA GGT CAC ATA CAC GGT TGC TGT	

Western blotting

Zebrafish brain and ear were homogenized in a lysis buffer (20 mM Tris, 150 mM NaCl, 1.0 mM EDTA, 1.0 mM EGTA, 2.5 mM NaPyrophosphate, 1.0 mM Na Vanadate, 1.0 mM betaglycerol phosphate, 1.0 mg/mL leupeptin, and 1.0% Triton X-100, pH 7.5) using a motor driven pestle (5 bursts of 10 s) on ice. The crude homogenate was centrifuged at 1.4×10^3 rpm (Eppendorf microfuge, Hauppauge, NY). The supernatant fraction was removed, saved and the pellet extracted again using lysis buffer plus 1.0% SDS. After centrifugation to remove insoluble material, the soluble pellet fraction was saved. Protein concentrations in each fraction were determined using a reagent (Pierce BCA, Pittsburgh, PA) as suggested by the manufacturer. Electrophoresis was conducted on 4 - 12% SDS Page minigels (Invitrogen, Grand Island, NY). A total of 25 - 30 μg of brain fractions, ear and heart fractions (10 - 12 μg) were loaded into separate lanes on the gel. After electrophoresis, the gel was blotted to PVDF membranes (Millipore, Billerica, MA) using a Biorad transfer cell and Tris-Glycine-20% methanol transfer buffer. Transfer was accomplished at a constant voltage (40 V) for 1.5 hrs at room temperature. Membranes were blocked in 5.0% nonfat dry milk in Trisbuffered saline (20 mM Tris -150 mM NaCl, pH 7.5) containing 0.1% Tween 20 (TBS-T). Blots were then treated with anti-Kcnq4 peptide antiserum (1:2000) in TBS-T with 5.0% nonfat dry milk at room temperature for 2.0 hrs. After washing 5x with TBS-T, the blots were then incubated with HRP-conjugated Goat anti-rabbit antibody (Bio-Rad, 1:5000) for 1.0 hr at room temperature. After washing 5x with TBS-T, the blot was developed with electrochemiluminescent substrate (Pierce West Pico, Pittsburgh, PA) and bands were detected on film (Kodak Biomax, Rochester, NY).

Data analysis

Expression intensity of gene transcripts was analyzed using Image J (NIH Image, Bethesda, MD). Data display was accomplished using Origin (v8.0 Origin Software, Northampton, MA).

Competing interests

The authors declare no financial or non-financial competing interests.

Authors' contributions

Conceived idea for research (EJM, TJL), designed research (EJM, TJL, CW), performed experiments (CW, KS, KL, MH, CT), data analysis (CW, TJL, EJM), wrote the paper (EJM, TJL, CW). All authors read and approved the final manuscript.

Acknowledgement

We are indebted to Allie Coffin for teaching us how to dissect the zebrafish inner ear. We thank Arthur Popper for introducing us to Allie. We received financial support from the Alliances for Graduate Education in the Professoriate (AGEP) (KS - EJM), American Society of Pharmacology & Experimental Therapeutics (ASPET) (KL - EJM), the Summer Research Opportunities Program (SROP) (MH, CT - EJM) of the Graduate School at

Northwestern University, the Montel Williams MS Foundation (EJM), and a UNT Research Opportunities Program grant (CW - EJM). We thank Nicole Calderon and Daniel Ledee for assistance with certain of the RT-PCR protocols.

Author details

[1]Department of Molecular Pharmacology & Biological Chemistry, Northwestern University, Chicago, IL 60611, USA. [2]Department of Biological Sciences, University of North Texas, Denton, TX 76203, USA. [3]Department of Speech & Hearing Sciences, University of North Texas, Denton, TX 76203, USA.

References

1. Jentsch TJ: **Neuronal KCNQ potassium channels: physiology and role in disease.** *Nat Rev Neurosci* 2000, **1:**21–30.
2. Holt JR, Stauffer EA, Abraham D, Géléoc GS: **Dominant-negative inhibition of M-like potassium conductances in hair cells of the mouse inner ear.** *J Neurosci* 2007, **27:**8940–8951.
3. Arnett J, Emery SB, Kim TB, Boerst AK, Lee K, Leal SM, Lesperance MM: **Autosomal dominant progressive sensorineural hearing loss due to a novel mutation in the KCNQ4 gene.** *Arch Otolaryngol Head Neck Surg* 2011, **137:**54–59.
4. Beisel KW, Nelson NC, Delimont DC, Fritzsch B: **Longitudinal gradients of KCNQ4 expression in spiral ganglion and cochlear hair cells correlate with progressive hearing loss in DFNA2.** *Brain Res Mol Brain Res* 2000, **82:**137–149.
5. Baek JI, Park HJ, Park K, Choi SJ, Lee KY, Yi JH, Friedman TB, Drayna D, Shin KS, Kim UK: **Pathogenic effects of a novel mutation (c.664_681del) in KCNQ4 channels associated with auditory pathology.** *Biochim Biophys Acta* 2011, **1812:**536–543.
6. Mackie AR, Byron KL: **Cardiovascular KCNQ (Kv7) potassium channels: physiological regulators and new targets for therapeutic intervention.** *Mol Pharmacol* 2008, **74:**1171–1179.
7. Chege SW, Hortopan GA, T Dinday M, Baraban SC: **Expression and function of KCNQ channels in larval zebrafish.** *Dev Neurobiol* 2012, **72:**186–198.
8. Whitfield TT: **Zebrafish as a model for hearing and deafness.** *J Neurobiol* 2002, **53:**157–171.
9. Kimmel CB, Ballard WW, Kimmel SR, Ullmann B, Schilling TF: **Stages of embryonic development of the zebrafish.** *Dev Dyn* 1995, **203:**253–310.
10. Bian JT, Yeh JZ, Aistrup GL, Narahashi T, Moore EJ: **Inhibition of K⁺ currents of outer hair cells in guinea pig cochlea by fluoxetine.** *Eur J Pharmacol* 2002, **453:**159–166.
11. Liang GH, Järlebark L, Ulfendahl M, Moore EJ: **Mercury (Hg²⁺) suppression of potassium currents of outer hair cells.** *Neurotoxicol Teratol* 2003, **25:**349–359.
12. Liang GH, Järlebark L, Ulfendahl M, Bian JT, Moore EJ: **Lead (Pb2+) modulation of potassium currents of guinea pig outer hair cells.** *Neurotoxicol Teratol* 2004, **26:**253–260.
13. Suh BC, Hille B: **Regulation of ion channels by phosphatidylinositol 4,5-bisphosphate.** *Curr Opin Neurobiol* 2005, **15:**370–378.
14. Hernandez CC, Zaika O, Tolstykh GP, Shapiro MS: **Regulation of neural KCNQ channels: signaling pathways, structural motifs and functional implications.** *J Physiol* 2008, **586:**1811–1821.
15. Gamper N, Shapiro MS: **Calmodulin mediates Ca²⁺-dependent modulation of M-type K⁺ channels.** *J Gen Physiol* 2003, **122:**17–31.
16. Ou HC, Santos F, Raible DW, Simon JA, Rubel EW: **Drug screening for hearing loss: using the zebrafish lateral line to screen for drugs that prevent and cause hearing loss.** *Drug Discov Today* 2010, **15:**265–271.
17. Grant KA, Raible DW, Piotrowski T: **Regulation of latent sensory hair cell precursors by glia in the zebrafish lateral line.** *Neuron* 2005, **45:**69–80.
18. Platt C: **Zebrafish inner ear sensory surfaces are similar to those in goldfish.** *Hear Res* 1993, **65:**133–140.
19. Wei AD, Butler A, Salkoff L: **KCNQ-like potassium channels in Caenorhabditis elegans. Conserved properties and modulation.** *J Biol Chem* 2005, **280:**21337–21345.
20. Brunak S, Engelbrecht J, Knudsen S: **Prediction of human mRNA donor and acceptor sites from the DNA sequence.** *J Mol Biol* 1991, **220:**49–65.
21. Krogh A: **Using database matches with for HMMGene for automated gene detection in Drosophila.** *Genome Res* 2000, **10:**523–528.
22. Phansuwan-Pujito P, Saleema L, Mukda S, Tongjaroenbuangam W, Jutapakdeegul N, Casalotti SO, Forge A, Dodson H, Govitrapong P: **The opioid receptors in inner ear of different stages of postnatal rats.** *Hear Res* 2003, **184:**1–10.
23. Howard RJ, Clark KA, Holton JM, Minor DL Jr: **Structural insight into KCNQ (Kv7) channel assembly and channelopathy.** *Neuron* 2007, **53:**663–675.
24. Søgaard R, Ljungstrøm T, Pedersen KA, Olesen SP, Jensen BS: **KCNQ4 channels expressed in mammalian cells: functional characteristics and pharmacology.** *Am J Physiol Cell Physiol* 2001, **280:**C859–C866.
25. Kubisch C, Schroeder BC, Friedrich T, Lütjohann B, El-Amraoui A, Marlin S, Petit C, Jentsch TJ: **KCNQ4, a novel potassium channel expressed in sensory outer hair cells, is mutated in dominant deafness.** *Cell* 1999, **96:**437–446.
26. Hill AS, Nishino A, Nakajo K, Zhang G, Fineman JR, Selzer ME, Okamura Y, Cooper EC: **Ion channel clustering at the axon initial segment and node of Ranvier evolved sequentially in early chordates.** *PLoS Genet* 2008, **4:**e1000317.
27. Rocha-Sanchez SM, Morris KA, Kachar B, Nichols D, Fritzsch B, Beisel KW: **Developmental expression of Kcnq4 in vestibular neurons and neurosensory epithelia.** *Brain Res* 2007, **1139:**117–125.
28. Nouvian R, Ruel J, Wang J, Guitton MJ, Pujol R, Puel JL: **Degeneration of sensory outer hair cells following pharmacological blockade of cochlear KCNQ channels in the adult guinea pig.** *Eur J Neurosci* 2003, **17:**2553–2562.
29. Kharkovets T, Dedek K, Maier H, Schweizer M, Khimich D, Nouvian R, Vardanyan V, Leuwer R, Moser T, Jentsch TJ: **Mice with altered KCNQ4 K⁺ channels implicate sensory outer hair cells in human progressive deafness.** *EMBO J* 2006, **25:**642–652.
30. Harris JA, Cheng AG, Cunningham LL, MacDonald G, Raible DW, Rubel EW: **Neomycin-induced hair cell death and rapid regeneration in the lateral line of zebrafish (Danio rerio).** *J Assoc Res Otolaryngol* 2003, **4:**219–234.
31. Murakami SL, Cunningham LL, Werner LA, Bauer E, Pujol R, Raible DW, Rubel EW: **Developmental differences in susceptibility to neomycin-induced hair cell death in the lateral line neuromasts of zebrafish (Danio rerio).** *Hear Res* 2003, **186:**47–56.
32. Behra M, Bradsher J, Sougrat R, Gallardo V, Allende ML, Burgess SM: **Phoenix is required for mechanosensory hair cell regeneration in the zebrafish lateral line.** *PLoS Genet* 2009, **5:**e1000455.
33. Millimaki BB, Sweet EM, Riley BB: **Sox2 is required for maintenance and regeneration, but not initial development, of hair cells in the zebrafish inner ear.** *Dev Biol* 2010, **338:**262–269.
34. Coffin AB, Ou H, Owens KN, Santos F, Simon JA, Rubel EW, Raible DW: **Chemical screening for hair cell loss and protection in the zebrafish lateral line.** *Zebrafish* 2010, **7:**3–11.
35. Tatulian L, Delmas P, Abogadie FC, Brown DA: **Activation of expressed KCNQ potassium currents and native neuronal M-type potassium currents by the anti-convulsant drug retigabine.** *J Neurosci* 2001, **21:**5535–5545.
36. Housley GD, Raybould NP, Thorne PR: **Fluorescence imaging of Na⁺ influx via P2X receptors in cochlear hair cells.** *Hear Res* 1998, **119:**1–13.
37. Mikkelsen JD: **The KCNQ channel activator retigabine blocks haloperidol-induced c-Fos expression in the striatum of the rat.** *Neurosci Lett* 2004, **362:**240–243.
38. Albert JT, Winter H, Schaechinger TJ, Weber T, Wang X, He DZ, Hendrich O, Geisler HS, Zimmermann U, Oelmann K, Knipper M, Göpfert MC, Oliver D: **Voltage-sensitive prestin orthologue expressed in zebrafish hair cells.** *J Physiol* 2007, **580:**451–461.
39. Zheng J, Madison LD, Oliver D, Fakler B, Dallos P: **Prestin, the motor protein of outer hair cells.** *Audiol Neurootol* 2002, **7:**9–12.
40. Schaechinger TJ, Oliver D: **Nonmammalian orthologs of prestin (SLC26A5) are electrogenic divalent/chloride anion exchangers.** *Proc Natl Acad Sci U S A* 2007, **104:**7693–7698.
41. Shapiro MS, Roche JP, Kaftan EJ, Cruzblanca H, Mackie K, Hille B: **Reconstitution of muscarinic modulation of the KCNQ2/KCNQ3 K (+) channels that underlie the neuronal M current.** *J Neurosci* 2000, **20:**1710–1721.
42. Ljungstrom T, Grunnet M, Jensen BS, Olesen SP: **Functional coupling between heterologously expressed dopamine D(2) receptors and KCNQ channels.** *Pflugers Arch* 2003, **446:**684–694.
43. Ricci AJ, Bai JP, Song L, Lv C, Zenisek D, Santos-Sacchi J: **Patch-clamp recordings from lateral line neuromast hair cells of the living zebrafish.** *J Neurosci* 2013, **33:**3131–3134.
44. Howe K, Clark MD, Torroja CF, Torrance J, Berthelot C, Muffato M, Collins JE, Humphray S, McLaren K, Matthews L, McLaren S, Sealy I, Caccamo M, Churcher C, Scott C, Barrett JC, Koch R, Rauch GJ, White S, Chow W, Kilian B,

Quintais LT, Guerra-Assunção JA, Zhou Y, Gu Y, Yen J, Vogel JH, Eyre T, Redmond S, Banerjee R, *et al*: The zebrafish reference genome sequence and its relationship to the human genome. *Nature* 2013, **469**:498–503.

45. Kettleborough RN, Busch-Nentwich EM, Harvey SA, Dooley CM, de Bruijn E, van Eeden F, Sealy I, White RJ, Herd C, Nijman IJ, Fényes F, Mehroke S, Scahill C, Gibbons R, Wali N, Carruthers S, Hall A, Yen J, Cuppen E, Stemple DL: A systematic genome-wide analysis of zebrafish protein-coding gene function. *Nature* 2013, **496**:494–497.

46. Westerfield M, Doerry E, Kirkpatrick AE, Douglas SA: Zebrafish informatics and the ZFIN database. *Methods Cell Biol* 1999, **60**:339–355.

47. Camacho C, Coulouris G, Avagyan V, Ma N, Papadopoulos J, Bealer K, Madden TL: BLAST+: architecture and applications. *BMC Bioinforma* 2009, **10**:421.

48. Miao H, Crabb AW, Hernandez MR, Lukas TJ: Modulation of factors affecting optic nerve head astrocyte migration. *Invest Ophthalmol Vis Sci* 2010, **51**:4096–4103.

9

Alteration in circulating metabolites during and after heat stress in the conscious rat: potential biomarkers of exposure and organ-specific injury

Danielle L Ippolito[1], John A Lewis[1], Chenggang Yu[2], Lisa R Leon[3] and Jonathan D Stallings[1]*

Abstract

Background: Heat illness is a debilitating and potentially life-threatening condition. Limited data are available to identify individuals with heat illness at greatest risk for organ damage. We recently described the transcriptomic and proteomic responses to heat injury and recovery in multiple organs in an *in vivo* model of conscious rats heated to a maximum core temperature of 41.8°C ($T_{c,Max}$). In this study, we examined changes in plasma metabolic networks at $T_{c,Max}$, 24, or 48 hours after the heat stress stimulus.

Results: Circulating metabolites were identified by gas chromatography/mass spectrometry and liquid chromatography/tandem mass spectrometry. Bioinformatics analysis of the metabolomic data corroborated proteomics and transcriptomics data in the tissue at the pathway level, supporting modulations in metabolic networks including cell death or catabolism (pyrimidine and purine degradation, acetylation, sulfation, redox alterations and glutathione metabolism, and the urea cycle/creatinine metabolism), energetics (stasis in glycolysis and tricarboxylic acid cycle, β-oxidation), cholesterol and nitric oxide metabolism, and bile acids. Hierarchical clustering identified 15 biochemicals that differentiated animals with histopathological evidence of cardiac injury at 48 hours from uninjured animals. The metabolic networks perturbed in the plasma corroborated the tissue proteomics and transcriptomics pathway data, supporting a model of irreversible cell death and decrements in energetics as key indicators of cardiac damage in response to heat stress.

Conclusions: Integrating plasma metabolomics with tissue proteomics and transcriptomics supports a diagnostic approach to assessing individual susceptibility to organ injury and predicting recovery after heat stress.

Keywords: Heat stress, Metabolomics, Systems biology, Energetics, Metabolic networks

Background

Heat illness and heat stroke, the most severe form of heat illness, are life-threatening conditions characterized by elevations in core temperature (T_c) resulting from an inability to adequately dissipate excess body heat to the environment. The intrinsic nature of military operations (i.e., heavy physical activity in extreme environments) places military personnel at greater risk of developing heat-related illnesses. Sustained military operations in the Middle East have been accompanied by an increase in the number of heat stroke cases on the battlefield and in training. During the past two decades alone the incidence of heat stroke has increased over seven-fold [1]. Moreover, the 30-year mortality rates from heart, kidney, and liver failure in US forces increases by 40% in individuals with a history of heat stroke [2,3]. In 2013, US forces sustained over 2000 heat-related injuries requiring hospitalization, including 324 cases of heat stroke [1]. The actual incidence is projected to be considerably higher when considering undocumented instances that never reach triage [4,5]. In a five-year retrospective study, 10,319 cases of heat injury required medical resources to treat, including 1872 cases of heat stroke [4]. The estimated cost to the military approaches $52 million per year (USD), assuming a cost of $6200 per

* Correspondence: jonathan.d.stallings.mil@mail.mil
[1]The United States Army Center for Environmental Health Research, Environmental Health Program, Bldg. 568 Doughten Drive, Fort Detrick, Frederick, MD 21702-5010, USA
Full list of author information is available at the end of the article

day, an average hospital stay of 3.2 days, and 2620 cases of heat injuries and heat stroke per year [6]. Other costs include duty days and salary lost during recovery (up to 5.5 months) and the loss in investment and training associated with service discharge for medical reasons [6]. Taken together, these statistics indicate that there is an urgent need for earlier indicators of organ injury and susceptibility and molecular based indicators to improve return to duty decisions [7].

The physiological responses to an excess heat load include elevations in heart rate, a drop in mean arterial pressure, attenuated sweating rates, stupor, and collapse. The molecular level alterations and influence of the physiological events preceding and contributing to the systemic inflammatory response associated with heat stroke remain largely unknown. Heat stroke compromises tight junction integrity in the gut, resulting in leakage of bacteria into the circulation [8]. If uncontrolled, the ensuing thermoregulatory and immune responses can progress to system inflammatory response syndrome (SIRS) and ultimately multi-organ failure and death [9-13]. Designing novel and effective treatment and detection strategies for heat stroke requires a better understanding of the physiological and molecular alterations that accompany heat stroke and characterize the SIRS event. However, in human studies $39.0 - 39.5°C$ is the highest ethically attainable maximal core temperature ($T_{c,Max}$), but these temperatures are insufficient to induce heat stroke. To overcome these ethical limitations, we recently described conscious rat and mouse models of heat illness [10,11,14-18]. The models use abdominally implanted radiotelemetry units to track T_c while supporting physiological and behavioral adjustments to heat stress. In a recent study, we used our physiological model of heat stress to conduct an integrated systems biology evaluation of transcriptomic and proteomic changes in heart, liver, kidney, and lung after heat stress, heat injury, and recovery [19]. We identified discriminatory gene and protein signatures in heat-injured cardiac tissue reflecting perturbations in oxidative phosphorylation, energy production, and inflammatory response.

These global changes in metabolic networks associated with energy production in target tissues suggest that more accessible biofluids (e.g., serum, plasma, urine, and saliva) are also likely to reflect changes in the physiological state of the heat-stressed and heat-injured organism. Metabolomic profiling of plasma in conjunction with proteomic and transcriptomic analysis has recently emerged as a powerful predictive tool reflecting the dynamic responses to genetic modification and physiological, pathophysioloigcal, and/or developmental stimuli. However, perturbation in metabolic networks has not been well studied in heat illness. Understanding the metabolic response to heat illness and subsequent organ injury

provides unique insight into understanding how mammalian systems react to heat illness and recovery. Further, methods to interrogate metabolites in accessible biofluids have been developed to allow a global assessment of organism response to environmental stressors [20]. One disadvantage of metabolomics is the likelihood of false positives given the metabolome's exquisite sensitivity to subtle changes in physiology (e.g., food intake, changes in temperature, stress, etc.). Therefore, any study of the metabolome must discriminate pathological changes in metabolic networks from changes inherent in normal physiological functioning. Integrating metabolic networks at the level of molecular function is one approach to differentiate changes related to heat-stress and/or heat-injury from physiological variation in the unperturbed system. Bioinformatics methods can be used to identify an integrated panel of multiple physiological networks and biomarkers.

In this study, we evaluate the metabolomic profile in response to heat stress and heat injury, and compare the results with the proteomic and transcriptomic profiles described previously. We demonstrate plasma metabolomics profiles unique to the physiological conditions of heat stress, heat injury in cardiac tissue, and heat stress without injury. Metabolomics network analysis demonstrates perturbations in biological processes associated with energy usage and cell death, similar to the transcriptomics and proteomics analyses conducted previously. Further, integrated analysis of variance (ANOVA) analysis, random forest analysis, and hierarchical clustering analysis identify panels of biochemicals differentiating controls from heat-stressed and heat-injured animals.

Results and discussion
Thermoregulation and histopathology
$T_{c,Max}$ was reached at 2–3 hours, as previously published by our laboratories in more detailed thermoregulation analyses conducted with these animals and other similar studies [19,21]. Animals in the 24 and 48 hour cohorts were allowed to recover for the specified time prior to termination. In thermoregulation studies with these animals, temperatures return to baseline by 24–48 hours, but cardiac-injured animals exhibit hypothermia before recovery, as published in detail by our laboratory [19].

Liver, kidney, and heart were assessed by histopathology and scored for evidence of injury as described previously [19]. The heart was the only tissue with treatment-related evidence for injury, with inflammation and cardiomyopathy in three out of six animals in the heated cohort as described in detail in a recent publication from our laboratory [19] (Additional file 1A). For the remainder of the study, animals in the 48 hour treatment group were sub-stratified into cohorts according to uninjured vs. injured.

The metabolomics heat stress response and recovery in plasma—biochemical networks

Overview of metabolic network changes

A total of 422 biochemicals were identified that matched 307 named/identified chemicals in Metabolon's reference library, with 115 unidentified biochemicals (Additional file 1). The largest change in number of biochemicals relative to controls occurred at $T_{c,Max}$, with fewer alterations at 24 and 48 hours. The key biochemicals represented pathways related to the following categories: cell death or catabolism (pyrimidine and purine degradation, acetylation, sulfation, redox alterations and glutathione metabolism, and the urea cycle/creatinine metabolism), energetics (stasis in glycolysis and tricarboxylic acid [TCA] cycle, β-oxidation), cholesterol and nitric oxide metabolism, and bile acids (Figure 1).

$T_{c,Max}$ showed the greatest percentage of biochemicals altered in response to heat injury in virtually all categories. At $T_{c,Max}$, nearly 100% of identified biochemicals associated with cell death in a given pathway were elevated, suggesting an overall increase in biosynthesis to combat an overt exposure to redox stress (Figure 1).

Biochemicals in all enriched metabolic pathways relating to cell death were up-regulated at $T_{c,Max}$, with progressively fewer biochemicals within each pathway elevated and/or reverting to down-regulation over time (Figure 1).

In a two-way ANOVA with contrasts evaluating changes across all time points, seven key biomarkers demarcated heat stress from control during recovery: 5,6-dihydrouracil, 3-ureidopropionate, GSSG, ornithine, creatinine, corticosterone and pyridoxal (Table 1).

Redox stress and cell death

The glutathione (GSH) metabolic network exhibited profound perturbation in response to heat stress (Figure 2). All three biochemicals involved in glutathione metabolism were elevated at $T_{c,Max}$, probably as a result of heat-initiated redox crisis (Figure 2). γ-Glutamylated amino acids (including alanine, glutamine, isoleucine, leucine, phenylalanine, tyrosine, and valine [Additional file 1]), 5-oxoproline, cysteine-GSH disulfide, and glutamate were significantly greater than control levels at $T_{c,Max}$. γ-Glutamylmethionine was slightly elevated at $T_{c,Max}$, but the difference did not reach statistical significance

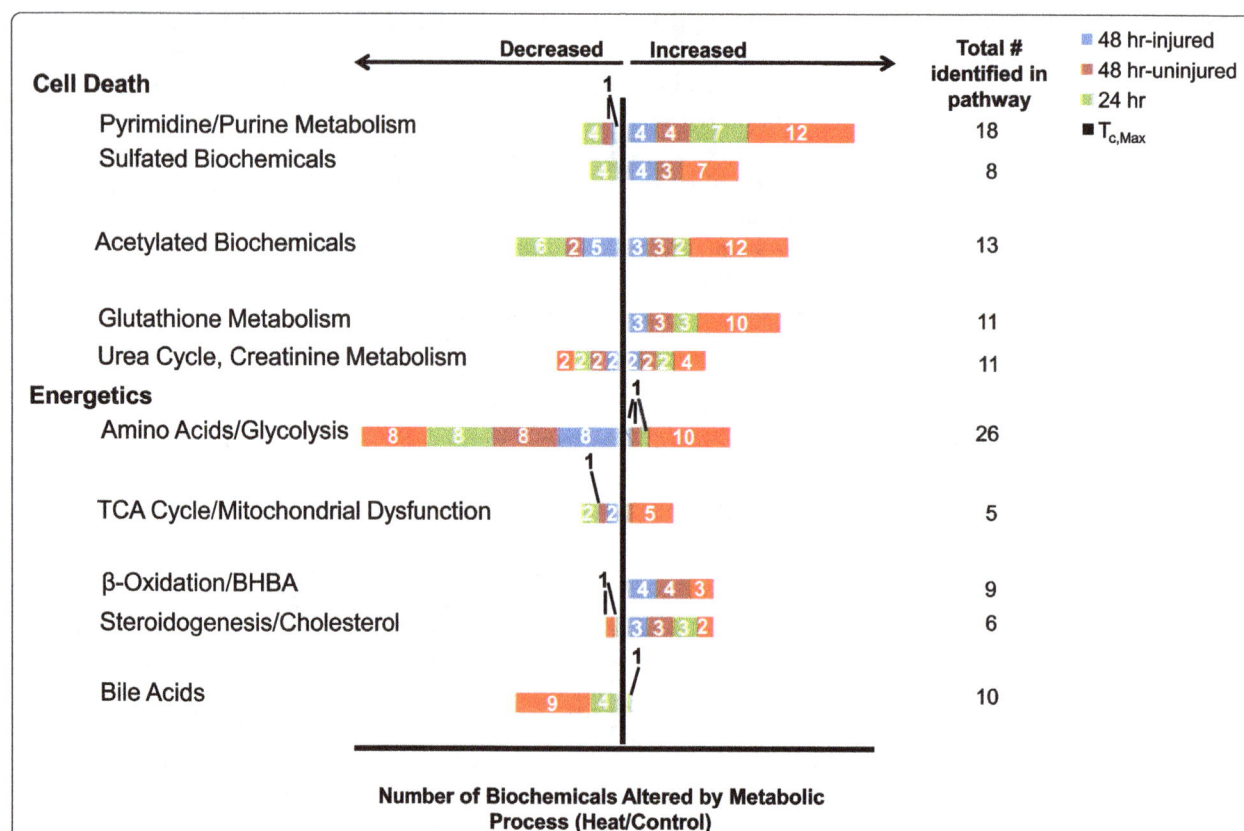

Figure 1 Altered metabolic pathways and process networks in plasma of rats after heat stress. Biochemicals were grouped by KEGG super-pathway and sub-pathway. Pathways meeting significance thresholds were plotted by number of affected metabolites per total number identified in the plasma (at right). Significance thresholds were determined by ANOVA, by ratio of heat/control at $T_{c,Max}$, 24 or 48 hours. The 48 hour endpoint was further subdivided into injured or uninjured animals by cardiac histopathology.

Table 1 List of seven key biochemical differentially expressed in heat-stressed and control animals*

Identified biochemical (pathway)	Literature review (biochemical and/or pathway)	References
5,6-Dihydrouracil (pyrimidine metabolism)	Early signal of apoptosis; DNA damage from reactive oxygen species elevation; deficiency	[22-25]
3-Ureidopropionate (alanine/aspartate metabolism)	Increased reactive oxygen species; inhibition of mitochondrial energy metabolism; neurotoxic/excitotoxic	[26]
Ornithine (urea cycle, arginine metabolism)	Production of arginine and increase in autophagy, cell death, removal of excess NH4+, energy metabolism; slight renal dysfunction	[27]
Glutathione disulfide, oxidized (redox)	Apoptosis, DNA damage, cell proliferation, survival, differentiation, metabolism; redox stress and/or crisis due to elevated reactive oxygen species	[28-30]
Corticosterone (steroid/sterol metabolism)	Mitochondrial conversion of acetyl-CoA to cholesterol and conversion of cholesterol to corticosterone; adrenal cortex production of cholesterol to pregnenalone, and ultimately cortisol; involved in glucocorticoid activity and stress response	[31]
7-α-Hydroxy-3-oxo-4-cholestenoate [7-HOCA] (steroid/sterol metabolism)	Bile acid synthesis from cholesterol; CYP7A1 activity in the liver; bile acid synthesis	[32]
Pyridoxal (vitamin B metabolism)	decreased renal function; Anabolism; cofactor for reaction releasing glucose from glycogen	[33]

*Not segregated based on cardiac injury.

(Additional file 1). At 24 and 48 hours, GSSG remained elevated. At 48 hours, three of the 11 biochemicals in GSH redox regulation remained elevated (γ-glutamylphenylalanine, 5-oxoproline, and oxidized glutathione [GSSG]).

Production of reactive oxygen species (ROS) and oxidative stress occur when the cell's protective mechanisms are saturated. ROS also play key signaling roles in cell proliferation, survival, disease and pathophysiology [28]. Increased ROS may lead to apoptosis, DNA damage, cell proliferation, survival, differentiation, and disruption in metabolism [34]. Heat exposure elevates free radicals [29]. Free radicals and other ROS are neutralized by GSH in redox regulation cycles. Deficient and/or dysfunctional GSH can disrupt cell processes and lead to cell death [30]. Oxidized GSH can be reduced back by glutathione reductase with NADPH (nicotinamide adenine dinucleotide phosphate) as an electron donor. GSH donates a reducing equivalent to unstable redox species. Under normal physiological conditions, more than 90% of the glutathione pool is in the GSH form and less than 10% is in the disulfide GSSG form. The ratio of GSH to GSSG is a metric of cellular toxicity, with elevated GSSG

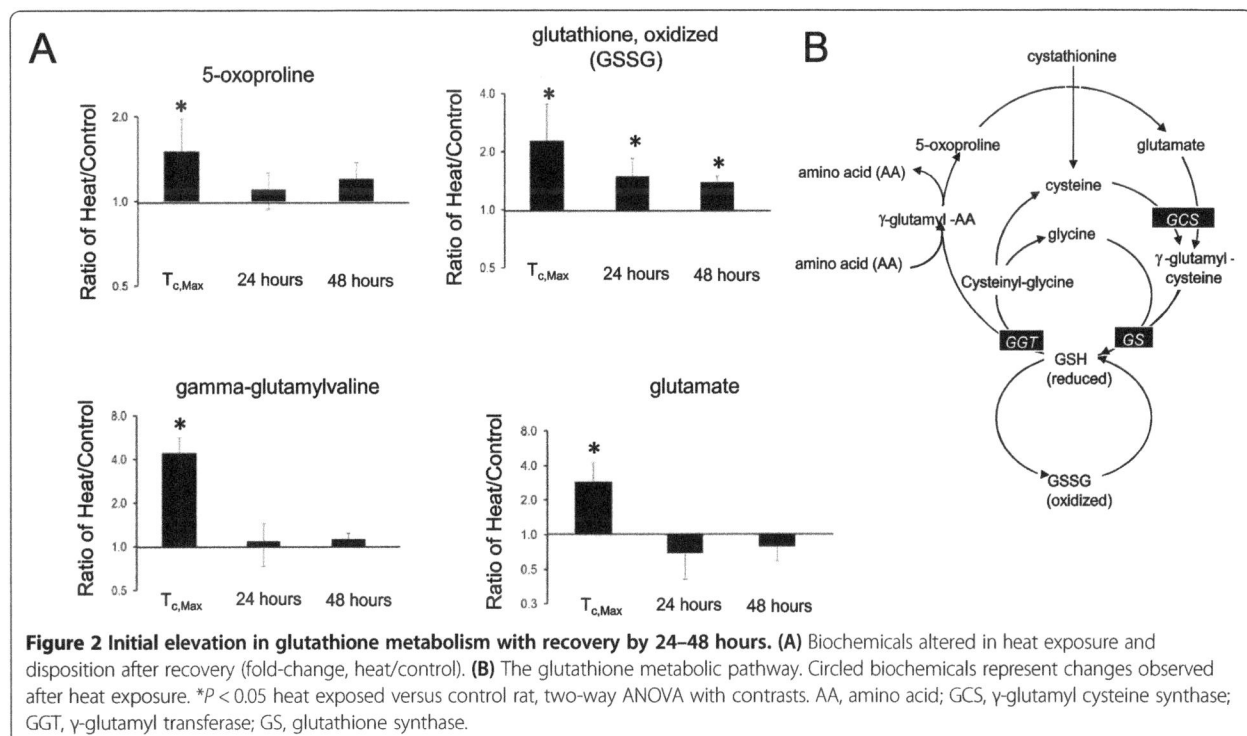

Figure 2 Initial elevation in glutathione metabolism with recovery by 24–48 hours. (A) Biochemicals altered in heat exposure and disposition after recovery (fold-change, heat/control). **(B)** The glutathione metabolic pathway. Circled biochemicals represent changes observed after heat exposure. *P < 0.05 heat exposed versus control rat, two-way ANOVA with contrasts. AA, amino acid; GCS, γ-glutamyl cysteine synthase; GGT, γ-glutamyl transferase; GS, glutathione synthase.

indicating oxidative stress [30]. Taken together, these results suggest that early perturbations in metabolic networks elicit persistent redox stress out to 48 hours after exposure. These persistent metabolic changes in heat-stressed individuals may affect performance during subsequent episodes of heat injury.

Arginine metabolism, nitric oxide metabolism, and cell death

Six biochemicals involved in arginine metabolism were altered after heat exposure (Figure 3). These biochemicals were involved in the urea cycle, which feeds creatine-to-creatinine production during metabolic mobilization of the muscle and/or brain energy reserves during energy crisis. Heat stress increased citrulline, decreased arginine, and increased urea in rat plasma at $T_{c,Max}$ (Figure 3A). Trans-4-hydroxyproline was not significantly changed in concentration after heat stress (Additional file 1).

Elevated citrulline levels suggest a concomitant increase in nitric oxide, a product of inflammatory signaling (Figure 3B) [27]. Increased urea may be associated with cell death, autophagy, and/or protein degradation. The combination of elevated urea and creatinine could also suggest renal dysfunction, consistent with the proteinosis observed in the renal histopathology as reported in the companion study. Elevated plasma creatinine at later time points could indicate continued use of skeletal muscle energy reserves and persistent renal dysfunction. Concomitantly decreased arginine and increased urea

may indicate slower kinetics of arginine metabolism with increased urea production (Figure 3B). Increased urea may also be the result of an increase in NH_4^+, a byproduct of cellular death [35].

At 24 and 48 hours, citrulline levels were no longer elevated, suggesting that nitric oxide (NO) production had decreased. Interestingly, however, ornithine levels increased at 24 and 48 hours, possibly reflecting slower arginine metabolism kinetics in general [36]. Taken together, these data suggest that a slight renal dysfunction was maintained during recovery, consistent with histopathologic evidence suggesting renal dysfunction.

Purine/Pyrimidine metabolism and cell death

Fourteen out of 18 identified biochemicals in the pyrimidine and purine metabolic pathways were significantly different at $T_{c,Max}$ relative to control (Figure 1 and Additional file 2). Exceptions were adenosine monophosphate (AMP), uridine, cytosine, and dihydroorotate. Uracil, 5,6-dihydrouracil, 3-ureidopropionate, β-alanine, and an acetylated form of β-alanine, N-acetyl-β-alanine, were all significantly increased at $T_{c,Max}$ compared to control rats, suggesting that a significant proportion of biochemicals involved in pyrimidine degradation was altered (Additional file 2). Significantly, nearly all the biochemicals immediately upstream of β-alanine metabolism in the pyrimidine metabolism reference Kyoto Encyclopedia of Genes and Genomes (KEGG) pathway are modulated, suggesting that a significant proportion of this biochemical network is affected by

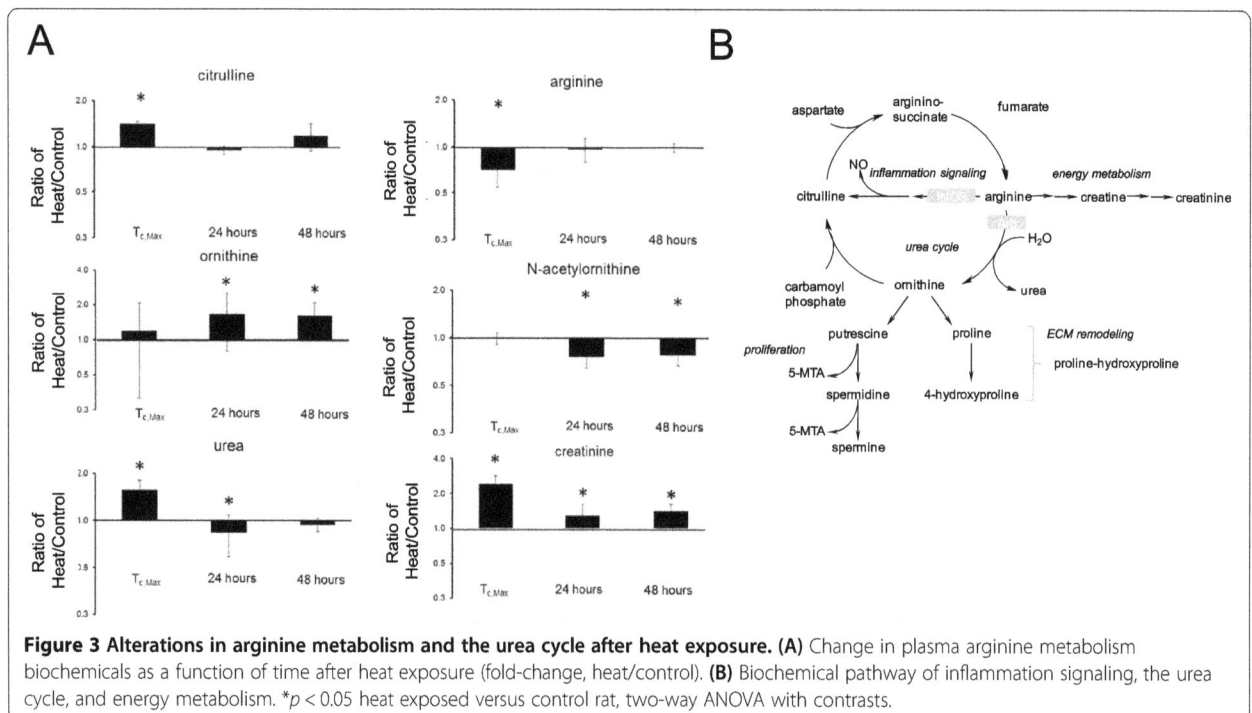

Figure 3 Alterations in arginine metabolism and the urea cycle after heat exposure. (A) Change in plasma arginine metabolism biochemicals as a function of time after heat exposure (fold-change, heat/control). **(B)** Biochemical pathway of inflammation signaling, the urea cycle, and energy metabolism. *$p < 0.05$ heat exposed versus control rat, two-way ANOVA with contrasts.

heat stress at $T_{c,Max}$. In plant cells, alterations in pyrimidine nucleotide metabolism are considered an early signal of apoptosis and often are induced by an increase in endogenous NO [22]. 3-ureidopropionate, the substrate of the enzyme dihydropyrimidinase, was elevated (Additional file 1) while the product, 5,6-dihydrouracil, was decreased (Additional file 2), suggesting a down-regulation in the level of dihydropyriminidase activity or 3-ureidopropionate. Further, carnosine is synthesized from L-histidine and β-alanine, with β-alanine as the rate-limiting precursor [37], and 3-ureidopropionate as the precursor to β-alanine production. The result of these alterations in pyrimidine degradation could suggest DNA damage by endogenous ROS over-riding cellular repair and protection mechanisms. Several altered biochemical pathways support elevated ROS.

Acetylation or sulfation and cell death

Of the N-acetylated biochemicals detected, 14 of 15 compounds were significantly elevated at $T_{c,Max}$ (Additional file 3). While 8 of 15 biochemicals were significantly changed at 24 hours, 6 remained altered at 48 hours. Heat exposure appeared to change in the activity of acetyltransferases or deacetylases, consistent with cellular damage. This initial response probably reflects hypoxia and initiation of cell death [38]. Acetyltransferases and deacetylases may allow an organism to adapt to recovery.

Eight sulfated compounds were detected and at $T_{c,Max}$, of which seven were significantly increased (Additional file 4). In addition, seven unnamed, putatively sulfated compounds also increased at $T_{c,Max}$ (X-12182, X-12183, X-12184, X-12185, X-12230 and X-12307; Additional file 1). At 24 hours, all biochemicals which had been higher than control at $T_{c,Max}$ were now significantly lower than controls, with a reversal of the trend after 48 hours (i.e., higher than controls; Additional file 4). Sulfotransferase enzymatic activity may have been induced or the activities of sulfatases may have reduced initially to facilitate clearance of cellular debris [35], then returned to control levels after recovery.

Amino acids and cell death

Of the 19 identified amino acids, seven were decreased and eight were increased relative to controls at $T_{c,Max}$, with a trend toward overall down-regulation at 24 hours and 48 hours. The exception was lysine, with a trend toward an increase at $T_{c,Max}$, with elevations at both 24 and 48 hours (Additional file 5). At $T_{c,Max}$, serine, threonine and alanine were lower than control. All three amino acids are synthesized from glycolytic intermediates. Although not definitive, these results may suggest a decrease in glycolysis [35]. Moreover, glutamate, which is consumed in the production of these amino acids, was increased at $T_{c,Max}$. Whether these amino acid changes are indicative of energetic alterations or increased autophagy is

unclear [39]. However, it is interesting to note that, at $T_{c,Max}$, amino acids used as anaplerotic contributors to the TCA cycle (i.e., glutamate and the branched-chain amino acids leucine, isoleucine, and valine) were increased and amino acids potentially synthesized as a consequence of glycolysis were decreased (serine, alanine, and threonine) (Additional file 5). These results may indicate perturbations in glycolysis and an overall slowing of energy production.

TCA cycle intermediates and energetics

All five of the TCA cycle intermediates identified at $T_{c,Max}$ were higher than controls (Figure 4), suggesting mitochondrial dysfunction and energy crisis. The concomitant increase in 2-hydroxybutyrate (AHB) further supported a perturbation in mitochondrial function [35]. By 24–48 hours, TCA metabolites in the plasma were no longer significantly elevated, suggesting restoration of the TCA cycle to homeostasis.

β-Oxidation, cholesterol synthesis, and bile acids

3-Hydroxybutyrate (BHBA) and carnitines were significantly increased at $T_{c,Max}$ (Additional file 6), supporting an increase in fatty acid β-oxidation for energy production. Increased β-oxidation is also implied from a trend toward lower plasma levels of the medium-chain fatty acids (e.g., palmitoylcarnitine, stearoylcarnitine, and oleoylcarnitine) relative to controls. These fatty acids can enter the mitochondria without requiring transporter activity (Additional file 6). Further, hexanoylcarnitine, a long-chain fatty acid conjugated to carnitine to facilitate entry into the mitochondria [35], is increased in heated animals. Increased β-oxidation may increase levels of acetyl coenzyme A (acetyl CoA) (Additional file 1, Additional file 6A), but the profound down-regulation in glycolysis, TCA cycle, and amino acid metabolism suggests that the acetyl CoA is not being used for adenosine triphosphate (ATP) production at $T_{c,Max}$.

β-Oxidation may also be up-regulated to facilitate cholesterol synthesis and corticosterone production [35]. At $T_{c,Max}$, corticosterone was significantly increased in heated animals relative to controls, and the increase persisted to 24–48 hours (Additional file 6). The increase in BHBA may reflect an increase in acetyl CoA for subsequent cholesterol metabolism and steroidogenesis, but functional mitochondria are required for this process. Alternatively, the elevated corticosterone could be released from the adrenal cortex during heat stress as part of a generalized stress response. Studies suggest prophylactic treatment with glucocorticoids protects against heat stress [40]. Changes in corticosterone levels could gauge severity of perturbations during heat and recovery [31].

Bile acids and steroids are generated from cholesterol. Following heat stress, plasma levels of steroids increased

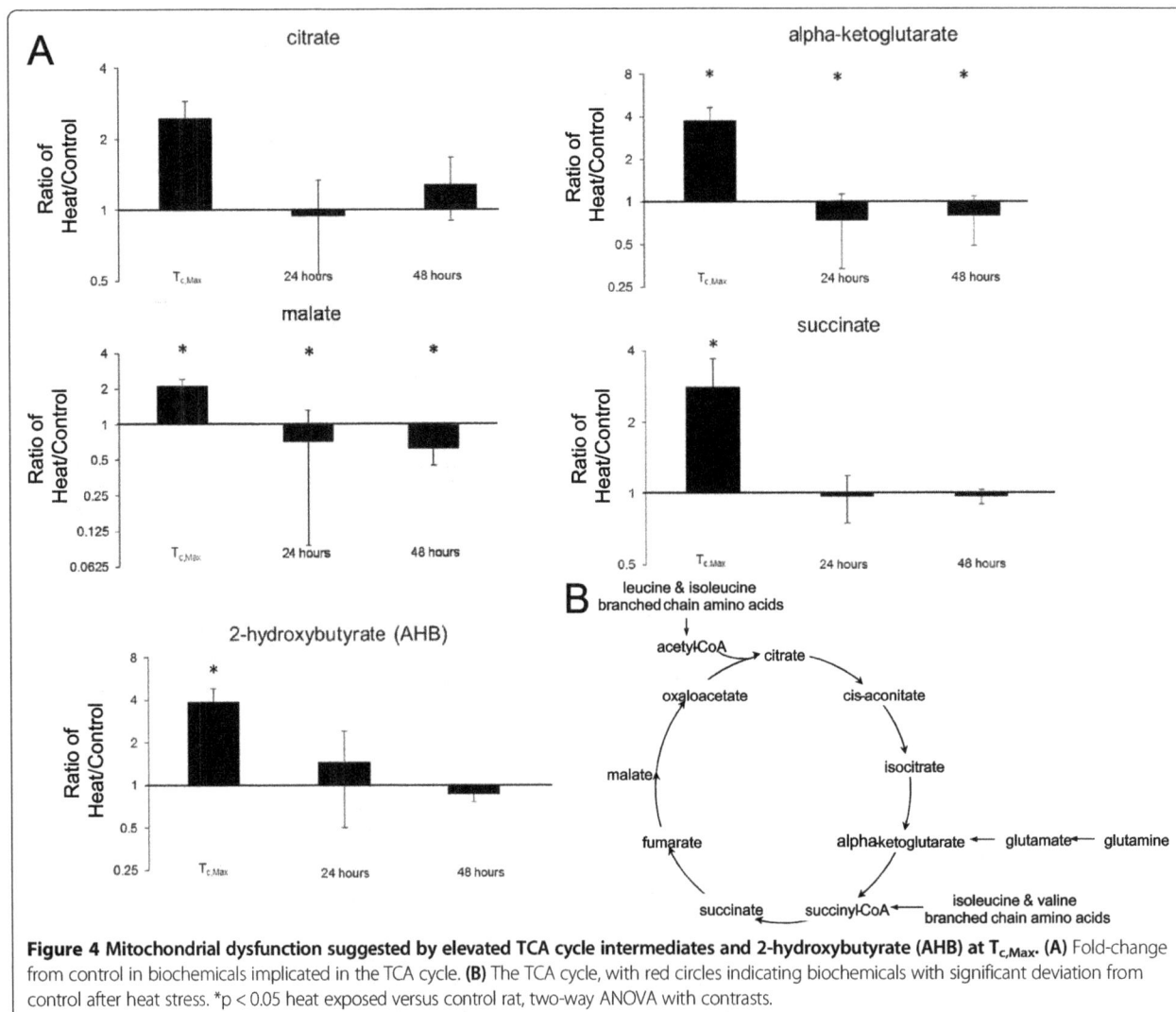

Figure 4 Mitochondrial dysfunction suggested by elevated TCA cycle intermediates and 2-hydroxybutyrate (AHB) at $T_{c,Max}$. (A) Fold-change from control in biochemicals implicated in the TCA cycle. **(B)** The TCA cycle, with red circles indicating biochemicals with significant deviation from control after heat stress. *$p < 0.05$ heat exposed versus control rat, two-way ANOVA with contrasts.

with a concomitant decrease in bile acids, suggesting *de novo* steroidogenesis (Additional file 7). Bile acid concentration is usually low in the normal systemic circulation. With heat stress, levels of nearly all bile acids detected were even lower at $T_{c,Max}$ (Additional file 7), possibly due to decreased reuptake within the small intestine and constricted intestinal circulation [41].

Co-factor metabolism

In addition to the broad categories of energetics and cell death, metabolites of Vitamin B_6 are altered by heat stress (Additional file 8). Heat stress resulted in an accumulation of pyridoxate (a breakdown product secreted in the urine), potentially reflecting renal dysfunction. Pyridoxal levels were increased in heated animals relative to controls at $T_{c,Max}$, possibly due to increased catabolism. In contrast, pyridoxal and pyridoxate levels were lower than control at 24–48 hours, possibly due to

increased anabolism (a process that requires B_6 as a cofactor) and return to homeostasis (Additional file 8).

Data integration—random forest analysis to identify biochemicals which discriminate heat exposure from unheated controls

Taken together, the results of the metabolic pathway analysis supports a model of heat stress perturbing metabolic networks affecting cell death and energetics. Ultimately, these metabolic network perturbations lead to disruption of cholesterol and bile acid synthesis, nitric oxide production and inflammatory signaling, and vitamin B_6 cofactor regulation (Figure 5). Performing integrated ANOVA analysis across biochemicals at all time points identified seven biomarkers within five metabolic networks which discriminated heat stressed individuals from controls at any time point (Figure 5).

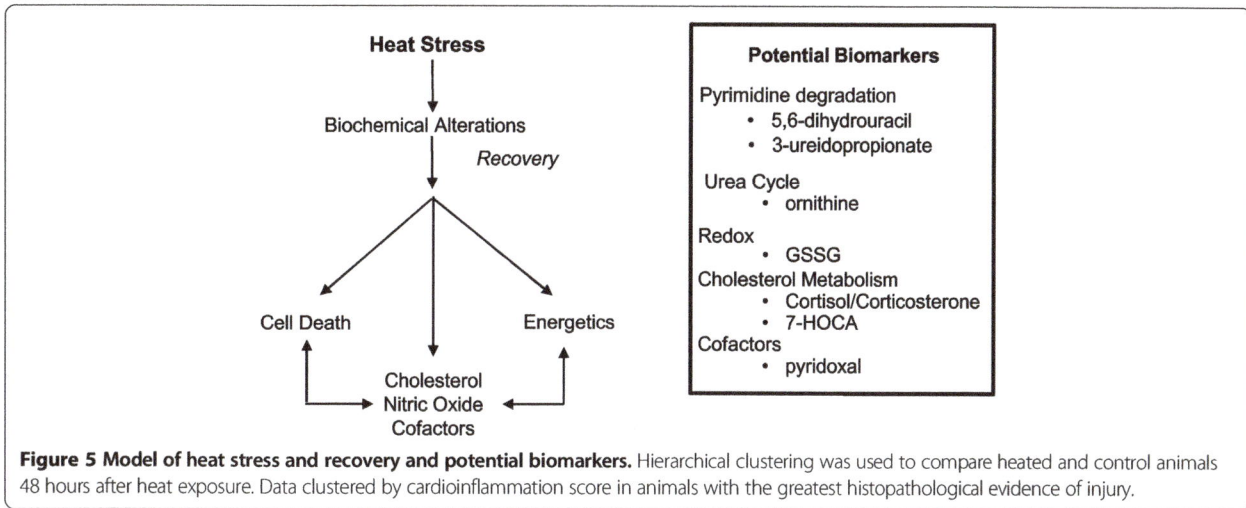

Figure 5 Model of heat stress and recovery and potential biomarkers. Hierarchical clustering was used to compare heated and control animals 48 hours after heat exposure. Data clustered by cardioinflammation score in animals with the greatest histopathological evidence of injury.

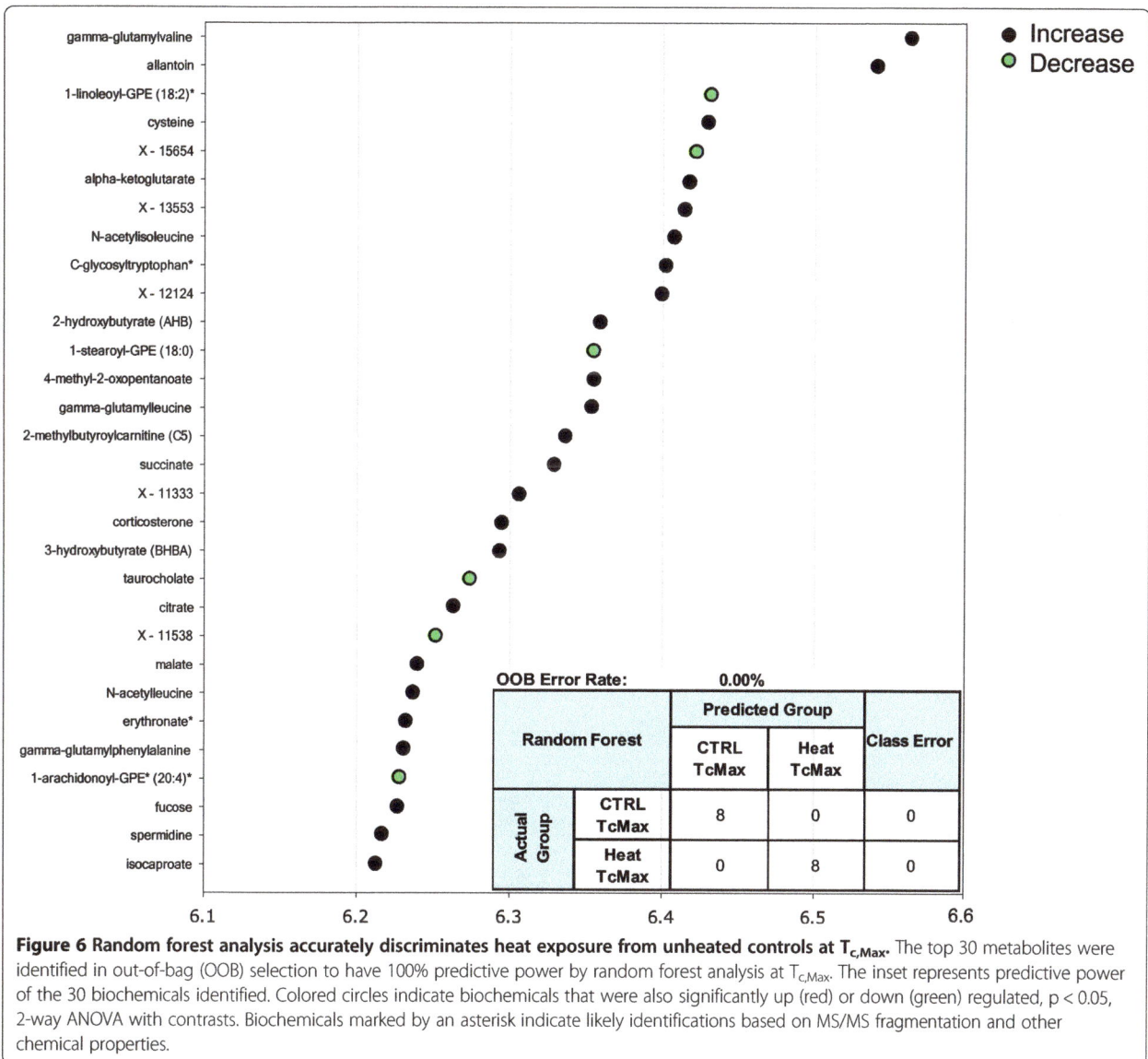

Figure 6 Random forest analysis accurately discriminates heat exposure from unheated controls at $T_{c,Max}$. The top 30 metabolites were identified in out-of-bag (OOB) selection to have 100% predictive power by random forest analysis at $T_{c,Max}$. The inset represents predictive power of the 30 biochemicals identified. Colored circles indicate biochemicals that were also significantly up (red) or down (green) regulated, $p < 0.05$, 2-way ANOVA with contrasts. Biochemicals marked by an asterisk indicate likely identifications based on MS/MS fragmentation and other chemical properties.

Random forest statistical analyses were used to determine sets of biomarkers capable of discriminating control from heat stress at $T_{c,Max}$ (Figure 6), 24 hours (Figure 7) and 48 hours (Figure 8) after exposure to heat. The out-of-bag (OOB) error rate for each forest plot was 0%, 6.25%, and 0%, respectively. The top predictive chemicals at $T_{c,Max}$ were γ-glutamylvaline and allantoin (Figure 6). Allantoin is not typically found in humans, but γ-glutamylvaline is elevated in response to perturbations in the redox cycle [28] (see also Figure 2). At 24 hours, the top predictive chemicals were C-glycosyltryptophan, N-acetyl-β-alanine, and asparagine (Figure 7). The predictive power of the model was slightly lower than $T_{c,Max}$, but still predicted with nearly 94% accuracy. At 48 hours, the most predictive biochemicals were 5-methyl-2'deoxycytidine, pyridoxate, 3-methylhistidine, palmitoylcarnitine (C16), erythritol, 3-(4-hydroxphenyl) lactate (HPLA), pseudouridine, oleoylcarnitine (C18), and X-12408 (Figure 8).

The degradation product of DNA (5-methyl-2'-deoxycytidine) and pseudouridine (a representative of RNA degradation) are both likely representative of continued cell death (see also Additional file 2) [22].

Identification of predictive indicators of persistent cardiac injury at 48 hours

At 48 hours, three out of six heated animals showed histopathological evidence of cardiac injury (see companion study). Segregating injured from uninjured animals did not result in significant differences at 48 hours for any biochemical pathway grouping except acetylation and sulfation (Additional files 1, 3, and 4). Using hierarchical clustering at 48 hours, we evaluated the global change in metabolites after heat exposure, segregating the 48 hour animals into injured and uninjured cohorts (n = 3 per cohort). A panel of 15 biochemicals discriminated animals with histopathologic evidence of heart

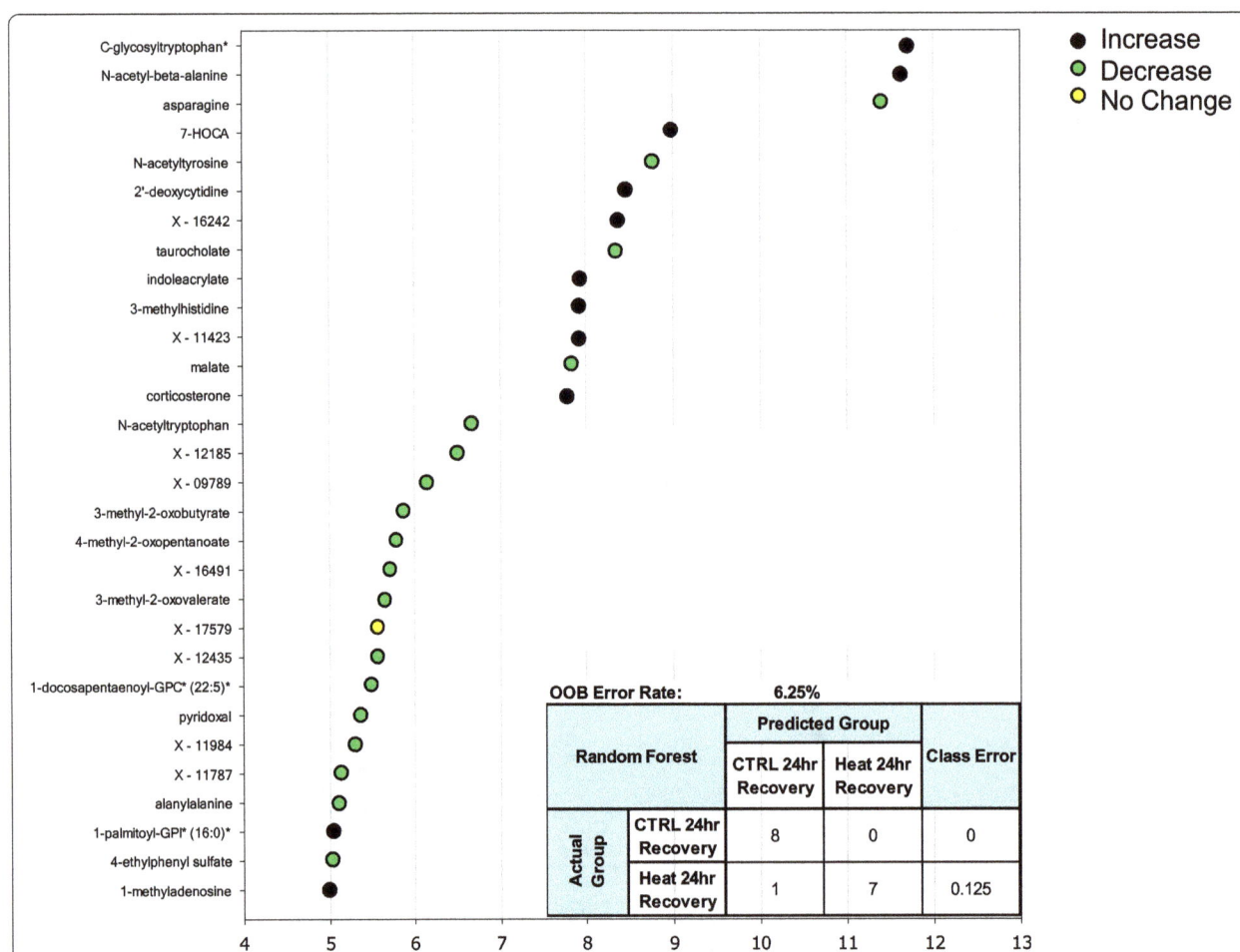

Figure 7 Random forest analysis accurately discriminates heat exposure from unheated controls at 24 hours. The top 30 metabolites were identified in OOB selection to have 94% predictive power by random forest analysis at $T_{c,Max}$. The inset represents predictive power of the 30 biochemicals identified. Colored circles indicate biochemicals that were also significantly up (red) or down (green) regulated, p < 0.05, 2-way ANOVA with contrasts. One biochemical was not significantly altered by ANOVA analysis (yellow). Biochemicals marked by an asterisk indicate likely identifications based on MS/MS fragmentation and other chemical properties.

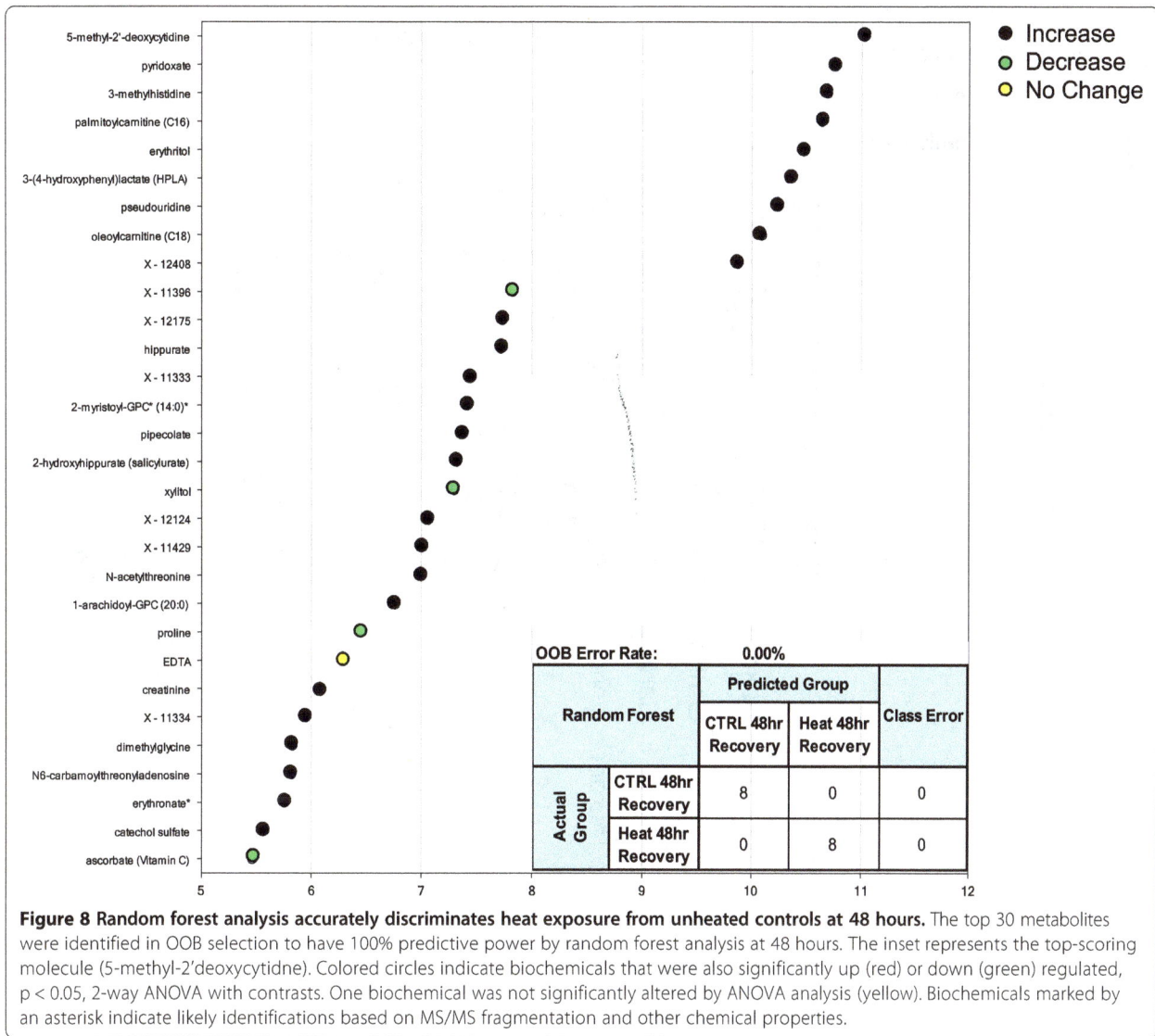

Figure 8 Random forest analysis accurately discriminates heat exposure from unheated controls at 48 hours. The top 30 metabolites were identified in OOB selection to have 100% predictive power by random forest analysis at 48 hours. The inset represents the top-scoring molecule (5-methyl-2'deoxycytidne). Colored circles indicate biochemicals that were also significantly up (red) or down (green) regulated, p < 0.05, 2-way ANOVA with contrasts. One biochemical was not significantly altered by ANOVA analysis (yellow). Biochemicals marked by an asterisk indicate likely identifications based on MS/MS fragmentation and other chemical properties.

injury from controls and uninjured, heated animals (Figure 9). Biochemicals in the panel were sub-categorized by metabolic pathway (Table 2). Ornithine and N1-methyladenosine and taurodeoxycholate have been associated with cardiac injury (summarized in Table 2).

The results of the random forest analyses at each time point were most concordant with the two-way ANOVA analysis at 24 hours (two of the seven biomarkers identified in both analyses—7-HOCA and corticosterone). At $T_{c,Max}$, only corticosterone was common to both analyses, and at 48 hours, only pyroxidate was common to both analyses. It is important to note, however, that 88 of the 90 biochemicals that were excellent classifiers of exposure were also significantly altered according to the ANOVA analyses (as indicated by the red and green circles in Figures 6, 7, 8). Thus, rather than the manual and somewhat arbitrary selection of the top seven biochemical

based on circulating levels, the random forest analysis pulls out a list of chemicals that in combination (whether up- or down-regulated) provide greater discriminatory power than a single biomarker, which may be a more powerful approach in populations that demonstrate significant individual variability in the metabolic response across time points.

Comparison of metabolic networks enriched in heat injury with complementary proteomics and transcriptomics pathway analysis

The strength of metabolomics is in its analysis of hundreds of analytes simultaneously. Multiple small changes (<2-fold) within a given biochemical pathway can signal a physiologically relevant perturbation of a physiological network regulating a metabolic function [58]. These physiologically relevant changes may be overlooked in

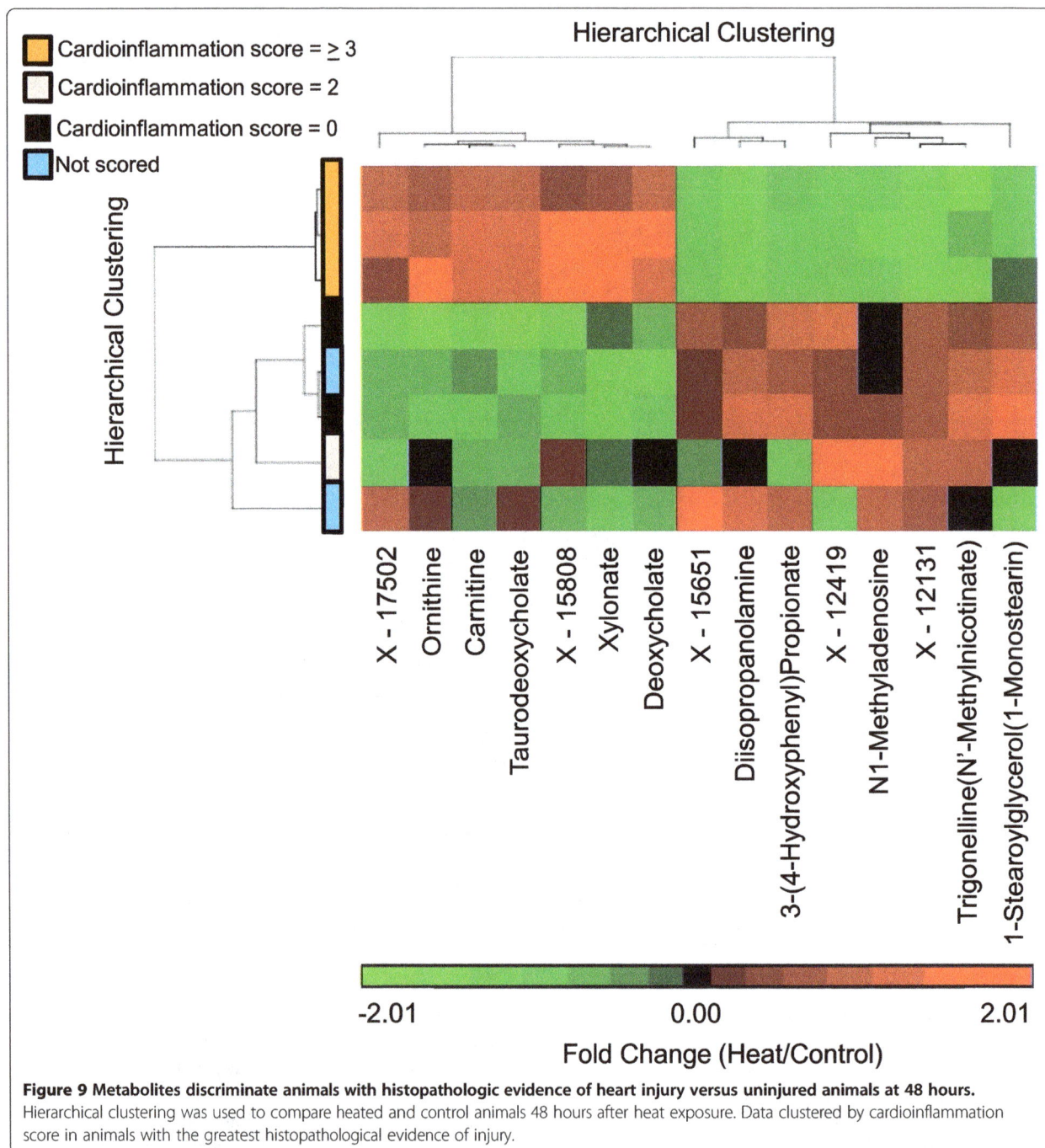

Figure 9 Metabolites discriminate animals with histopathologic evidence of heart injury versus uninjured animals at 48 hours. Hierarchical clustering was used to compare heated and control animals 48 hours after heat exposure. Data clustered by cardioinflammation score in animals with the greatest histopathological evidence of injury.

the analysis of single analytes. The network-wide comparison of plasma metabolites complements the transcriptomic and proteomic profiles observed in cardiac tissue in our recently published study [19]. The greatest concordance was observed in down-regulated biomolecules among KEGG pathways enriched in the three data sets (Figure 10). Metabolomics, proteomics, and transcriptomics data integration suggests concurrence in the transcripts, proteins, and metabolites supporting a down-regulation of oxidative phosphorylation and the TCA cycle. Taken together, these results support energy crisis and oxidative stress at 48 hours in cardiac-injured animals. Importantly, the metabolomics data obtained in plasma are concordant with tissue-based proteomics and transcriptomics profiles at the pathway level. Sampling blood (an accessible biofluid) indicates cardiac distress at the tissue level in this study. The metabolomics data were more discordant than the proteomics and the transcriptomics data, especially when comparing up-regulated genes and proteins with metabolites in the corresponding KEGG

Table 2 Review of 15 metabolites differentiating animals with histopathological evidence of cardioinflammation from uninjured animals

Identified biochemical (pathway)	Literature review (biochemical and/or pathway)	References
Ornithine (phenylalanine and tyrosine metabolism)	inhibition of nitric oxide; relationship between nitric oxide modulation of the Frank-Starling response in heart; nitric oxide and nitric oxide synthase are sensitive to thermal stress in fish	[42]
3-(4-Hydroxyphenyl) propionate (phenylalanine and tyrosine metabolism)	Biological nitrification inhibition (in plants); phenylalanine and tyrosine concentrations are reduced after Hsp70 increase and heat stress (in yeast)	[43,44]
N1-Methyladenosine (purine metabolism, adenine containing)	N1-methyladenosine analogues are cardioprotective agents in ischemic reperfusion model; decreased infarction; purine metabolism associated with myocardial steatosis and down-regulation of adipose triglyceride In heart	[45,46]
Xylonate (nucleotide sugars, pentose metabolism)	Deficiency in pentose metabolism produces a protective effect through decreased cholesterol synthesis, superoxide production, and reductive stress	[47]
1-Stearoylglycerol (1-Monostearin) (monoacylglycerol)	Associated with increased lipid catabolism and remodeling mitochondrial oxidation to aerobic glycolysis (hepatocellular carcinoma)	[48]
Carnitine (carnitine metabolism)	Disrupted carnitine metabolism is associated with mitochondrial dysfunction and increased pulmonary flow (lamb model); cardioprotective by increasing heat shock protein synthesis in adriamycin-induced cardiomyopathy	[49-51]
Taurodeoxycholate (bile acid metabolism)	Bile acids exert a protective effect after ischemic injury in porcine hearts; cause endoplasmic reticulum mitochondrial stress; deoxycholate and taurodeoxycholate affect heart mitochondria by decreasing respiration, affecting membrane potential, inducing mitochondrial permeability transition, and altering mitochondrial bioenergetics; impaired cardiac mitochondrial function may cause cardiac alterations in cholestasis	[52-55]
Deoxycholate (bile acid metabolism)	(see above)	(see above)
Trigonelline (N′-Methylnicotinate) (nicotinate and nicotinamide metabolism)	Cardioprotective effects after isoproterenol induced myocardial dysfunction (reduction in Hsp27, αB-crystallin and calcium/calmodulin dependent kinase-II-δ)	[56]
Diisopropanolamine (xenobiotics - chemical metabolism)	Increases choline uptake without affecting phospholipid synthesis (Chinese hamster ovary cells)	[57]
X – 17502 (Unknown)	n/a	n/a
X – 12419 (unknown)	n/a	n/a
X – 15808 (unknown)	n/a	n/a
X – 12131 (unknown)	n/a	n/a
X – 15651 (unknown)	n/a	n/a

pathways. However, amino acid/nucleotide sugar metabolism were modulated at the transcript, protein, and metabolite level, supporting a stasis of energy production/energy crisis (Figure 11). Combined with the panel of potential cardiac injury markers (Figure 9), these results suggest a plasma-based series of metabolic indicators for tissue damage induced by heat stress. Detecting biomarkers predictive of cardiac injury in an accessible biofluid supports further studies investigating whether these metabolites represent viable biomarker candidates for predicting cardiac injury and recovery.

Conclusion

In this work, we present a plasma metabolomic profile of heat stress and heat injury in an *in vivo* rodent model of heat stress. The metabolomic profile in plasma is concordant with tissue proteomics and transcriptomic profiles indicating energy crisis and oxidative stress, suggesting that metabolic indicators in the plasma may provide surrogate markers for tissue injury in an accessible biofluid. Coupled with the earlier work in tissue transcriptomics

and proteomics in the heat-stressed rodent model [19], the global metabolomic profiles identified the basis for future work for modeling the response to heat stress and heat injury [18]. Integration of metabolomics, proteomics, and transcriptomics in a top-down manner will provide the foundation for network analysis and computational based experiments in a human 3D thermoregulation model [59]. Anchoring these systemic stress responses to the physiological model of heat stroke will provide further insight into forecasting risk of disease, timing of disease onset, and intensity of disease at the organ level. As a result, we anticipate that such a model would accelerate the development of tools to improve disease prevention, classification, and ultimately treatment.

Methods
Materials and methods
Animal model
In vivo rat experiments were performed at the US Army Research Institute of Environmental Medicine (USARIEM). The Institutional Animal Care and Use Committee

Transcriptomics*			Proteomics (iTRAQ)*			Metabolomics**			
Pathways enriched in animals with cardiac injury	Count	P-value	Pathways enriched in animals with cardiac injury	Count	P-value	Pathways enriched in animals with cardiac injury	Complementary KEGG designation (DAVID)	# identified	# changed
rno00190:Oxidative phosphorylation	63	2.1E-37	rno05012:Parkinson's disease	46	4.6E-44	Oxidative phosphorylation	rno00190:Oxidative phosphorylation	2	1
rno05012:Parkinson's disease	61	4.3E-34	rno00190:Oxidative phosphorylation	44	9.0E-42				
rno05016:Huntington's disease	63	1.1E-27	rno05016:Huntington's disease	47	4.4E-39				
rno05010:Alzheimer's disease	62	7.6E-26	rno05010:Alzheimer's disease	45	1.3E-35				
rno04260:Cardiac muscle contraction	33	4.9E-18	rno00020:Citrate cycle (TCA cycle)	17	4.0E-20	Citrate cycle (TCA cycle)	rno00020:Citrate cycle (TCA cycle)	4	4
rno00280:Valine, leucine and isoleucine degradation	23	2.0E-14	rno04260:Cardiac muscle contraction	23	5.2E-20	Ketone bodies	rno00072:Synthesis and degradation of ketone bodies	2	2
rno00020:Citrate cycle (TCA cycle)	18	5.3E-13	rno00280:Valine, leucine and isoleucine degradation	13	7.0E-11	Fatty acid, dicarboxylate	rno00630:Glyoxylate and dicarboxylate metabolism	2	7
rno05414:Dilated cardiomyopathy	28	1.6E-11	rno00071:Fatty acid metabolism	11	7.8E-09	Nicatinate and nicotinamide metabolism	rno00760:Nicotinate and nicotinamide metabolism	2	1
rno05410:Hypertrophic cardiomyopathy (HCM)	26	1.1E-10	rno00640:Propanoate metabolism	10	1.2E-08				
rno00071:Fatty acid metabolism	17	4.9E-09	rno00650:Butanoate metabolism	9	2.3E-07				
rno00640:Propanoate metabolism	14	8.9E-08	rno00062:Fatty acid elongation in mitochondria	5	1.1E-05				
rno05412:Arrhythmogenic right ventricular cardiomyopathy (ARVC)	19	1.4E-06	rno05410:Hypertrophic cardiomyopathy (HCM)	9	3.0E-04				
rno00650:Butanoate metabolism	12	6.1E-06	rno05414:Dilated cardiomyopathy	9	4.8E-04				
rno03320:PPAR signaling pathway	17	1.5E-05							
rno00620:Pyruvate metabolism	12	3.7E-05							
rno00760:Nicotinate and nicotinamide metabolism	8	6.0E-04							
rno00230:Purine metabolism	20	7.8E-03							
rno00062:Fatty acid elongation in mitochondria	4	1.3E-02							
rno04920:Adipocytokine signaling pathway	11	1.4E-02							
rno00072:Synthesis and degradation of ketone bodies	4	1.9E-02							
rno00360:Phenylalanine metabolism	5	2.0E-02							
rno00380:Tryptophan metabolism	8	2.4E-02							
rno00630:Glyoxylate and dicarboxylate metabolism	4	4.3E-02							

Figure 10 Down-regulated biomarkers predictive of cardiac injury. KEGG pathways negatively enriched in animals with cardiac injury were compared across transcriptomics, proteomics, and metabolomics studies in cardiac tissue. For metabolomics results, the Metabolon pathway designation is listed along with the complementary KEGG designation (in DAVID). The metabolomics studies are described in this study and the proteomics and transcriptomics results were described in detail in a previous study. *, previous study; **, this study; red text, common to at least two data sets, with the same direction in all data sets (up-regulated or down-regulated); blue text, common to at least two data sets, but direction (up-regulated or down-regulated) differs.

approved all experimental procedures, which were performed in accordance with the American Physiological Society's guiding principles for research involving animals and adhered to the high standard (best practice) of veterinary care as stipulated in the Guide for Care and Use of Laboratory Animals. Research was conducted in compliance with the Animal Welfare Act, and other Federal statutes and regulations relating to animals and experiments involving animals and adheres to principles stated in the "Guide for Care and Use of Laboratory Animals" (NRC 2011) as prepared by the Committee on Care and Use of Laboratory Animals of the Institute of Laboratory Animal Resources, National Research Council in facilities that are fully accredited by the Association for Assessment and Accreditation of Laboratory Animal Care, International. As previously described [18], male Fischer 344 (F344; n = 48; Charles River Laboratories, Stone Ridge, NY) rats weighing 234–336 g (~2–3 months old) were used. Briefly, rats were housed under standard laboratory conditions (22°C, 12:12 hour light:dark cycle, lights on at 6:00 AM) in an Association for Assessment and Accreditation of Laboratory Animal Care-accredited facility. A relatively cool housing temperature was chosen to support survival during heat-stress recovery [18], during which chow (Harlan Teklad, LM-485; Madison, WI) and water were provided *ad libitum* [60]. Rats were implanted with TL11M2-C50-PXT PhysioTel® Multiplus Transmitters (Data Sciences International, St. Paul, MN) to measure core temperature (T_c; ±0.25°C), heart rate, and mean arterial pressure (±3 mmHg). Physiological response and temperature regulation after heat stress has been published in recent studies by our laboratories [18,21,59].

All experiments were conducted in conscious, free-moving animals, as previously described [18]. Briefly, rats were placed in a floor-standing incubator (Thermo Scientific, Ashville, NC) set at room temperature (RT, 22°C) 24 hours prior to initiation of heat stress experiments. Non-heated rats were not introduced to the incubator environment. Heat-stress experimentation was initiated after T_c of the control and experimental rats reached values of approximately 37.3°C. The following day, food and water were removed from the animal

Transcriptomics*			Proteomics (iTRAQ)*			Metabolomics**			
Pathways enriched in animals with cardiac injury	Count	P-value	Pathways enriched in animals with cardiac injury	Count	P-value	Pathways enriched in animals with cardiac injury	Complementary KEGG designation (DAVID)	# identified	# changed
rno04110:Cell cycle	34	1.43E-18	rno04612:Antigen processing and presentation	10	2.7E-05	Fatty acid metabolism	rno00071:Fatty acid metabolism	4	2
rno03030:DNA replication	16	1.51E-09	rno04610:Complement and coagulation cascades	7	1.6E-03	Valine, leucine, and isoleucine metabolism	rno00280:Valine, leucine and isoleucine degradation	17	16
rno04114:Oocyte meiosis	19	6.24E-08	rno04722:Neurotrophin signaling pathway	9	2.0E-03	Butanoate metabolism	rno00650:Butanoate metabolism	1	1
rno05322:Systemic lupus erythematosus	21	3.96E-07	rno00010:Glycolysis / Gluconeogenesis	7	4.1E-03	Glycolysis, gluconeogenesis, pyruvate metabolism	rno00010:Glycolysis / Gluconeogenesis, rno00620:Pyruvate metabolism	7	2
rno04666:Fc gamma R-mediated phagocytosis	18	2.22E-06	rno04810:Regulation of actin cytoskeleton	11	4.5E-03	Nucleotide sugars, pentose metabolism	rno00030:Pentose phosphate pathway	3	2
rno04142:Lysosome	19	2.89E-05	rno00030:Pentose phosphate pathway	4	9.0E-03	Phenylalanine and tyrosine	rno00360:Phenylalanine metabolism	16	10
rno04650:Natural killer cell mediated cytotoxicity	17	8.51E-05	rno03010:Ribosome	5	6.4E-02	Tryptophan metabolism	rno00380:Tryptophan metabolism	11	9
rno00240:Pyrimidine metabolism	15	2.00E-04				Purine metabolism	rno00230:Purine metabolism	5	4
rno04914:Progesterone-mediated oocyte maturation	14	3.85E-04				Pyrimidine metabolism	rno00240:Pyrimidine metabolism		
rno03010:Ribosome	14	7.41E-04				Aminosugars metabolism; Nucleotide sugars, pentose metabolism	rno00520:Amino sugar and nucleotide sugar metabolism	6	5
rno03440:Homologous recombination	7	7.97E-04							
rno04662:B cell receptor signaling pathway	12	9.06E-04							
rno04115:p53 signaling pathway	12	0.0032091							
rno00520:Amino sugar and nucleotide sugar metabolism	9	0.0032557							
rno04810:Regulation of actin cytoskeleton	22	0.011394							
rno04672:Intestinal immune network for IgA production	8	0.0156864							
rno03420:Nucleotide excision repair	6	0.0201							
rno03430:Mismatch repair	5	0.0409884							
rno04620:Toll-like receptor signaling pathway	10	0.045185							

Figure 11 Up-regulated biomarkers predictive of cardiac injury. KEGG pathways positively enriched in animals with cardiac injury were compared across transcriptomics, proteomics, and metabolomics studies in cardiac tissue. For metabolomics results, the Metabolon pathway designation is listed along with the complementary KEGG designation (in DAVID). The metabolomics studies are described in this study and the proteomics and transcriptomics results were described in detail in a previous study. *, previous study; **, this study; red text, common to at least two data sets, with the same direction in all data sets (up-regulated or down-regulated); blue text, common to at least two data sets, but direction (up-regulated or down-regulated) differs.

cages; the incubator temperature was increased to 37.0 ± 0.2°C; and the rats were heated until a T_c of 41.8°C ($T_{c,Max}$) was reached, at which time they were removed from the incubator, weighed, placed in a new cage, and returned to normal housing temperature (22.0 ± 0.2°C). Animals in the 24 and 48 hour cohorts were allowed to recover for the specified time prior to termination. Time-matched control rats experienced the same experimental procedures as the heat-stressed rats, but remained at the normal housing temperature of 22.0°C throughout experimentation. Control and experimental animals were provided food and water ad libitum throughout recovery. Plasma, heart, liver, lung, and kidney were harvested at $T_{c,Max}$, 24, or 48 hours with T_c, mean arterial pressure, and heart rate monitored continuously throughout recovery.

Histopathology

At necropsy, tissues (heart, liver, lung, kidney) were fixed in paraformaldehyde, mounted, sectioned, and stained with hematoxylin and eosin (IHC World, Woodstock, MD). Twenty serial sections were cut per tissue, with three to five sections per slide. Inflammatory or degenerative lesions were graded on a scale of 1 to 5 (grade 1, minimal; grade 5, severe) by a board-certified pathologist (Experimental Pathology Laboratories® [Sterling, VA]).

The results of the histopathological evaluation have been previously published [19].

Metabolomics

Metabolomic analysis was conducted by Metabolon (Durham, NC). Briefly, frozen plasma samples (150 μl) were thawed, and extracts were prepared according to Metabolon's standard protocol, which is designed to remove protein, dislodge small molecules bound to protein or physically trapped in the precipitated protein matrix and recover a wide range of chemically diverse metabolites. Samples were extracted and split into equal parts for analysis on the gas chromatography mass spectrometer and liquid chromatography mass spectrometer platforms. Proprietary software was used to match ions to an in-house library of standards for metabolite identification and for metabolite quantitation by peak area integration.

Data analysis—metabolomics

Two-way ANOVA with contrasts was used to analyze the data (See Additional file 1). For all analyses, missing values (if any) were inputted with the observed minimum for that particular compound (inputted values were added after block-normalization). The statistical analyses were performed on natural log-transformed data to reduce the effect of any potential outliers in the data. Two-way ANOVA and contrast comparisons were made between the means of each biochemical from the groups and were calculated using either or both of the statistical analysis software programs Array Studio (Omicsoft, Inc.) or 'R' (R Foundation for Statistical Computing, Vienna, Austria). Statistical cut-offs are typically used to detemine physiological significance in metabolomics studies. Conservative criteria of $p < 0.05$ and $q < 0.1$ are routinely used in metabolomic studies [61], allowing for the identification of significantly altered responses between groups with a false discovery rate of no more than 10%. Because we analyzed a constellation of metabolites in conjunction with biochemical pathways rather than single analytes, we considered $p < 0.05$ significant, regardless of the q value. Using this approach, we could be more inclusive of data that did not meet strict cut-off values, taking both p-value and number of metabolites changing in a given biochemical pathway.

Random forest, a supervised classification technique based on an ensemble of decision trees [62,63] was used to determine the predictive value of multiple biochemicals for both exposure and health effect. For a given decision tree, a random subset of the data with identifying true class information was selected to build the tree ("bootstrap sample" or "training set"), and then the remaining data, the OOB variables, were passed down the tree to obtain a class prediction for each sample, then repeated thousands of times to produce the forest. The final classification of each sample was determined by computing the class prediction frequency for the OOB variables over the whole forest. Class predictions were compared to the true classes, generating the "OOB error rate" as a measure of prediction accuracy. To determine which variables (biochemicals) made the largest contribution to the classification, a variable importance measure was computed, termed the mean decrease accuracy (MDA). The MDA was determined by randomly permuting a variable, running the observed values through the trees, and then reassessing the prediction accuracy. If a variable is not important, then this procedure had little change in the accuracy of the class prediction (permuting random noise gave random noise). By contrast, if a variable is important to the classification, the prediction accuracy will drop after such a permutation, which we record as the MDA. Thus, the random forest analysis provided an importance rank-ordering of biochemical, and the top 30 biochemicals were reported.

Additional files

> **Additional file 1: Is the raw metabolomics data and ANOVA with contrasts for each biochemical analyzed in the study.**

Additional file 2: Heat stress persistently increases metabolites controlling pyrimidine and purine degradation. (A) Eighteen biochemicals were identified in the purine and pyrimidine metabolism sub-pathways: at $T_{c,Max}$, fold changes (heat/control) were significantly increased for 12 biochemicals and significantly decreased for 1 biochemical; at 24 hours, 8 biochemicals were increased and 2 decreased; and at 48 hours, 4 were elevated and 2 decreased in both uninjured and heat-injured animals. **(B)** Biochemical pathway for pyrimidine degradation. Red, increased over control; green, decreased relative to control; green and red, $p < 0.05$; light red, $0.05 < p < 0.1$.

Additional file 3: Acute increase in acetylated biochemicals followed by a decrease at 24 hours and significant differences between uninjured animals and animals with cardiac injury at 48 hours. Of the 13 acetylated biochemicals at $T_{c,Max}$, 12 were greater in heated animals than controls; at 24 hours, 5 were significantly lower and 2 were significantly higher; at 48 hours in uninjured animals, 3 were significantly higher and 2 were significantly lower; in heat-injured animals, 3 were higher and 5 were lower than controls. Red, fold change significantly higher; green, fold change significantly lower than control ($p < 0.05$ by ANOVA); light green, fold change lower compared to controls ($0.05 < p < 0.1$ by ANOVA).

Additional file 4: Acute increase in sulfated biochemicals followed by a decrease at 24 hours and significant differences between uninjured animals and animals with cardiac injury at 48 hours. Of the 8 sulfated biochemicals at $T_{c,Max}$, 7 were greater in heated animals than controls; at 24 hours, 4 were significantly lower and none were significantly higher; at 48 hours in uninjured animals, 3 were significantly higher and none were significantly lower; and in heat-injured animals, 4 were higher and none were lower than controls. Red, fold change significantly higher; green, fold change significantly lower than control ($p < 0.05$ by ANOVA); light green, fold change slightly lower compared to controls with $0.05 < p < 0.1$ by ANOVA.

Additional file 5: Altered amino acids and mediators of glycolysis, gluconeogenesis, and pyruvate metabolism after heat stress and recovery. (A) Of the 19 identified amino acids, at $T_{c,Max}$ 7 were significantly lower and 8 were significantly greater; 4 were lower at 24 hours; at 48 hours, 5 were lower and 1 was greater in both uninjured and cardiac-injured animals. Metabolites contributing to glycolysis were initially greater than control, then either returned to normal or were lower than control at 24 and 48 hours. Red, fold change significantly higher; green, fold change significantly lower than control ($p < 0.05$ by ANOVA); light green, fold change slightly lower compared to controls; light red, fold change lightly higher than control ($0.05 < p < 0.1$ by ANOVA). **(B)** Three amino acids that contribute to the tricarboxylic acid (TCA) cycle for energy production were decreased.

Additional file 6: Increased fatty acid β-Oxidation modulates acetyl CoA production and cholesterol synthesis in energy production. (A) Metabolic network illustrating how elevations in fatty acid β-oxidation compensates for compromised TCA cycle, glycolysis, and amino acid metabolism in the production of cellular energy. **(B)** Alterations in medium chain fatty acids in response to heat stress and recovery. **(C)** Alterations in biochemicals involved in carnitine metabolism after heat stress. Green cells represent significant decrease. Red cells represent a significant increase in heat-stressed individuals over control cases ($0.05 < p < 0.10$ heat exposed versus control rat, 2-way ANOVA with contrasts).

Additional file 7: Decrease in bile acids and increase in associated metabolites of bile acid biosynthesis at $T_{c,Max}$ and 24–48 hours after heat exposure. (A) Tabulation of bile acids and associated metabolites at $T_{c,Max}$ and 24–48 hours as fold-change from control after heat exposure. **(B)** Circulation of bile acids. **(C)** Trend in bile acid and associated metabolites over time after heat stress. Green cells represent significant decrease. Pink reflects a trending increase and light green represents a trending decrease ($0.05 < p < 0.10$ heat exposed versus control rat, 2-way ANOVA with contrasts); *, $p < 0.05$, 2-way ANOVA with contrasts.

Additional file 8: Change in vitamin B6 cofactor activity at $T_{c,Max}$ and 24–48 hours after heat exposure. (A) Role of vitamin B6 metabolism in amino acid, serotonin/norepinephrine, and sphingolipid synthesis. Trend in **(B)** pyridoxal and **(C)** pyridoxate after heat stress. *, $p < 0.05$, 2-way ANOVA with contrasts.

Abbreviations
7-HOCA: 7-α-hydroxy-3-oxo-4-cholestenoate; AA: Amino acid; acetyl CoA: Acetyl coenzyme A; AHB: 2-hydroxybutyrate; AMP: Adenosine monophosphate; ANOVA: Analysis of variance; ATP: Adenosine triphosphate; GCS: γ-glutamyl cysteine synthase; GGT: γ-glutamyl transferase; GSH: Glutathione; GS: Glutathione synthase; GSSG: Glutathione disulfide, oxidized; KEGG: Kyoto encyclopedia of genes and genomes; MDA: Mean decrease accuracy; NADPH: Nicotinamide adenine dinucleotide phosphate; NO: Nitric oxide; OOB: Out-of-bag; ROS: Reactive oxygenated species; SIRS: System inflammatory response syndrome; $T_{c,Max}$: Maximum core temperature; TCA: Tricarboxylic acid; USACEHR: US Army Center for Environmental Health Research; USAMRMC: US Army Medical Research and Materiel Command; USARIEM: US Army Research Institute of Environmental Medicine.

Competing interests
The authors declare that they have no competing interests to declare. Research was conducted in compliance with the Animal Welfare Act, and other Federal statutes and regulations relating to animals and experiments involving animals and adheres to principles stated in the "Guide for Care and Use of Laboratory Animals" (NRC 2011) as prepared by the Committee on Care and Use of Laboratory Animals of the Institute of Laboratory Animal Resources, National Research Council in facilities that are fully accredited by the Association for Assessment and Accreditation of Laboratory Animal Care, International. The views, opinions, assertions, and/or findings contained herein are those of the authors and should not be construed as official US Department of Defense or Department of the Army position, policy, or decision, unless so designated by other official documentation. Citations of commercial organizations or trade names in this report do not constitute an official Department of the Army endorsement or approval of the products or services of these organizations. This paper has been approved for public release with unlimited distribution. This research was supported in part by an appointment to the Research Participation Program at the US Army Center for Environmental Health Research (USACEHR) administered by the Oak Ridge Institute for Science and Education through an interagency agreement between USACEHR, the US Department of Energy, and the US Army Medical Research and Materiel Command (USAMRMC). The research was supported by the Military Operational Medicine Research Program, USAMRMC, MD.

Authors' contributions
The initiation and conception of this study involved JDS, JAL, and LRL. CY and JAL provided critical methods review, random forest analyses, hierarchical clustering. DLI (overall) and JDS were responsible for writing the manuscript, which was edited by CY, JAL, and LRL. All authors reviewed the final manuscript.

Acknowledgements
We would like to thank Dr. Roy Vigneulle (Military Operational Medicine Research Program), CAPT Carroll D. Forcino (Director, Military Operational Medicine Research Program), Dr. David A. Jackson (Director, Pulmonary Health, USACEHR), and LTC Thomas C. Timmes (current Commander, USACEHR) for their programmatic support, encouragement, and insightful discussion. We also thank Dr. Bryan Helwig, J. Ward, S. Dineen, M. Blaha, and R. Duran for access to biofluids and technical support with the rat heat stress experiments. We thank Dr. Andrea Eckhart and Dr. Rob Mohney from Metabolon, Inc., for the report and data analysis of the metabolomics data.

Author details
[1]The United States Army Center for Environmental Health Research, Environmental Health Program, Bldg. 568 Doughten Drive, Fort Detrick, Frederick, MD 21702-5010, USA. [2]Biotechnology High Performance Computing Software Applications Institute, Frederick, MD 21702-5010, USA. [3]Thermal Mountain Medicine Division, US Army Research Institute of Environmental Medicine, Natick, MA 01760-5007, USA.

References
1. Armed Forces Health Surveillance C: **Update: heat injuries, active component, U.S. Armed Forces, 2013.** *Msmr* 2014, **21**(3):10–13.
2. Wallace RF, Kriebel D, Punnett L, Wegman DH, Wenger CB, Gardner JW, Gonzalez RR: **The effects of continuous hot weather training on risk of exertional heat illness.** *Med Sci Sports Exerc* 2005, **37**(1):84–90.
3. Wallace RF, Kriebel D, Punnett L, Wegman DH, Wenger CB, Gardner JW, Kark JA: **Risk factors for recruit exertional heat illness by gender and training period.** *Aviat Space Environ Med* 2006, **77**(4):415–421.
4. Armed Forces Health Surveillance Center: **Update: heat injuries, active component, U.S. Armed Forces, 2011.** *MSMR* 2012, **19**(3):14–16.
5. Armed Forces Health Surveillance Center: **Update: heat injuries, active component, U.S. Armed Forces, 2012.** *MSMR* 2013, **20**(3):17–20.
6. Merrill CT, Miller M, Steiner C: **Hospital stays resulting from excessive heat and cold exposure due to weather conditions in U.S. Community Hospitals, 2005: statistical brief #55.** In: *Healthcare Cost and Utilization Project (HCUP) Statistical Briefs.* Agency for Health Care Policy and Research (US): Rockville (MD); 2006.
7. United States Army: *Army Regulation 40–501: Standards of Medical Fitness.* 2011. http://www.armypubs.army.mil/epubs/pdf/r40_501.pdf.
8. Liu ZF, Sun XG, Tang J, Tang YQ, Tong HS, Wen Q, Liu YS, Su L: **Intestinal inflammation and tissue injury in response to heat stress and cooling treatment in mice.** *Mol Med Rep* 2011, **4**(3):437–443.
9. Leon LR: **The thermoregulatory consequences of heat stroke: are cytokines involved?** *J Therm Biol* 2006, **31**(1–2):67–81.
10. Leon LR, Helwig BG: **Heat stroke: role of the systemic inflammatory response.** *J Appl Physiol* 2010, **109**(6):1980–1988.
11. Leon LR, Helwig BG: **Role of endotoxin and cytokines in the systemic inflammatory response to heat injury.** *Front Biosci* 2010, **2**:916–938.
12. Zeller L, Novack V, Barski L, Jotkowitz A, Almog Y: **Exertional heatstroke: clinical characteristics, diagnostic and therapeutic considerations.** *Eur J Intern Med* 2011, **22**(3):296–299.
13. Zhou FH, Song Q, Peng ZY, Pan L, Kang HJ, Tang S, Yue H, Liu H, Xie F: **Effects of continuous venous-venous hemofiltration on heat stroke patients: a retrospective study.** *J Trauma-Injury Infect Crit Care* 2011, **71**(6):1562–1568.
14. Grosman B, Shaik OS, Helwig BG, Leon LR, Doyle FJ: **A physiological systems approach to modeling and resetting of mouse thermoregulation under heat stress.** *J Appl Physiol* 2011, **111**(3):938–945.
15. Leon LR, Dineen SM, Clarke DC: **Early Activation of liver apoptotic signaling pathways during heat stroke recovery in mice.** *Faseb J* 2013, **27**:1201.7
16. Leon LR, Duran RM, Helwig BG: **Complementing heat stroke: activation and amplification of the IL-6 and complement system during heat stroke recovery in F344 rats.** *Faseb J* 2013, **27**:1201.6.
17. Leon LR, Eustis HL, Urso ML: **Skeletal muscle is a potential source of cytokines during heat stroke recovery in mice.** *Faseb J* 2012, **26**:1084.17.
18. Rakesh V, Stallings JD, Helwig BG, Leon LR, Jackson DA, Reifman J: **A 3-D mathematical model to identify organ-specific risks in rats during thermal stress.** *J Appl Physiol* 2013, **115**(12):1822–1837.
19. Stallings JD, Ippolito DL, Rakesh V, Baer CE, Dennis WE, Helwig BG, Jackson DA, Leon LR, Lewis JA, Reifman J: **Patterns of gene expression associated with recovery and injury in heat-stressed rats.** *BMC Genomics* 2014, **15**(1):1058.
20. Malmendal A, Overgaard J, Bundy JG, Sorensen JG, Nielsen NC, Loeschcke V, Holmstrup M: **Metabolomic profiling of heat stress: hardening and recovery of homeostasis in Drosophila.** *Am J Physiol Regul Integr Comp Physiol* 2006, **291**(1):R205–R212.
21. Quinn CM, Duran RM, Audet GN, Charkoudian N, Leon LR: **Cardiovascular and thermoregulatory biomarkers of heat stroke severity in a conscious rat model.** *J Appl Physiol* 2014, **117**(9):971–978.
22. Stasolla C, Loukanina N, Yeung EC, Thorpe TA: **Alterations in pyrimidine nucleotide metabolism as an early signal during the execution of programmed cell death in tobacco BY-2 cells.** *J Exp Bot* 2004, **55**(408):2513–2522.
23. Piskur J, Schnackerz KD, Andersen G, Bjornberg O: **Comparative genomics reveals novel biochemical pathways.** *Trends Genet* 2007, **23**(8):369–372.
24. Lu Z, Zhang R, Diasio RB: **Dihydropyrimidine dehydrogenase activity in human peripheral blood mononuclear cells and liver: population characteristics, newly identified deficient patients, and clinical implication in 5-fluorouracil chemotherapy.** *Cancer Res* 1993, **53**(22):5433–5438.
25. van Lenthe H, van Kuilenburg AB, Ito T, Bootsma AH, van Cruchten A, Wada Y, van Gennip AH: **Defects in pyrimidine degradation identified by HPLC-electrospray tandem mass spectrometry of urine specimens or urine-soaked filter paper strips.** *Clin Chem* 2000, **46**(12):1916–1922.

26. Kolker S, Okun JG, Horster F, Assmann B, Ahlemeyer B, Kohlmuller D, Exner-Camps S, Mayatepek E, Krieglstein J, Hoffmann GF: **3-Ureidopropionate contributes to the neuropathology of 3-ureidopropionase deficiency and severe propionic aciduria: a hypothesis.** *J Neurosci Res* 2001, **66**(4):666–673.

27. Kellogg DL Jr, Crandall CG, Liu Y, Charkoudian N, Johnson JM: **Nitric oxide and cutaneous active vasodilation during heat stress in humans.** *J Appl Physiol* 1998, **85**(3):824–829.

28. Ray PD, Huang BW, Tsuji Y: **Reactive Oxygen Species (ROS) homeostasis and redox regulation in cellular signaling.** *Cell Signal* 2012, **24**(5):981–990.

29. Hall DM, Baumgardner KR, Oberley TD, Gisolfi CV: **Splanchnic tissues undergo hypoxic stress during whole body hyperthermia.** *Am J Physiol* 1999, **276**(5 Pt 1):G1195–G1203.

30. Wu G, Fang YZ, Yang S, Lupton JR, Turner ND: **Glutathione metabolism and its implications for health.** *J Nutr* 2004, **134**(3):489–492.

31. Lim CL, Wilson G, Brown L, Coombes JS, Mackinnon LT: **Pre-existing inflammatory state compromises heat tolerance in rats exposed to heat stress.** *Am J Physiol Regul Integr Comp Physiol* 2007, **292**(1):R186–R194.

32. Meaney S, Babiker A, Lutjohann D, Diczfalusy U, Axelson M, Bjorkhem I: **On the origin of the cholestenoic acids in human circulation.** *Steroids* 2003, **68**(7–8):595–601.

33. Moccand C, Boycheva S, Surriabre P, Tambasco-Studart M, Raschke M, Kaufmann M, Fitzpatrick TB: **The pseudoenzyme PDX1.2 boosts vitamin B6 biosynthesis under heat and oxidative stress in Arabidopsis.** *J Biol Chem* 2014, **289**(12):8203–8216.

34. Trachootham D, Lu W, Ogasawara MA, Nilsa RD, Huang P: **Redox regulation of cell survival.** *Antioxid Redox Signal* 2008, **10**(8):1343–1374.

35. Nelson DL, Lehninger AL, Cox MM: *Lehninger Principles of Biochemistry.* W. H. Freeman and Company New York, NY; 2008.

36. Colleuori DM, Ash DE: **Classical and slow-binding inhibitors of human type II arginase.** *Biochemistry* 2001, **40**(31):9356–9362.

37. Derave W, Everaert I, Beeckman S, Baguet A: **Muscle carnosine metabolism and beta-alanine supplementation in relation to exercise and training.** *Sports Med* 2010, **40**(3):247–263.

38. Evans DA: **N-acetyltransferase.** *Pharmacol Ther* 1989, **42**(2):157–234.

39. Ezaki J, Matsumoto N, Takeda-Ezaki M, Komatsu M, Takahashi K, Hiraoka Y, Taka H, Fujimura T, Takehana K, Yoshida M, Iwata J, Tanida I, Furuya N, Zheng DM, Tada N, Tanaka K, Kominami E, Ueno T: **Liver autophagy contributes to the maintenance of blood glucose and amino acid levels.** *Autophagy* 2011, **7**(7):727–736.

40. Gathiram P, Wells MT, Brockutne JG, Gaffin SL: **Prophylactic corticosteroid increases survival in experimental heat-stroke in primates.** *Aviat Space Environ Med* 1988, **59**(4):352–355.

41. Hofmann AF, Molino G, Milanese M, Belforte G: **Description and simulation of a physiological pharmacokinetic model for the metabolism and enterohepatic circulation of bile acids in man. cholic acid in healthy man.** *J Clin Invest* 1983, **71**(4):1003–1022.

42. Amelio D, Garofalo F, Capria C, Tota B, Imbrogno S: **Effects of temperature on the nitric oxide-dependent modulation of the Frank-Starling mechanism: the fish heart as a case study.** *Comp Biochem Physiol A Mol Integr Physiol* 2013, **164**(2):356–362.

43. Waagner D, Heckmann LH, Malmendal A, Nielsen NC, Holmstrup M, Bayley M: **Hsp70 expression and metabolite composition in response to short-term thermal changes in Folsomia candida (Collembola).** *Comp Biochem Physiol A Mol Integr Physiol* 2010, **157**(2):177–183.

44. Zakir HA, Subbarao GV, Pearse SJ, Gopalakrishnan S, Ito O, Ishikawa T, Kawano N, Nakahara K, Yoshihashi T, Ono H, Yoshida M: **Detection, isolation and characterization of a root-exuded compound, methyl 3-(4-hydroxyphenyl) propionate, responsible for biological nitrification inhibition by sorghum (Sorghum bicolor).** *New Phytol* 2008, **180**(2):442–451.

45. Inoue T, Kobayashi K, Inoguchi T, Sonoda N, Maeda Y, Hirata E, Fujimura Y, Miura D, Hirano K, Takayanagi R: **Downregulation of adipose triglyceride lipase in the heart aggravates diabetic cardiomyopathy in db/db mice.** *Biochem Biophys Res Commun* 2013, **438**(1):224–229.

46. Kasiganesan H, Wright GL, Chiacchio MA, Gumina G: **Novel l-adenosine analogs as cardioprotective agents.** *Bioorg Med Chem* 2009, **17**(14):5347–5352.

47. Hecker PA, Leopold JA, Gupte SA, Recchia FA, Stanley WC: **Impact of glucose-6-phosphate dehydrogenase deficiency on the pathophysiology of cardiovascular disease.** *Am J Physiol Heart Circ Physiol* 2013, **304**(4):H491–H500.

48. Beyoglu D, Imbeaud S, Maurhofer O, Bioulac-Sage P, Zucman-Rossi J, Dufour JF, Idle JR: **Tissue metabolomics of hepatocellular carcinoma: tumor energy metabolism and the role of transcriptomic classification.** *Hepatology* 2013, **58**(1):229–238.

49. Sharma S, Aramburo A, Rafikov R, Sun X, Kumar S, Oishi PE, Datar SA, Raff G, Xoinis K, Kalkan G, Fratz S, Fineman JR, Black SM: **L-carnitine preserves endothelial function in a lamb model of increased pulmonary blood flow.** *Pediatr Res* 2013, **74**(1):39–47.

50. Strauss M, Anselmi G, Hermoso T, Tejero F: **Carnitine promotes heat shock protein synthesis in adriamycin-induced cardiomyopathy in a neonatal rat experimental model.** *J Mol Cell Cardiol* 1998, **30**(11):2319–2325.

51. Sun X, Sharma S, Fratz S, Kumar S, Rafikov R, Aggarwal S, Rafikova O, Lu Q, Burns T, Dasarathy S, Wright J, Schreiber C, Radman M, Fineman JR, Black SM: **Disruption of endothelial cell mitochondrial bioenergetics in lambs with increased pulmonary blood flow.** *Antioxid Redox Signal* 2013, **18**(14):1739–1752.

52. Dai BH, Geng L, Wang Y, Sui CJ, Xie F, Shen RX, Shen WF, Yang JM: **microRNA-199a-5p protects hepatocytes from bile acid-induced sustained endoplasmic reticulum stress.** *Cell Death Dis* 2013, **4**:e604.

53. Ejiri S, Eguchi Y, Kishida A, Ishigami F, Kurumi Y, Tani T, Kodama M: **Cellular distribution of thrombomodulin as an early marker for warm ischemic liver injury in porcine liver transplantation: protective effect of prostaglandin I2 analogue and tauroursodeoxycholic acid.** *Transplantation* 2001, **71**(6):721–726.

54. Ferreira M, Coxito PM, Sardao VA, Palmeira CM, Oliveira PJ: **Bile acids are toxic for isolated cardiac mitochondria: a possible cause for hepatic-derived cardiomyopathies?** *Cardiovasc Toxicol* 2005, **5**(1):63–73.

55. Gao X, Fu L, Xiao M, Xu C, Sun L, Zhang T, Zheng F, Mei C: **The nephroprotective effect of tauroursodeoxycholic acid on ischaemia/reperfusion-induced acute kidney injury by inhibiting endoplasmic reticulum stress.** *Basic Clin Pharmacol Toxicol* 2012, **111**(1):14–23.

56. Panda S, Biswas S, Kar A: **Trigonelline isolated from fenugreek seed protects against isoproterenol-induced myocardial injury through down-regulation of Hsp27 and alphaB-crystallin.** *Nutrition* 2013, **29**(11–12):1395–1403.

57. Stott WT, Kleinert KM: **Effect of diisopropanolamine upon choline uptake and phospholipid synthesis in Chinese hamster ovary cells.** *Food Chem Toxicol* 2008, **46**(2):761–766.

58. Khatri P, Sirota M, Butte AJ: **Ten years of pathway analysis: current approaches and outstanding challenges.** *PLoS Comput Biol* 2012, **8**(2):e1002375.

59. Rakesh V, Stallings JD, Reifman J: **A virtual rat for simulating environmental and exertional heat stress.** *J Appl Physiol* 2014, **117**(11):1278–1286.

60. Davies B, Morris T: **Physiological parameters in laboratory animals and humans.** *Pharm Res* 1993, **10**(7):1093–1095.

61. Bartel J, Krumsiek J, Theis FJ: **Statistical methods for the analysis of high-throughput metabolomics data.** *Comput Struct Biotechnol J* 2013, **4**:e201301009.

62. Breiman L: **Using iterated bagging to debias regressions.** *Mach Learn* 2001, **45**(3):261–277.

63. Goldstein BA, Hubbard AE, Cutler A, Barcellos LF: **An application of random forests to a genome-wide association dataset: methodological considerations & new findings.** *BMC Genet* 2010, **11**:49.

cAMP-stimulated Cl⁻ secretion is increased by glucocorticoids and inhibited by bumetanide in semicircular canal duct epithelium

Satyanarayana R Pondugula[1], Suresh B Kampalli[1], Tao Wu[1], Robert C De Lisle[2], Nithya N Raveendran[1], Donald G Harbidge[1] and Daniel C Marcus[1*]

Abstract

Background: The vestibular system controls the ion composition of its luminal fluid through several epithelial cell transport mechanisms under hormonal regulation. The semicircular canal duct (SCCD) epithelium has been shown to secrete Cl⁻ under β_2-adrenergic stimulation. In the current study, we sought to determine the ion transporters involved in Cl⁻ secretion and whether secretion is regulated by PKA and glucocorticoids.

Results: Short circuit current (I_{sc}) from rat SCCD epithelia demonstrated stimulation by forskolin (EC_{50}: 0.8 μM), 8-Br-cAMP (EC_{50}: 180 μM), 8-pCPT-cAMP (100 μM), IBMX (250 μM), and RO-20-1724 (100 μM). The PKA activator N6-BNZ-cAMP (0.1, 0.3 & 1 mM) also stimulated I_{sc}. Partial inhibition of stimulated I_{sc} individually by bumetanide (10 & 50 μM), and [(dihydroindenyl)oxy]alkanoic acid (DIOA, 100 μM) were additive and complete. Stimulated I_{sc} was also partially inhibited by CFTR$_{inh}$-172 (5 & 30 μM), flufenamic acid (5 μM) and diphenylamine-2,2'-dicarboxylic acid (DPC; 1 mM). Native canals of CFTR$^{+/-}$ mice showed a stimulation of I_{sc} from isoproterenol and forskolin+IBMX but not in the presence of both bumetanide and DIOA, while canals from CFTR$^{-/-}$ mice had no responses. Nonetheless, CFTR$^{-/-}$ mice showed no difference from CFTR$^{+/-}$ mice in their ability to balance (rota-rod). Stimulated I_{sc} was greater after chronic incubation (24 hr) with the glucocorticoids dexamethasone (0.1 & 0.3 μM), prednisolone (0.3, 1 & 3 μM), hydrocortisone (0.01, 0.1 & 1 μM), and corticosterone (0.1 & 1 μM) and mineralocorticoid aldosterone (1 μM). Steroid action was blocked by mifepristone but not by spironolactone, indicating all the steroids activated the glucocorticoid, but not mineralocorticoid, receptor. Expression of transcripts for CFTR; for KCC1, KCC3a, KCC3b and KCC4, but not KCC2; for NKCC1 but not NKCC2 and for WNK1 but only very low WNK4 was determined.

Conclusions: These results are consistent with a model of Cl⁻ secretion whereby Cl⁻ is taken up across the basolateral membrane by a Na⁺-K⁺-2Cl⁻ cotransporter (NKCC) and potentially another transporter, is secreted across the apical membrane via a Cl⁻ channel, likely CFTR, and demonstrate the regulation of Cl⁻ secretion by protein kinase A and glucocorticoids.

Keywords: Chloride secretion, Rat, Knockout mouse, Primary culture, Epithelium, Inner ear, Bumetanide, DIOA, Glucocorticoid, NKCC, KCC

---

* Correspondence: marcus@vet.k-state.edu
[1]Dept. Anatomy & Physiology, Cellular Biophysics Laboratory, Kansas State University, Manhattan, KS 66506, USA
Full list of author information is available at the end of the article

Background

The inner ear controls the ion composition of its luminal fluid, endolymph, through a multiplicity of transepithelial transport mechanisms in different cell types bounding the lumen. The high-K^+, low Na^+, low Ca^{2+} endolymph composition is needed for proper auditory and vestibular function [1-3]. K^+ secretion by both strial marginal cells and vestibular dark cells is stimulated by β-adrenergic receptors via cytosolic cAMP as second messenger [4,5]. Secretion of the primary anion, Cl^-, is known to also be under adrenergic control in semicircular canal duct (SCCD) epithelium [6].

Cl^- transport by several epithelia has been shown to be under control of a cAMP signal pathway that is mediated by apical CFTR Cl^- channels via protein kinase A (PKA) [7]. Vectorial transport in those epithelia depends also on basolateral Na^+-K^+-ATPase and K^+ channels as well as basolateral Cl transporters such as the Na^+-K^+-$2Cl^-$ cotransporter (NKCC1/Slc12a2) [6,8-10]. Cellular cAMP levels and cAMP-mediated processes, including ion transport, depend on cAMP metabolism regulated by the enzymatic activity of anabolic adenylyl cyclase and catabolic phosphodiesterase [11-13].

Glucocorticoids can modify cellular responses via genomic and non-genomic pathways, including regulation of ion transport processes [14-17]. Na^+ absorption by SCCD has already been demonstrated to be stimulated by glucocorticoids [17,18]. There is considerable evidence in various tissues, including epithelia, that glucocorticoids have long-term (genomic) effects on cAMP metabolism and potentiate cAMP-mediated responses, including ion transport by activation of the glucocorticoid receptor [19-21].

We therefore sought to determine in SCCD a) whether there is a basal constitutive adenylyl cyclase activity driving cAMP-mediated Cl^- secretion, b) whether Cl^- secretion is enhanced by glucocorticoid hormones via activation of glucocorticoid receptors, c) whether Cl^- secretion is mediated through PKA action and d) whether Cl^- secretion is mediated by a basolateral NKCC and/or KCC and an apical CFTR Cl^- channel. Our findings establish that the SCCD is a site in the inner ear for PKA-mediated Cl^- transport, that this transport depends on NKCC1 and another Cl^- uptake process (perhaps KCC), that apical CFTR is likely involved and that it is enhanced by glucocorticoid-receptor activation.

Results

Adenylyl cyclase activator, cAMP analogs, and phosphodiesterase inhibitors stimulate I_{sc}

The SCCD epithelium actively contributes to endolymph homeostasis by Cl^- secretion under control of $β_2$-adrenergic receptors via a cAMP pathway [6], like other epithelia that are known to secrete Cl^- upon stimulation by β-adrenergic

receptor activation [22-26]. Forskolin (adenylyl cyclase activator) [6] (Figure 1A & B), cell permeable cAMP analogs (8-Br-cAMP and 8-pCPT-cAMP [100 μM]) (Figure 2A & B), the non-selective phosphodiesterase inhibitor 3-isobutyl-1-methylxanthine (IBMX; 250 μM) (Figure 2C), and the cAMP-specific phosphodiesterase-4 (PDE4) inhibitor RO-20-1724 (100 μM) (Figure 2D) increased I_{sc} in the presence of apical amiloride (10 μM), an inhibitor of the epithelial Na^+ channel. The maximal forskolin-stimulated I_{sc} was 0.58 ± 0.06 μA/cm2 (n=38) (Figure 1B). In the present series of experiments (Figures 2B,C,D), amiloride produced no significant changes in I_{sc} in the absence of steroids, although in a previous larger series of experiments there was a small (15%) but significant decrease in I_{sc} [17]. The initial

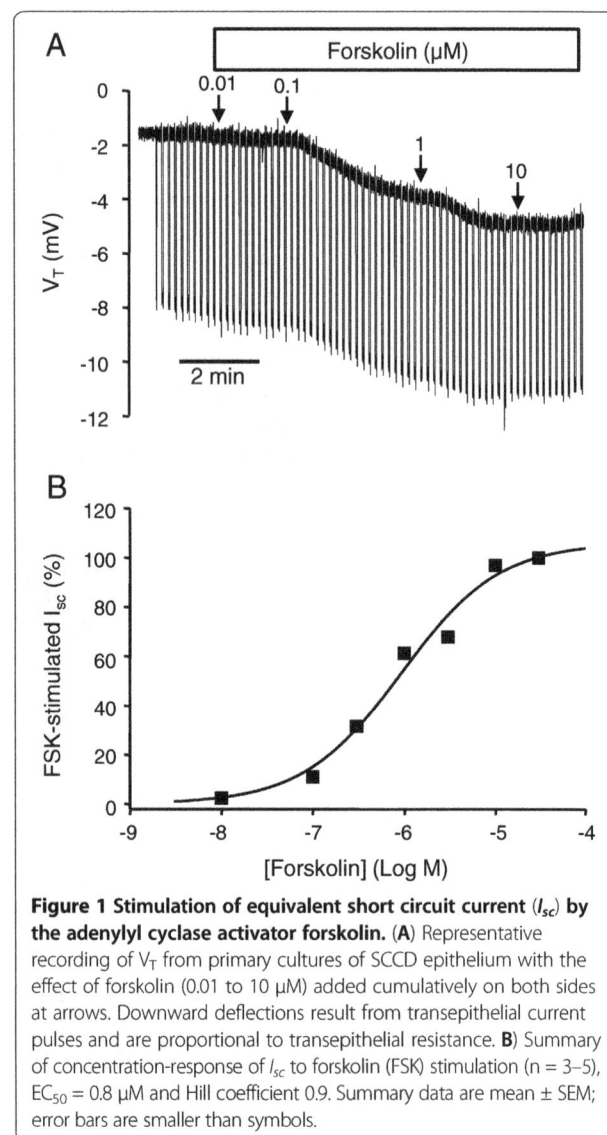

Figure 1 Stimulation of equivalent short circuit current (I_{sc}) by the adenylyl cyclase activator forskolin. (A) Representative recording of V_T from primary cultures of SCCD epithelium with the effect of forskolin (0.01 to 10 μM) added cumulatively on both sides at arrows. Downward deflections result from transepithelial current pulses and are proportional to transepithelial resistance. **B)** Summary of concentration-response of I_{sc} to forskolin (FSK) stimulation (n = 3–5), EC_{50} = 0.8 μM and Hill coefficient 0.9. Summary data are mean ± SEM; error bars are smaller than symbols.

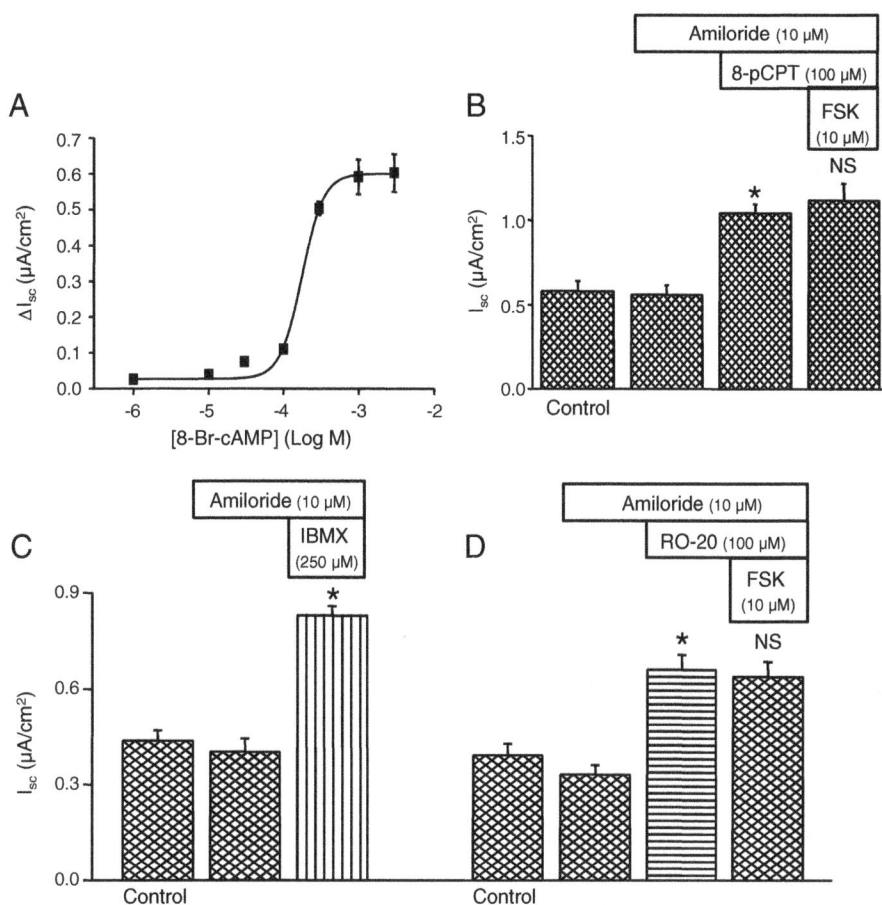

Figure 2 Membrane-permeable cAMP analogs and phosphodiesterase inhibitors increase I_{sc}. A) Summary of concentration-response of I_{sc} to 8-Br-cAMP (n = 3–4) on both sides after prior application of 10 μM apical amiloride, EC_{50} = 180 μM and Hill coefficient 3.0. **B)** Summary of response of I_{sc} to 8-pCPT-cAMP (8-pCPT; 100 μM; n = 4) on both sides in the presence of apical amiloride (10 μM); no further stimulation by subsequent forskolin (FSK, 10 μM). **C)** Summary of response of I_{sc} to 3-isobutyl-1-methylxanthine (IBMX; 250 μM; n = 3) on both sides and **D)** RO-20-1720 (RO-20; 100 μM; n = 3) on both sides after prior application of apical amiloride (10 μM). Summary data are mean ± SEM; *, P < 0.05; NS, not significant; compared to bar immediately to the left.

transepithelial resistance (Figure 1B) was 4.7 ± 0.6 kΩ-cm^2 (n=3) and decreased significantly with 30 μM forskolin to 3.1 ± 0.3 kΩ-cm^2 (n=3).

The lipid-soluble drugs forskolin, 8-pCPT-cAMP, RO-20-1724, 3-isobutyl-1-methylxanthine (IBMX), were added to both the apical and basolateral baths. Amiloride was added to only the apical side and bumetanide to the basolateral side. Amiloride had no significant effect on I_{sc}, whereas subsequent addition of both forskolin (Figure 1) and 8-Br-cAMP (Figure 2A) increased I_{sc} in a concentration dependent manner with an EC_{50} of about 0.8 μM and 180 μM respectively. Forskolin showed no additional effect after prior stimulation by either 8-pCPT-cAMP (100 μM) (Figure 2B) or by RO-20-1724 (100 μM) (Figure 2D), demonstrating constitutive activity of adenylyl cyclase in SCCD epithelium.

Glucocorticoids increase forskolin-stimulated I_{sc}

We investigated whether forskolin-stimulated Cl⁻ secretion was altered by glucocorticoid treatment (24 hr). As in the absence of dexamethasone, increasing intracellular cAMP in dexamethasone-treated epithelia by exposure to 8-pCPT-cAMP in the presence of amiloride (10 μM) led to an increased I_{sc} (representative recording in Figure 3). Similar responses were seen with forskolin (10 μM), 8-Br-cAMP (100 μM) and IBMX (250 μM) (data not shown). The glucocorticoid-stimulated Na⁺ absorption via apical sodium channels (ENaC) was blocked by amiloride, which decreased I_{sc} by 81 − 92% [17]; the remaining current was due to Cl⁻ secretion [6].

The concentration-dependence of natural and synthetic glucocorticoids was determined (Figure 4). Interestingly, the stimulation by forskolin was significantly

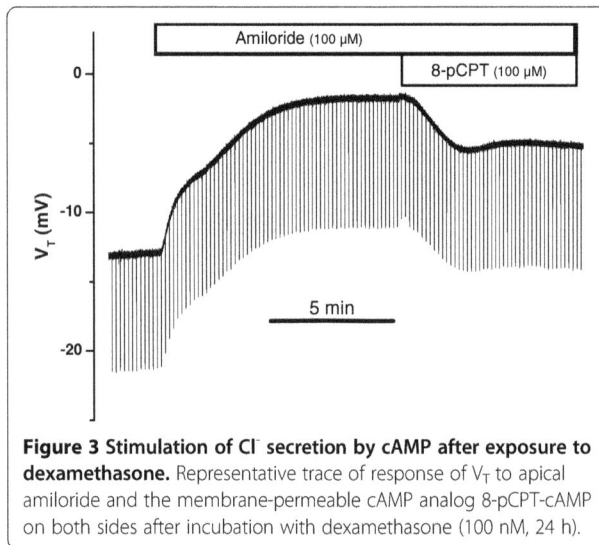

Figure 3 Stimulation of Cl⁻ secretion by cAMP after exposure to dexamethasone. Representative trace of response of V_T to apical amiloride and the membrane-permeable cAMP analog 8-pCPT-cAMP on both sides after incubation with dexamethasone (100 nM, 24 h).

greater after treatment with 100 or 300 nM dexamethasone, as observed previously with single concentrations of dexamethasone and forskolin [17]. Similarly, the stimulation of I_{sc} by forskolin was significantly greater after 24 hr treatment with the other glucocorticoids (hydrocortisone, corticosterone, and prednisolone) and the mineralocorticoid aldosterone in the continued presence of amiloride (Figure 4). The transepithelial resistance was significantly reduced by about one third after exposure to effective concentrations of glucocorticoids (ANOVA analysis of Table two in [17]), as would be expected after insertion of a conductive pathway (epithelial sodium channels) in the apical membrane.

The natural and synthetic glucocorticoids stimulated within their respective physiologic and therapeutic ranges [17], while aldosterone was only effective at concentrations much higher than found under normal physiologic conditions [17].

Glucocorticoids increase forskolin-stimulated I_{sc} by activation of glucocorticoid receptor

We investigated whether dexamethasone, hydrocortisone, and aldosterone increased FSK-stimulated I_{sc} by activation of glucocorticoid receptors and/or mineralocorticoid receptors. SCCD epithelia were incubated in the presence of dexamethasone (100 nM), hydrocortisone (1 μM) or aldosterone (1 μM) alone or in the presence of receptor antagonists. Mifepristone significantly reduced the effects of dexamethasone, hydrocortisone and aldosterone (Figure 4A,D,E), consistent with action of all of these corticosteroids at the glucocorticoid receptor. Mifepristone is also known to be an antagonist of the progesterone receptor; however, progesterone (10–1000 nM) had no effect on forskolin stimulation (Figure 4F). The mineralocorticoid receptor antagonist spironolactone had no significant effect on dexamethasone-, hydrocortisone- or

aldosterone-treated epithelia (Figure 4A,D,E), consistent with a lack of involvement of mineralocorticoid receptor in the increase of the FSK-stimulated I_{sc} in these cells. These findings suggest that corticosteroids increase forskolin-stimulated I_{sc} (cAMP-mediated Cl⁻ secretion) solely by activation of glucocorticoid receptors in SCCD epithelia.

PKA activator stimulates I_{sc}

It is known that cAMP-dependent Cl⁻ secretion in many epithelia is mostly mediated through activation of protein kinase A (PKA) [7]. We therefore investigated whether PKA activation increases I_{sc} in SCCD. Indeed, apical and basolateral addition of PKA activator N6-BNZ-cAMP stimulated I_{sc} at 30, 100, 300 and 1000 μM after prior inhibition of Na⁺ transport with apical amiloride (10 μM) (Figure 5).

Blockers of basolateral Na⁺-K⁺-2Cl⁻ and K⁺-Cl⁻ cotransporters inhibit forskolin and/or forskolin + IBMX-stimulated I_{sc}

We have previously shown that both Ba²⁺-sensitive K⁺ channels and ouabain-sensitive Na⁺-K⁺-ATPase are involved in Cl⁻ secretion by SCCD [6]. However, the participation of Na⁺-K⁺-2Cl⁻ and K⁺-Cl⁻ cotransporters is not known. Therefore, we investigated whether these transport proteins are involved in cAMP-mediated Cl⁻ secretion. Untreated and dexamethasone (100 nM; 24 hr)-treated SCCD epithelia were stimulated with apical and basolateral forskolin and forskolin + IBMX respectively, followed by application of blockers of ion transporters to the basolateral side. Na⁺-K⁺-2Cl⁻ cotransporter inhibitor bumetanide (50 μM) partially decreased the magnitude of forskolin (5 μM) + IBMX (125 μM)-stimulated I_{sc} (Figure 6A). Bumetanide (10 & 50 μM) also decreased the forskolin (10 μM)-stimulated I_{sc} by 20 ± 2% (10 μM; n = 8) and 18 ± 5% (50 μM; n = 3) (data not shown). Similarly, the K⁺-Cl⁻ cotransporter blocker [(dihydroindenyl)oxy]alkanoic acid (DIOA, 100 μM) partially inhibited the forskolin + IBMX-stimulated I_{sc} (Figure 6B). Interestingly, DIOA and bumetanide, when added to the bath cumulatively, completely inhibited all of the forskolin + IBMX-stimulation, returning I_{sc} to the level observed with amiloride (Figure 6C). These findings are consistent with the presence of Na⁺-K⁺-2Cl⁻ and K⁺-Cl⁻ cotransporters at the basolateral membrane and their participation in Cl⁻ secretion by SCCD epithelium, although DIOA is lipophilic and could cross to a KCC on the apical membrane. However, the observed effect is not likely a result of action of DIOA on an apical KCC since transport of Cl⁻ by an apical KCC would also result in a similar rate of K⁺ secretion, and no transepithelial K⁺ (Rb⁺) flux was detected from cAMP-stimulated SCCD [6].

Expression of KCC and WNK isoforms

Additive inhibition of I_{sc} by bumetanide and DIOA suggested dependence of electrogenic Cl⁻ transport in SCCD

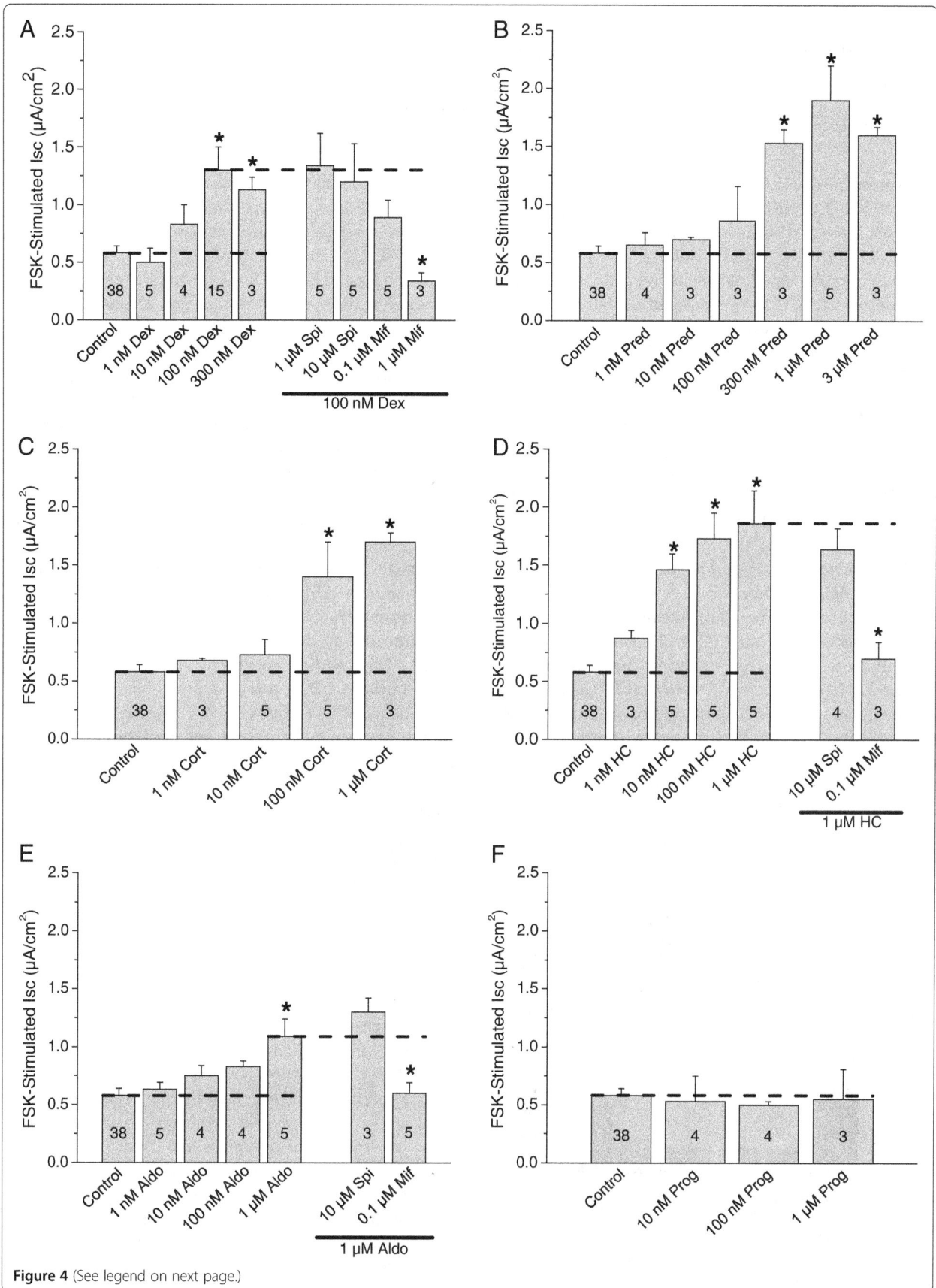

Figure 4 (See legend on next page.)

(See figure on previous page.)
Figure 4 Response of forskolin-stimulated I_{sc} to corticosteroids. Summary data of responses to forskolin (10 μM) after incubation (24 h) in steroids or steroids + receptor antagonists at the concentrations shown. **A)** dexamethasone (Dex) ± spironolactone (Spi) or mifepristone (mif); **B)** prednisolone (Pred); **C)** corticosterone (Cort); **D)** hydrocortisone (HC) ± spironolactone (Spi) or mifepristone (mif); **E)** aldosterone (Aldo) ± spironolactone (Spi) or mifepristone (mif); **F)** progesterone (Prog). The horizontal dashed lines show the reference levels for statistical comparisons.

on expression of NKCC and KCC. The basolateral isoform of NKCC, (NKCC1/Slc12a2 Affymetrix probe set 1367853_at), was shown to be present in a gene array of SCCD and the apical isoform (NKCC2/Slc12a1 Affymetrix probe set 1368548_at) is absent [27]. Not all isoforms of KCC were identified on the gene chips; we tested for expression of transcripts with RT-PCR and observed expression of KCC1, KCC3a, KCC3b and KCC4; but, KCC2 was absent (Table 1).

It is known that genetic mutations in the kinase WNK1 and WNK4 cause a disease featuring hypertension and hyperkalemia and the etiology appears to be related to regulation of NKCC and KCC (reviewed in [49]). We observed that SCCD expresses WNK1 but only very low or absent WNK4 (Table 2).

Blockers of apical Cl⁻ transport inhibit forskolin and/or forskolin + IBMX-stimulated I_{sc}

Cl⁻ secretion across the apical membrane in many epithelia is mediated by the CFTR Cl⁻ channel [8,10]. Na⁺ currents were blocked by amiloride (100 μM) in dexamethasone (100 nM, 24 hr)-treated SCCD epithelia. I_{sc} was then stimulated with apical and basolateral forskolin (5 μM) + IBMX (125 μM), followed by apical addition of blockers of Cl⁻ transporters. Non-selective Cl⁻ channel inhibitors DPC (1 mM) and flufenamic acid (5 μM) (Figure 7A) partially inhibited the stimulated I_{sc}. The CFTR Cl⁻ channel blocker CFTR$_{inh}$-172 (5 μM or 30 μM)

[28] partially inhibited the forskolin (10 μM) and forskolin (5 μM) + IBMX (125 μM)-stimulated I_{sc} in both the absence and presence of dexamethasone (100 nM, 24 hr; Figure 7B, *left* and *right* panels). Taken together, these results suggest that CFTR Cl⁻ channels are functionally expressed at the apical membrane and account for at least part of the Cl⁻ secretion by SCCD epithelium, although CFTR appears to not be essential for vestibular function under normative conditions (see below). The observation of the presence of mRNA transcripts of CFTR in gene arrays of rat primary cultures (Affymetrix Probe set 1384960_at [27]) is consistent with that interpretation.

SCCD from CFTR⁺/⁻ mice showed an increase in response of I_{sc} to a β₂-adrenergic receptor agonist isoproterenol (100 nM) and a mixture of forskolin and IBMX (Figure 8, *top panel*). Heterozygous CFTR mice are known to have an ion transport profile similar to wild-type mice [29]. A mixture of DIOA (KCC inhibitor) and bumetanide (NKCC inhibitor) completely inhibited the increased I_{sc} by forskolin + IBMX (Figure 8, *top panel*). This result is consistent with the results shown above in rat SCCD primary cultures (Figure 6C). On the other hand, SCCD from CFTR⁻/⁻ mice lacked response to both isoproterenol (10 μM) and a mixture of forskolin and IBMX, suggesting that all of the cAMP-stimulated I_{sc} is mediated by, or dependent on, CFTR in mouse SCCD (Figure 8, *top panel*). The vestibular functional phenotype, as assessed by Rota-Rod, of the CFTR⁻/⁻ mice did not differ significantly from the CFTR⁺/⁻ mice (Figure 8, *bottom panel*), in spite of the profound difference in stimulated I_{sc} (above).

Discussion

Sensory transduction of acceleration in the vestibular labyrinth is mediated by modulation of K⁺ currents through sensory cells, where the K⁺ originates from the high-[K⁺] luminal fluid. Secretion of K⁺ is controlled by β-adrenergic stimulation (among other signal pathways) [30,31] and it is to be expected that secretion of the primary anion would also be regulated by the same agonists. Movements of anions would be expected to be transcellular since the paracellular pathway must be extremely tight in this epithelium to support the large ion concentration gradients. Cl⁻ secretion by the semicircular canal duct (SCCD) in the vestibular labyrinth is stimulated by cAMP as second messenger [6] and similar mechanisms have been proposed in the cochlea [32,33],

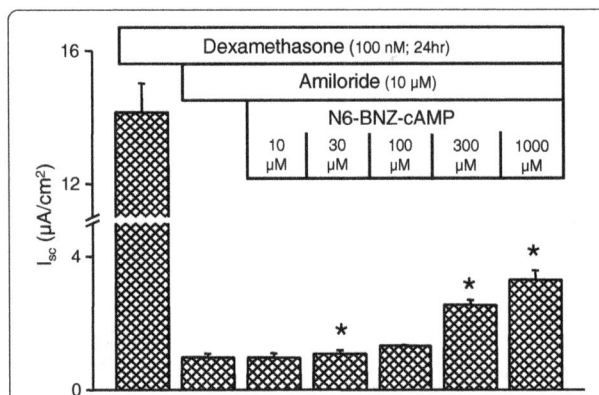

Figure 5 PKA activation of I_{sc}. Summary of response of I_{sc} to the PKA activator N6-BNZ-cAMP (n = 3) after treatment with dexamethasone in the presence of apical amiloride (10 μM). Summary data are mean ± SEM; *, P < 0.05; compared to bar prior to addition of activator. Note a break in the Y-axis.

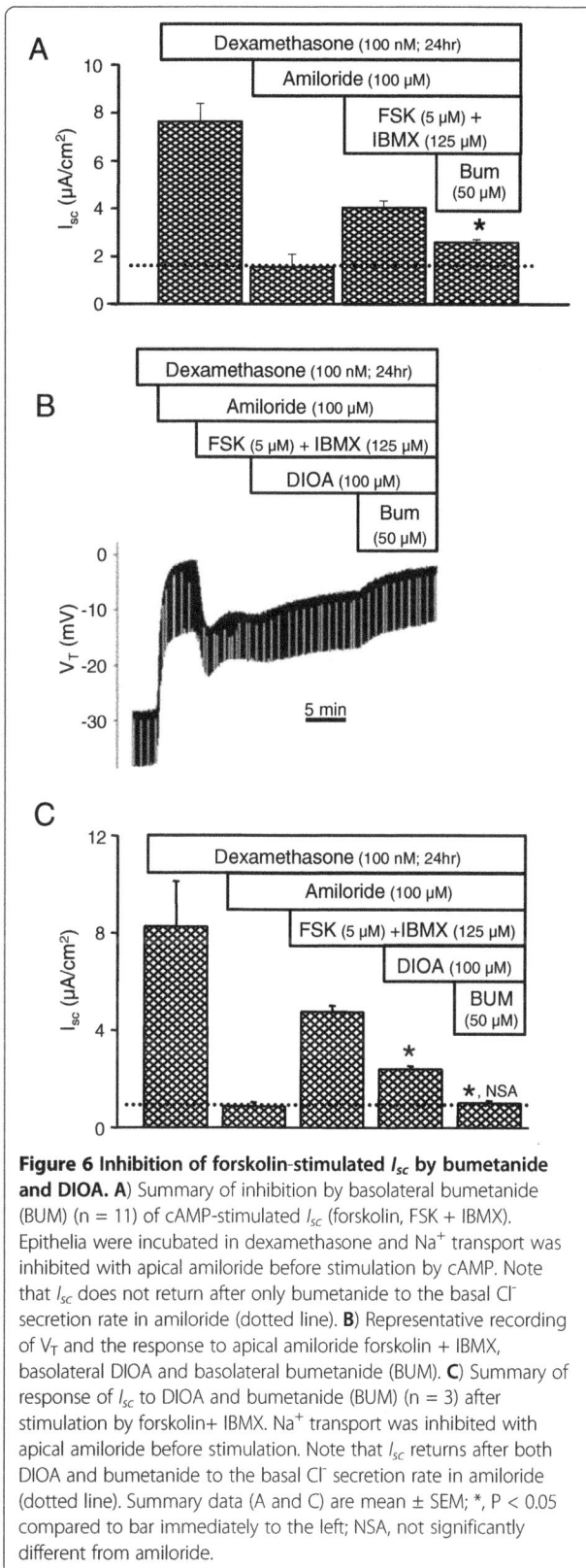

Figure 6 Inhibition of forskolin-stimulated I_{sc} by bumetanide and DIOA. A) Summary of inhibition by basolateral bumetanide (BUM) (n = 11) of cAMP-stimulated I_{sc} (forskolin, FSK + IBMX). Epithelia were incubated in dexamethasone and Na^+ transport was inhibited with apical amiloride before stimulation by cAMP. Note that I_{sc} does not return after only bumetanide to the basal Cl⁻ secretion rate in amiloride (dotted line). **B**) Representative recording of V_T and the response to apical amiloride forskolin + IBMX, basolateral DIOA and basolateral bumetanide (BUM). **C**) Summary of response of I_{sc} to DIOA and bumetanide (BUM) (n = 3) after stimulation by forskolin+ IBMX. Na^+ transport was inhibited with apical amiloride before stimulation. Note that I_{sc} returns after both DIOA and bumetanide to the basal Cl⁻ secretion rate in amiloride (dotted line). Summary data (A and C) are mean ± SEM; *, P < 0.05 compared to bar immediately to the left; NSA, not significantly different from amiloride.

Table 1 RT-PCR demonstration of the presence of KCC1, KCC3a, KCC3b, KCC4 and absence of KCC2 in rat SCCD primary cultures

Tissue	18S	KCC1	KCC2	KCC3a	KCC3b	KCC4
			Ct, average			
rSCCD		26.4	BT	25.0	27.3	26.7
rat kidney	14.2	25.9	–	23.3	24.5	26.3
rat brain	–	–	22.6	–	–	–
blank	35.0	30.2	BT	BT	32.3	35.8

BT, Below Threshold fluorescence at end of 38 thermocycles. Ct values are based on duplicate runs of 4 samples SCCD and duplicates of control tissue total RNA. The difference between Ct values of duplicates varied by 0.3 ± 0.04 (n=26) with a range from 0.0 to 0.8.

although the cell types responsible in the cochlea have not yet been unambiguously determined (see [34]).

The SCCD is an epithelial domain that has a high ratio of surface area to endolymph volume and would therefore be a strong candidate for a site of effective ion homeostasis. Indeed, it was recently shown that these cells also absorb Na^+ via the epithelial sodium channel (ENaC) under glucocorticoid receptor control [17,18] and absorb Ca^{2+} via an epithelial Ca^{2+} channel [35], in addition to their role in Cl⁻ secretion.

We determined in the present study that cAMP acts via PKA, whose target may be an apical CFTR Cl channel [6]. Evidence supporting the involvement of CFTR include inhibition of Cl⁻ secretion (cAMP-stimulated I_{sc}) by the poorly-specific inhibitors flufenamic acid and DPC and by the specific inhibitor CFTR$_{inh}$-172. Partial inhibition in rSCCD by CFTR$_{inh}$-172 is consistent with reports of significant but only partial inhibition in avian proximal tubule at 20 μM [36]. In addition, mRNA message for CFTR was found to be present in the rat primary cultures of SCCD (GEO database, Accession GSE6196, [27]). The observation of cAMP-stimulated I_{sc} in mouse canals extends the findings in gerbil and rat [6] to another rodent species. The absence of cAMP-stimulated I_{sc} in CFTR knockout mice is consistent with an essential role of CFTR in canal Cl⁻ secretion, although there is no strict proof ruling out the unlikely occurrence of dissection damage to only the knockout mouse canals.

Table 2 RT-PCR demonstration of the presence of WNK1 and absence of WNK4 in rat SCCD primary cultures

Tissue	18S	WNK1	WNK4
rSCCD	13.4	24.7	31.6
rat kidney	14.7	25.0	26.0
blank	34.4	BT	35.2

Ct, average. BT, Below Threshold fluorescence at end of 38 thermocycles. Ct values are based on duplicate runs of 4 samples SCCD and duplicates of rat kidney as a control tissue. The difference between Ct values of duplicates varied by 0.6 ± 0.09 (n=36) with a range from 0.0 to 2.1.

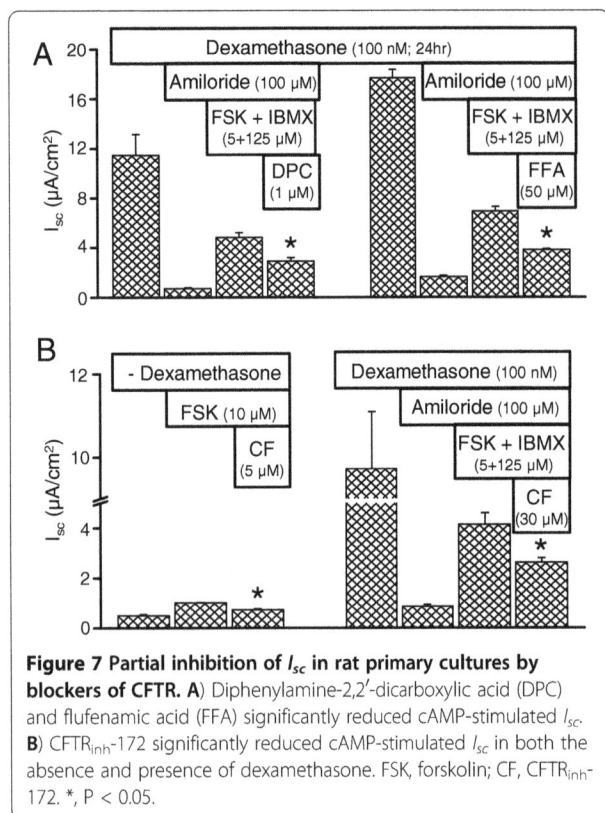

Figure 7 Partial inhibition of I_{sc} in rat primary cultures by blockers of CFTR. A) Diphenylamine-2,2'-dicarboxylic acid (DPC) and flufenamic acid (FFA) significantly reduced cAMP-stimulated I_{sc}. **B)** CFTR$_{inh}$-172 significantly reduced cAMP-stimulated I_{sc} in both the absence and presence of dexamethasone. FSK, forskolin; CF, CFTR$_{inh}$-172. *, P < 0.05.

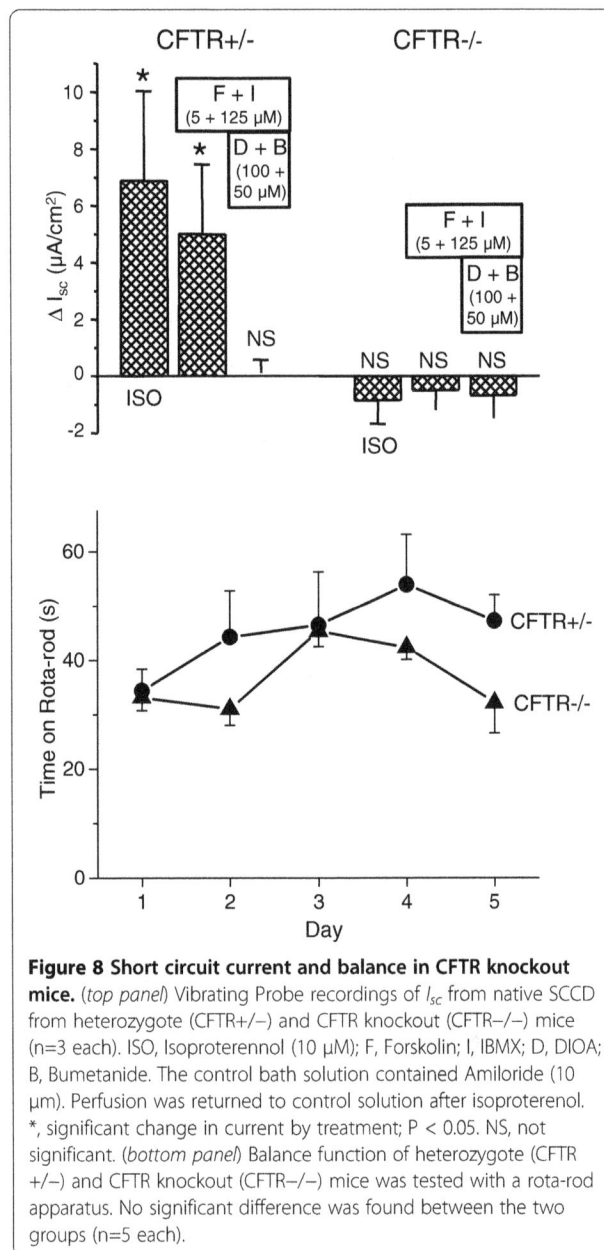

Figure 8 Short circuit current and balance in CFTR knockout mice. (*top panel*) Vibrating Probe recordings of I_{sc} from native SCCD from heterozygote (CFTR+/−) and CFTR knockout (CFTR−/−) mice (n=3 each). ISO, Isoproterennol (10 μM); F, Forskolin; I, IBMX; D, DIOA; B, Bumetanide. The control bath solution contained Amiloride (10 μm). Perfusion was returned to control solution after isoproterenol. *, significant change in current by treatment; P < 0.05. NS, not significant. (*bottom panel*) Balance function of heterozygote (CFTR +/−) and CFTR knockout (CFTR−/−) mice was tested with a rota-rod apparatus. No significant difference was found between the two groups (n=5 each).

Interestingly, there is no correlation of deafness in persons with dysfunctional CFTR (cystic fibrosis) [37,38] and no reports of vertigo in this population. Our results with vestibular tests of CFTR knockout mice are consistent with that observation. It may be, however, that this anion transport system is not by itself essential for normal inner ear function, but may be necessary in times of systemic stress when β-adrenergic agonist levels are elevated, but this proposition remains to be tested.

The results here demonstrated increased I_{sc} by stimulation of the cAMP signal pathway in several ways: through increased cAMP production (forskolin stimulation of adenylyl cyclase), addition of exogenous cAMP analogs (8-Br-cAMP and 8-pCPT-cAMP), and inhibition of cAMP catabolism (IBMX and RO-20-1724 inhibition of phosphodiesterase). The action of all of these agents has been well-documented in other cells [11-13,19-21]. Increased Cl⁻ secretion by inhibition of phosphodiesterase implies that the adenylyl cyclase is constitutively active in the SCCD epithelium in the absence of β-adrenergic agonists, and is therefore consistent with the earlier observation of constitutive low-level Cl⁻ secretion [6]. Stimulation of Cl⁻ secretion has been reported in mouse jejunum, guinea pig distal colon, T84 monolayers and human colonic epithelial cells by phosphodiesterase inhibition [39-42]. Of particular interest is the finding that phosphodiesterase inhibition did not elevate Cl⁻

secretion in the absence of exogenous stimulation of adenylyl cyclase in T84 epithelial monolayers [41]. This is in contradistinction to our observations in rat semicircular canal primary cultures (vide infra and [6]).

The responsiveness of adenylyl cyclase and phosphodiesterase to multiple physiological challenges is related to the presence of multiple families of isoforms with tissue-specific localization [11-13]. Ten isoforms of adenylyl cyclase (AC; membranous AC1-9 and soluble AC) have been identified in mammalian cells [11]. In SCCD, the non-selective adenylyl cyclase activator forskolin, which is known to activate all identified adenylyl cyclase isoforms with varying sensitivity [11,43,44], stimulated Cl⁻ secretion. Gene array results showed expression of transcripts for AC2 and AC4 in SCCD among the genes that were tested (AC2, AC3, AC4, AC5, AC6, and AC8) using Affymetrix Rat Genome 230 2.0 Array chips [27]. However, it is not known whether other isoforms that were not represented on the gene array are expressed in SCCD.

Eleven families of phosphodiesterases (PDE1 to PDE11) have been identified in mammalian cells, with each family having several isoforms [13]. Phosphodiesterases show three types of substrate specificity [13]. The PDE4, PDE7, and PDE8 families hydrolyze cAMP specifically. PDE5, PDE6, and PDE9 are cGMP specific and PDE1, PDE2, PDE3, PDE10, and PDE11 are dual substrate phosphodiesterases i.e. they hydrolyze both cAMP and cGMP. In SCCD, both the non-selective phosphodiesterase inhibitor IBMX and the selective PDE4 inhibitor RO-20-1724 [19] stimulated Cl⁻ secretion. Gene array results showed expression of the transcripts for PDE4 and PDE7 isoforms but not PDE8 in SCCD [27]. Expression of PDE4 at the transcript level is consistent with RO-20-1724 stimulation of I_{sc}.

Glucocorticoids are known to affect cAMP metabolism and potentiate cAMP-mediated responses, including salt and water transport by activation of the glucocorticoid receptor [16,19-21]. It is known that glucocorticoids stimulate anion transport, including Cl⁻ in mammalian ileal mucosa, by increasing the concentration of cyclic nucleotides [16]. Glucocorticoids elevate cellular cAMP levels by regulating the activity of both adenylyl cyclases and phosphodiesterases, predominantly by suppressing the activity of phosphodiesterases [19,20]. It is not known if glucocorticoids increase cAMP-mediated Cl⁻ secretion in SCCD epithelium by a similar mechanism.

Glucocorticoids increase cAMP-mediated Cl⁻ secretion in SCCD epithelium by activation of exclusively the glucocorticoid receptor. However, the exact mechanism of potentiation of cAMP response is not known. The stimulation of cAMP-mediated I_{sc} could not have been a result of the increase in glucocorticoid-activated ENaC function [17], since increased Na⁺ conductance would depolarize the cell, which in turn would reduce the outward driving force for Cl⁻ across the apical membrane, in contrast to observations. In addition, Na⁺ absorption was blocked by amiloride in these experiments. Another putative mechanism of action of glucocorticoids in SCCD is regulation of NKCC expression, as observed in vascular smooth muscle and trabecular meshwork cells [45,46]. However, there was no change in expression of NKCC1 in SCCD after incubation with 100 nM dexamethasone for 24 h [27]. The molecular mechanism for glucocorticoid-increased cAMP-mediated Cl⁻ secretion in SCCD epithelium has not yet been resolved.

One pathway of corticosteroid action is via the kinases SGK1 and WNK1 [47] among other kinases involved in regulation of ion transport such as SPAK and OSR1 [48]. Our gene array of rat SCCD cultures [27] showed SPAK or Stk39 to be present (1387059_at based on Genbank NM_019362) and minimally down-regulated 1.2-fold by dexamethasone. There were no probe sets identified on the chips for OSR1. WNK1 is downstream from SGK1 and is implicated in the control of both NKCC and KCC transporters and thereby their roles in Cl⁻ transport [49]. The expression of WNK1 in the SCCD may therefore be involved in the regulation of Cl⁻ secretion in SCCD through these two transporters. The transcript expression for WNK4 was nearly absent.

Complete additive inhibition of the cAMP-stimulated I_{sc} by bumetanide and DIOA is consistent with the participation of both Na⁺-K⁺-2Cl⁻ and K⁺-Cl⁻ cotransporter in Cl⁻ cotransport. The concentration of bumetanide used fully inhibits NKCC1 but has no effect on KCC1 and KCC4 [50,51]. Similarly, DIOA is a potent well-established KCC transport inhibitor (IC50 = 10–40 μM) that is without effect on NKCC [52,53] and has been used as a specific KCC inhibitor in the range 30 – 100 μM [53-55]. However, DIOA has also been observed in several epithelia to have diverse effects [56-59].

The canonical interpretation that the effect of DIOA is a result of inhibition of a KCC, however, is problematic. Foremost, the KCC would be operating "backwards" from its most-commonly observed mode and if this were indeed the case it would necessitate an extremely low intracellular [Cl⁻]. A low intracellular concentration of the secreted ion species (Cl⁻) would not favor a strong efflux across the apical membrane. Although most cells operate KCC transporters as cellular *efflux* pathways, Payne calculates that some neuronal cells have sufficiently-low intracellular [Cl⁻] to thermodynamically drive *influx* of KCl [60]. The membrane potential, intracellular [K⁺] and [Cl⁻] of SCCD epithelial cells is not known, so it is not possible at this time to evaluate whether these cells are able to support concurrent basolateral KCC electroneutral influx and apical electrogenic Cl⁻ secretion. The discussion by Payne [60] shows that at the normal extracellular [K⁺] of about 4 mM, the intracellular [Cl⁻] would need to be about 5 mM or less; a highly unlikely constellation. An elevation of extracellular [K⁺] at the canal epithelium due to hair cell stimulation is also highly unlikely since the hair cells are located remotely from the canals and excess K⁺ would be removed from perilymph by vestibular dark cells recycling the K⁺ back into the lumen.

The observation that basolateral bumetanide causes only a partial inhibition of cAMP-stimulated Cl⁻ secretion at 50 μM suggests the existence of a parallel Cl⁻ uptake mechanism. Block of the remaining secretion by DIOA points to a KCC, subject to the caveats given above. An alternative explanation is that DIOA is not a specific inhibitor for KCC in SCCD and either blocks another Cl⁻ uptake mechanism that operates under thermodynamically-favorable conditions or acts broadly on active transport through inhibition of metabolic processes. This last suggestion has been observed with another lipid-soluble weak acid, the Cl⁻ channel blocker NPPB, restricting its use to <100 μM [61]. In addition, DIOA has been shown to interfere with ATP recovery after metabolic insult and to release cytochrome c from isolated mitochondria at the concentration used here [62]. Nonetheless, if this is the basis for action of DIOA in the semicircular canal epithelium, the metabolic interference is not complete (Figure 6) and the likely involvement of a parallel Cl⁻ uptake pathway in rat canal remains.

In summary, our results are consistent with the following cell transport model of regulated Cl⁻ secretion by SCCD (Figure 9). A basolateral Na⁺-K⁺-ATPase removes Na⁺ from the cell and brings in K⁺, which is energized by ATP. The resulting Na⁺ concentration gradient drives the basolateral influx of K⁺ and Cl⁻ along with the recirculating Na⁺ ions via the bumetanide-sensitive NKCC1. Cl⁻ would be secreted across the apical membrane through Cl⁻ channels that may include CFTR as a channel or transport modulator. The rate of secretion is controlled by glucocorticoids and β₂-adrenergic signalling via cAMP and PKA.

Conclusions

The rat semicircular canal duct epithelium expresses three major ion transport systems, including a β₂-adrenergic receptor-stimulated Cl⁻ secretion [6]. We have demonstrated here that Cl⁻ secretion is under control of a PKA-mediated signal pathway that depends on

basolateral Cl⁻ uptake via NKCC and (KCC?) transporters and that it is enhanced by activation of glucocorticoid receptors. Interestingly, NKCC does not appear to contribute to ENaC-mediated Na⁺ absorption [17] in the same cells. The role of the β₂-adrenergic receptor/cAMP pathway in inner ear function remains unknown but is likely activated under stress.

Methods

All experiments were performed on primary cultures of rat SCCD, except the measurements of short circuit current from native canals and vestibular function that were performed on CFTR mutant mice.

Cell cultures of rat SCCD epithelium

Primary cultures of neonatal Wistar rat SCCD epithelium were produced as described previously [6]. Briefly, animals were anesthetized and sacrificed according to a protocol approved by the Kansas State University Institutional Animal Care and Use Committee. SCCD epithelial cells were microdissected from isolated temporal bones. Isolated cells, exclusive of connective tissue and common crus, were seeded on 6.5 mm diameter permeable (4 μm) Costar (#3470) Transwell supports and cultured in DMEM/F12 medium (Invitrogen 12500–062; http://www.invitrogen.com/site/us/en/home/support/Product-Technical-Resources/media_formulation.60.html) supplemented with 5% fetal bovine serum, 26.8 mM NaHCO₃, penicillin (100 U/ml) and streptomycin (100 μg/ml). Cultures treated with steroids, in the

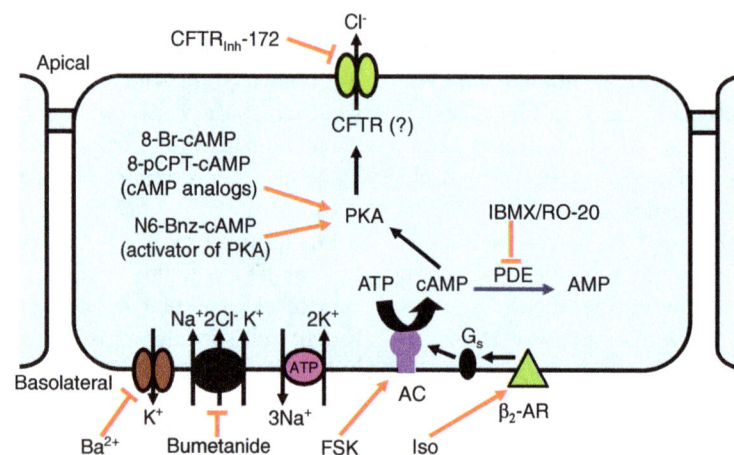

Figure 9 Proposed cell model for cAMP/PKA-mediated Cl⁻ secretion by SCCD epithelium. Cl⁻ is taken up across the basolateral membrane by NKCC (Na⁺-K⁺-2Cl⁻ cotransporter). A Na⁺-K⁺-ATPase and Ba²⁺-sensitive K⁺ conductance in the basolateral membrane is thought to create a negative cell membrane potential that drives Cl⁻ exit across the apical membrane via a Cl⁻ channel, likely CFTR. Cl⁻ secretion is stimulated by PKA from activation of a basolateral β₂-adrenergic receptor (β₂-AR; activated by agonists such as isoproterenol, ISO) coupled to a cAMP second messenger pathway (Gₛ-protein activation of adenylyl cyclase (AC) which can also be directly activated by forskolin (FSK). Phosphodiesterase (PDE) catabolizes cAMP and can be inhibited by IBMX and RO-20-1720 (RO-20). The cAMP-dependent Cl⁻ secretion pathway is further stimulated by activation of intracellular glucocorticoid receptors (not shown) after chronic exposure to glucocorticosteroids.

presence and absence of antagonists, were exposed for 24 h unless otherwise stated.

Reagents

Amiloride (#A-7410, Sigma), forskolin (#F-6886, Sigma), spironolactone (#S-3378, Sigma), mifepristone (#M-8046, Sigma), corticosterone (#C-2505, Sigma), prednisolone (#6004, Sigma), bumetanide (#B-3023, Sigma), RO-20-1724 (#557502, Calbiochem), 3-isobutyl-1-methylxanthine (IBMX; #I-7018, Sigma), flufenamic acid (#F-9005, Sigma), CFTR $_{inh}$-172 ([28](gift from Dr. Bruce Schultz), and [(dihydroindenyl) oxy]alkanoic acid (DIOA; # D-129, Sigma) were dissolved in DMSO. Progesterone (#P-8783, Sigma), and aldosterone (#215360050, Acros Organics, New Jersey) were dissolved in absolute ethanol. DMSO or ethanol alone had no effect on electrical parameters in Ussing chamber experiments.

Cyclodextrin-encapsulated dexamethasone (#D-2915, Sigma), hydrocortisone (#H-0396, Sigma), isoproterenol (#I-6504, Sigma), 8-Br-cAMP (#203800, Calbiochem), 8-pCPT-cAMP (#C-3912, Sigma), and N^6-Benzoyl-Adenosine 3',5'-cyclic Monophosphate, Sodium Salt (N6-BNZ-cAMP; #116802, Calbiochem) were dissolved in water.

Mice breeding and maintenance

CFTR heterozygous parents in a C57BL/6 background were bred and the offspring were genotyped for $CFTR^{+/+}$, $CFTR^{+/-}$ or $CFTR^{-/-}$ All the animals were maintained on Colyte in water to avoid intestinal impaction [63].

Dissection of mouse SCCD

$CFTR^{+/-}$ and $CFTR^{-/-}$ mice (34–39 days old) [63] were anesthetized with sodium pentobarbital (50–100 mg/kg; i.p.) and sacrificed under a protocol approved by the Institutional Animal Care and Use Committee of Kansas State University. The temporal bones were removed and SCCD without common crus were dissected in HEPES-buffered saline. The SCCD were mounted in a 200 µl perfusion chamber on the stage of an inverted microscope (Nikon ECLIPSE TE 300) and continuously perfused at 37°C with HEPES-buffed solution at an exchange rate of 180 µl/sec.

Electrophysiological measurements

I_{sc} from Primary cultures of rat SCCD

SCCD epithelia were bathed in HEPES-buffered solution equilibrated with air. The composition was (in mM) 150 NaCl, 3.6 KCl, 1 $MgCl_2$, 0.7 $CaCl_2$, 5 glucose, and 10 HEPES, pH 7.4. Transepithelial voltage (V_T) and resistance (R_T) were measured from confluent monolayers of SCCD in an Ussing chamber under current clamp ($\Delta I = 1$ µA) mode as described previously [17,18]. The equivalent I_{sc} was calculated from $I_{sc} = V_T/R_T$. I_{sc} was measured either in the absence of steroids (Figure 1, 2, 7B *left*) or after 24 h incubation with steroid. Steroid-stimulated Na^+ current was blocked with amiloride before measurement of cAMP-stimulated I_{sc}. Cytosolic cAMP levels were raised by stimulation of adenylyl cyclase with forskolin, block of phosphodiesterase with IBMX or RO-20-1724 or a combination of forskolin and IBMX,

Table 3 Gene-specific primers

Gene	Primers 5′—3′	GenBank # (species)	Amplicon size (bp)	Source
18S	S: GAG GTT CGA AGA CGA TCA GA	BK000964 (many)	316	[65]
	AS: TCG CTC CAC CAA CTA AGA AC			
KCC1	S: GTT CGC CTC ACT CTT CCT GGC	U55815 (rat)	419	[66]
	AS: TGG GCC ACC ACA TAC AGG GA			
KCC2	S: CAT CAC AGA TGA ATC TCG GG	U55816 (rat)	213	[66]
	AS: TTC TCT GGG TCT GTC TCC C			
KCC3a	S: CCT CGC CTC CTC ACC TTT GC	AF211854 (mouse)	284	This study
	AS: TCA CTC TGA CGC CAG CCA TTG			
KCC3b	S: AGT AAA AGC CCG GAT TCA GG	AF211855 (mouse)	330	[66]
	AS: ATG AAA GTA CCC ATT TGG GG			
KCC4	S: AGG AAG CTG CTG AGC GCA C	AF087436 (mouse)	443	[66]
	AS: CAG CAT TGT ACA GGT GCA GC			
WNK1	S: ACC AGA AAG CCT CAT GTA AGC C	NM_053794 (rat)	301	This study
	AS: GTC CGC AGG GAA CGT CAT TG			
WNK4	S: CAC CTC CCG CCG CAA CAG	NM_175579 (rat)	347	This study
	AS: TCC ACA CAG CAA AGA GCA CCC			

Primers designed on mouse sequences also specifically recognized and amplified the corresponding rat genes. All primer sets were validated to specifically recognize their targets.

as indicated. The lipid-soluble drugs dexamethasone, hydrocortisone, aldosterone, forskolin, 8-pCPT-cAMP, N6-BNZ-cAMP, spironolactone, mifepristone, corticosterone, prednisolone, progesterone and [(dihydroindenyl) oxy]alkanoic acid (DIOA) were added to both the apical and basolateral baths. Amiloride was added to only the apical side and bumetanide to the basolateral side.

I_{sc} from mouse native canal ducts; Voltage-sensitive vibrating probe recordings

The vibrating probe technique was identical to that previously described [34,64]. Briefly, the current density was monitored from mouse SCCD by vibrating (200–400 Hz) a platinum-iridium wire microelectrode with a platinum-black tip positioned 20 μm from the basolateral surface of the SCCD with computer-controlled stepper-motor manipulators (Applicable Electronics, Forest Dale, MA) and probe software (ASET version 2.00, Science Wares, East Falmouth, MA). The bath references were 26-gauge Pt-black electrodes. The phase-locked signal from the electrode was detected by phase-sensitive amplifiers, digitized y (0.5 Hz, 16 bit), and the output was expressed as current density at the electrode. HEPES-buffered solution was used as the bath.

Vestibular function test

4 sets of littermate-matched CFTR$^{+/-}$ and CFTR$^{-/-}$ mice (mean age = 56 d) were tested 4 times/day (with a five minute rest between tests) over five days. The RotaRod (Series 8, IITC, Woodland Hills, CA) used a 32 mm diameter rod and was programmed to start at 4 RPM, increasing to 40 RPM over 1 minute. All mice were placed on the rod before rotation was initiated and the time until falling was recorded. The instrument was modified by placing a landing cushion on the platform of the timer stop switch. The daily mean time for each mouse was used to calculate the mean and standard error of each group. After the last run of each day, all homozygous mice were given a 1 ml saline injection to prevent dehydration.

RNA isolation and RT-PCR

Total RNA was extracted from SCCD primary cultures using RNeasy Micro Kit and the quality and quantity were determined as described previously [18]. RT-PCR was performed on total RNA as described previously using a One Step RT-PCR Kit following the manufacturer's protocol (#210210, Qiagen) [18].

Gene-specific primers for KCC and WNK isoforms were based on GenBank sequences (Table 3) and were verified to amplify the intended targets. Reverse transcription (RT) was performed on 10 ng of total RNA for 30 min at 50°C and 15 min at 95°C. RT was followed by 38 PCR cycles. Each PCR cycle consisted of 95°C for 1

min, 55°C for 1 min and 72°C for 1 min. To exclude the possibility of genomic DNA amplification during the PCR reaction, RT negative controls were performed (−RT). PCR products were run on 2% agarose gels and detected by ethidium bromide. Purified PCR products were sequenced to verify the identity of the RT- PCR products.

Statistical analyses

Electrophysiology data are presented as original recordings and as mean values ± SE from n observations. Student's t-test was used to determine statistical significance of paired and unpaired samples. The Hill equation was fitted to concentration-response curves by using individual data points in order to retain appropriate weighting and presented here plotted with the mean and SEM. Differences were considered significant for $P < 0.05$.

Competing interests
The authors declare that they have no competing interests.

Authors' contributions
SRP contributed to the design and analysis of the experiments, to performance of many of the electrophysiological measurements and to writing the manuscript. SBK contributed to the design and analysis of the experiments, and to performance of many of the electrophysiological measurements. TW performed the vibrating probe experiments on the CFTR mutant mice. RCD provided the CFTR mutant mice and consulted on their breeding, care and genotyping. NNR designed PCR primers and performed the RT-PCR measurements. DGH contributed to the electrophysiological measurements. DCM contributed to the design and analysis of the experiments and to writing the manuscript. All authors read and approved the final manuscript.

Authors' information
Current address for SRP: 112 Greene Hall, Department of Anatomy, Physiology and Pharmacology, College of Veterinary Medicine, Auburn University, Auburn, AL 36849.

Acknowledgements
This work was supported by NIH-NIDCD grant R01-DC00212 and NIH-NCRR grant P20-RR017686 to DCM and by the Cystic Fibrosis Foundation to RCD. Publication of this article was funded in part by the Kansas State University Open Access Publishing Fund. We thank Dr. Bruce Schultz for the gift of CFTR$_{inh}$-172.

Author details
^{1}Dept. Anatomy & Physiology, Cellular Biophysics Laboratory, Kansas State University, Manhattan, KS 66506, USA. ^{2}Dept. Anatomy & Cell Biology, University of Kansas Medical Center, Kansas City, KS 66160, USA.

References
1. Marcus DC, Acoustic Transduction, In Cell Physiology Source Book: *Acoustic Transduction*. San Diego: Academic Press: Essentials of Membrane Biophysics. Edited by Sperelakis N; 2012:649–668.
2. Marcus DC, Wangemann P, In The Oxford Handbook of Auditory Science: *Inner ear fluid homeostasis*. Oxford: Oxford University Press: The Ear. Edited by Fuchs PA; 2010:213–230.
3. Marcus DC, Wangemann P, In Physiology and Pathology of Chloride Transporters and Channels in the Nervous System--From molecules to diseases: *Cochlear and Vestibular Function and Dysfunction*. New York: Elsevier: Edited by Alvarez-Leefmans FJ, Delpire E; 2009:425–437.

4. Sunose H, Liu J, Shen Z, Marcus DC: cAMP increases apical I_{sK} channel current and K^+ secretion in vestibular dark cells. *J Membr Biol* 1997, **156**:25–35.

5. Sunose H, Liu J, Shen Z, Marcus DC: cAMP increases K^+ secretion via activation of apical I_{sK}/KvLQT1 channels in strial marginal cells. *Hear Res* 1997, **114**:107–116.

6. Milhaud PG, Pondugula SR, Lee JH, Herzog M, Lehouelleur J, Wangemann P, Sans A, Marcus DC: Chloride secretion by semicircular canal duct epithelium is stimulated via b2-adrenergic receptors. *Am J Physiol, Cell Physiol* 2002, **283**:C1752–C1760.

7. Bradbury NA: cAMP signaling cascades and CFTR: is there more to learn? *Pflugers Arch* 2001, **443**(Suppl 1):S85–S91.

8. Hryciw DH, Guggino WB: Cystic fibrosis transmembrane conductance regulator and the outwardly rectifying chloride channel: a relationship between two chloride channels expressed in epithelial cells. *Clin Exp Pharmacol Physiol* 2000, **27**:892–895.

9. Schultz BD, Singh AK, Devor DC, Bridges RJ: Pharmacology of CFTR chloride channel activity. *Physiol Rev* 1999, **79**:S109–S144.

10. Kurihara K, Nakanishi N, Moore-Hoon ML, Turner RJ: Phosphorylation of the salivary Na^+-K^+-2Cl$^-$ cotransporter. *Am J Physiol, Cell Physiol* 2002, **282**:C817–C823.

11. Sunahara RK, Dessauer CW, Gilman AG: Complexity and diversity of mammalian adenylyl cyclases. *Annu Rev Pharmacol Toxicol* 1996, **36**:461–480.

12. Cooper DM: Regulation and organization of adenylyl cyclases and cAMP. *Biochem J* 2003, **375**:517–529.

13. Wheeler MA, Ayyagari RR, Wheeler GL, Weiss RM: Regulation of cyclic nucleotides in the urinary tract. *J Smooth Muscle Res* 2005, **41**:1–21.

14. Dagenais A, Denis C, Vives MF, Girouard S, Masse C, Nguyen T, Yamagata T, Grygorczyk C, Kothary R, Berthiaume Y: Modulation of alpha-ENaC and alpha$_1$-Na^+-K^+-ATPase by cAMP and dexamethasone in alveolar epithelial cells. *Am J Physiol Lung Cell Mol Physiol* 2001, **281**:L217–L230.

15. Wehling M: Specific, nongenomic actions of steroid hormones. *Annu Rev Physiol* 1997, **59**:365–393.

16. Sellin JH, Field M: Physiologic and pharmacologic effects of glucocorticoids on ion transport across rabbit ileal mucosa in vitro. *J Clin Invest* 1981, **67**:770–778.

17. Pondugula SR, Sanneman JD, Wangemann P, Milhaud PG, Marcus DC: Glucocorticoids stimulate cation absorption by semicircular canal duct epithelium via epithelial sodium channel. *Am J Physiol Renal Physiol* 2004, **286**:F1127–F1135.

18. Pondugula SR, Raveendran NN, Ergonul Z, Deng Y, Chen J, Sanneman JD, Palmer LG, Marcus DC: Glucocorticoid Regulation of Genes in the Amiloride-Sensitive Sodium Transport Pathway by Semicircular Canal Duct Epithelium of Neonatal Rat. *Physiol Genomics* 2006, **24**:114–123.

19. Yingling JD, Fuller LZ, Jackson BA: Modulation of cyclic AMP metabolism by glucocorticoids in PC18 cells. *J Neurochem* 1994, **63**:1271–1276.

20. Jackson BA, Braun-Werness JL, Kusano E, Dousa TP: Concentrating defect in the adrenalectomized rat. Abnormal vasopressin-sensitive cyclic adenosine monophosphate metabolism in the papillary collecting duct. *J Clin Invest* 1983, **72**:997–1004.

21. Plee-Gautier E, Grober J, Duplus E, Langin D, Forest C: Inhibition of hormone-sensitive lipase gene expression by cAMP and phorbol esters in 3T3-F442A and BFC-1 adipocytes. *Biochem J* 1996, **318**(Pt 3):1057–1063.

22. Reddy MM, Bell CL: Distinct cellular mechanisms of cholinergic and beta-adrenergic sweat secretion. *Am J Physiol* 1996, **271**:C486–C494.

23. Chan HC, Liu CQ, Fong SK, Law SH, Wu LJ, So E, Chung YW, Ko WH, Wong PY: Regulation of Cl$^-$ secretion by extracellular ATP in cultured mouse endometrial epithelium. *J Membr Biol* 1997, **156**:45–52.

24. Barker PM, Brigman KK, Paradiso AM, Boucher RC, Gatzy JT: Cl$^-$ secretion by trachea of CFTR (+/–) and (–/–) fetal mouse. *Am J Respir Cell Mol Biol* 1995, **13**:307–313.

25. Liu W, Sato Y, Hosoda Y, Hirasawa K, Hanai H: Effects of higenamine on regulation of ion transport in guinea pig distal colon. *Jpn J Pharmacol* 2000, **84**:244–251.

26. Reinach P, Holmberg N: Inhibition of calcium of beta adrenoceptor mediated cAMP responses in isolated bovine corneal epithelial cells. *Curr Eye Res* 1989, **8**:85–90.

27. Pondugula SR, Raveendran NN, Marcus DC: Ion transport regulation by P2Y receptors, protein kinase C and phosphatidylinositol 3-kinase within the semicircular canal duct epithelium. *BMC Res Notes* 2010, **3**:100.

28. Ma T, Thiagarajah JR, Yang H, Sonawane ND, Folli C, Galietta LJ, Verkman AS: Thiazolidinone CFTR inhibitor identified by high-throughput screening blocks cholera toxin-induced intestinal fluid secretion. *J Clin Invest* 2002, **110**:1651–1658.

29. Clarke LL, Harline MC: CFTR is required for cAMP inhibition of intestinal Na^+ absorption in a cystic fibrosis mouse model. *Am J Physiol* 1996, **270**:G259–G267.

30. Wangemann P, Liu J, Shimozono M, Scofield MA: b$_1$-adrenergic receptors but not b$_2$-adrenergic or vasopressin receptors regulate K^+ secretion in vestibular dark cells of the inner ear. *J Membr Biol* 1999, **170**:67–77.

31. Wangemann P, Liu J, Shimozono M, Schimanski S, Scofield MA: K^+ secretion in strial marginal cells is stimulated via b1-adrenergic receptors but not via b2-adrenergic or vasopressin receptors. *J Membr Biol* 2000, **175**:191–202.

32. Doi K, Mori N, Matsunaga T: Effects of adenylate cyclase activation on electrical resistance of scala media. *Acta Otolaryngol Suppl* 1993, **501**:76–79.

33. Kitano I, Doi K, Mori N, Umemoto M, Sakagami M, Fukazawa K, Matsunaga T: Failure of forskolin to elevate the endocochlear potential in kanamycin-poisoned animals. *Hear Res* 1994, **78**:58–64.

34. Lee JH, Marcus DC: Endolymphatic sodium homeostasis by Reissner's membrane. *Neuroscience* 2003, **119**:3–8.

35. Yamauchi D, Raveendran NN, Pondugula SR, Kampalli SB, Sanneman JD, Harbidge DG, Marcus DC: Vitamin D upregulates expression of ECaC1 mRNA in semicircular canal. *Biochem Biophys Res Commun* 2005, **331**:1353–1357.

36. Laverty G, Anttila A, Carty J, Reddy V, Yum J, Arnason SS: CFTR mediated chloride secretion in the avian renal proximal tubule. *Comp Biochem Physiol A Mol Integr Physiol* 2012, **161**:53–60.

37. Cipolli M, Canciani M, Cavazzani M, Uras P, Zampieri P, Mastella G: Ear disease is not a common complication in cystic fibrosis. *Eur J Pediatr* 1993, **152**:265–266.

38. Forman-Franco B, Abramson AL, Gorvoy JD, Stein T: Cystic fibrosis and hearing loss. *Arch Otolaryngol* 1979, **105**:338–342.

39. Chao PC, Hamilton KL: Genistein stimulates electrogenic Cl$^-$ secretion via phosphodiesterase modulation in the mouse jejunum. *Am J Physiol, Cell Physiol* 2009, **297**:C688–C698.

40. Halm ST, Zhang J, Halm DR: beta-Adrenergic activation of electrogenic K+ and Cl- secretion in guinea pig distal colonic epithelium proceeds via separate cAMP signaling pathways. *Am J Physiol Gastrointest Liver Physiol* 2010, **299**:G81–G95.

41. Liu S, Veilleux A, Zhang L, Young A, Kwok E, Laliberte F, Chung C, Tota MR, Dube D, Friesen RW, Huang Z: Dynamic activation of cystic fibrosis transmembrane conductance regulator by type 3 and type 4D phosphodiesterase inhibitors. *J Pharmacol Exp Ther* 2005, **314**:846–854.

42. O'Grady SM, Jiang X, Maniak PJ, Birmachu W, Scribner LR, Bulbulian B, Gullikson GW: Cyclic AMP-dependent Cl secretion is regulated by multiple phosphodiesterase subtypes in human colonic epithelial cells. *J Membr Biol* 2002, **185**:137–144.

43. Seifert R, Lushington GH, Mou TC, Gille A, Sprang SR: Inhibitors of membranous adenylyl cyclases. *Trends Pharmacol Sci* 2012, **33**:64–78.

44. Cumbay MG, Watts VJ: Novel regulatory properties of human type 9 adenylate cyclase. *J Pharmacol Exp Ther* 2004, **310**:108–115.

45. Jiang G, Cobbs S, Klein JD, O'Neill WC: Aldosterone regulates the Na-K-2Cl cotransporter in vascular smooth muscle. *Hypertension* 2003, **41**:1131–1135.

46. Putney LK, Brandt JD, O'Donnell ME: Effects of dexamethasone on sodium-potassium-chloride cotransport in trabecular meshwork cells. *Invest Ophthalmol Vis Sci* 1997, **38**:1229–1240.

47. Kim SH, Kim KX, Raveendran NN, Wu T, Pondugula SR, Marcus DC: Regulation of ENaC-mediated sodium transport by glucocorticoids in Reissner's membrane epithelium. *Am J Physiol, Cell Physiol* 2009, **296**:C544–C557.

48. Gagnon KB, Delpire E: Molecular physiology of SPAK and OSR1: two Ste20-related protein kinases regulating ion transport. *Physiol Rev* 2012, **92**:1577–1617.

49. Kahle KT, Rinehart J, Ring A, Gimenez I, Gamba G, Hebert SC, Lifton RP: WNK protein kinases modulate cellular Cl$^-$ flux by altering the phosphorylation state of the Na-K-Cl and K-Cl cotransporters. *Physiology (Bethesda)* 2006, **21**:326–335.

50. Marcus DC, Marcus NY, Greger R: Sidedness of action of loop diuretics and ouabain on nonsensory cells of utricle: a micro-Ussing chamber for inner ear tissues. *Hear Res* 1987, **30**:55–64.

51. Mercado A, Song L, Vazquez N, Mount DB, Gamba G: **Functional comparison of the K$^+$-Cl$^-$ cotransporters KCC1 and KCC4.** *J Biol Chem* 2000, **275**:30326–30334.

52. Garay RP, Nazaret C, Hannaert PA, Cragoe EJ Jr: **Demonstration of a [K+, Cl-]-cotransport system in human red cells by its sensitivity to [(dihydroindenyl)oxy]alkanoic acids: regulation of cell swelling and distinction from the bumetanide-sensitive [Na+, K+, Cl-]-cotransport system.** *Mol Pharmacol* 1988, **33**:696–701.

53. Saitta M, Cavalier S, Garay R, Cragoe E Jr, Hannaert P: **Evidence for a DIOA-sensitive [K+, Cl-]-cotransport system in cultured vascular smooth muscle cells.** *Am J Hypertens* 1990, **3**:939–942.

54. Capo-Aponte JE, Iserovich P, Reinach PS: **Characterization of regulatory volume behavior by fluorescence quenching in human corneal epithelial cells.** *J Membr Biol* 2005, **207**:11–22.

55. Coull JA, Boudreau D, Bachand K, Prescott SA, Nault F, Sik A, De Koninck P, De Koninck Y: **Trans-synaptic shift in anion gradient in spinal lamina I neurons as a mechanism of neuropathic pain.** *Nature* 2003, **424**:938–942.

56. Anfinogenova YJ, Rodriguez X, Grygorczyk R, Adragna NC, Lauf PK, Hamet P, Orlov SN: **Swelling-induced K(+) fluxes in vascular smooth muscle cells are mediated by charybdotoxin-sensitive K(+) channels.** *Cell Physiol Biochem* 2001, **11**:295–310.

57. Koltsova SV, Luneva OG, Lavoie JL, Tremblay J, Maksimov GV, Hamet P, Orlov SN: **HCO3-dependent impact of Na+, K+,2Cl- cotransport in vascular smooth muscle excitation-contraction coupling.** *Cell Physiol Biochem* 2009, **23**:407–414.

58. Kurbannazarova RS, Bessonova SV, Okada Y, Sabirov RZ: **Swelling-activated anion channels are essential for volume regulation of mouse thymocytes.** *Int J Mol Sci* 2011, **12**:9125–9137.

59. Lauf PK, Misri S, Chimote AA, Adragna NC: **Apparent intermediate K conductance channel hyposmotic activation in human lens epithelial cells.** *Am J Physiol, Cell Physiol* 2008, **294**:C820–C832.

60. Payne JA: **Functional characterization of the neuronal-specific K-Cl cotransporter: implications for [K+]o regulation.** *Am J Physiol* 1997, **273**:C1516–C1525.

61. Wangemann P, Wittner M, Di SA, Englert HC, Lang HJ, Schlatter E, Greger R: **Cl(–)-channel blockers in the thick ascending limb of the loop of Henle. Structure activity relationship.** *Pflugers Arch* 1986, **407**(Suppl 2):S128–S141.

62. Pond BB, Galeffi F, Ahrens R, Schwartz-Bloom RD: **Chloride transport inhibitors influence recovery from oxygen-glucose deprivation-induced cellular injury in adult hippocampus.** *Neuropharmacology* 2004, **47**:253–262.

63. De Lisle RC, Isom KS, Ziemer D, Cotton CU: **Changes in the exocrine pancreas secondary to altered small intestinal function in the CF mouse.** *Am J Physiol Gastrointest Liver Physiol* 2001, **281**:G899–G906.

64. Lee JH, Marcus DC: **Nongenomic effects of corticosteroids on ion transport by stria vascularis.** *Audiol Neurootol* 2002, **7**:100–106.

65. Wangemann P, Itza EM, Albrecht B, Wu T, Jabba SV, Maganti RJ, Lee JH, Everett LA, Wall SM, Royaux IE, Green ED, Marcus DC: **Loss of KCNJ10 protein expression abolishes endocochlear potential and causes deafness in Pendred syndrome mouse model.** *BMC Med* 2004, **2**:30.

66. Davies SL, Roussa E, Le Rouzic P, Thevenod F, Alper SL, Best L, Brown PD: **Expression of K$^+$-Cl$^-$ cotransporters in the alpha-cells of rat endocrine pancreas.** *Biochim Biophys Acta* 2004, **1667**:7–14.

11

Identification of uterine ion transporters for mineralisation precursors of the avian eggshell

Vincent Jonchère, Aurélien Brionne, Joël Gautron and Yves Nys[*]

Abstract

Background: In *Gallus gallus*, eggshell formation takes place daily in the hen uterus and requires large amounts of the ionic precursors for calcium carbonate ($CaCO_3$). Both elements (Ca^{2+}, HCO_3^-) are supplied by the blood via trans-epithelial transport. Our aims were to identify genes coding for ion transporters that are upregulated in the uterine portion of the oviduct during eggshell calcification, compared to other tissues and other physiological states, and incorporate these proteins into a general model for mineral transfer across the tubular gland cells during eggshell formation.

Results: A total of 37 candidate ion transport genes were selected from our database of overexpressed uterine genes associated with eggshell calcification, and by analogy with mammalian transporters. Their uterine expression was compared by qRTPCR in the presence and absence of eggshell formation, and with relative expression levels in magnum (low Ca^{2+}/HCO_3^- movement) and duodenum (high rates of Ca^{2+}/HCO_3^- trans-epithelial transfer). We identified overexpression of eleven genes related to calcium movement: the TRPV6 Ca^{2+} channel (basolateral uptake of Ca^{2+}), 28 kDa calbindin (intracellular Ca^{2+} buffering), the endoplasmic reticulum type 2 and 3 Ca^{2+} pumps (ER uptake), and the inositol trisphosphate receptors type 1, 2 and 3 (ER release). Ca^{2+} movement across the apical membrane likely involves membrane Ca^{2+} pumps and Ca^{2+}/Na^+ exchangers. Our data suggests that Na^+ transport involved the SCNN1 channel and the Na^+/Ca^{2+} exchangers SLC8A1, 3 for cell uptake, the Na^+/K^+ ATPase for cell output. K^+ uptake resulted from the Na^+/K^+ ATPase, and its output from the K^+ channels (KCNJ2, 15, 16 and KCNMA1).

We propose that the HCO_3^- is mainly produced from CO_2 by the carbonic anhydrase 2 (CA2) and that HCO_3^- is secreted through the HCO_3^-/Cl^- exchanger SLC26A9. HCO_3^- synthesis and precipitation with Ca^{2+} produce two H^+. Protons are absorbed via the membrane's Ca^{2+} pumps ATP2B1, 2 in the apical membrane and the vacuolar (H+)-atpases at the basolateral level. Our model incorporate Cl^- ions which are absorbed by the HCO_3^-/Cl^- exchanger SLC26A9 and by Cl^- channels (CLCN2, CFTR) and might be extruded by Cl^-/H^+ exchanger (CLCN5), but also by Na^+ K^+ 2 Cl^- and K^+ Cl^- cotransporters.

Conclusions: Our *Gallus gallus* uterine model proposes a large list of ion transfer proteins supplying Ca^{2+} and HCO_3^- and maintaining cellular ionic homeostasis. This avian model should contribute towards understanding the mechanisms and regulation for ionic precursors of $CaCO_3$, and provide insight in other species where epithelia transport large amount of calcium or bicarbonate.

Keywords: Ion, Mineral, Calcium, Transporter, Uterus, Eggshell, Chicken

* Correspondence: yves.nys@tours.inra.fr
INRA, UR83 Recherches Avicoles, F-37380, Nouzilly, France

Background

Biomineralisation is a process by which living organisms develop mineral structures to perform a variety of roles related to support, defence and feeding. Amongst these, a large number of animals (birds, molluscs, foraminifera, corals, sea urchins) mineralises by co-precipitation of calcium (Ca^{2+}) and carbonates (CO_3^{-}) to form a protective shell or a skeleton. The prerequisite for shell mineralisation is the supply of large amounts of Ca^{2+} and CO_3^{2-} in a limited extracellular milieu by trans-cellular transport, requiring the presence of ion channels, ion pumps and ion exchangers. In *Gallus gallus*, eggshell formation takes place daily in the hen uterus and is one of the most rapid mineralisation processes [1]. It requires large amount of calcium carbonate ($CaCO_3$) as the hen exports the equivalent of her body weight as eggshell in one year of egg production (>1.5 kg). Both elements (Ca^{2+} and HCO_3) are not stored in the uterus but are continuously supplied during eggshell formation by the blood plasma via trans-epithelial transport taking place across the uterine glandular cells [2-4]. Early studies determined the ion concentrations of the uterine fluid, which bathes the eggshell and changes during the sequential stages of calcification (Table 1) [5], identified several proteins involved in ion transport [3,6,7], and recorded changes in ion fluxes across the uterine epithelium in response to ion transporter inhibitors [8-10]. These classic approaches led to a hypothesis concerning the mechanisms of ion transfer through the uterine glandular cells (Figure 1; [1]). In hens, the Ca^{2+} blood (1.2 mM) and epithelial cell concentrations (10^{-4} mM), suggest that Ca^{2+} entry in cell is passive via a Ca^{2+} channel, which remains unidentified. The intracellular Ca^{2+} transport through the cell involves 28 kDa calbindin [3,11,12]. The 28 kDa calbindin expression is greatly upregulated during eggshell formation and falls after suppression of calcification (by premature egg expulsion), suggesting a very close relationship between

uterine calbindin levels and Ca^{2+} flux [11,13,14]. This protein could also take part in maintaining low intracellular Ca^{2+} to avoid cell death as observed in other species and tissues [15]. Ca^{2+} secretion from epithelial cells to the uterine fluid is active involving a Ca^{2+} ATPase, the activity of which varies with the stage of eggshell calcification [4,7]. A recent study [16] identified and localized the plasma membrane Ca^{2+} ATPase isoform 4 (PMCA4) in the apical membrane of epithelial cells of king quail. The disruption of sodium (Na^+) reabsorption by specific inhibitors in perfused uterus or *in vitro* reduced Ca^{2+} secretion by 50% [9,17], revealing a strong relationship between Na^+ and Ca^{2+} transfers and therefore the putative presence of Na^+/Ca^{2+} exchangers in uterine cells. The Na^+/K^+ ATPase responsible for Na^+ re-absorption in the plasma membrane is characterised and is upregulated during the period of shell calcification [18].

The second essential component of eggshell mineralisation is carbonate. Blood carbon dioxide (CO_2) is provided in cells by passive diffusion through the plasma membrane [2,19]. In the uterine tubular gland cells, a family of key enzymes, the carbonic anhydrases (CA) [6] catalyses the hydration of CO_2 to HCO_3 as confirmed by inhibition of HCO_3 production and secretion by acetazolamide, a CA inhibitor [9]. Chloride (Cl^-) is absorbed by the uterus and any perturbation of Na^+ flux by ouabain [9] reverses both the Na^+ and Cl^- fluxes, but reduces also HCO_3^- secretion suggesting that its transfer is dependent on Cl^- via a Cl^-/HCO_3^- exchanger which has not been identified. Finally, the production of HCO_3^- in tubular gland cells and of CO_3^{2-} in the uterine fluid generates high levels of protons (H^+) ions. The concomitant decrease in uterine and plasma pH during calcification reflects the reabsorption of H^+ [5].

Only a few genes and related proteins involved in uterine ion transfer have been identified to date. Our objective therefore was to use the recent information issuing from the chicken genome sequencing [20] and subsequent enrichment in the chicken gene/protein databases to identify uterine ion transport proteins. Use of a recent transcriptomic study revealing uterine genes related to eggshell calcification [21] and of the analogies with transporters previously described in mammalian tissues transferring large quantities of ions (intestine, kidney, pancreas) allows the identification of putative genes encoding proteins involved in uterine trans-epithelial ion transports. Confirmation of their presence in birds and evaluation of their involvement have been analysed by comparing gene expression in the uterus compared to the magnum (the oviduct segment responsible for the synthesis and secretion of egg white proteins) and the duodenum (Ca^{2+} uptake and neutralization of stomach acid), where both Ca^{2+} and HCO_3 trans-epithelial

Table 1 PH and ion concentrations in blood plasma, uterine fluid and epithelial cells during eggshell mineralisation[5]

	Blood plasma	Epithelial cells	Uterine fluid	
			8 h PO	18 h PO
Ions	[mM]	[mM]	[mM]	[mM]
Ca^{2+}	1.2	<0.0002	6	10
Na^+	140	12	144	80
K^+	4	139	12	60
HCO_3^-	23	12	60	110
pH	7.4	7.0-7.4	7.6	7.1
Cl^-	130	4	71	45

The eggshell precursors are secreted in the uterine fluid where the eggshell mineralization daily takes place from 10 hours to 22 hours post ovulation (yolk entry in the oviduct). PO: post ovulation.

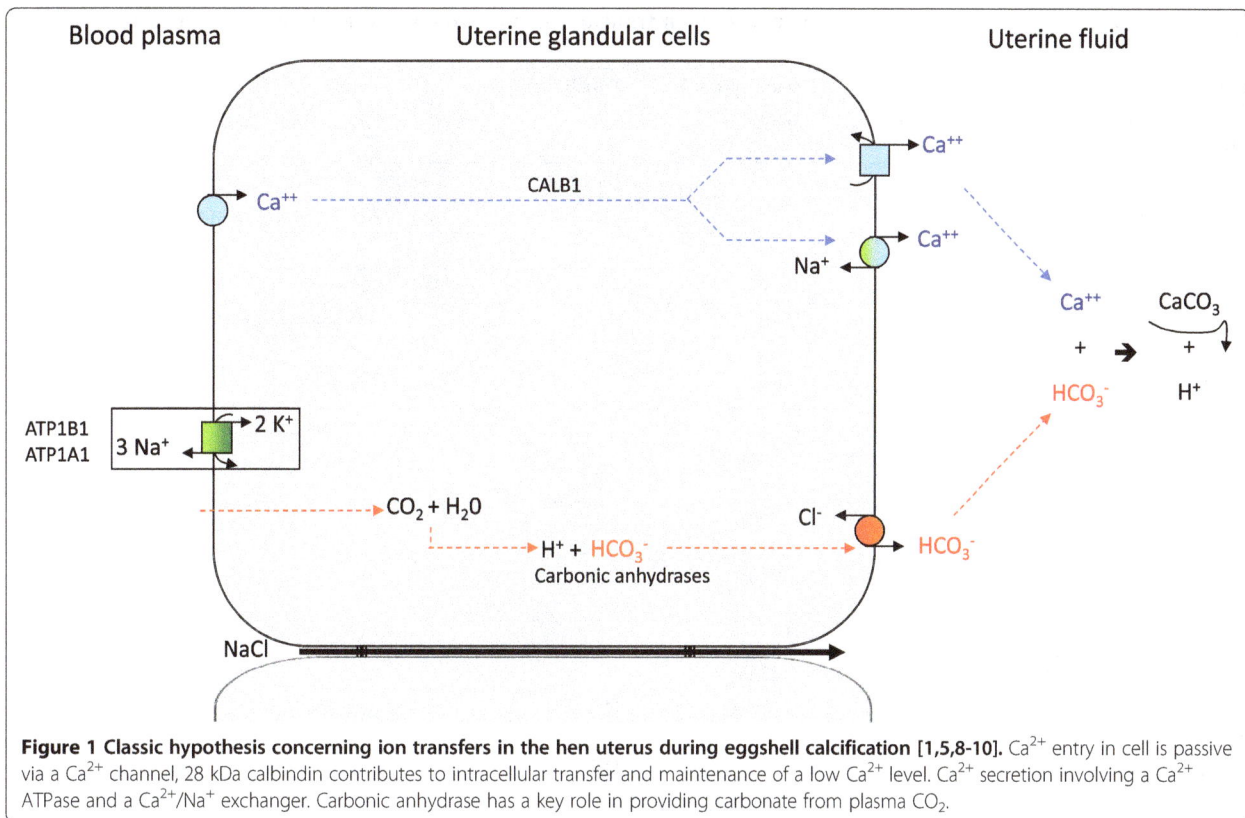

Figure 1 Classic hypothesis concerning ion transfers in the hen uterus during eggshell calcification [1,5,8-10]. Ca^{2+} entry in cell is passive via a Ca^{2+} channel, 28 kDa calbindin contributes to intracellular transfer and maintenance of a low Ca^{2+} level. Ca^{2+} secretion involving a Ca^{2+} ATPase and a Ca^{2+}/Na^{+} exchanger. Carbonic anhydrase has a key role in providing carbonate from plasma CO_2.

transfers are respectively low and high. The magnum and the uterus secrete a large amount of water, Na^{+} and Cl^{-} during the phase of hydration of egg albumen which takes place before the active phase of eggshell formation in the uterus [5,22]. By contrast, the duodenum is the proximal region of the intestine with a high capacity for Ca^{2+} absorption [23] and secretes a large amount of HCO_3^- for neutralization of gastric acidity [24,25]. An additional experimental approach was the comparison of gene expression in the uterus isolated from hens at the stage of eggshell formation, to those for which eggshell formation was suppressed by premature egg expulsion. We identified a large number of genes coding for ion transport and propose a general model describing the putative contribution and localisation of the ion transporters in the tubular gland cell of the hen's uterus.

Results

Identification of uterine ion transporters

The first step of this work was to establish a list of ion transporters potentially involved in supplying eggshell minerals. The ion transfer model established in the *Gallus gallus* uterus (Figure 1) using physiological data [5,8,9] was used to produce a first list of genes encoding ionic transporter proteins. This approach was completed by using a recent transcriptomic study revealing genes overexpressed in the uterus (shell formation) compared

to the magnum (egg white protein secretion) [21] and analogies with transporters previously described in mammalian tissues at the intestinal and kidney level [24,26]. A list of 37 genes was therefore selected as candidates possibly involved in uterine trans-epithelial ion transfers (Table 2). To facilitate identification of candidates in the manuscript, we have only used the gene symbol for describing both genes and proteins.

Uterine expression of the 37 genes encoding ion transporters

The mRNA expression of 37 transporters was analysed by RT-PCR in the uterus, and three other ion secreting or absorbing epithelia (magnum, duodenum and kidney) and in muscle where no trans-epithelial ion transfer occurs (Additional file 1: Table 1). Amongst these 37 genes, mRNA expression was observed in the uterus for 34 genes. Three genes (the endoplasmic Ca^{2+} pump type 1(ATP2A1), two exchangers Na^{+} dependent (SLC4A8) or independent (SLC4A9) Cl^{-}/HCO_3^- were not expressed in the uterus and were not further studied.

A large majority of these 34 genes were also revealed in the duodenum. Conversely, SLC4A8 was expressed only in duodenum. Four genes were revealed only in the uterus and were not present in the magnum (TRPV6, CALB1, SCNN1B and SLC26A9) or in muscle (CALB1, SCNN1B, SLC4A10 and CLCN2). The 34 genes revealed

Table 2 Function of genes potentially involved in the ion transfer for supplying eggshell mineral precursors in hen uterus

Name	Gene symbol	Functional data	Transfer type
Transient receptor potential cation channel subfamily V member 6	TRPV6		Ca^{2+} channel (plasma membrane)
Calbindin 28 K	CALB1	[11,14,28]	Ca^{2+} intracellular transporter (intracellular)
Endoplasmic reticulum calcium ATPase 1	ATP2A1		Ca^{2+}ATPases (endoplasmic & plasma membrane)
Endoplasmic reticulum calcium ATPase 2	ATP2A2		
Endoplasmic reticulum calcium ATPase 3)	ATP2A3		
IP3 receptor1	ITPR1		Ca^{2+} channels (endoplasmic membrane)
IP3 receptor2	ITPR2		
IP3 receptor3	ITPR3		
Ryanodine receptor 1	RYR1		Ca^{2+} channel (endoplasmic membrane)
Plasma membrane calcium-transporting ATPase 1 (PMCA1)	ATP2B1		Ca^{2+}/H^+ exchanger (plasma membrane)
Plasma membrane calcium-transporting ATPase 2 (PMCA2)	ATP2B2		
Plasma membrane calcium-transporting ATPase 4 (PMCA4)	ATP2B4	[16]	
Sodium/calcium exchanger 1	SLC8A1		Na^+/Ca^{2+} exchanger (plasma membrane)
Sodium/calcium exchanger 3	SLC8A3		
Amiloride-sensitive sodium channel subunit alpha	SCNN1A	[31]	Na^+ channels (plasma membrane)
Amiloride-sensitive sodium channel subunit beta	SCNN1B	[31]	
Amiloride-sensitive sodium channel subunit gamma	SCNN1G	[31]	
Sodium/potassium-transporting ATPase subunit alpha-1	ATP1A1	[18]	Na^+/K^+ exchanger (plasma membrane)
Sodium/potassium-transporting ATPase subunit beta-1	ATP1B1	[18]	
Solute carrier family 4 member 4	SLC4A4		Na^+/HCO_3 co-transporters (plasma membrane)
Solute carrier family 4 member 5	SLC4A5		
Solute carrier family 4 member 7	SLC4A7		
Solute carrier family 4 member 10	SLC4A10		
Inward rectifier potassium channel 2	KCNJ2		Inward rectifiers K^+ channels (plasma membrane)
Inward rectifier potassium channel 5	KCNJ15		
Inward rectifier potassium channel 16	KCNJ16		
Calcium-activated potassium channel subunit alpha-1	KCNMA1		K^+ channel (plasma membrane)
Carbonic anhydrase 2	CA2	[6]	Catalyse HCO_3^- formation (plasma membrane)
Carbonic anhydrase 4	CA4		
Carbonic anhydrase 7	CA7		
Solute carrier family 4 member 8	SLC4A8		HCO_3/Cl^- exchangers (plasma membrane)
Solute carrier family 4 member 9	SLC4A9		
Solute carrier family 26 member 9	SLC26A9		
Vacuolar H ATPase B subunit osteoclast isozyme	ATP6V1B2		H^+ pump (organelles and plasma membrane
Cystic fibrosis transmembrane conductance regulator	CFTR		Cl^- channel (plasma membrane)
Chloride channel protein 2	CLCN2		Cl^- channel (plasma membrane)
H(+)/Cl(−) exchange transporter 5	CLCN5		Cl^-/H^+ exchanger (plasma membrane)

in the uterus are candidates for supplying ions in the uterus.

Comparative expression of ion transfer genes between uterus and other secreting tissues

The expression of the 34 genes encoding proteins potentially involved in uterine ion transfer were quantitatively evaluated by comparing their gene expression in the uterus to those of two other tissues (magnum, duodenum) where Ca^{2+} and HCO_3^- trans-epithelial transport are at low and high levels, respectively. After normalisation, the fold changes in gene expression between uterus vs magnum and uterus vs duodenum was statistically analysed (Figure 2).

Amongst the 34 comparisons of gene expression between the uterus and the magnum, only one gene (the ryanodine receptor 1) was not differentially expressed. The 33 other genes showed higher levels of gene expression in the uterus than in the magnum (fold change of Ut/Ma up to 12 ln). Amongst these 33 genes, 16 genes (underlined in the following list) are not differentially expressed between uterus and duodenum suggesting they are equally important in both tissues able to absorb or secrete large amounts of Ca^{2+} and HCO_3^-. These 33 gene candidates suspected to be involved in uterine ionic transfer corresponded to:

(1) Ca^{2+} transfer: TRPV Ca^{2+} channel (TRPV6), calbindin 28 kDa (CALB1), endoplasmic Ca^{2+} pump type 2 and 3 (ATP2A2, 3), inositol trisphosphate receptor type 1, 2, 3 (ITPR1, 2, 3), Ca^{2+} pumps PMCA type 1, 2 and 4 (ATP2B1, 2, 4) and Ca^{2+}/Na^+ exchanger type 1, 3 (SLC8A1, 3).

(2) Na^+ transfer: amiloride-sensitive Na^+ channel subunit α, β, and γ (SCNN1A, B, G), Na^+/K^+ transporting ATPase subunit α and β (ATP1A1, B1), Ca^{2+}/Na^+ exchanger type 1 and 3 (SLC8A1, 3), several Na^+/HCO_3^- co-transporters (SLC4A4, 5, 7, 10).

(3) K^+ transfer: Na^+/K^+ transporting ATPase subunit α and β (ATP1A1, B1) and several K^+ channels (KCNJ2, 15, 16, KCNMA1).

(4) HCO_3^- production and transfer: CAs type 2, 4, 7, (CA2, 4, 7), an HCO_3^-/Cl^- exchanger (SLC26A9), and several Na^+/HCO_3^- co-transporters (SLC4A4, 5, 7, 10).

(5) H^+ transfer: VH$^+$ ATPase pump subunit B (ATP6V1B2), and Cl^-/H^+ exchanger (CLCN5).

(6) Cl^- transfer: CFTR channel (CFTR), Cl^- channel protein 2 (CLCN2), an HCO_3^-/Cl^- exchanger (SLC26A9) and a Cl^-/H^+ exchanger (CLCN5).

Fourteen genes amongst the 33 were overexpressed in the uterus compared with the duodenum. This overexpression of transporters in the uterus relative to the

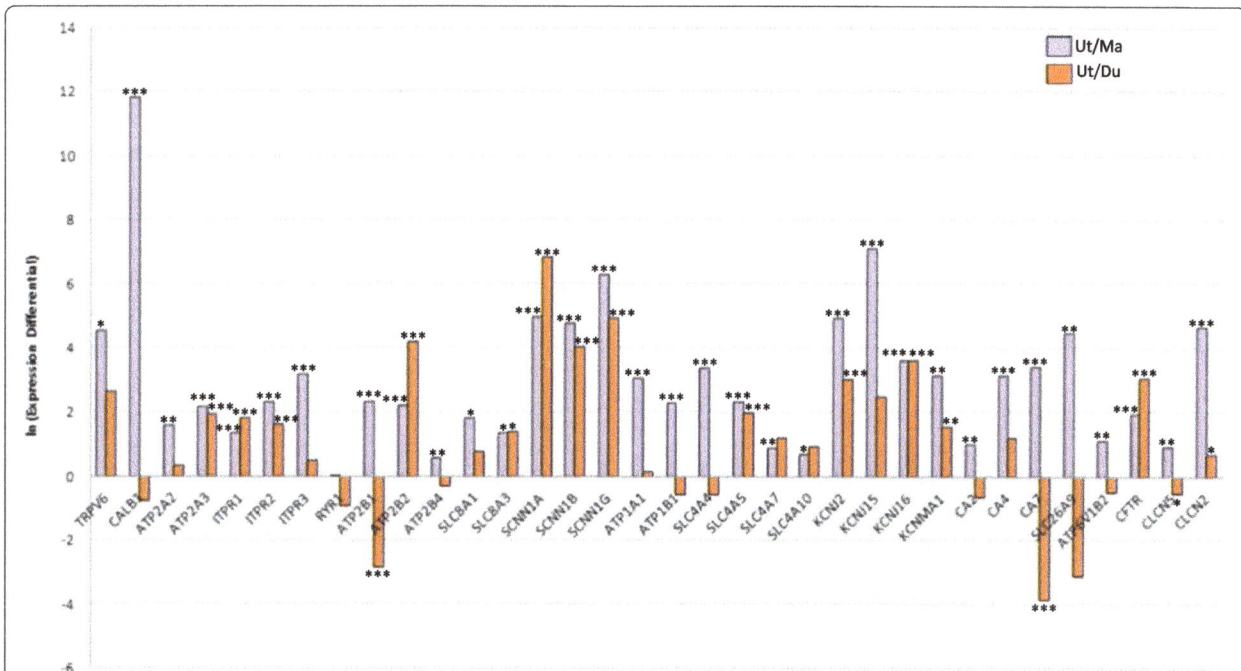

Figure 2 Relative expression of genes coding ion transporters in chicken uterus compared to magnum or duodenum. Gene expression of ion transporters for eggshell mineralisation were quantitatively evaluated by qRT-PCR in the uterus (eggshell formation) and compared to those of magnum and duodenum where Ca^{2+} and HCO_3^- trans-epithelial transport are at low and high levels, respectively.

duodenum is indicative of genes whose function is more uterine specific. They corresponded to:

(1) Ca^{2+} transfer: endoplasmic Ca^{2+} pump type 3 (ATP2A3), inositol trisphosphate receptors (ITPR1, 2), Ca^{2+} pumps PMCA2 (ATP2B2) and Ca^{2+}/Na^+ exchanger type 3 (SLC8A3).
(2) Na^+ transfer: amiloride-sensitive Na^+ channel subunit α, β, and γ (SCNN1A, B, G), Ca^{2+}/Na^+ exchanger type 3 (SLC8A3), Na^+/HCO_3^- co-transporters (SLC4A5).
(3) K^+ transfer: several K^+ channels (KCNJ2, 16 and KCNMA1).
(4) HCO_3^- production and transfer: Na^+/HCO_3^- co-transporters (SLC4A5).
(5) Cl^- transfer: Cl^- channel protein 2 (CLCN2) and CFTR channel (CFTR).

Three genes are underexpressed in the uterus compared with the duodenum suggesting that their function is more specific to the duodenum:

(1) Ca^{2+} transfer: Ca^{2+} pumps PMCA1 (ATP2B1).
(2) HCO_3^- production and transfer: CA type 7 (CA7).
(3) H^+ transfer and (4) Cl^- transfer: H^+/Cl^- exchanger (CLCN5).

Comparative expression of genes in the presence or absence of eggshell formation

This model was explored to reveal regulation of gene expression associated with the process of shell formation and to discern some of the ionic transport proteins more likely to be involved in supplying shell mineral precursors. We compared expression of these genes in the uterus when calcification takes place or after its suppression due to premature expulsion of the eggs for 3–4 consecutive days. The early egg expulsion eliminates the Ca^{2+} and HCO_3^- requirement for shell formation, and eliminates the mechanical stimulation of the uterine wall due to the presence of the egg, which is known to upregulate expression of certain genes. Fold changes in gene expression between the calcifying or inactive uterus are presented in Figure 3.

Twelve genes amongst 33 were overexpressed in the presence of eggshell calcification compared to hens in which shell formation had been suppressed (67 fold change):

(1) Ca^{+2+} transfer: 28 kDa calbindin (CALB1), endoplasmic Ca^{2+} pump type 3 (ATP2A3), and Ca^{2+} pumps PMCA2 (ATP2B1, 2).
(2) Na^+ transfer: amiloride-sensitive Na^+ channel subunit γ (SCNN1G) and Na^+/K^+ transporting ATPase subunit α (ATP1A1).
(3) K^+ transfer: Na^+/K^+ transporting ATPase subunit α (ATP1A1) and the K^+ channels (KCNJ2, KCNJ15 and KCNMA1).
(4) HCO_3^- production and transfer: carbonic anhydrase CA type 2 (CA2), an HCO_3^-/Cl^- exchanger (SLC26A9).
(5) Cl^- transfer: the Cl^- channel (CFTR) and an HCO_3^-/Cl^- exchanger (SLC26A9).

In contrast, 2 genes corresponding to a Ca^{2+}/H^+ exchanger (ATP2B4) and to a Na^+/HCO_3^- co-transporter (SLC4A7) showed an underexpression when eggshell calcification takes place.

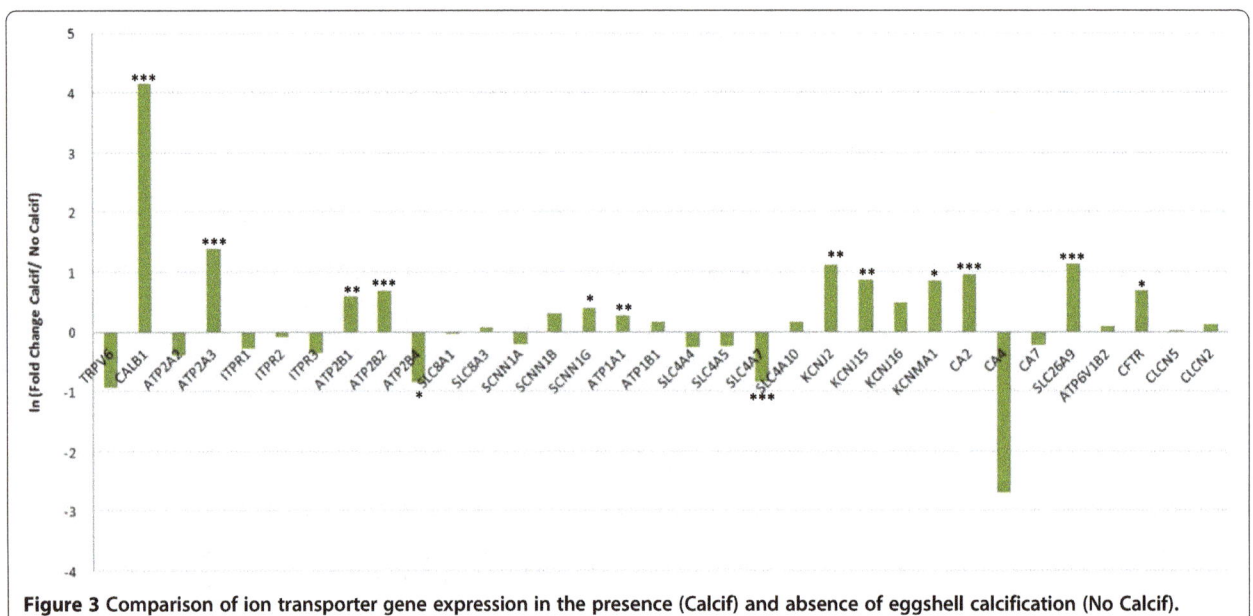

Figure 3 Comparison of ion transporter gene expression in the presence (Calcif) and absence of eggshell calcification (No Calcif).

Nineteen of the 33 uterine genes did not show any fold change between these two physiological conditions:

(1) Ca^{2+} transfer: TRPV Ca^{2+} channel (TRPV6), endoplasmic Ca^{2+} pump type 2 (ATP2A2), inositol trisphosphate receptors (ITPR1, 2, 3), and Ca^{2+}/Na^+ exchanger type 1 and 3 (SLC8A1, 3).

(2) Na^+ transfer: amiloride-sensitive Na^+ channel subunit α and γ (SCNN1A, B), Na^+/K^+ transporting ATPase subunit β (ATP1B1), Ca^{2+}/Na^+ exchanger type 1 and 3 (SLC8A1, 3), Na^+/HCO_3^- co-transporters (SLC4A4, 5, 10).

(3) K^+ transfer: Na^+/K^+ transporting ATPase subunit β (ATP1B1) and a K^+ channel (KCNJ16).

(4) HCO_3^- production and transfer: CA type 4, 7 (CA4, 7), several Na^+/HCO_3^- co-transporters (SLC4A4, 5, 10).

(5) Cl^- transfer: Cl^- channel protein 2 (CLCN2) and H^+/Cl^- exchanger (CLCN5).

(6) H^+ transfer: VH^+ ATPase pump subunit B (ATP6V1B2) and H^+/Cl^- exchanger (CLCN5).

Discussion

Eggshell calcification in the avian uterus is one of the fastest mineralisation processes in the living world. The Ca^{2+} metabolism is intense in *Gallus gallus* hens which export a large amount of Ca^{2+} (2 g daily) and consequently there are numerous physiological adaptations to support this function [1,27-30]. In fact, an egg-producing hen shows a specific appetite for Ca^{2+} a few hours before shell calcification is initiated and its capacity to absorb Ca^{2+} in the intestine increases by 6-fold due to large stimulation of the active metabolite of vitamin D at the kidney level. The uterus acquires the capacity to transfer a great quantity of Ca^{2+} and HCO_3^- for supplying mineral precursors of the eggshell during less than 14 hours. This model is therefore particularly relevant to explore the mechanisms of mineral transport needed for the extracellular biomineralisation of the eggshell. In this study, we focused on intracellular ionic transporters and did not explore the proteins involved in their regulation. This process has been the object of many physiological and pharmacological works as reviewed by Nys [1] and Bar [30]. However, the molecular identification of ionic transporters remains incomplete in the uterus. Genome sequencing in human and other mammalian species has contributed to the molecular identification of genes and related proteins involved in ionic trans-epithelial transfer in the intestine and kidneys [24,26]. By using this literature and data provided by a recent high throughput analysis of chicken uterine genes related to eggshell calcification [21], we identified 37 putative genes encoding ion trans-epithelial transporters and tested their involvement in providing

mineral precursors in the hen's uterus. Analysis of their expression by RT-PCR, showed that 34 of these genes were expressed at the uterine level. In order to study their involvement in providing both Ca^{2+} and HCO_3^- for eggshell formation, the expression of these 34 genes in the uterus was quantified by qRT-PCR and compared with two other epithelia (magnum and duodenum) where Ca^{2+} and HCO_3^- transfers are respectively low and high. In addition, the expression of these genes was compared in the uterus during two situations: during eggshell calcification and when Ca^{2+} and HCO_3^- secretions were suppressed due to premature egg expulsion. These approaches allowed the identification of numerous transporting proteins providing minerals for shell formation in the hen's uterus.

Ca^{2+} transfer

Ca^{2+} is not stored in the uterus before eggshell calcification but comes from blood plasma by trans-epithelial transport. This Ca^{2+} export is extremely rapid during calcification and corresponds to a consumption of the total plasmatic Ca^{2+} pool every 12 min. Studies of Ca^{2+} transfer *in vivo* using perfusion of uterus [8,9] and *in vitro* exploring the effects of inhibitors of ion ATPases or carbonic anhydrase [10,31], and ionic analysis of uterine fluid during eggshell formation [5], made it possible to build a first model of Ca^{2+} transfer in the uterus (Figure 1): Ca^{2+}, HCO_3^- secretion and Na^+ reabsorption was considered to occur against their electrochemical gradient, to involve active intracellular transfer as shown by specific inhibitors [8-10] and to occur in the uterine glandular cells as revealed by immunohistochemistry of transport proteins [32]. Trans-epithelial transfer of Ca^{2+} occurs in three steps as observed in all transporting epithelia: Ca^{2+} influx through a downhill gradient, an intracellular Ca^{2+} transport involving calbindin 28 kDa protein [33] and active output into the lumen through a Ca^{2+} pump [4]. The high plasma Ca^{2+} concentration (1.2 mM free Ca^{2+}) relative to the uterine cell interior (10^{-4} mM free Ca^{2+}) (Table 1) suggests that the Ca^{2+} entry into cells passively occurs via Ca^{2+} selective channels present in the basolateral plasma membrane. In other tissues, such as intestine, kidney and plasma, TRPVs 5, 6 (Transient Receptor Potential Vanilloid) are epithelial channels that represent the principal pathway for Ca^{2+} uptake into the cell [26,34]. Our study showed that in *Gallus gallus*, only one gene [NCBI Gene ID: 418307; Swiss-Prot: TRPV6] is present. This channel is significantly overexpressed in the uterus compared with the magnum, where Ca^{2+} transfer is low. Its uterine expression is similar to that of the duodenum where Ca^{2+} absorption is also large. Cellular Ca^{2+} influx might use a similar Ca^{2+} channel, TRPV6, at the intestinal and uterine level but their localisation is hypothesized to differ according to the site of Ca^{2+} influx, being located in the basal membrane in the uterus but in the apical membrane in the intestine. The uterine expression of TRPV6 is not however modified according to whether calcification takes place. The presence of other Ca^{2+} channels cannot be ruled out as additional putative candidates. A recent transcriptomic study in our laboratory comparing uterine gene expression in hens with or without shell calcification revealed the presence of high expression of TRPC1, TRPP, TRPM7, TRPML1 and ORAI 1 (unpublished data, Brionne A, Nys Y and Gautron J).

An intracellular Ca^{2+} buffer is crucial to keep the free cytosolic Ca^{2+} concentration below toxic levels. Following Ca^{2+} entry into the uterine glandular cell, several systems could contribute to intracellular transport of Ca^{2+}, while maintaining the low but essential free Ca^{2+} concentration for survival of the cell. In certain tissues, calbindin proteins, 9 kDa and 28 kDa in mammals [15] or 28 kDa in birds [3,35], are present at high cytosolic concentration and possess high Ca^{2+} binding capacity. Direct correlation has been demonstrated between their mucosal concentration and the efficiency of Ca^{2+} transfer in intestine and uterus under numerous experimental conditions [26,28,30]. It is generally accepted that calbindins facilitate the diffusion of intracellular Ca^{2+} and serve as a Ca^{2+} buffer needed for cell protection against Ca^{2+} stress and accompanying apoptotic cellular degradation that is induced by a high intracellular Ca^{2+} concentration [15,36,37]. In our study, we observed an elevated expression of calbindin 28 kDa in the uterus during calcification of an eggshell compared to the magnum (Figure 2) and compared to the uterus with no shell in formation (fold difference in expression: 67) in agreement with previous studies [11,14,28]. This uterine calbindin 28 kDa is therefore associated with intracellular Ca^{2+} transport from the basal membrane of the glandular cells to the apical membrane where Ca^{2+} is extruded into the uterine fluid.

An alternative system in mammals to maintain a low intracellular Ca^{2+} concentration relies on the endoplasmic reticulum which contributes to Ca^{2+} homeostasis through its capacity for Ca^{2+} uptake and storage [38,39]. The endoplasmic reticulum Ca^{2+} ATPases (ATP2A1, 2, 3) play an active role in Ca^{2+} uptake by this organelle (reaching 10 to 100 mM free Ca^{2+}), while maintaining the cytoplasmic concentration at low concentrations of 10^{-4} mM free Ca^{2+}. Amongst the three isoenzymes (Table 2), only ATP2A2 and ATP2A3 were overexpressed in the uterus compared to the magnum. The absence of ATP2A1 expression fits with its predominant localisation in mammalian muscle in contrast to ATP2A2 and ATP2A3 which are expressed in numerous tissues [40]. The overexpression of ATP2A3 in the uterus compared to duodenum suggests a more crucial role of this transporter, the regulation of which remained to be explored.

The inositol 1, 4, 5-trisphosphate receptors (ITPR) are intracellular Ca^{2+} channels, localised mainly in the endoplasmic reticulum [41,42] and allowing the release of Ca^{2+} from this organelle. The three isoforms (ITPR1, 2 3) were overexpressed in the uterus compared to the magnum but were not modified when comparing the presence or absence of calcification. The higher expression of ITPR1 and ITPR 2 in the uterus compared to the duodenum supports our hypothesis concerning their contribution to the regulation of intra-cellular Ca^{2+}. The ryanodine receptors which are involved in muscle excitation-contraction coupling in mammalian tissues [38] are alternative channels for Ca^{2+} release from the endoplasmic reticulum. RYR1 expression was revealed in the uterus, but there was no difference between the uterus, magnum or duodenum, suggesting a weak involvement in endoplasmic reticulum Ca^{2+} release. In conclusion, these observations of high expression of genes encoding ATP2A pumps and ITPR Ca^{2+} channels involved in Ca^{2+} uptake and release in endoplasmic reticulum suggest the involvement of this organelle in intracellular Ca^{2+} buffering in uterine glandular cells.

The last step of uterine Ca^{2+} trans-epithelial transport is output from the glandular cells, which occurs against a concentration gradient. Ca^{2+} secretion towards the uterine fluid occurs via an active process, involving the Ca^{2+} ATPase [7,32,43]. This has recently been associated with the PMCA4 (plasma membrane ATPase Ca^{2+}) [16]. Four isoenzymes (ATP2B1, B2, B3 and B4) of PMCAs pumps are identified in mammals [44]. Only three (ATP2B1, B2, B4) are conserved in birds. Each of these were overexpressed in the uterus compared to the magnum (Figure 2). ATP2B2 was also overexpressed in the uterus compared to the duodenum, and in presence of the eggshell mineralisation (Figure 3) suggesting a more active role in Ca^{2+} secretion at the uterine level. In contrast, ATP2B1 and ATP2B4 were underexpressed in the uterus compared to duodenum and for ATP2B4 in presence of shell formation. In mammals, it is ATP2B1 which plays a more important role in intestinal Ca^{2+} absorption [26,45]. In other bird species, Parker et al. [16] localized the plasma membrane Ca^{2+}-transporting ATPase 4 (ATP2B4) in the apical membrane of uterine epithelial cells but did not explore the presence of ATP2B2 and its differential expression during calcification. In human osteoblasts, the isoforms 1 and 2 take part in the Ca^{2+} supply necessary for bone mineralisation whereas the isoform 4 is not detected [46].

It was observed thirty years ago that the inhibition of Na^+ transfer by Na^+/K^+ ATPase inhibitors considerably reduced Ca^{2+} secretion into the uterine lumen [9,17], showing a coupling between uterine Ca^{2+} secretion and Na^+ re-absorption. The uterine absorption of Na^+ is revealed by the decreased Na^+ concentrations in the uterine fluid observed between the early stage of shell calcification and the end of calcification (Table 1). These observations support the hypothesis that Na^+/Ca^{2+} exchangers participate in the uterine Ca^{2+} secretion. The role of these transporters is clearly established at the mammalian intestinal and renal level [47]. Our study supported this mechanism for Ca^{2+} secretion in the chicken uterus, as both Na^+/Ca^{2+} exchangers (SLC8A1 and 3) were overexpressed in the uterus compared to the magnum, whereas their expression did not change in the presence or absence of eggshell mineralisation (Figures 2 and 3). The mammalian exchangers allow the cell output of one Ca^{2+} ion against three Na^+ ions at the basolateral membrane level. This transport is facilitated by the Na^+ gradient, which provides the energy necessary for the Ca^{2+} output against its gradient [34,47]. Similarly, the respective Na^+ gradient between the cell (12 mM) and the uterine fluid (80 to 144 mM, Table 1) may provide the bird uterus with the energy needed for the Ca^{2+} output towards the uterine fluid at the apical membrane of the glandular cells. Conversely, the unfavourable gradient of Na^+ concentrations between blood (140 mM) and glandular cells at the basal membrane level will prevent Ca^{2+} uptake in the cells by exchange with Na^+. Both Na^+/Ca^{2+} exchangers (SLC8A1 and 3) are therefore predicted to be present only in the apical membrane of the uterine glandular cells. The co-expression of the SLC8A1 and 3 genes and of ATP2BX is observed in numerous Ca^{2+} transporting epithelia [48-51] but their respective involvements in Ca^{2+} flux has been questioned. Na^+/Ca^{2+} exchangers have a weak affinity for Ca^{2+}, but strong Ca^{2+} conductance. On the other hand, the Ca^{2+} ATP2BX pumps have a strong affinity for Ca^{2+}, but a weaker conductance [26]. These data suggest that Ca^{2+} transport is mainly assured by the Na^+/Ca^{2+} exchangers. In the hen uterus, the inhibition of the Na^+/K^+ ATPase led to a 60% decrease in Ca^{2+} transport *in vitro* or during uterine perfusion [9,17]. This observation underlines the importance of the Na^+/Ca^{2+} exchangers in the avian uterus.

The information on uterine Ca^{2+} transport is summarized in the model described in Figure 4.

Na$^+$ transfer

During eggshell calcification, Na^+ is absorbed from the uterine fluid into the blood plasma. This absorption resulting from the predominance of apical to basolateral flux relative to basolateral to apical flux, is partly due to the presence of the Na^+/Ca^{2+} exchangers (SLC8A1 and 3), but a complementary system has been demonstrated by using epithelial Na^+ channel blockers [31]. Amiloride-sensitive Na^+ channels are essential in various epithelia [52]. Three subunits (SCNN1A, 1B, 1 G) of the Na^+ channel are overexpressed in the uterus compared to the magnum and to the duodenum (Figure 2), suggesting the involvement of these transporters in Na^+ uptake

by the uterine glandular cells at the apical membrane. The γ subunit (SCNN1G) was overexpressed during shell calcification in contrast to the α and β subunits (SCNN1A, 1B) suggesting its predominant involvement in the uterus.

In the basolateral membrane, the Na^+ glandular cell output towards plasma is active and occurs against a large electrochemical gradient (Table 1). This is provided by the Na^+/K^+ ATPase, which is crucial in all animals for actively transporting Na^+ out and K^+ into the cell, and for maintaining the membrane potential and active transport of other solutes in intestine, kidney or placenta [34,53]. Its presence in the avian uterus and crucial role in ionic transfer during shell formation has been demonstrated [8-10,17]. *In situ* hybridization in the chicken uterus [18] showed that only the α1 subunit of Na^+/K^+ ATPase (ATP1A1), is present in the uterus whereas the α2 and α3 subunits (ATP1A2, A3) are absent. In this study, the α1 subunit (ATP1A1), but also the β1 subunit of Na^+/K^+ ATPase (ATP1B1), were overexpressed in the uterus compared to the magnum. We also confirmed the overexpression of α1 subunit of Na^+/K^+ ATPase during the phase of calcification in contrast to the β1subunit of Na^+/K^+ ATPase, in agreement with Lavelin et al. [18].

The possibility of an uptake of Na^+ from plasma into the uterine glandular cells at the basal membrane via Na^+/HCO_3^- co-transporters (SLC4A4, 5, 7, 10) is discussed in the section addressing HCO_3^- transfer.

K$^+$ secretion

In the gastrointestinal or kidney epithelia, K^+ channels provide the driving force for electrogenic transport processes across membranes and are involved in cell volume regulation or in secretory and reabsorptive processes. K^+ channels are crucial for maintenance of body homeostasis and form the largest group of ion channels in mammals as more than one hundred thirty genes have been identified in human [54,55]. The chicken database revealed more than 80 such genes in birds. We explored only a limited number of K^+ channel candidates in chicken uterus by selecting 4 K^+ channels overexpressed in uterus compared to their expression in magnum, as revealed in our hen transcriptomic study [21]. The increased K^+ concentrations in uterine fluid between early (8 hours) and late stages of calcification (Table 1), demonstrates that uterine K^+ net flow corresponds to a secretion into uterine fluid. A portion of K^+ secretion might be associated with the passive component of water secretion which occurs during the egg plumping at the early stage of shell calcification (up to 10 hours) but no experimental data has explored this contribution through a putative paracellular pathway. K^+ uptake at the basolateral membrane, from the blood plasma

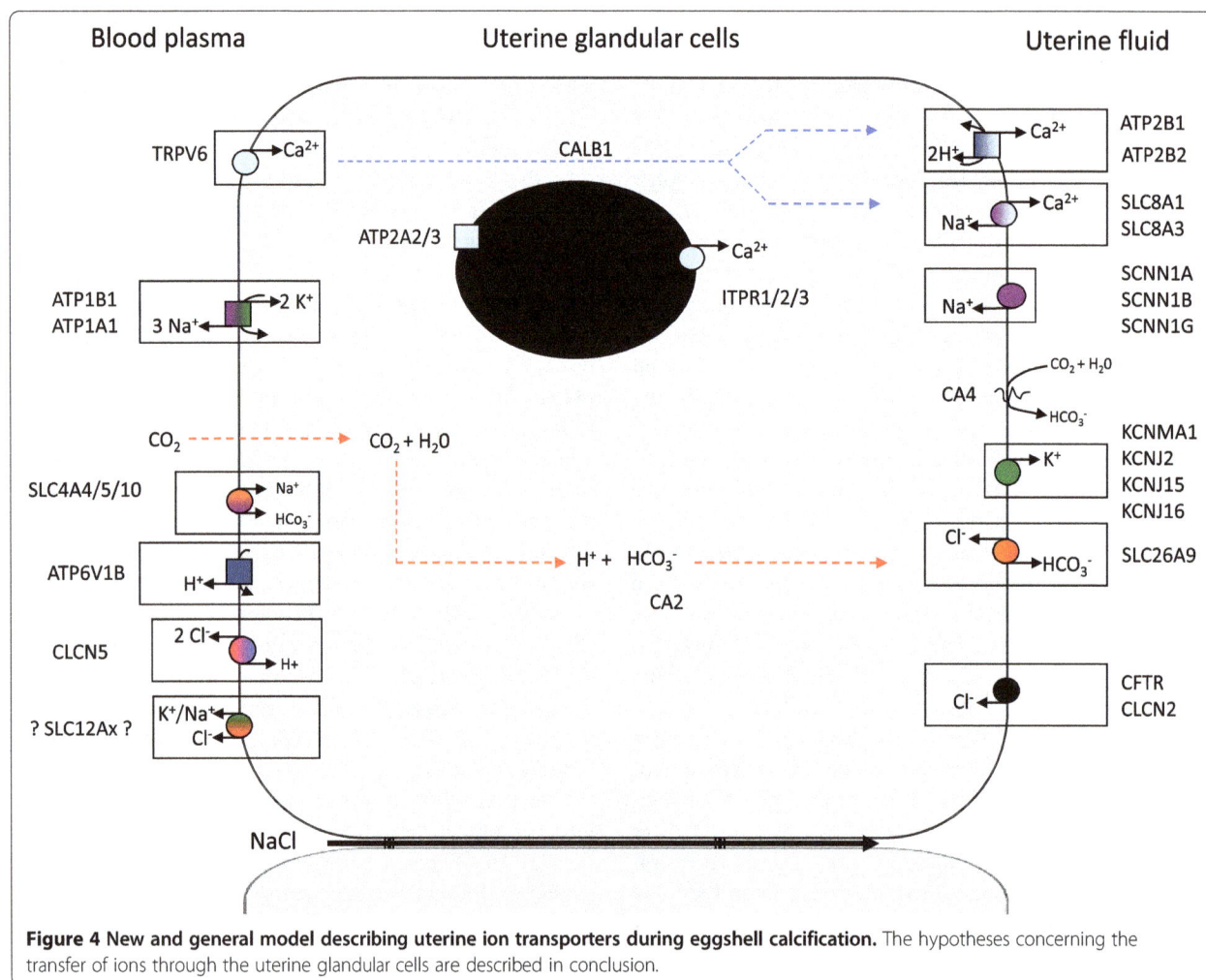

Figure 4 New and general model describing uterine ion transporters during eggshell calcification. The hypotheses concerning the transfer of ions through the uterine glandular cells are described in conclusion.

towards the uterine glandular cells, should result from activities of the Na^+/K^+ ATPases (ATP1A1, B1). By analogy with other intestinal, kidney, pancreatic, placenta, mammary glands or blood cells, we expect that K^+ channels present in the glandular cell will recycle K^+ to allow functioning of the active Na^+/K^+ ATPases. We tested 4 genes: three coding K^+ channels (KCNJ2, 15, 16) and one K^+ large conductance Ca^{2+} activated channel (KCNMA1), which could be involved in K^+ cell output (Tables 1 and 3). The KCNJ2, 15, 16 channels belong to the KCNJ family (potassium inwardly-rectifying channel, subfamily J) which are stimulated by external K^+ concentration. Their expressions are observed in numerous epithelia where K^+ secretion occurs [54-56]. The KCNMs (K^+ large conductance Ca^{2+} activated channels, subfamily M) participate in K^+ output in a large range of tissues and epithelia and are regulated by Ca^{2+} cellular levels [54-56]. Our results showed that the expression of KCNJ2, 15, 16 and KCNMA1 K^+ channels were higher in the uterus compared with the magnum. Moreover, the expression of KCNJ2, 15 and KCNMA1 (KCNM

subunit α) was stimulated during calcification (Figure 3). These results showed that KCNJ2, 15, 16, and KCNM K^+ channels are involved in the maintenance of potential membrane and K^+ recycling during eggshell calcification and have therefore been introduced in the model (Figure 4). We propose to localize them in the apical membrane but we have no evidence that they are absent from the basolateral membranes.

HCO_3^- production and transfer

Eggshell mineralisation results from the co-precipitation of Ca^{2+} and HCO_3^-. The bicarbonate precursor of the eggshell calcite is mainly derived from the blood carbon dioxide (CO_2) which penetrates the uterine glandular cells by simple diffusion through the plasma membrane [2,19]. Carbonic anhydrases (CAs) [6] catalyse the hydration of intracellular CO_2 to HCO_3^-, which is secreted into the uterine fluid. In the mammalian gastrointestinal tract, including pancreas, the cellular and membrane bound CAs are key enzymes allowing secretion or reabsorption of large amount of acid across the mucosa or protect epithelial cells from acid injury by secreting bicarbonate [24,25,57]. In all mammalian species, the duodenum buffers gastric acid secretion by producing intracellular HCO_3^- from CO_2 at a higher rate than the stomach or distal small intestine. The CO_2 originates from intestinal lumen at the duodenal level but is provided from blood plasma via the respiratory system to the uterine tissue [1]. This study showed a larger expression of the cytosolic CA2 and 7 and of the membrane bound CA4 in the chicken uterus than in magnum (Figure 2). No difference in expression was observed between the uterus and the duodenum for CA2 and 4. Cytoplasmic CA2 is the predominant CA in the duodenum, playing a major function in the hydration of CO_2 to produce HCO_3^- [25]. Similarly, we propose that CA2 plays a major role in the uterus to provide the carbonate precursor for the eggshell. CA7 is significantly underexpressed in the uterus compared to the duodenum, suggesting a secondary rule in HCO_3^- uterine production. A major role for CA2 is supported by the overexpression of this CA gene in the presence of eggshell mineralisation, in contrast to CA4 and 7 (Figure 3).

The HCO_3^- produced by CA2 in uterine glandular cells must be then secreted into the uterine fluid to build the eggshell. In mammalian pancreas [57] and in duodenum [25] which secrete large amounts of HCO_3^- towards the lumen, anion HCO_3^-/Cl^- exchangers (SLC4AX) have been located in apical membrane and Na^+/HCO_3^- co-transporters (SLC26AX) at the basolateral membrane [58,59]. In the bird uterus, there is a strong association between HCO_3^- secretion and Cl^- transport [9,31] which supports the involvement of HCO_3^-/Cl^- exchangers. The HCO_3^- flow through the uterine apical membrane is an electrogenic process which is facilitated by output of intracellular Cl^-, via an exchanger of the SLC26 electrogenic family [31,57]. Our study confirmed the expression of a HCO_3^-/Cl^- exchanger (SLC26A9) in the uterus as shown in other epithelial cells [59]. SLC26A9 is suspected to have a role in intestinal HCO_3^- secretion, in particular to neutralise gastric acidity [60,61]. Our results showed an overexpression of SLC26A9 exchanger in the uterus compared to the magnum or when the calcification takes place, whereas no variation of expression was observed between the duodenum and the uterus (Figure 2). These observations suggest a common mechanism between both tissues and support the hypothesis of the involvement of this transporter in the supply of HCO_3^- for eggshell calcification. Na^+/HCO_3^- co-transporter genes (SLC4A4, 5, 7, 10; [58,62]) are also expressed in the uterus and likely contribute to HCO_3^- transport. SLC4A4, 5, 7 and 10 showed higher expression in the uterus than in the magnum. An overexpression relative to the duodenum is observed only for SLC4A5, the three others being similarly expressed

(Figure 2). SLC4A7 is underexpressed in the uterus during calcification compared to its absence (Figure 3) suggesting that involvement of this transporter is limited during the eggshell calcification process. In mammals, Na^+/HCO_3^- co-transporters mediate the electroneutral movement of Na^+ and HCO_3^- across the plasma membrane [58]. The ionic concentrations in the plasma and uterine glandular cells (Table 1) show a favourable concentration gradient for uptake of these ions, supporting the localisation of these transporters in the basolateral membrane of uterine glandular cells to allow HCO_3^- entry. However, previous studies [2,19] showed that the majority of HCO_3^- used for the eggshell came from blood CO_2 and only for a minor part from plasma HCO_3^-. Na^+/HCO_3^- co-transporters (SLC4A4, 5, 10) are likely to have a minor role in HCO_3^- supply to the uterine glandular cells. The cystic fibrosis transmembrane conductance regulator (CFTR) contributes to fluid secretion from epithelial cells of the lung, pancreas and intestine, as shown in pathological situations associated with impaired fluid production, Cl^- and HCO_3^- secretion due to defective CFTR [63,64] or in pharmacological studies of reproductive epithelium [65]. Its contribution to HCO_3^- secretion is unlikely because of the unfavourable gradient or it is possibly indirect through regulation of HCO_3^- transporters [65]. Its role as a Cl^- channel is discussed in the following section on Cl^-. Studies using specific inhibitors and measuring Cl^- and HCO_3^- flows are needed to quantify the contribution of HCO_3^-/Cl^- exchangers in HCO_3^- uterine secretion.

H^+ transfer

HCO_3^- production in the glandular epithelial cells, its secretion into uterine fluid and the co-precipitation of CO_3^{2-} with Ca^{2+} leads to a progressive acidification of the uterine fluid and of glandular cells [1,5]. In fact, two H^+ are produced for each $CaCO_3$ formed. This metabolic acidosis is partially compensated by hyperventilation by the hen and by an increased renal H^+ excretion [22].

The plasma membrane Ca^{2+}-transporting ATPases (ATP2B1, 2) of the apical membrane actively extrude Ca^{2+}, as previously mentioned. However several lines of evidence have established that these pumps contribute to H^+ re-absorption coupled to Ca^{2+} secretion [66,67]. The present study highlights their crucial role in Ca^{2+} secretion by uterine glandular cells during eggshell formation and therefore in H^+ re-absorption from the uterine fluid through the apical membrane. Alternatively, the Na^+/H^+ exchangers have been shown to contribute to H^+ output in the pancreatic duct which also secretes large amount of HCO_3^-. In a recent transcriptomic study of the uterus (unpublished data, Brionne A, Nys Y and Gautron J), we detected expression of various Na^+/H^+

exchangers (SLC9A 1, 2, 6, 7, 8, 9), supporting this possibility.

In this study, RT-PCR shows that the V H^+ ATPase pump (VAT) is expressed in the bird uterus during calcification. In mammals, this VAT complex is made up of at least 14 subunits and allows transfer of H^+ by hydrolysis of ATP [68,69]. This VAT is present in many membranes of organelles and also frequently in the plasma membranes of renal cells or osteoclasts [70]. VAT is therefore a good candidate for transferring protons to plasma in the hen uterine glandular cell, especially as this VAT was revealed in other species producing $CaCO_3$ biominerals and shown to export H^+ during mineralisation [71,72]. This proton ATPase extrudes H^+ across the basolateral membrane of pancreatic duct epithelium [57] which is secreting high amounts of HCO_3^- using mechanisms quite similar to uterine glandular cells. Our study reveals overexpression of the VAT subunit B in the uterus, which transfers large amounts of H^+ compared with the magnum, where limited amounts of H^+ are transferred. The VAT is likely to participate in H^+ export from cytoplasm of the uterine cells to the blood plasma across the plasma membrane. The role of CLCN5 in H^+ transfer is discussed in the ensuing Cl^- section.

Cl^- transfer

The Cl^- concentrations decrease from 71 to 45 mM in the uterine fluid (Table 1) when comparing the initial and late stage of eggshell calcification in parallel with changes of larger magnitude in Na^+ concentrations. The high concentration of these ions observed at the early stage of calcification might result from the large secretions of water, Na^+ and Cl^- which occurs during the plumping period (hydration of the egg white proteins), 6 to 10 h after ovulation possibly through a paracellular pathway [1]. These water and saline secretions are completed at the initiation of the rapid phase of shell formation, when Na^+ and Cl^- net fluxes are inversed. The net flux of Cl^- is inhibited by acetazolamide, demonstrating the relationship between Cl^- transport and HCO_3^- secretion derived from CAs activity [8,9,31], and the involvement of HCO_3^-/Cl^- exchangers of the SLC4 or SLC26 family [57,62,73]. Amongst the SLC4Ax HCO_3^-/Cl^- exchangers, we observed no expression of SLC4A8 and there is no evidence of any expression of SLC4A1, 2 or 3 in avian uterine transcriptomic study [21]. The role of SLC26A9 exchanger was previously discussed in the HCO_3^- section. This exchanger is predicted to be located in the apical membrane of the uterine glandular cells and to contribute to Cl^- cell uptake during eggshell calcification as suggested in hens subjected to acetazolamide inhibitors [31] or in other species [57,59].

The CLCN2 channel, a family member of the CLCN (Cl^- channel), is relatively ubiquitous in epithelial cells and other cellular types [74,75]. It is considered to participate in various functions such as cellular volume regulation [76,77], cardiac activity regulation [78,79] and Cl^- trans-epithelial transfer [80,81]. Our study revealed that the CLCN2 channel is overexpressed in the uterus compared to the magnum or the duodenum (Figure 2). The uterine fluid (>45 mM) and intracellular (4 mM) Cl^- concentrations are favourable to a Cl^- passive entry in uterine glandular cells. In parallel, another Cl^- channel, the cystic fibrosis transmembrane conductance regulator (CFTR) could also contribute to Cl^- entry in the cell as observed in numerous tissues [74]. In the chicken uterus, the CFTR channel is expressed at a higher level than in the magnum and the duodenum (Figure 2). It is also overexpressed in the uterus during eggshell calcification (Figure 3). The CLCN2 and CFTR channel are therefore probably expressed in the apical membrane and might contribute to Cl^- entry in the cell.

On the other hand, Cl^- output could be carried out by CLCN5, another member of CLCN family. Renal proximal tubule cells highly express the V H^+ ATPase for acidification of endosomes and electroneutrality is ensured by transfer of Cl^- by CLCN5 [74]. The CLCN5 H^+/Cl^- exchanger [75] has been localised mainly in organelle membranes but also in the plasma membrane. Our study revealed an overexpression of CLCN5 H^+/Cl^- in the uterus compared to the magnum, so this channel might contribute to Cl^- output through the basal membrane. An alternative would be that Cl^- output relies on cation-coupled cotransport as observed in fish or mammals. The SLC12 family consists of Na^+-K^+-$2Cl^-$ cotransporters and of K^+-Cl^- electroneutral cotransporters, and are expressed either in kidney where they contribute to salt reabsorption, or more ubiquitously being involved in cell volume regulation [82-84]. In the chicken uterus, one Na^+-K^+-$2Cl^-$ cotransporter (SLC12A2) and 4 K^+-Cl^- cotransporters (SLC12A4, 7, 8, 9) are putative candidate, as expression of these genes is revealed in the chicken uterus transcriptome (unpublished data, Brionne A, Nys Y and Gautron J). In addition, furosemide, a blocker of Na^+-K^+-$2Cl^-$ cotransporters, has been shown to decrease egg shell thickness [85].

Conclusions

Initial studies on ion transfer in the uterus using physiological and pharmacological approaches provided a preliminary model of ion transfer contributing to the uterine Ca^{2+} and HCO_3^- necessary for shell mineralisation (Figure 1) [1,5,8-10,17]. The current approaches using knowledge gleaned from the chicken genome sequence and uterine transcriptomic expression data [21] identified numerous genes encoding putative transporters

Table 3 Primers used for RT-PCR and qRT-PCR of ion transporter genes

Gene symbol	RefSeq accession	Forward primer	Reverse primer
TPRV6	XM_416530	AACACCTGTGAAGGAGCTGGTGAG	TCTGCTGCTTGTTTTGTTGCC
CALB1	NM_205513	CAGGGTGTCAAAATGTGTGC	GCCAGTTCTGCTCGGTAAAG
ATP2A1	NM_205519	AAGGGGGGGTCTTTAAGGATGG	CAAACTGCTCCACCACCAACTC
ATP2A2	XM_415130	GCAGCTTGCATATCTTTTGTGCTG	CATTTCTTTCCTGCCACACTCC
ATP2A3	NM_204891	CAACCCCAAGGAGCCTCTTATC	GGTCCCTCAGCGTCATACAAGAAC
ITPR1	XM_414438	AATGGCAAAAGGCGAGGAAAGC	GGAGCAGCAGCAAGCGGG
ITPR2	XM_001235612	TGAGCATTGTGAGTGGCTTC	GTTGACCTGGCTGTCCAAAT
ITPR3	XM_418035	AGTACAACGTGGCCCTCATC	GTCGTGTCTGCTCTCCATGA
RYR1	X95266	GTTCCTCTGCATCATCGGCTAC	AATTGCTGGGGAAGGACTGTG
ATP2B1	XM_416133	CTGCACTGAAGAAAGCAGATGTTG	GCTGTCATATACGTTTCGTCCCC
ATP2B2	XM_001231767	TTACTGTACTTGTGGTTGCTGTCCC	GGTTGTTAGCGTCCCTGTTTTG
ATP2B4	XM_418055	GCTGGTGAAGTTGTCATCCGTC	TGCTCTGAAGAAAGCTGATGTTGG
SLC8A1	NM_001079473	GGATTGTGGAGGTTTGGGAAGG	CTGTTTGCCAGCTCGGTATTTC
SLC8A3	XM_001231413	GGAGAGACCACAACAACAACCATTC	AGCTACGAATCCATGCCCACAC
SCNN1A	NM_205145	GCTTGCCAGAAAACAGTCCCTC	AGTCAGACTCATCCAGGTCTTTGG
SCNN1B	XM_425247	ATGGAAGTAGACCGCAGT	GTTGTATGGCAGCACAGT
SCNN1G	XM_414880	CAAAAGGCACTTCACCCGTTTC	GGACAATGATCTTGGCTCCTGTC
ATP1A1	NM_205521	GCACAAAGAAGAAAAAGGCGAAGG	GGGTGGAGGTGTAAGGGTATTTG
ATP1B1	NM_205520	TCTGGAACTCGGAGAAGAAGGAG	GACGGTGAGCAACATCACTTGG
SLC4A4	XM_420603	GGAAAGCACCATTCTTCGCC	CCTCCAAAAGTGATAGCATTGGTC
SLC4A5	XM_423797	TGAACGTCTCCGCTACATCCTG	ACTTTATCCACCTGGCTGACTCC
SLC4A7	XM_418757	AAATTGCCAAGTTCGTGGTGG	GCGAAGCAAATGAGAAGTTACGG
SLC4A9	XM_001232427	TCCTGACTGGAGTCTCTGTCTTCC	AGGTGATCTGGCTGGTGTTTTG
SLC4A10	XR_026836	CGCTGATGACAGATGAGGTGTTC	GGTGGTTCTATTCGGATTGTTGG
KCNJ2	NM_205370	CCATTGCTGTTTTCATGGTG	TCCTGGACTTGAGGAGCTGT
KCNJ15	XM_425554	TGAGGGAAGGGAGACTCTGA	GCTTCCATCCTCACTGCTTC
KCNJ16	XM_425383	CATTCCTGTTCTCCCTGGAA	CATTTTAGCCAAGGCTGCTC
KCNMA1	NM_204224	GGGATGATGCGATCTGTCTT	GACAAACCCACAAAGGCACT
CA2	NM_205317	ATCGTCAACAACGGGCACTCCTTC	TGCACCAACCTGTAGACTCCATCC
CA4	XM_415893	GCTAACACATTTTTCCCCCTTCC	CTTTATAGCACATCGCATCAGCC
CA7	XM_414152	GCACAAGTCTTATCCCATTGCC	GCCGTTGTTGGAGATGTTGAGAG
SLC4A8	XM_001235579	AGAAGAAGAAGTTGGACGATGCC	GGTCAGTTCTGTCCTTGCTGTTCTG
SLC26A9	XM_425821	GCCTCTTCGATGAGGAGTTTGAG	CTGACCCCACCAAGAACATCAG
ATP6V1B2	XM_424534	ATTCTCTGCTGCTGGTTTGCCC	CATGGACCCATTTTCCTCAAAGTC
CFTR	NM_001105666	AAGAGGGCAGGGAAGATCAACGAG	CGGGTTAGCTTCAGTTCAGTTTCAC
CLCN2	XM_423073	CCTGGACACCAATGTGATGCTG	CACGAAGGTCTTCAGGGTGAGATAC
CLCN5	XM_420265	CGATTGGAGGAGTGCTCTTTAGTC	CAAAAGGATTGATGGAACGCAG

supplying the mineral precursors of eggshell mineralisation. We have used this information to build a model describing the ion supply mechanisms in the uterus, following a logical sequence for ion transfers for secretion of large amounts of Ca^{2+} and HCO_3^- to form the eggshell (Figure 4). This work identified 31 genes and related proteins involved in this process. It is consistent with preliminary hypotheses. Our analysis also revealed that analogies exist in the mechanisms of HCO_3^- secretion by pancreatic duct cells and by duodenum, and to a lower extent with

intestinal epithelial cells for Ca^{2+} movement, even if the Ca^{2+} flux is reversed between both uterus and duodenum.

The main steps of ion transfer in the hen's uterus can be summarised (as presented in Figure 4):

(1) Ca^{2+} secretion through epithelial glandular cells involves TRPV6 Ca^{2+} channel in the basolateral membrane (cell uptake entry), 28 kDa calbindin (CALB1, intracellular transfer), endoplasmic Ca^{2+} pumps type 2, 3 (ATP2A2, 3, uptake by endoplasmic

reticulum), and inositol trisphosphate receptors type 1, 2, 3 (ITPR1, 2, 3, output from the reticulum). Ca^{2+} is then extruded from the glandular cells by the membrane's Ca^{2+} pumps (ATP2B1, 2) and Ca^{2+}/Na^+ exchangers (SLC8A1, 3). The endoplasmic Ca^{2+} pumps, inositol trisphosphate receptors, and 28 kDa calbindin contribute to maintain a low intracellular free Ca^{2+} concentration essential for cell survival.

(2) Na^+ transport involves three Na^+ channels (subunits SCNN1A, 1B, 1 G; uptake in the cell), Na^+/Ca^{2+} exchangers SLC8A1 and 3 (uptake in the cell) and the Na^+/K^+ ATPase (ATP1A1, ATP1B1, output from the cell).

(3) K^+ uptake entry into the cell results from the Na^+/K^+ ATPase; the K^+ channels (KCNJ2, 15, 16 and KCNMA1) contribute to its output release at the apical membrane.

(4) HCO_3^- is mainly produced from CO_2 by CA2 and to a lesser extent by CA4, and is also provided at a low level from plasma by the Na^+/HCO_3^- co-transporters (SLC4A4, 5, 10). HCO_3^- is exported from the cell through the HCO_3^-/Cl^- exchanger SLC26A9.

(5) HCO_3^- synthesis in the cell and co-precipitation of HCO_3^- with Ca^{2+} in the uterine fluid produces two H^+ which are transferred to plasma via the membrane Ca^{2+} pumps ATP2B1, 2 in the apical membrane and the VAT pump at the basolateral level.

(6) Cl^- ions in the uterine fluid enter the cell by the HCO_3^-/Cl^- exchanger SLC26A9 and by Cl^- channels (CLCN2, CFTR uptake in the cells), and might be extruded by Cl^-/H^+ exchanger (CLCN5), but also by $Na^+-K^+-2Cl^-$ and K^+-Cl^- cotransporters (SLC12Ax).

This model proposes a large but not exhaustive list of ionic transfer proteins involved in the supply of Ca^{2+} and HCO_3^- or in maintaining cellular homeostasis (volume, electroneutrality). The model qualitatively describes putative mechanisms and cellular localisation of the candidates. These hypotheses relying on expression of the genes and on analogies with other tissues that transfer large amount of ions, need to be confirmed using immunochemistry for their cell localisation or by specific inhibition, to establish their relative contribution and understand their interaction and regulation. This avian model where huge amounts of Ca^{2+} and HCO_3^- are exported daily following a precise spatial and temporal sequence should contribute to understanding the mechanism and regulation of ionic precursors of $CaCO_3$ and provide insight for other species secreting a

$CaCO_3$ biomineral such as coral, molluscs, foraminifera or sea urchins.

Methods
Animals handling and housing
The experiment was conducted at the Unité Expérimentale Pôle d'Expérimentation Avicole de Tours (UEPEAT - INRA, Tours, France) according to the legislation on research involving animal subjects set by the European Community Council Directive of November 24, 1986 (86/609/EEC) and under the supervision of an authorized scientist (Authorization # 7323, J Gautron). Forty week old laying hens (ISA brown strain) were caged individually and subjected to a light/dark cycle of 14 hour light and 10 hour darkness (14 L:10D). The hens were fed a layer of mash as recommended by the Institut National de la Recherche Agronomique (INRA). Each cage was equipped with a device for automatic recording of oviposition time.

Collection of laying hens oviduct tissues
Tissue samples (magnum, uterus, duodenum, kidney and *gastrocnemius*) were harvested in 8 hens while the egg was in the uterus during the active phase of calcification (16–18 hour post-ovulation). Additionally, uterine tissues were collected from 8 birds injected with 50 μg of F2-α prostaglandin during 4 consecutive days to expel the egg before mineralisation had begun (6 to 8 hours post ovulation). All tissue samples were quickly frozen in liquid nitrogen and stored at −80°C until RNA extraction.

Determination of *Gallus gallus* cDNA sequences involved in mineral supply and design of primers
The list of ion transporters was established using recent transcriptomic data and *Gallus gallus* databases when available. The transporters not yet identified in chicken were identified using human orthologs in Swiss-Prot/TrEMBL and RefSeq databases. The corresponding human sequences were aligned to *Gallus gallus* Refseq database using BlastN algorithm an e-value cut-off of 10^{-20}. Primers (Table 3), were designed from the *Gallus gallus* using Mac vector software (MacVector, Cambridge, U.K.). The quality of the primers was tested by virtual PCR for dimerization and specificity using Amplify 3X software [86].

RNA isolation, reverse transcription and classical
Total RNA was extracted from frozen tissue samples using a commercial kit (RNeasy Mini kit, Qiagen; Courtaboeuf, France) and simultaneously treated with DNase (RNase-free DNase set, Qiagen; Courtaboeuf, France) according to the manufacturer's procedure. RNA concentrations were measured at 260 nm using

a NanodropND 1000 (Thermo Fischer, Wilmington, Delaware, USA). The integrity of RNA was evaluated on a 2% agarose gel and with an Agilent 2100 Bioanalyser (Agilent Technologies, Massy, France). Only RNA samples with a 28S/18S ratio > 1.3 were considered for RT-PCR and qRT-PCR experiments. Total RNA samples (5 μg) were subjected to reverse-transcription using RNase H-MMLV reverse transcriptase (Superscript II, Invitrogen, Cergy Pontoise, France) and random hexamers (Amersham, Orsay, France). PCR was performed using primers (Table 3) for 30 cycles at 60°C. The specificity of the PCR reaction was assessed by sequencing of PCR products (Cogenics, Meylan, France), and alignment of the sequences using BLASTN algorithm against the *Gallus gallus* RefSeq nucleic data bank.

Quantitative RT-PCR (qRT-PCR)

Alternatively, cDNA sequences were amplified in real time using the qPCR Master mix plus for SYBR® Green I assay (Eurogentec, Seraing, Belgium) with the ABI PRISM 7000 Sequence Detection System (Applied Biosystems, France). To account for variations in mRNA extraction and reverse transcription reaction between samples, mRNA levels were normalized either to ribosomal 18S rRNA levels for each sample in the first series of comparison (magnum, uterus, and duodenum) or to TBP (TATA box binding protein) for each samples in the second series of comparison (comparison of expression in the uterus with and without mineralisation). The expression levels of 18S rRNA were measured using TaqMan Universal PCR Master Mix and developed TaqMan assay for human 18S rRNA (Applied Biosystems, Courtaboeuf, France) as previously validated [87]. The PCR conditions consisted of an uracil-N-glycosylase pre-incubation step at 50°C for 2 min, followed by a denaturation step at 95°C for 10 min, and 40 cycles of amplification (denaturation for 15 sec at 95°C, annealing and elongation for 1 min at 60°C). A melting curve was carried out from 60 to 95°C for each sample amplified with SYBR® Green. Each run included triplicates of no template controls, standards and samples. Standards correspond respectively to a pool of the magnum, uterus, and duodenum RT products for the first series of experiments and of the uterus with and without mineralisation for the second series of comparison. The threshold cycle (Ct), defined as the cycle at which fluorescence rises above a defined base line, was determined for each sample and cDNA control. A calibration curve was calculated using the Ct values of the cDNA control samples and relative amount of unknown samples were deduced from this curve. The ratio value was calculated for each sample as sample/18 S rRNA in the first comparison (magnum, uterus, and duodenum) or sample/TBP in the

second comparison (uterus with and without calcification). The log of the ratio was used for statistical analysis using the 5th version of StatView, software (SAS Institute Inc. Cary, NC). A one-way analysis of variance was performed to detect differences (P < 0.05; 8 replicates/treatment) in gene expression amongst different conditions.

Competing interests

The authors declare that they have no competing interests.

Authors' contributions

VJ, JG contributed to the strategy, the experimental design, and planning of the study. VJ carried out the experiments and analyses, interpreted data and wrote the first draft of the paper. JG is the supervisor of VJ (Ph.D. student). AB contributed to the interpretation of data and to the writing of the paper. YN conceived the research program focused on identification of egg proteins. He was involved in the strategy, the experimental design, data interpretation and was fully involved in the writing of the paper. All authors have read and approved the final manuscript.

Acknowledgements

The authors gratefully acknowledge the European Community for its financial support through the RESCAPE project (RESCAPE Food CT 2006–036018), and SABRE program (European Integrating project Cutting-Edge Genomics for Sustainable Animal Breeding Project 016250). VJ thanks the Region Centre and INRA for financial support. We also thank Magali Berges for her technical assistance and Jean Didier Terlot-Brysinne for care of experimental birds. We wish to thank Prof. Maxwell Hincke, Department of Cellular & Molecular Medicine, University of Ottawa, 451 Smyth Road, Ottawa K1H 8 M5, Canada, for his critical reading of the manuscript and constructive remarks.

References

1. Nys Y, Hincke MT, Arias JL, Garcia-Ruiz JM, Solomon SE: **Avian eggshell mineralization.** *Poult Avian Biol Rev* 1999, **10**(3):143–166.
2. Hodges R, Lörcher K: **Possible sources of the carbonate fraction of egg shell calcium carbonate.** *Nature* 1967, **216**:606–610.
3. Lippiello L, Wasserman RH: **Fluorescent-antibody localization of vitamin-D-dependent calcium-binding protein in oviduct of laying hen.** *J Histochem Cytochem* 1975, **23**(2):111–116.
4. Coty WA, McConkey CL: **A high-affinity calcium-stimulated atpase activity in the hen oviduct shell gland.** *Arch Biochem Biophys* 1982, **219**(2):444–453.
5. Sauveur B, Mongin P: **Comparative study of uterine fluid and egg albumen in shell gland of hen.** *Ann Biol Anim Biochim Biophys* 1971, **11**(2):213–224.
6. Common RH: **The carbonic anhydrase activity of the hen oviduct.** *J Agri Soc Univ Coll Wales* 1941, **31**:412–414.
7. Pike JW, Alvarado RH: **Ca2 + −Mg2 +−activated atpase in shell gland of japanese-quail (Coturnix-coturnix-japonica).** *Comp Biochem Physiol B* 1975, **51**(1):119–125.
8. Eastin WC, Spaziani E: **Control of calcium secretion in avian shell gland (Uterus).** *Biol Reprod* 1978, **19**(3):493–504.
9. Eastin WC, Spaziani E: **On the mechanism of calcium secretion in the avian shell gland (Uterus).** *Biol Reprod* 1978, **19**(3):505–518.
10. Pearson TW, Goldner AM: **Calcium-transport across avian uterus - Effects of electrolyte substitution.** *Am J Physiol* 1973, **225**(6):1508–1512.
11. Nys Y, Mayel-Afshar S, Bouillon R, Vanbaelen H, Lawson DEM: **Increases in calbindin D-28 k messenger-Rna in the uterus of the domestic-fowl induced by sexual maturity and shell formation.** *Gen Comp Endocrinol* 1989, **76**(2):322–329.

12. Striem S, Bar A: Modulation of quail intestinal and egg-shell gland calbindin (Mr 28000) gene-expression by vitamin-D3, 1,25-dihydroxyvitamin-D3 and egg-laying. *Mol Cell Endocrinol* 1991, 75(2):169–177.

13. Nys Y, Zawadzki J, Gautron J, Mills AD: Whitening of brown-shelled eggs: mineral composition of uterine fluid and rate of protoporphyrin deposition. *Poult Sci* 1991, 70(5):1236–1245.

14. Bar A, Striem S, Mayel-afshar S, Lawson DEM: Differential regulation of calbindin-D28K mRNA in the intestine and eggshell gland of the laying hen. *J Mol Endocrinol* 1990, 4(2):93–99.

15. Christakos S, Barletta F, Huening M, Dhawan P, Liu Y, Porta A, Peng X: Vitamin D target proteins: Function and regulation. *J Cell Biochem* 2003, 88(2):238–244.

16. Parker SL, Lindsay LA, Herbert JF, Murphy CR, Thompson MB: Expression and localization of Ca2 + –ATPase in the uterus during the reproductive cycle of king quail (Coturnix chinensis) and zebra finch (Poephila guttata). *Comp Biochem Physiol A* 2008, 149(1):30–35.

17. Pearson TW, Goldner AM: Calcium-transport across avian uterus.II. Effects of inhibitors and nitrogen. *Am J Physiol* 1974, 227(2):465–468.

18. Lavelin I, Meiri N, Genina O, Alexiev R, Pines M: Na + –K + –ATPase gene expression in the avian eggshell gland: distinct regulation in different cell types. *Am J Physiol Regul Integr Comp Physiol* 2001, 281(4):R1169–R1176.

19. Lörcher K, Zscheile C, Bronsch K: Rate of CO2 and C14 exhalation in laying hens resting and during egg-shell mineralisation after a single injection of NaHC1403. *Ann Biol Anim Biochim Biophys* 1970, 10:133–139.20.

20. Consortium ICGS: Sequence and comparative analysis of the chicken genome provide unique perspectives on vertebrate evolution. *Nature* 2004, 432(7018):695–716.

21. Jonchère V, Rehault-Godbert S, Hennequet-Antier C, Cabau C, Sibut V, Cogburn LA, Nys Y, Gautron J: Gene expression profiling to identify eggshell proteins involved in physical defense of the chicken egg. *BMC Genomics* 2010, 11:57.

22. Sauveur B: Electrolyte composition of different zones of egg albumen in 2 breeds of hen. *Ann Biol Anim Biochim Biophys* 1969, 9(4):563–573.

23. Bronner F, Pansu D: Nutritional aspects of calcium absorption. *J Nutr* 1999, 129(1):9–12.

24. Kaunitz JD, Akiba Y: Duodenal carbonic anhydrase: Mucosal protection, luminal chemosensing, and gastric acid disposal. *Keio J Med* 2006, 55(3):96–106.

25. Flemström G, Allen A: Gastroduodenal mucus bicarbonate barrier: protection against acid and pepsin. *Am J Physiol Cell Physiol* 2005, 288(1):1–19.

26. Bouillon R, Van Cromphaut S, Carmeliet G: Intestinal calcium absorption: Molecular vitamin D mediated mechanisms. *J Cell Biochem* 2003, 88(2):332–339.

27. Hurwitz S: Calcium homeostasis in birds. *Vitam Horm* 1989, 45:173–221.

28. Nys Y: Regulation of plasma 1,25 (OH)2D3, of osteocalcin and of intestinal and uterine calbindin in hens. In *Avian Endocrinology*. Edited by Sharp PJ. Bristol: Society for Endocrinology; 1993:345–357. 408p.

29. Nys Y: *Régulation endocrinienne du metabolisme calcique chez la poule et calcification de la coquille*. 6th edition. Paris: Thèse de Docteur de l'université en Physiologie animale; 1990:162p.

30. Bar A: Calcium transport in strongly calcifying laying birds: Mechanisms and regulation. *Comp Biochem Physiol A* 2009, 152(4):447–469.

31. Vetter AE, O'Grady SA: Sodium and anion transport across the avian uterine (shell gland) epithelium. *J Exp Biol* 2005, 208(3):479–486.

32. Wasserman RH, Smith CA, Smith CM, Brindak ME, Fullmer CS, Krook L, Penniston JT, Kumar R: Immunohistochemical localization of a calcium-pump and calbindin-D28k in the oviduct of the laying hen. *Histochemistry* 1991, 96(5):413–418.

33. Wasserman RH, Taylor AN: Vitamin D3-induced calcium-binding protein in chick intestinal mucosa. *Science* 1966, 152(3723):791–793.

34. Hoenderop JGJ, Nilius B, Bindels RJM: Calcium absorption across epithelia. *Physiol Rev* 2005, 85(1):373–422.

35. Jande S, Tolnai S, Lawson D: Immunohistochemical localization of vitamin D-dependent calcium-binding protein in duodenum, kidney, uterus and cerebellum of chickens. *Histochemistry* 1981, 71(1):99–116.

36. Lambers TT, Mahieu F, Oancea E, Hoofd L, de Lange F, Mensenkamp AR, Voets T, Nilius B, Clapham DE, Hoenderop JG, et al: Calbindin-D-28 K dynamically controls TRPV5-mediated Ca2+ transport. *EMBO J* 2006, 25(13):2978–2988.

37. Christakos S, Dhawan P, Benn B, Porta A, Hediger M, Oh GT, Jeung EB, Zhong Y, Ajibade D, Dhawan K, et al: Vitamin D molecular mechanism of action. *Ann N Y Acad Sci* 2007, 1116:340–348.

38. Gorlach A, Klappa P, Kietzmann T: The endoplasmic reticulum: Folding, calcium homeostasis, signaling, and redox control. *Antioxid Redox Signal* 2006, 8(9–10):1391–1418.

39. Rossi D, Barone V, Giacomello E, Cusimano V, Sorrentino V: The sarcoplasmic reticulum: An organized patchwork of specialized domains. *Traffic* 2008, 9(7):1044–1049.

40. Periasamy M, Kalyanasundaram A: SERCA pump isoforms: Their role in calcium transport and disease. *Muscle Nerve* 2007, 35(4):430–442.

41. Vermassen E, Parys JB, Mauger JP: Subcellular distribution of the inositol 1,4,5-trisphosphate receptors: functional relevance and molecular determinants. *Biol Cell* 2004, 96(1):3–17.

42. Patterson RL, van Rossum DB, Kaplin AI, Barrow RK, Snyder SH: Inositol 1,4,5-trisphosphate receptor/GAPDH complex augments Ca2+ release via locally derived NADH. *Proc Natl Acad Sci USA* 2005, 102(5):1357–1359.

43. Lundholm CE: DDE-induced eggshell thinning in birds: Effects of p, p'-DDE on the calcium and prostaglandin metabolism of the eggshell gland. *Comp Biochem Physiol C* 1997, 118(2):113–128.

44. Strehler EE, Zacharias DA: Role of alternative splicing in generating isoform diversity among plasma membrane calcium pumps. *Physiol Rev* 2001, 81(1):21–50.46.

45. Howard A, Legon S, Walters JRF: Human and rat intestinal plasma-membrane calcium-pump isoforms. *Am J Physiol* 1993, 265(5):G917–G925.47.

46. Kumar R, Haugen JD, Penniston JT: Molecular-cloning of a plasma-membrane calcium-pump from human osteoblasts. *J Bone Miner Res* 1993, 8(4):505–513.

47. Philipson KD, Nicoll DA: Sodium-calcium exchange: A molecular perspective. *Annu Rev Physiol* 2000, 62:111–133.

48. Belkacemi L, Bedard I, Simoneau L, Lafond J: Calcium channels, transporters and exchangers in placenta: a review. *Cell Calcium* 2005, 37(1):1–8.

49. Herchuelz A, Kamagate A, Ximenes H, Van Eylen F: Role of Na/Ca exchange and the plasma membrane Ca2 + –ATPase in beta cell function and death. *Ann N Y Acad Sci* 2007, 1099:456–467.

50. Ruknudin AM, Lakattaa EG: The regulation of the Na/Ca exchanger and plasmalemmal Ca2+ ATPase by other proteins. *Ann N Y Acad Sci* 2007, 1099:86–102.

51. Blaustein MP, Juhaszova M, Golovina VA, Church PJ, Stanley EF: Na/Ca exchanger and PMCA localization in neurons and astrocytes - Functional implications. *Ann N Y Acad Sci* 2002, 976:356–366.

52. Garty H: Molecular-properties of epithelial, amiloride-blockable Na + channels. *FASEB J* 1994, 8(8):522–528.

53. Jorgensen PL, Hakansson KO, Karlish SJD: Structure and mechanism of Na, K-ATPase: Functional sites and their interactions. *Annu Rev Physiol* 2003, 65:817–849.

54. Heitzmann D, Warth R: Physiology and pathophysiology of potassium channels in gastrointestinal epithelia. *Physiol Rev* 2008, 88(3):1119–1182.

55. Hebert SC, Desir G, Giebisch G, Wang WH: Molecular diversity and regulation of renal potassium channels. *Physiol Rev* 2005, 85(1):319–371.

56. Warth R: Potassium channels in epithelial transport. *Pflugers Arch* 2003, 446(5):505–513.

57. Steward MC, Ishiguro H, Case RM: Mechanisms of bicarbonate secretion in the pancreatic duct. *Annu Rev Physiol* 2005, 67:377–409.

58. Romero MF, Fulton CM, Boron WF: The SLC4 family of HCO3- transporters. *Pflugers Arch* 2004, 447(5):495–509.

59. Dorwart MR, Shcheynikov N, Yang D, Muallem S: The solute carrier 26 family of proteins in epithelial ion transport. *Physiol* 2008, 23(2):104–114.

60. Xu J, Henriksnas J, Barone S, Witte D, Shull GE, Forte JG, Holm L, Soleimani M: SLC26A9 is expressed in gastric surface epithelial cells, mediates Cl-/HCO3- exchange, and is inhibited by NH4+. *Am J Physiol Cell Physiol* 2005, 289(2):C493–C505.

61. Xu J, Song PH, Miller ML, Borgese F, Barone S, Riederer B, Wang ZH, Alper SL, Forte JG, Shull GE, et al: Deletion of the chloride transporter Slc26a9 causes loss of tubulovesicles in parietal cells and impairs acid secretion in the stomach. *Proc Natl Acad Sci USA* 2008, 105(46):17955–17960.

62. Alper SL: Molecular physiology of SLC4 anion exchangers. *Exp Physiol* 2006, 91(1):153–161.

63. Choi JY, Muallem D, Kiselyov K, Lee MG, Thomas PJ, Muallem S: **Aberrant CFTR-dependent HCO3- transport in mutations associated with cystic fibrosis.** *Nature* 2001, **410**(6824):94–97.

64. Hug MJ, Tamada T, Bridges RJ: **CFTR and bicarbonate secretion to epithelial cells.** *News Physiol Sci* 2003, **18**:38–42.

65. Chan HC, Shi QX, Zhou CX, Wang XF, Xu WM, Chen WY, Chen AJ, Ni Y, Yuan YY: **Critical role of CFTR in uterine bicarbonate secretion and the fertilizing capacity of sperm.** *Mol Cell Endocrinol* 2006, **250**(1–2):106–113.

66. Niggli V, Sigel E, Carafoli E: **The Purified Ca-2+ Pump of Human-Erythrocyte Membranes Catalyzes an Electroneutral Ca-2+–H+ Exchange in Reconstituted Liposomal Systems.** *J Biol Chem* 1982, **257**(5):2350–2356.

67. Smallwood JI, Waisman DM, Lafreniere D, Rasmussen H: **Evidence That the Erythrocyte Calcium-Pump Catalyzes a Ca-2+–Nh+ Exchange.** *J Biol Chem* 1983, **258**(18):1092–1097.

68. Beyenbach KW, Wieczorek H: **The V-type H+ATPase: molecular structure and function, physiological roles and regulation.** *J Exp Biol* 2006, **209**(4):577–589.

69. Marshansky V, Futai M: **The V-type H+–ATPase in vesicular trafficking: targeting, regulation and function.** *Curr Opin Cell Biol* 2008, **20**(4):415–426.

70. Nishi T, Forgac M: **The vacuolar (H+)-atpases - Nature's most versatile proton pumps.** *Nat Rev Mol Cell Biol* 2002, **3**(2):94–103.

71. Furla P, Galgani I, Durand I, Allemand D: **Sources and mechanisms of inorganic carbon transport for coral calcification and photosynthesis.** *J Exp Biol* 2000, **203**(22):3445–3457.

72. Bertucci A, Tambutte E, Tambutte S, Allemand D, Zoccola D: **Symbiosis-dependent gene expression in coral-dinoflagellate association: cloning and characterization of a P-type H(+)-ATPase gene.** *Proc Biol Sci* 2010, **277**(1678):87–95.

73. Chang MH, Plata C, Zandi-Nejad K, Sindic A, Sussman CR, Mercado A, Broumand V, Raghuram V, Mount DB, Romero MF: **Slc26a9-Anion exchanger, channel and Na+transporter.** *J Membr Biol* 2009, **228**(3):125–140.

74. Jentsch TJ, Stein V, Weinreich F, Zdebik AA: **Molecular structure and physiological function of chloride channels.** *Physiol Rev* 2002, **82**(2):503–568.

75. Duran C, Thompson CH, Xiao Q, Hartzell HC: **Chloride Channels: Often Enigmatic, Rarely Predictable.** *Annu Rev Physiol* 2010, **72**:95–121.

76. Furukawa T, Ogura T, Katayama Y, Hiraoka M: **Characteristics of rabbit ClC-2 current expressed in Xenopus oocytes and its contribution to volume regulation.** *Am J Physiol* 1998, **274**(2):C500–C512.

77. Britton FC, Hatton WJ, Rossow CF, Duan D, Hume JR, Horowitz B: **Molecular distribution of volume-regulated chloride channels (ClC-2 and ClC-3) in cardiac tissues.** *Am J Physiol Heart Circ Physiol* 2000, **279**(5):H2225–H2233.

78. Britton FC, Wang GL, Huang ZM, Ye LD, Horowitz B, Hume JR, Duan DY: **Functional characterization of novel alternatively spliced ClC-2 chloride channel variants in the heart.** *J Biol Chem* 2005, **280**(27):25871–25880.

79. Huang ZM, Prasad C, Britton FC, Ye LL, Hatton WJ, Duan D: **Functional role of CLC-2 chloride inward rectifier channels in cardiac sinoatrial nodal pacemaker cells.** *J Mol Cell Cardiol* 2009, **47**(1):121–132.

80. Bosl MR, Stein V, Hubner C, Zdebik AA, Jordt SE, Mukhopadhyay AK, Davidoff MS, Holstein AF, Jentsch TJ: **Male germ cells and photoreceptors, both dependent on close cell-cell interactions, degenerate upon ClC-2Cl(–) channel disruption.** *EMBO J* 2001, **20**(6):1289–1299.

81. Nehrke K, Arreola J, Nguyen HV, Pilato J, Richardson L, Okunade G, Baggs R, Shull GE, Melvin JE: **Loss of hyperpolarization-activated Cl- current in salivary acinar cells from Clcn2 knockout mice.** *J Biol Chem* 2002, **277**(26):23604–23611.

82. Hebert SC, Mount DB, Gamba G: **Molecular physiology of cation-coupled Cl- cotransport: the SLC12 family.** *Pflugers Arch* 2004, **447**(5):580–593.

83. Adragna NC, Di Fulvio M, Lauf PK: **Regulation of K-Cl cotransport: from function to genes.** *J Membr Biol* 2004, **201**(3):109–137.

84. Gamba G: **Molecular physiology and pathophysiology of electroneutral cation-chloride cotransporters.** *Physiol Rev* 2005, **85**(2):423–493.

85. Lundholm CE, Bartonek M: **Furosemide decreases eggshell thicjness and inhibits 45Ca^{2+} uptake by asubcellular fraction of eggshell gland mucosa of the domestic-Fowl.** *Comp Biochem Physiol C* 1992, **101**(2):317–320.

86. Engels WR: **Contributing software to the internet - the amplify program.** *Trends Biochem Sci* 1993, **18**(11):448–450.

87. Gautron J, Murayama E, Vignal A, Morisson M, McKee MD, Rehault S, Labas V, Belghazi M, Vidal ML, Nys Y: **Cloning of ovocalyxin-36, a novel chicken eggshell protein related to lipopolysaccharide-binding proteins, bactericidal permeability-increasing proteins, and plunc family proteins.** *J Biol Chem* 2007, **282**(8):5273–5286.

12

Effects of postnatal growth restriction and subsequent catch-up growth on neurodevelopment and glucose homeostasis in rats

Erica E. Alexeev[1], Bo Lönnerdal[1] and Ian J. Griffin[2*]

Abstract

Background: There is increasing evidence that poor growth of preterm infants is a risk factor for poor long-term development, while the effects of early postnatal growth restriction are not well known. We utilized a rat model to examine the consequences of different patterns of postnatal growth and hypothesized that early growth failure leads to impaired development and insulin resistance. Rat pups were separated at birth into normal (N, n = 10) or restricted intake (R, n = 16) litters. At d11, R pups were re-randomized into litters of 6 (R-6), 10 (R-10) or 16 (R-16) pups/dam. N pups remained in litters of 10 pups/dam (N-10). Memory and learning were examined through T-maze test. Insulin sensitivity was measured by i.p. insulin tolerance test and glucose tolerance test.

Results: By d10, N pups weighed 20 % more than R pups ($p < 0.001$). By d15, the R-6 group caught up to the N-10 group in weight, the R-10 group showed partial catch-up growth and the R-16 group showed no catch-up growth. All R groups showed poorer scores in developmental testing when compared with the N-10 group during T-Maze test ($p < 0.05$). Although R-16 were more insulin sensitive than R-6 and R-10, all R groups were more glucose tolerant than N-10.

Conclusion: In rats, differences in postnatal growth restriction leads to changes in development and in insulin sensitivity. These results may contribute to better elucidating the causes of poor developmental outcomes in human preterm infants.

Keywords: Growth restriction, Catch-up growth, Development, Insulin sensitivity

Background

In term infants, *in utero* growth restriction or small-for-gestational-age status at birth (SGA) are associated with the development of increased adiposity and impaired insulin sensitivity in later life [1], that may be exacerbated by more rapid catch-up growth in the first 1–2 years of life [1, 2]. In comparison, preterm infants grow much more poorly after birth, a term coined *ex utero* growth restriction, and by term corrected age most are below the 5th weight-for-age centile [3]. This *ex utero*, postnatal, growth failure is common in preterm infants, [3, 4] and is associated with poorer neurocognitive outcomes in later life [5, 6]. Further, it has been shown that neonatal leptin deficiency may contribute to adverse neurodevelopmental outcomes associated with postnatal growth restriction [7]. Subsequently, preterm infants have variable amounts of catch-up growth, especially during the first 1–3 years of life [8, 9]. This pattern of small body size at term corrected age, followed by increased rates of growth is similar to that seen in SGA term infants, and there has been concern that this may lead to increased risk of obesity and metabolic disorders arising from impaired glucose tolerance, such as type II diabetes, in preterm infants, similar to the increased risk in term SGA infants [10–12].

We have previously described a rodent model of *ex utero* growth restriction and the effects of variable amounts of

* Correspondence: ijgriffin@ucdavis.edu
[2]Department of Pediatrics, University of California, Davis Medical Center, Sacramento, CA 95817, USA
Full list of author information is available at the end of the article

catch-up growth on early metabolic and neurocognitive outcomes [13]. Changes in litter size lead to *ex utero* growth restriction (EUGR), and in turn, changes in body composition and poorer neurodevelopment. However, no differences in fasting insulin or glucose in early life were seen [13]. In the present study, we used the same model to assess the effects of *ex utero* growth restriction and subsequent catch-up growth on longer-term metabolic outcomes including glucose tolerance and insulin sensitivity.

The objectives of our study were to examine the effects of early postnatal growth restriction, followed by varying degrees of postnatal catch-up growth on growth (both body size and body composition), insulin sensitivity, glucose tolerance, neurodevelopment, and brain myelination. We hypothesized that early postnatal growth restriction would result in poorer neurodevelopment and lead to improved glucose tolerance and insulin sensitivity. We further hypothesized that in EUGR rats, early catch-up growth would lead to improved neurodevelopment but reduced insulin sensitivity and glucose tolerance compared to EUGR rats that did not have early catch-up growth.

Results

Growth

Growth differed significantly between the normal (N) and restricted (R) intake groups by d5 (14.2 ± 0.19 g vs. 11.4 ± 0.10 g, $p < 0.001$) onwards. By d10 the R groups were approximately 20 % smaller than the N groups ($p < 0.001$, Fig. 1).

On d10, R animals were re-randomized to litters of 6 (R-6), 10 (R-10) or 16 (R-16), while N pups remained in litters of 10 (N-10). The R-16 group remained significantly smaller than the N-10 group throughout the study. The weight of the R-6 pups "caught-up" with the N-10 pups by d15 and were statistically indistinguishable from them for the rest of the study.

The R-10 group grew intermediate to the N-10 and R-16 animals until d21 (Fig. 2), and was similar to the N-10 and R-6 groups thereafter.

By d40, the R-16 group remained significantly smaller than the three other groups, which were all statistically similar. On d60, the R-16 rats remained significantly smaller than the other three groups. This was seen for both males and females (Fig. 3).

Body composition

Body composition was assessed in a subset of animals (N-10 = 10, R-10 = 10, R-6 = 6, R-16 = 16) at d60. There were no significant differences in percentage water, protein, fat, or ash between the four groups (Fig. 4).

Serum hormones

On d10, serum leptin was significantly higher in the N group (3.93 ± 0.33 ng/ml) than the R group (1.09 ± 0.31; $p < 0.0001$). Serum triglycerides on d10 were similar in the N (1370 ± 330 mg/L) and R (860 ± 360 mg/L; $p = 0.77$) groups.

Serum leptin on d60 differed significantly between groups, with the R-16 group having the lowest levels (Table 1). Serum triglycerides on d60 were similar among groups, but hepatic triglycerides on d60 differed with the lowest level in the R-10 and R-16 groups and the highest in the R-6 group. Serum insulin values did not differ between groups.

Insulin sensitivity

Fasting blood glucose on d50 was similar in all four groups ($p = 0.07$). When expressed as the area under the curve (AUC), the two catch-up groups, R-6 (7635 ± 189, n = 23) and R-10 (7531 ± 147, n = 38), had significantly higher AUC than the R-16 group (6870 ± 119, n = 58), while the N-10 group was intermediate between the others (7229 ± 132, n = 47) (Fig. 5). Similar patterns were seen for the AUC between 0 and 30 min and between 30 and 120 min. When individual time-points were considered, the R-6 and R-10 groups had higher blood glucose concentrations than the other groups (N-10 and R-16) at 30, 45 and 60 min.

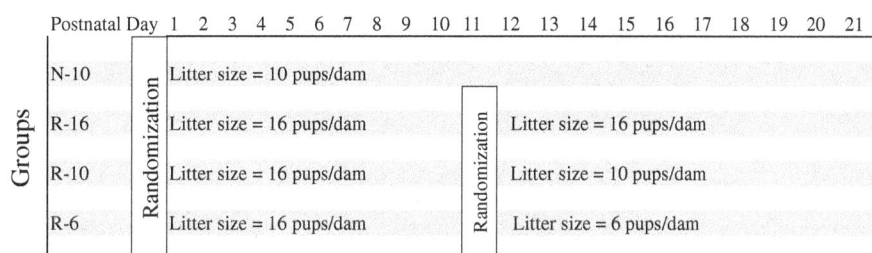

Fig. 1 Design of the animal study. On d2, rat pups were randomized to litters of 10/dam (Normal growth (N), five males and five females) or 16/dam (Restricted growth (R), eight males and eight females). On d11, R pups were re-randomized into litters creating catch-up (R-6, 6 pups/dam), normal (R-10, 10 pups/dam) or reduced growth (R-16, 16 pups/dam) groups. N pups remained in litters of 10 pups/dam (N-10)

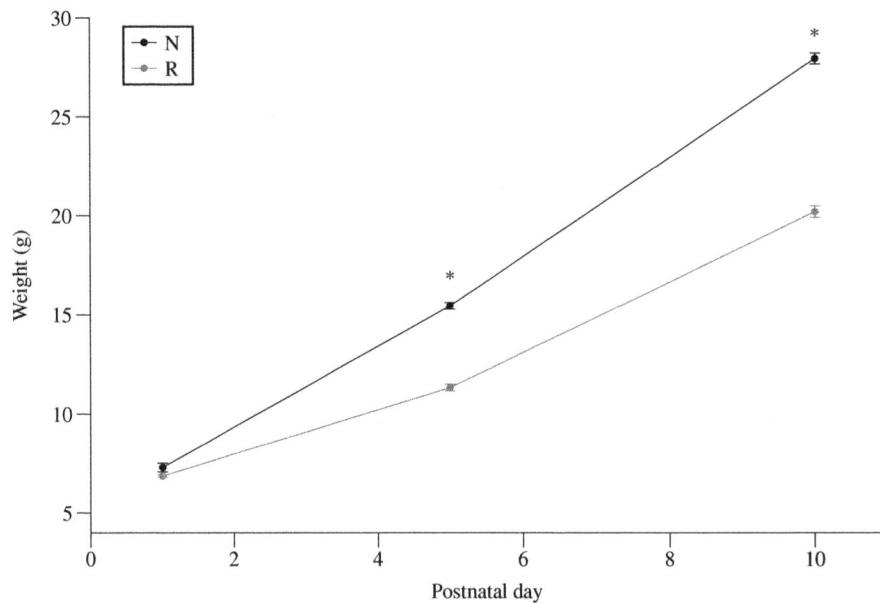

Fig. 2 Postnatal weight (g) from d1-10. By d5, R pups were ~ 20 % smaller than N pups. Values are means ± SEM. *Different from N litters, $p < 0.05$

When the data were examined as change in glucose concentration from baseline, the area under baseline (AUB) between 0 and 30 min was significantly greater for the N-10 group (593 ± 43, n = 47) than for the R-6 group (387 ± 61, n = 58), while the R-10 (428 ± 48, n = 38) and R-16 groups (489 ± 37, n = 58) were intermediate between the two. There were no differences in AUB among the groups for the time period 30 min to 120 min.

Glucose tolerance

Fasting blood glucose on d55 was significantly affected by sex (M > F; $p = 0.0061$) and by group ($p = 0.0022$). Fasting glucose was lower in the N-10 (99.0 ± 1.4 mg/L) and the R-16 (99.1 ± 1.3 mg/L) groups than in the R-10 group (105.3 ± 1.5 mg/L), with the R-6 group being intermediate between them (102.8 ± 2.0 mg/L).

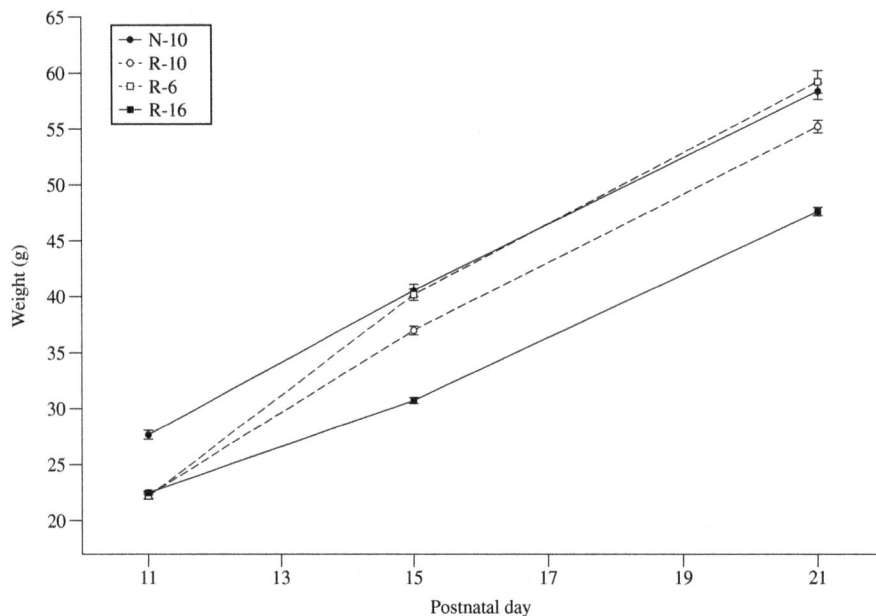

Fig. 3 Postnatal weight (g) from d11-21. All R groups diverged by d12. By d15, the N-10 and R-6 groups were similar, the R-16 group showed no catch-up growth, and the R-10 group caught-up half-way between the N-10 and R-16 groups. Error bars represent ± 1 SEM, if not visible they are smaller than the plot symbol

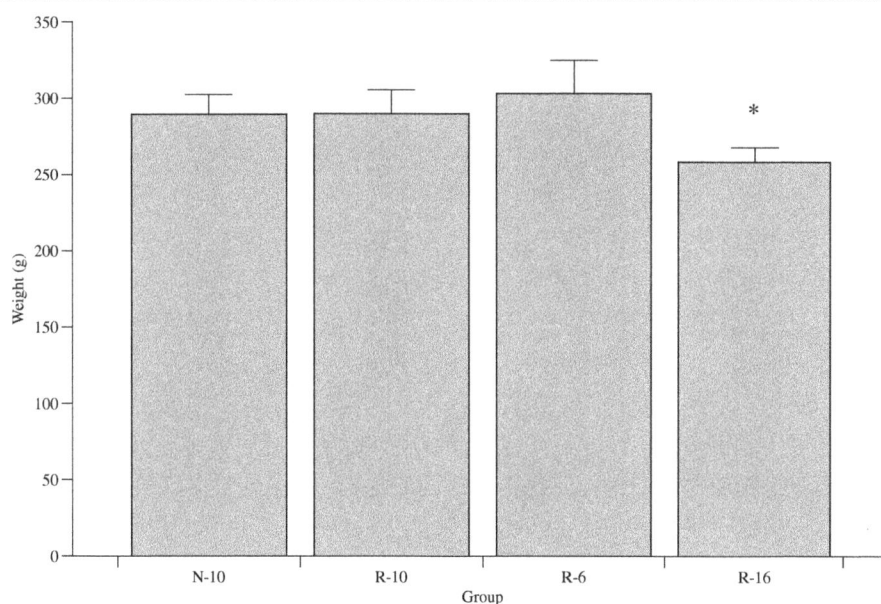

Fig. 4 Postnatal weight (g) at d60. The R-16 rats were significantly smaller than the other three groups, and this was seen in males and females. *$P < 0.05$. Error bars represent $\pm$ 1 SEM

The AUC was significantly different between groups ($p = 0.0079$) and was greater in males than females ($p = 0.06$). The AUC for the N-10 group (10778 ± 413, n = 47) was significantly greater than both the R-16 (9210 ± 368, n = 59) and the R-10 (8819 ± 453, n = 39) groups, with the R-6 group being intermediate (9620 ± 577, n = 24) (Fig. 6). There were no significant group effects between 0 and 30 min, but were seen subsequently during the remainder of the GTT for the time period 30 to 180 min. A similar pattern was seen in AUB among the groups.

T-Maze test

Memory and learning was assessed using spontaneous alternation in a T-maze. The N-10 group scored significantly better (6.86 ± 0.13 successes (n = 69); $p < 0.05$) than any of the other groups (R-6 5.6 ± 0.18 (n = 36), R-10 5.6 ± 0.26 (n = 50), R-16, 5.14 ± 0.15 successes (n = 96)). The effects of group were similar in both sexes (Fig. 7).

Brain histology

The area of MBP-positive fibers in the R-16 group appeared smaller than that in the N-10 group on d60, but no significant differences could be detected. These results suggest that myelination within the hypothalamus and corpus callosum may have been completed by d60 (Fig. 8).

Discussion

Since poor growth in preterm infants occurs postnatally, we aimed to produce a postnatal model of growth restriction in neonatal rats. Many animal models have been used to examine effects of *in utero* growth restriction with or without catch-up growth on metabolic outcomes, and though these models have provided great insight into infants born small for gestational age or who experience intrauterine growth restriction [14, 15], they do not represent the type of growth that is experienced by most preterm infants. Further, the effects of growth restriction and subsequent catch-up growth on cognition and metabolism have not been examined concurrently.

Table 1 Fasting glucose, insulin, leptin, and triglycerides in the four groups on d60

Group	N-10	R-10	R-6	R-16	P value
Fasting glucose (mg/L)	1084.7 ± 34.4	1057.3 ± 19.3	1080 ± 31.8	1075.2 ± 22.0	NS
Serum insulin (ng/mL)	2.24 ± 0.43	2.41 ± 0.26	2.36 ± 0.61	2.46 ± 0.71	NS
Leptin (ng/mL)	3.74 ± 0.37	4.13 ± 1.12	4.27 ± 0.77	2.79 ± 0.58^a	P = 0.0037
Serum TG (mg/L)	1603 ± 307	1220 ± 238	1794 ± 487	1450 ± 373	NS
Hepatic TG (mg/L)	1550 ± 263	1100 ± 139^a	2130 ± 270	$1138 \pm 194*$	P = 0.0203
n	20	20	12	32	

Data are expressed as mean $\pm$ SEM. *P*-values represent the overall ANOVA p-values. [a]Denote significant difference from the N-10 group, $p < 0.05$

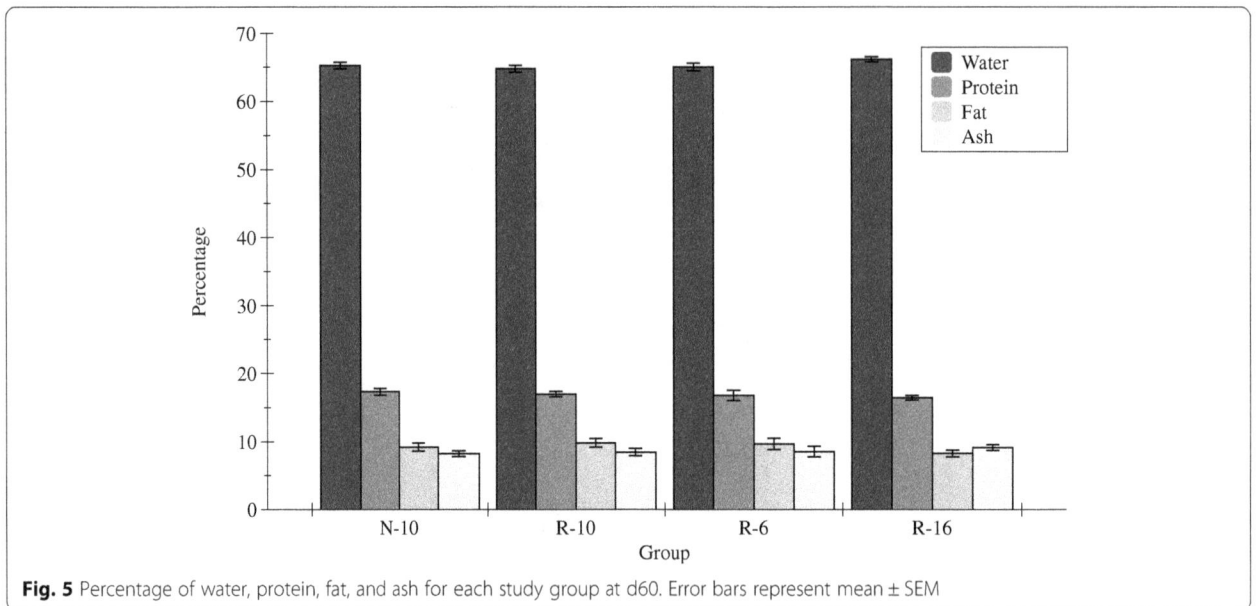

Fig. 5 Percentage of water, protein, fat, and ash for each study group at d60. Error bars represent mean ± SEM

We therefore developed a model of post-natal growth restriction in rat pups based on manipulations in litter size, that we have shown leads to reproducible levels of *ex utero* growth restriction and catch-up growth [13]. This model leads to changes in both milk intake and in growth. However, it is possible that other factors may also be changed by modifications in litter size, for example dam-pup interactions and pup-pup interactions, as seen in other rodents [16, 17].

The initial intervention in our study was carried out from birth until d10 of age, as this period in rats is believed to be equivalent to the third trimester of pregnancy in humans [18], or the period when reduced intake and poor growth are common in premature infants. The increased milk volume intake that occurs as litter size is decreased in the second intervention represents the increased volume intake that preterm infants who experience catch-up growth encounter after hospital discharge.

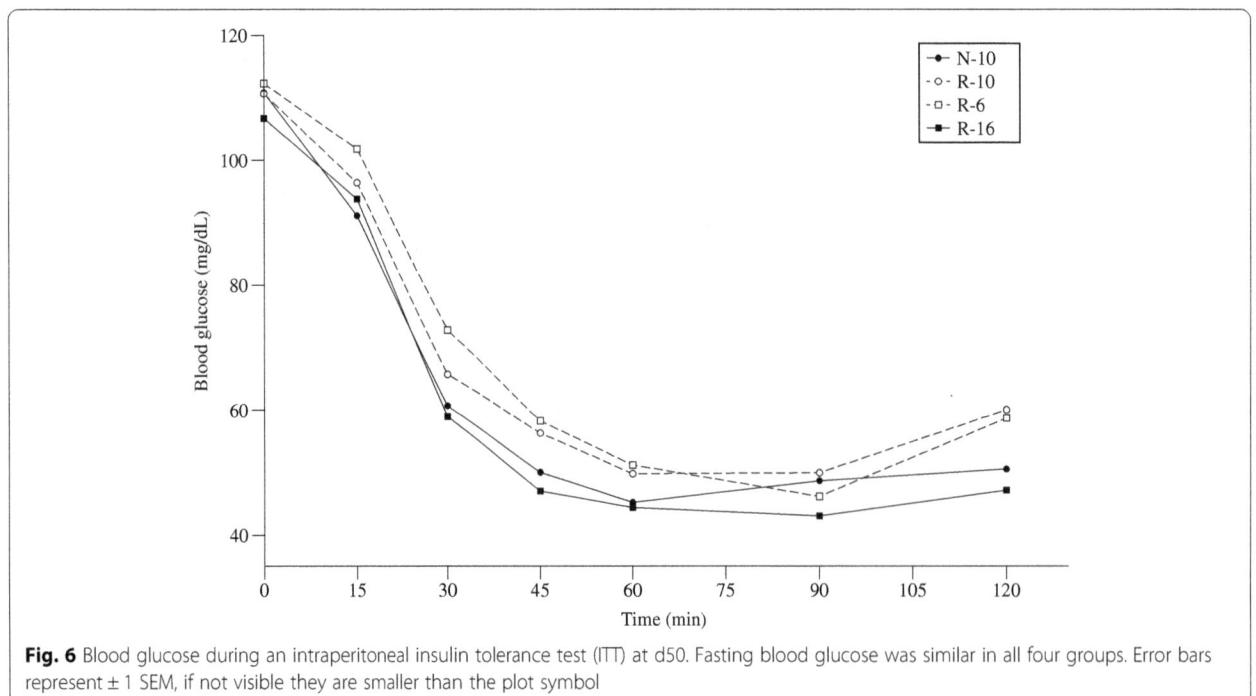

Fig. 6 Blood glucose during an intraperitoneal insulin tolerance test (ITT) at d50. Fasting blood glucose was similar in all four groups. Error bars represent ± 1 SEM, if not visible they are smaller than the plot symbol

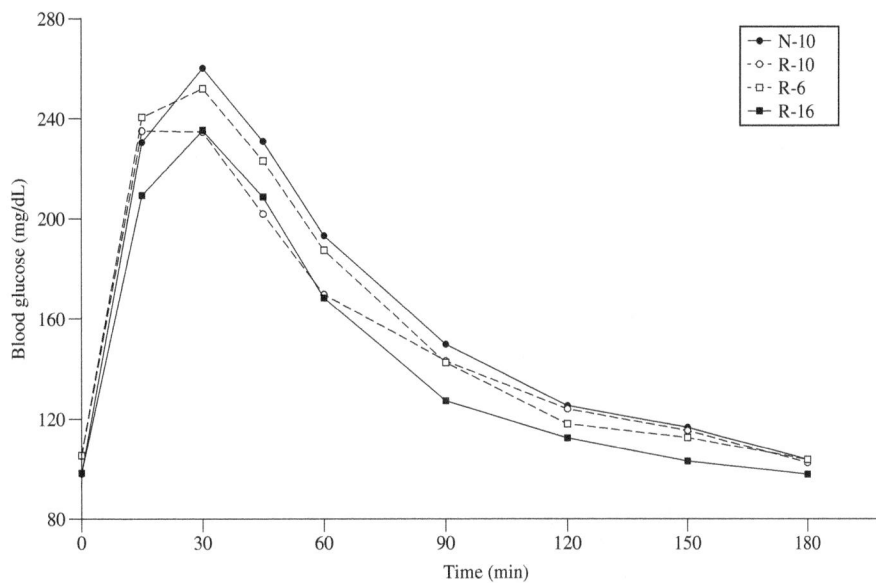

Fig. 7 Blood glucose during an intraperitoneal glucose tolerance test (GTT) at d55. Fasting blood glucose was significantly affected by sex (M > F; $p = 0.0061$) and by group ($p = 0.0022$). Error bars represent ± 1 SEM, if not visible they are smaller than the plot symbol

Further, dams of large litters have been shown to produce milk with unaltered protein composition, and thus litter size manipulation results in modified volume intake without altered milk composition [19].

The current study confirms our previous findings that R-6 pups catch-up with N-10 pups by d21, R-10 pups show partial catch-up by d21, and R-16 pups remain smaller than the other three groups [13]. The current study confirms this, but also demonstrates that the R-10 group does ultimately show complete catch-up in body weight by d60. The R-16 group, however, remained significantly smaller than the N-10 group until at least d60.

We have previously shown that catch-up growth in R-6 pups comes at the cost of changes in body composition with R-6 pups having significantly greater percentage body fat, and significantly lower percent lean mass on d21 [13]. The current study demonstrates that by d60, body composition in the R-6 pups has normalized, and is similar to the N-10 pups. Furthermore, although the R-10 pups catch-up to the N-10 pups by d60, the two groups have similar body composition on d60, just as they have at d21. The early changes in body composition related to catch-up group are therefore not maintained over time.

We have previously shown that the R-16 group has lower percentage body fat in d21. By d60, however, the differences in body composition are lost, and all groups have similar percent body fat despite the fact that the R-16 rats remain smaller. Once again, early differences in body composition are not sustained over time. These findings are consistent with the human data, which suggests that although preterm infants with catch-up growth have increased adiposity at term corrected age, those changes are not maintained during the rest of the first year of life [20].

In our previous study there were no differences between groups in fasting insulin or glucose of d21. In the current study we carried out more detailed investigations of glucose homeostasis in older animals. Fasting blood glucose prior to the glucose tolerance test (after a 12 h fast) was significantly greater in the two catch-up groups (R-6 and R-10) than in the groups without catch-up growth (N-10 and R-16). The difference in fasting blood glucose prior to the insulin tolerance test (after a 4 h fast) failed to reach statistical significance. Insulin sensitivity was higher in the groups without catch-up growth (N-10 and R-16) than in the groups that changed their dietary intakes on d10 (R-6 and R-10) and experienced catch-up growth, as shown by their higher AUC values. This occurred even though all groups had similar body composition at the end of the study. It is possible that early changes in body composition may be responsible for the poorer insulin sensitivity seen in the R-6 and R-10 groups in later life, or that changes in early dietary intake or growth lead to long-term changes in insulin sensitivity, possibly via epigenetic mechanisms. Growth restriction may result in improved insulin sensitivity in adulthood since it has been suggested that early undernourishment may enhance insulin sensitivity, as well as fatty acid oxidation [21]. It has been shown that children born prematurely have decreased insulin sensitivity immediately after birth, and those who experience greater weight gain remain having lower insulin sensitivity compared to infants born at term [22].

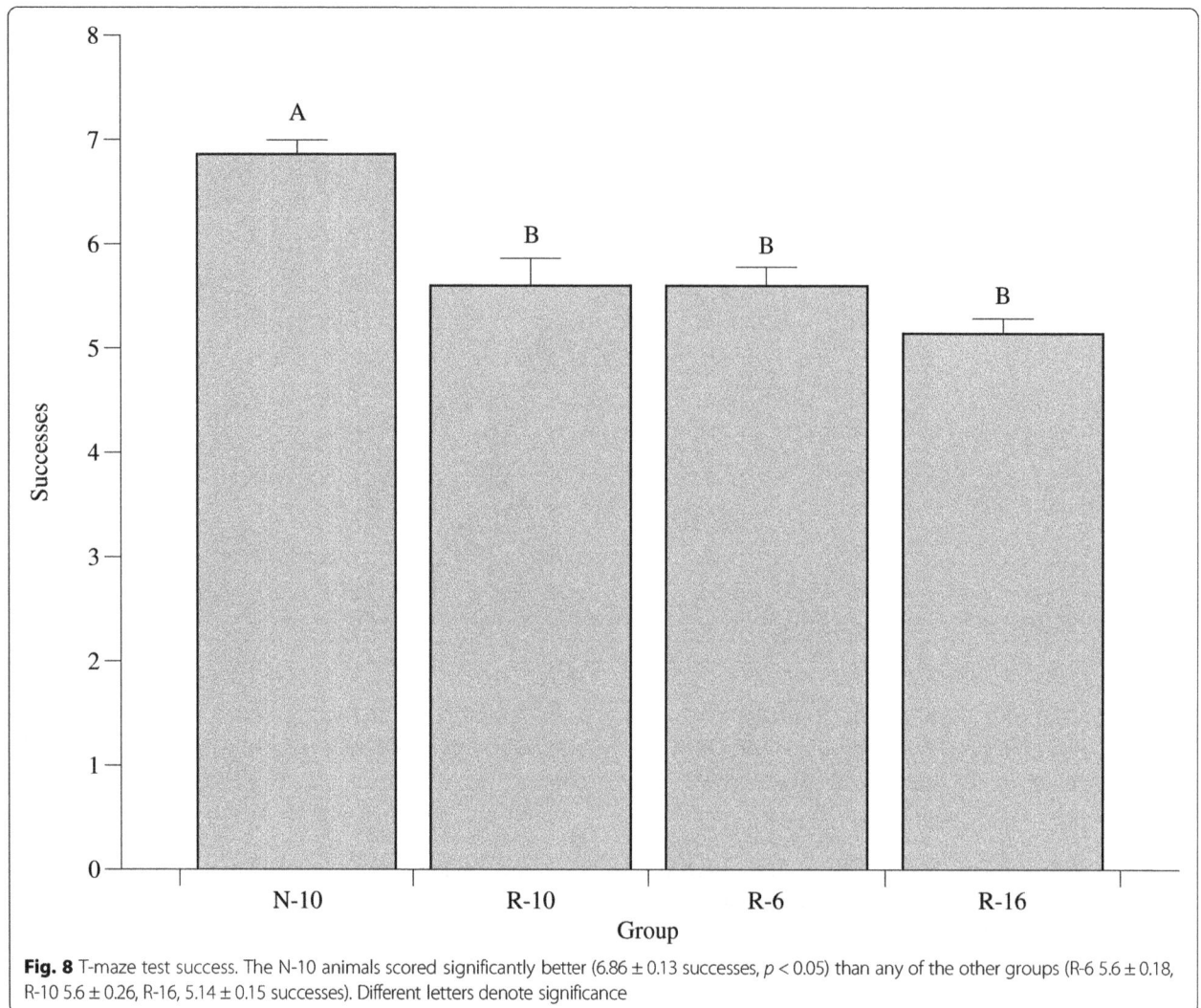

Fig. 8 T-maze test success. The N-10 animals scored significantly better (6.86 ± 0.13 successes, $p < 0.05$) than any of the other groups (R-6 5.6 ± 0.18, R-10 5.6 ± 0.26, R-16, 5.14 ± 0.15 successes). Different letters denote significance

Conversely, glucose tolerance by GTT was significantly worse in the N-10 group than the R-16 group, as shown by AUC. The two catch-up groups were intermediate between the N-10 and R-16 groups. The differences in fasting blood glucose among the groups is consistent with the findings that mice who are small at birth and have postnatal catch-up growth are at high risk of glucose intolerance [23]; however, there was no significant group effect in AUC for the first 30 min of the GTT, and differences in glucose tolerance were only apparent after 30 min.

Growth before weaning, specifically before d11, could be a critical window for later programming. The developmental origins of disease hypothesis suggests that prenatal development is critical to metabolic adaptation later in life [24]. However, the postnatal environment may be "mismatched" to the early *in utero* environment, creating a disadvantageous phenotype [25]. Cognitive outcomes were worse in the three groups with early growth restriction (R-6, R-10, R-16), and highest in the group with

greater early growth (N-10). We thus show that growth restriction, despite catch-up growth, may predispose poor cognition. Though there were no differences in MBP expression at d60, this may be due to the fact that the maximum rate of myelin accumulation in the rat occurs around d20 [26, 27]. Myelin accumulation does continue into adulthood in the rat, though it occurs at a decreasing rate [28]. Several animal studies have shown that dietary restriction during the suckling period results in decreased myelination in early life [29–31]. In our study, early postnatal growth restriction and possible undernutrition due to large litter size may be a cause for the developmental impairments seen in the R groups.

We also examined the effects of growth restriction and catch-up growth on serum hormones, specifically insulin and leptin. Neonatal overfeeding of pups by litter size manipulation has been shown to result in a significant elevation of serum insulin concentration and alterations in hepatic enzymes involved in carbohydrate and lipid metabolism [32]. However, we did not find a significant difference in serum insulin concentrations. Interestingly, serum leptin at d22 and d60 differed significantly between groups, with the R-16 group having the lowest levels. This is consistent with our previous data on d21 [13]. The association of low leptin concentrations in the R litters and poor T-maze score suggests that reduced leptin levels may be a mechanism behind the differences seen in cognition. Leptin has recently been proposed to play a role in brain development during the prenatal and neonatal periods [33]. Administration of leptin to *ob/ob* mice, which are leptin deficient, has been shown to increase brain weight, total brain DNA, and increase MBP-mRNA expression in rodents [34, 35], further suggesting a role for leptin in brain development.

Finally, we demonstrated that hepatic triglyceride content was highest in the group with early catch-up growth (R-6). Hepatic lipid accumulation may be one of the earliest findings in the metabolic syndrome in humans. This, combined with the differences in fasting glucose and in insulin sensitivity, suggests that catch-up growth in this model may be associated with increased risk of metabolic syndrome.

Conclusion

In summary, we have demonstrated that early growth restriction leads to profound and long-lasting adverse effects on neurodevelopment. Catch-up growth occurs after early postnatal growth restriction, and complete catch-up in weight can occur if it begins before d21 in the rat (equivalent to the first 2–3 years in humans). Postnatal growth restriction without catch-up growth (R-16) leads to short-term reductions in body adiposity, while postnatal growth restriction with catch-up growth (R-6) leads to short-term increases in body adiposity. Neither of these changes in body composition is maintained long-term. Postnatal growth restriction without catch-up growth leads to improved glucose tolerance. However, insulin sensitivity is reduced if catch-up growth occurs after postnatal growth restriction. These finding reinforce the concerns that *ex utero* growth restriction in preterm infants reduces long-term neurocognitive outcomes, and that subsequent catch-up growth may impair insulin sensitivity without improving development.

Methods
Animals
Timed pregnant CD dams were obtained from Charles River (Wilmington, MA) at 14 d of gestation. Rats were housed in solid plastic hanging cages under constant conditions (temperature, 22 °C; humidity, 62 %) with a 12-h dark–light cycle and were allowed to consume food and water *ad libitum*. On d2, rat pups were randomized to litters of 10 pups per dam (Normal growth, N) or 16 pups per dam (Restricted growth, R). On d11, R pups were

re-randomized into litters creating catch-up (R-6, 6 pups/dam), normal (R-10, 10 pups/dam) or reduced growth (R-16, 16 pups/dam) groups. N pups remained in litters of 10 pups/dam (N-10). Equal numbers of males and females were included in all litters (Fig. 9). Pups were weaned at d21 to a standard, non-purified rodent diet (LabDiet 5001, Purina, Hayward, CA) fed *ad libitum*. Weights were monitored until d60. The University of California Institutional Animal Care and Use Committee approved all animal procedures.

The period from d2-10 in rats is typically taken to represent the period between the early third trimester and term in humans, and therefore represents early *ex utero* life in preterm infants. The period from d11-21 in the rat is broadly representative of the first 2 years of life in humans, and therefore reflects the period where catch-up growth is common in human preterm infants [18].

Body composition
A subset of animals had body composition assessed at d60 by carcass analysis. Frozen carcasses were cut and freeze-dried for 24 h to determine water content, calculated from change in weight before and after freeze-drying. Fat content was measured from the change in weight after diethyl ether (Fisher Scientific, Pittsburgh, PA) extraction for 7 d using a Soxhlet apparatus, followed by acetone (Fisher Scientific, Pittsburg, PA) extraction for an additional 7 d. Total ash content was determined following muffle furnace incineration for 72 h at 540 °C and desiccation for 24 h. Protein was calculated as the difference between post-fat extraction weight and ash content. Water, protein, fat and ash content of each animal were expressed as a percentage of total body weight.

Biochemical analysis
Blood samples were collected at time of sacrifice on d22 and d60. Specimens were centrifuged at $1000 \times g$ for 15 min at 4 °C, and serum samples stored at −80 °C until analysis. Serum insulin and serum leptin were measured using ELISA kits (Millipore, Billerica, MA). Serum and hepatic triglycerides were measured with Triglyceride Reagent (Fisher Scientific, Pittsburg, PA) and read at 540 nm at 37 °C.

Insulin and glucose tolerance tests
An intraperitoneal insulin tolerance test (ITT) was performed on d50 after 4 h of food deprivation. Insulin (0.5 U/kg body weight [36]) was injected intraperitoneally and blood glucose levels were measured in tail vein blood using a glucometer (Easy Plus, Home Aid Diagnostics, Deerfield Beach, FL) at 0, 15, 30, 45, 60, 90, and 120 min after insulin injection. The area under the blood glucose curve (AUC) was calculated using a rhomboid rule. The primary comparison between groups was the total AUC

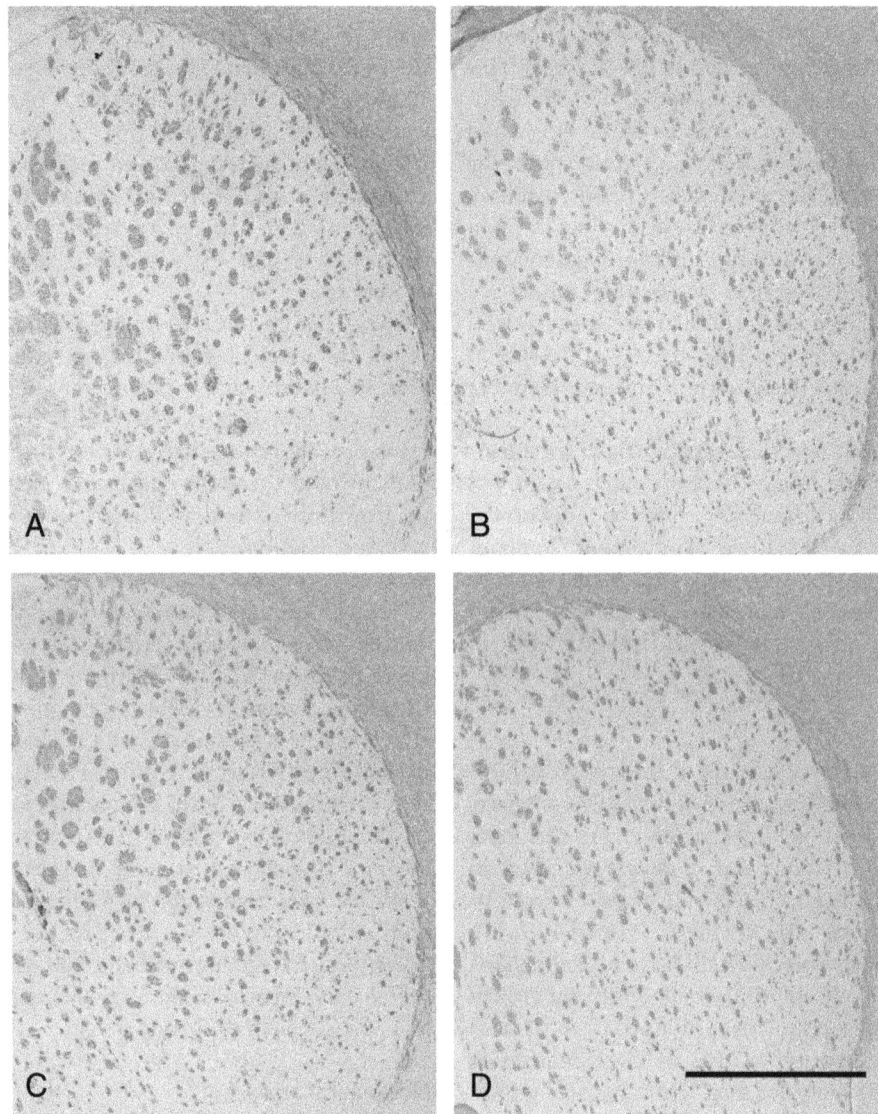

Fig. 9 Myelin basic protein (MBP) staining at d60 of (**a**) N-10, (**b**) R-10, (**c**) R-6, and (**d**) R-16 groups. No significant differences in MBP-positive fibers could be detected. Scale bar = 1000 μm

for the entire study (120 min); secondary comparisons were for the AUC between 0 min and 30 min, and between 30 min and 120 min. Larger values for AUC denote poorer insulin sensitivity. In addition, the change in blood glucose from baseline (0 min) was examined. The area under baseline (AUB) was calculated for the entire period, and for the first 30 min and last 90 min separately.

After a 3-days recovery period, an intraperitoneal glucose tolerance test (GTT) was performed after 12 h of food deprivation. Rats were injected intraperitoneally with 2 g/kg of glucose solution (Sigma, St. Louis, MO) and blood glucose was measured at 0, 15, 30, 45, 60, 90, 120, 150, and 180 min after glucose injection [37]. As before,

the blood glucose concentrations were used to calculate the area under the blood glucose versus time curve (AUC) for the entire study (0 min to 180 min), as well as for the first 30 min and the last 150 min. Changes in blood glucose from the 0 min baseline were also calculated and the area over the baseline (0 min) value calculated using a rhomboid rule for the time periods 0–180 min, 0–30 min, and 30–180 min.

T-Maze

Memory and learning were examined by spontaneous alternation in a T-maze on d35. In the T-maze test, rats were tested on their capability to alternate between two directions of an enclosed apparatus in the form of a T placed horizontally, as previously described [38]. Upon successful alternation of direction, animals were given a score of 1. This was repeated ten times, with the maximum score being 9.

Brain Histology and Immunohistochemistry

For brain histology studies, rats (d60) were deeply anaesthetized with pentobarbital (100 mg/kg) and fixed by transcardial perfusion with 4 % paraformaldehyde. Total brains were removed and placed in 4 % paraformaldehyde solution overnight at 4 °C. Samples were next placed in serial dilutions until fixed in 100 % ethanol and embedded in paraffin. Coronal sections were cut into 8–10 μm sections and immunohistochemically stained with goat polyclonal anti-MBP antibody (sc-13914, Santa Cruz Biotechnology, Santa Cruz, CA) at 1:100 dilution in blocking buffer and donkey anti-goat secondary antibody (sc-2020, Santa Cruz, Biotechnology, Santa Cruz, CA) at 1:500 in 1 % BSA. The staining was developed with DAB substrate (Vector Laboratories, Burlingame, pt]?>CA) and sections were counterstained with toluidine (0.1 %) blue. Images were acquired under microscope at 40X magnification (DP Olympus BX51). Areas of MBP fibers were assessed as MPB-positive per high power field and quantified using ImageJ software (NIH, Bethesda, MD).

Data analysis
Glucose homeostasis

Blood glucose data for the glucose tolerance test are expressed as area under the curve (AUC), calculated using a rhomboid rule. AUC was calculated for the entire study period (AUC_{0-180}), for the first 30 min (0–30 min, AUC_{0-30}) of the study and for the last 150 min (30–180 min, AUC_{30-180}) of the study. Changes in blood glucose from the time-0 baseline are expressed as the area over the time-0 baseline (AOB) for the same time intervals.

Blood glucose data for the insulin tolerance test were converted to AUC, and are expressed for the entire study period (AUC_{0-120}), for the first 30 min (AUC_{0-30}), and for 30–120 min (AUC_{30-120}). Changes in blood glucose data for the insulin tolerance test are expressed as the area under the baseline (AUB) for the same time intervals.

The primary outcome measure for the glucose tolerance test and for the insulin tolerance tests was the area under the curve (AUC) for the entire study period (AUC_{0-120}).

Secondary outcomes for the glucose tolerance test and for the insulin tolerance test was the area under the curve (AUC) for the first 30 min, and for the rest of the study, and the changes in glucose from baseline.

Statistical analysis

Weight data were analyzed by repeated-measures ANOVA with age, sex, and group as independent variables.

The effect of group on other continuously distributed outcomes was assessed by ANOVA with sex as a covariant. If main effects ANOVA showed a significant effect of "group", post-hoc testing to assess differences between the groups was carried out when needed using Tukey's HSD. All statistical analyses were performed using JMP Pro 11.0 (SAS Institute, Cary, NC) and statistical significance was accepted at $P < 0.05$.

Data are expressed as means ± SEM.

Competing interests
The authors declare that they have no competing interests.

Authors' contributions
EEA carried out the animal experiments and assays, interpreted data, and drafted the manuscript. BL participated in the study design, data interpretation, and revised the manuscript. IJG conceived the study and performed the statistical analysis, participated in data interpretation, and also revised the manuscript. All authors read and approved the final manuscript.

Acknowledgements
This work was supported by funds from the Allen Foundation and the Department of Pediatrics at the University of California, Davis Medical Center.

Author details
[1]Department of Nutrition, University of California, Davis, CA 95616, USA. [2]Department of Pediatrics, University of California, Davis Medical Center, Sacramento, CA 95817, USA.

References
1. Ibanez L, Ong K, Dunger DB, de Zegher F. Early development of adiposity and insulin resistance after catch-up weight gain in small-for-gestational-age children. J Clin Endocrinol Metab. 2006;91(6):2153–8.
2. Soto N, Bazaes RA, Pena V, Salazar T, Avila A, Iniguez G, et al. Insulin sensitivity and secretion are related to catch-up growth in small-for-gestational-age infants at age 1 year: results from a prospective cohort. J Clin Endocrinol Metab. 2003;88(8):3645–50.
3. Ehrenkranz RA, Younes N, Lemons JA, Fanaroff AA, Donovan EF, Wright LL, et al. Longitudinal growth of hospitalized very low birth weight infants. Pediatrics. 1999;104(2 Pt 1):280–9.
4. Embleton NE, Pang N, Cooke RJ. Postnatal malnutrition and growth retardation: an inevitable consequence of current recommendations in preterm infants? Pediatrics. 2001;107(2):270–3.
5. Ehrenkranz RA, Dusick AM, Vohr BR, Wright LL, Wrage LA, Poole WK. Growth in the neonatal intensive care unit influences neurodevelopmental and growth outcomes of extremely low birth weight infants. Pediatrics. 2006;117(4):1253–61.
6. Johnson S. Cognitive and behavioural outcomes following very preterm birth. Semin Fetal Neonat M. 2007;12(5):363–73.
7. Meyer LR, Zhu V, Miller A, Roghair RD. Growth restriction, leptin, and the programming of adult behavior in mice. Behav Brain Res. 2014;275:131–5.
8. Altigani M, Murphy JF, Newcombe RG, Gray OP. Catch up growth in preterm infants. Acta Paediatr Scand Suppl. 1989;357:3–19.
9. Bertino E, Di Nicola P, Varalda A, Occhi L, Giuliani F, Coscia A. Neonatal growth charts. Journal Matern Fetal Neonatal Med. 2012;25 Suppl 1:67–9.
10. Thureen P, Heird WC. Protein and energy requirements of the preterm/low birthweight (LBW) infant. Pediatr Res. 2005;57(5 Pt 2):95R–8R.
11. Greer FR. Long-term adverse outcomes of low birth weight, increased somatic growth rates, and alterations of body composition in the premature infant: review of the evidence. J Pediatr Gastroenterol Nutr. 2007;45 Suppl 3:S147–151.
12. Ong KK, Ahmed ML, Emmett PM, Preece MA, Dunger DB. Association between postnatal catch-up growth and obesity in childhood: prospective cohort study. BMJ. 2000;320(7240):967–71.

13. Jou MY, Lonnerdal B, Griffin IJ. Effects of early postnatal growth restriction and subsequent catch-up growth on body composition, insulin sensitivity, and behavior in neonatal rats. Pediatr Res. 2013;73(5):596–601.

14. Vuguin PM. Animal models for small for gestational age and fetal programing of adult disease. Horm Res. 2007;68(3):113–23.

15. Holemans K, Aerts L, Van Assche FA. Fetal growth restriction and consequences for the offspring in animal models. J Soc Gynecol Invest. 2003;10(7):392–9.

16. Guerra RF, Nunes CR. Effects of litter size on maternal care, body weight and infant development in golden hamsters (Mesocricetus auratus). Behav Processes. 2001;55(3):127–42.

17. Chiang CF, Johnson RK, Neilsen MK. Maternal behavior in mice selected for large litter size. Appl Anim Behav Sci. 2002;79(1):63–73.

18. Dobbing J, Sands J. Comparative aspects of the brain growth spurt. Early Hum Dev. 1979;3(1):79–83.

19. Fiorotto ML, Burrin DG, Perez M, Reeds PJ. Intake and use of milk nutrients by rat pups suckled in small, medium, or large litters. Am J Physiol. 1991;260(6):R1104–13.

20. Griffin IJ, Cooke RJ. Development of whole body adiposity in preterm infants. Early Hum Dev. 2012;88 Suppl 1:S19–24.

21. Prior LJ, Velkoska E, Watts R, Cameron-Smith D, Morris MJ. Undernutrition during suckling in rats elevates plasma adiponectin and its receptor in skeletal muscle regardless of diet composition: a protective effect? Int J Obes (Lond). 2008;32(10):1585–94.

22. Regan FM, Cutfield WS, Jefferies C, Robinson E, Hofman PL. The impact of early nutrition in premature infants on later childhood insulin sensitivity and growth. Pediatrics. 2006;118(5):1943–9.

23. Jimenez-Chillaron JC, Hernandez-Valencia M, Lightner A, Faucette RR, Reamer C, Przybyla R, et al. Reductions in caloric intake and early postnatal growth prevent glucose intolerance and obesity associated with low birthweight. Diabetologia. 2006;49(8):1974–84.

24. Hales CN, Barker DJ. The thrifty phenotype hypothesis. Br Med Bull. 2001;60:5–20.

25. Godfrey KM, Lillycrop KA, Burdge GC, Gluckman PD, Hanson MA. Epigenetic mechanisms and the mismatch concept of the developmental origins of health and disease. Pediatr Res. 2007;61(5 Pt 2):5R–10R.

26. Wiggins RC. Myelin development and nutritional insufficiency. Brain Res. 1982;257(2):151–75.

27. Downes N, Mullins P. The Development of Myelin in the Brain of the Juvenile Rat. Toxicol Pathol. 2013.

28. Doretto S, Malerba M, Ramos M, Ikrar T, Kinoshita C, De Mei C, et al. Oligodendrocytes as regulators of neuronal networks during early postnatal development. PLoS One. 2011;6(5):e19849.

29. Egwim PO, Cho BH, Kummerow FA. Effects of postnatal protein undernutrition on myelination in rat brain. Comp Biochem Physiol A Comp Physiol. 1986;83(1):67–70.

30. Sima A, Sourander P. The effect of pre- and postnatal undernutrition on axonal growth and myelination of central motor fibers. A morphometric study on rat cortico-spinal tract. Acta Neuropathol. 1978;42(1):15–8.

31. Royland JE, Konat G, Wiggins RC. Abnormal upregulation of myelin genes underlies the critical period of myelination in undernourished developing rat brain. Brain Res. 1993;607(1–2):113–6.

32. Duff DA, Snell K. Effect of altered neonatal nutrition on the development of enzymes of lipid and carbohydrate metabolism in the rat. J Nutr. 1982;112(6):1057–66.

33. Udagawa J, Hatta T, Hashimoto R, Otani H. Roles of leptin in prenatal and perinatal brain development. Congenit Anom. 2007;47(3):77–83.

34. Steppan CM, Swick AG. A role for leptin in brain development. Biochem Biophys Res Commun. 1999;256(3):600–2.

35. Hashimoto R, Matsumoto A, Udagawa J, Hioki K, Otani H. Effect of leptin administration on myelination in ob/ob mouse cerebrum after birth. Neuroreport. 2013;24(1):22–9.

36. Reid MA, Latour MG, Legare DJ, Rong N, Lautt WW. Comparison of the rapid insulin sensitivity test (RIST), the insulin tolerance test (ITT), and the hyperinsulinemic euglycemic clamp (HIEC) to measure insulin action in rats. Can J Physiol Pharmacol. 2002;80(8):811–8.

37. Andrikopoulos S, Blair AR, Deluca N, Fam BC, Proietto J. Evaluating the glucose tolerance test in mice. Am J Physiol Endocrinol Metab. 2008;295(6):E1323–1332.

38. Deacon R. T-Maze alteration in the rodent. Nature. 2006;1(1):7–12.

13

Dynamically regulated miRNA-mRNA networks revealed by exercise

Alexander G Tonevitsky[1,2], Diana V Maltseva[3], Asghar Abbasi[4], Timur R Samatov[3*], Dmitry A Sakharov[3], Maxim U Shkurnikov[2], Alexey E Lebedev[1], Vladimir V Galatenko[1], Anatoly I Grigoriev[5] and Hinnak Northoff[4*]

Abstract

Background: MiRNAs are essential mediators of many biological processes. The aim of this study was to investigate the dynamics of miRNA-mRNA regulatory networks during exercise and the subsequent recovery period.

Results: Here we monitored the transcriptome changes using microarray analysis of the whole blood of eight highly trained athletes before and after 30 min of moderate exercise followed by 30 min and 60 min of recovery period. We combined expression profiling and bioinformatics and analysed metabolic pathways enriched with differentially expressed mRNAs and mRNAs which are known to be validated targets of differentially expressed miRNAs. Finally we revealed four dynamically regulated networks comprising differentially expressed miRNAs and their known target mRNAs with anti-correlated expression profiles over time. The data suggest that hsa-miR-21-5p regulated TGFBR3, PDGFD and PPM1L mRNAs. Hsa-miR-24-2-5p was likely to be responsible for *MYC* and *KCNJ2* genes and hsa-miR-27a-5p for *ST3GAL6*. The targets of hsa-miR-181a-5p included ROPN1L and SLC37A3. All these mRNAs are involved in processes highly relevant to exercise response, including immune function, apoptosis, membrane traffic of proteins and transcription regulation.

Conclusions: We have identified metabolic pathways involved in response to exercise and revealed four miRNA-mRNA networks dynamically regulated following exercise. This work is the first study to monitor miRNAs and mRNAs in parallel into the recovery period. The results provide a novel insight into the regulatory role of miRNAs in stress adaptation.

Keywords: Exercise, Regulation, miRNA-mRNA networks

Background

MiRNAs are one family of small (20–22 nucleotides) non-coding RNAs. They regulate gene expression post-transcriptionally through binding to the complementary sites of target mRNAs in the 3′-UTR, and play an important role in regulating diverse biological processes [1].

Recently, miRNA have been demonstrated as regulators of processes involved in physiological stress adaptation, including inflammation [2], angiogenesis [3], mitochondrial metabolism [4], muscle force generation [5]. However, just a few studies were published to date describing the changes in miRNA expression during exercise of different intensity [6-12]. They did not include the analysis of post-

exercise recovery period and thus provided no information concerning dynamics of the predicted miRNA-mRNA regulatory pairs. Detailed investigation of miRNA-mRNA networks specifically regulated by exercise could reveal important biomarkers of exercise physiology and would provide for deep insight into the molecular control of the stress response.

MiRNAs regulate target gene expression in different ways including mRNA degradation and translation inhibition [1]. The target genes which were regulated by miRNAs through mRNA degradation are anti-correlated with the miRNA regulators. In this study, for the first time whole transcriptome changes were monitored during exercise followed by 30 min and 60 min of recovery period and differentially expressed mRNAs and miRNAs were analysed resulting in identification of four dynamically regulated miRNA-mRNA networks.

* Correspondence: timur.samatov@gmail.com;
Hinnak.Northoff@med.uni-tuebingen.de
[3]SRC Bioclinicum, Ugreshskaya str 2/85, Moscow 115088, Russia
[4]Institute of Clinical and Experimental Transfusion Medicine (IKET), University of Tübingen, Otfried-Müller-str. 4/1, Tübingen 72076, Germany
Full list of author information is available at the end of the article

Results and discussion

Anthropometric and physiological data

To exclude possible effects of gender, only male subjects were recruited for this study. Anthropometric and physiological parameters of athletes are presented in Table 1. Before exercise the serum lactate level was 1.7 ± 0.4 mM. After exercise, it was mildly elevated, but still below 4.0 mM, confirming that the exercise performed was moderate without transgression of the anaerobic threshold.

Branched-chain amino acids (BCAA) include three structurally related amino acids Leucine (Leu), Isoleucine (Ile), and Valine (Val). The initial steps of their degradation are catalyzed by the same set of mitochondrial enzymes, and therefore, the BCAA behave as a very homogenous group. Their regulation is performed by short-term metabolic control reflecting consuming of energy sources. It has been shown previously that an acute bout of prolonged exercise increases the rate of BCAA oxidation by skeletal muscle [13]. We observed a slight increase in the BCAA level immediately after exercise followed by a decline below base level during recovery (Table 2). The ratio of citrulline (Cit) to ornithine (Orn) is indicative of the ornithine carbamoylphosphate transferase activity and characterizes the regulation of the urea cycle pathway [14]. This ratio had a tendency to increase (Table 2). The ratios of methionine sulfoxide (Met-SO) to methionine (Met) and tyrosine (Tyr) to phenylalanine (Phe) indicate oxidative stress [15,16]. We found a decrease in Met-SO/Met and a slight increase in Tyr/Phe (Table 2).

The data summarized in Table 2 confirmed that the exercise was moderate and athletes reacted as normal healthy subjects [17].

Flow cytometry analysis

Changes in white blood cell subpopulations in response to exercise are presented in Table 3. Total white blood cell counts revealed the expected exercise-induced leukocytosis. NK lymphocytes (defined as CD3−, CD16/56+) substantially contributed to the observed changes which was consistent with the published data [18]. However NK-specific mRNAs (e.g., coding for KIR receptors) in the whole

Table 1 Anthropometric and physiological data

Parameter	Value
Age (year)	21.7 ± 2.6
Body mass (kg)	74.9 ± 2.3
Height (cm)	185.3 ± 3.5
Body mass index (kg/m^2)	21.8 ± 1.2
Heart rate before exercise(bpm)	57.3 ± 1.9
Heart rate after exercise (bpm)	179.4 ± 3.2
Blood pressure before exercise (mmHg)	$120/66 \pm 3/2$
VO$_{2max}$ (ml min^{-1} kg^{-1})	74.8 ± 3.3

Values are mean ± SD.

Table 2 Aminoacids before and in response to exercise

	BCAA, µM	Cit/Orn	Met-SO/Met	Tyr/Phe
Pre	567.63 ± 172.16	0.35 ± 0.09	2.28 ± 1.73	0.83 ± 0.15
Post (E)	612.83 ± 99.68	0.34 ± 0.11	0.92 ± 0.21	0.91 ± 0.18
Rest 30 min (R1)	496.89 ± 128.31	0.42 ± 0.09	1.71 ± 0.92	0.91 ± 0.19
Rest 60 min (R2)	417.75 ± 58.2	0.5 ± 0.15	1.21 ± 0.47	0.9 ± 0.16

Abbreviations: *BCAA* Branched-Chain Amino Acids, *Cit* Citrulline, *Orn* ornithine, *Met-SO* Methionine Sulfoxide, *Met* Methionine, *Tyr* Tyrosine, *Phe* Phenylalanine.

blood did not demonstrate similar nearly 3-fold increase (see Additional file 1) thus confirming that our subsequent microarray analysis showed true changes in RNA expression.

miRNA and mRNA differential expression profiles

The miRNA and mRNA expression profiles in the whole blood for each time point and each athlete were determined using microarray analysis. PAXgene RNA tubes enable the isolation of intracellular RNA of circulating leukocytes, including B cells, T cells, neutrophils, monocytes, and other less abundant cell types. Furthermore, a large proportion of reticulocyte-derived globin mRNA is prepared from PAXgene blood RNA tubes, as it has been demonstrated previously [19]. Affymetrix GeneChip Human Gene 1.0 ST arrays contain both miRNA and mRNA probes and are capable of measuring about 20,000 mRNAs and 200 miRNAs.

The data are presented in Additional file 1. 298 mRNAs and 5 miRNAs were changed significantly (at least 40% change with the adjusted P-value threshold of 0.05), including hsa-miR-21-5p, hsa-miR-24-2-5p, hsa-miR-27a-5p, hsa-miR-181a-5p and hsa-miR-181b-5p. Remarkably, hsa-miR-24-2-5p is clustered with hsa-miR-27a-5p, and hsa-miR-181a-5p is clustered with hsa-miR-181b-5p. Consistently, the clustered miRNAs exhibited similar expression profiles over time (see Additional file 1 and Figures 1, 2, 3 and 4).

Pathway analysis of differentially expressed mRNAs

All 298 differentially expressed mRNAs were analysed for enriched metabolic pathways. Table 4 indicates the revealed pathways including immune response and glycoproteins. As expected, they were previously reported to be associated with exercise [6,8] thus confirming the relevance of our experimental model.

Pathway analysis of mRNA targets of differentially expressed miRNAs

All 5 differentially expressed miRNAs have 1136 validated target mRNAs in total. We performed pathway enrichment analysis for these mRNAs (Table 5). Again, the revealed pathways are highly relevant to exercise, e.g. transcription regulation, apoptosis, response to stress etc.

It has been demonstrated that the same mRNAs can be targeted by more than one miRNA which provides

Table 3 Changes in white blood cell subpopulations in response to an exercise

	Pre		Post (E)		Fold change relative
	Absolute, cells/ul	Relative, %	Absolute, cells/ul	Relative, %	
WBC	5710 ± 1170		7705 ± 2000		
LY	2387 ± 674	41.8 ± 11.8	3989 ± 932	69.9 ± 12.1	1.67
CD3+	1616 ± 549	28.3 ± 9.6	2349 ± 901	41.1 ± 11.7	1.45
CD3 + CD4+	1020 ± 413	17.9 ± 7.2	1189 ± 419	20.8 ± 5.4	1.17
CD3 + CD8+	596 ± 265	10.4 ± 4.6	1124 ± 532	19.7 ± 6.9	1.89
CD3-CD16+	494 ± 203	8.7 ± 3.6	1380 ± 523	24.2 ± 6.8	2.79
CD3-CD56+	393 ± 217	6.9 ± 3.8	1111 ± 468	19.5 ± 6.1	2.83
CD19+	227 ± 124	4.0 ± 2.2	308 ± 221	5.4 ± 2.9	1.36

Values are mean ± SD.

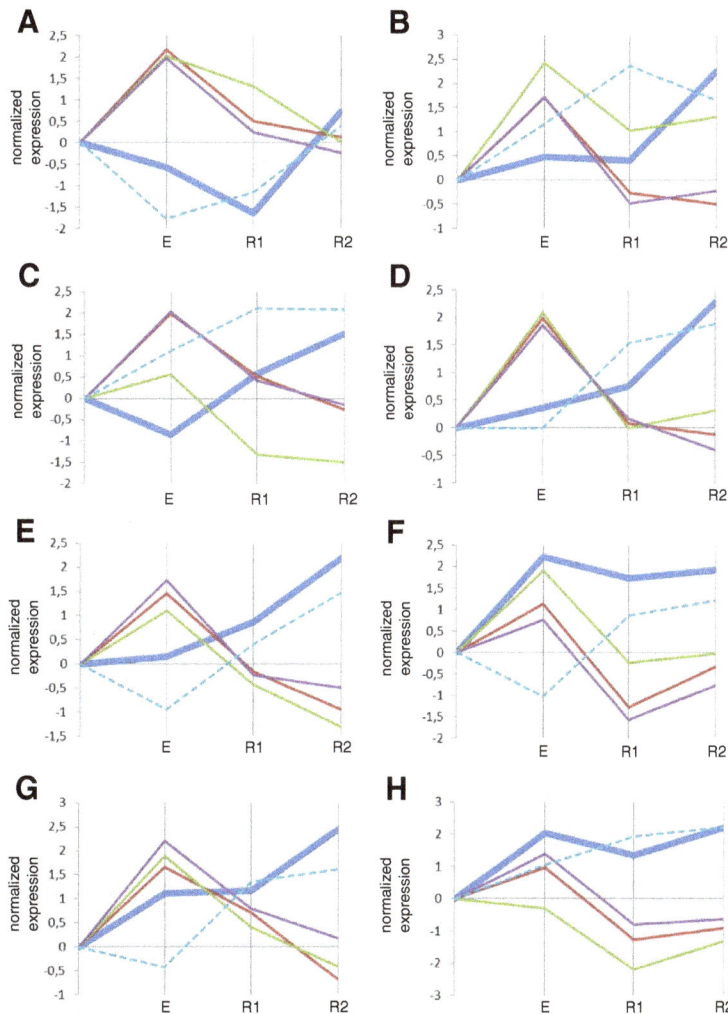

Figure 1 Expression profiles of hsa-miR-21-5p and its target mRNAs. (A-H) the tested athletes. **E**, after 30 min of exercise; R1, after 30 min relaxation; R2, after 60 min relaxation. Bold blue, hsa-miR-21-5p; brown, TGFBR3; green, PDGFD; violet, PPM1L; light blue, RHOBTB3. Solid lines indicate validated mRNA targets and dashed line indicates predicted potential mRNA target.

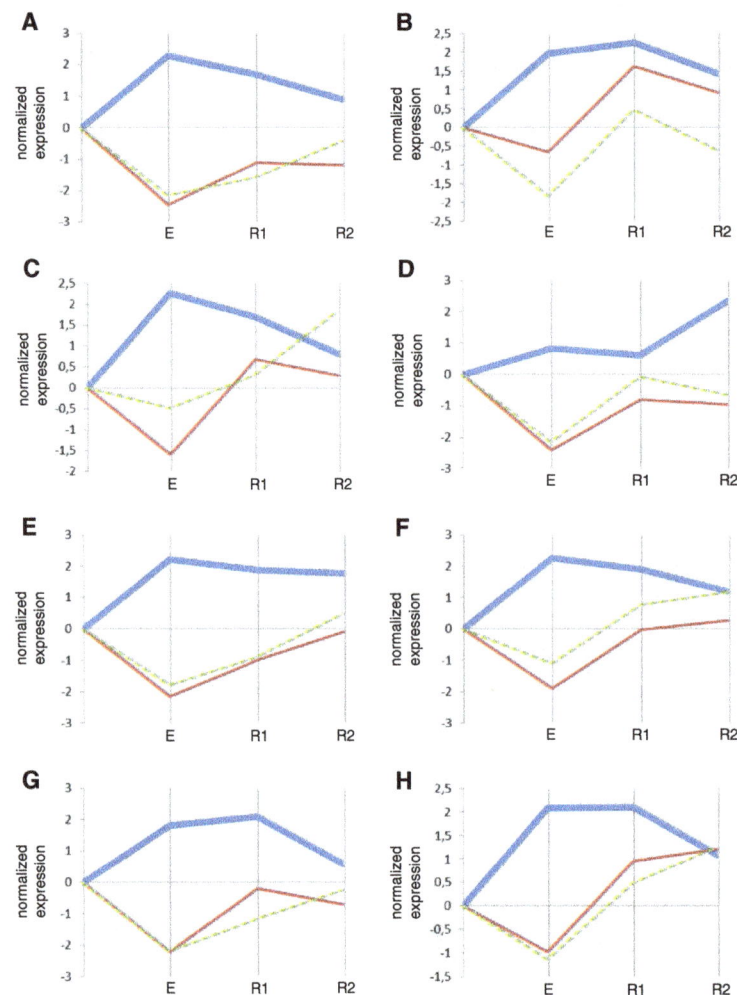

Figure 2 Expression profiles of hsa-miR-24-2-5p and its target mRNAs. (A-H) the tested athletes. **E**, after 30 min of exercise; R1, after 30 min relaxation; R2, after 60 min relaxation. Bold blue, hsa-miR-24-2-5p; brown, MYC; green, KCNJ2. Solid line indicates validated mRNA target and dashed line indicates predicted potential mRNA target.

for more efficient and specific regulation [20,21]. We found 49 mRNAs which are known to be validated targets for 2 or even 3 differentially expressed miRNAs. They have higher potential to be involved in exercise-induced regulation. Table 6 shows the pathways enriched with some of these mRNAs. Notably, these exercise-relevant pathways (cell death, stress response, proliferation) comprise significant number of intersecting mRNAs. Figure 5 presents the identified regulatory miRNA-mRNA network for all 3 revealed pathways. Interestingly, some of these genes are known to interact with each other. Namely transcription factor MYC was reported to be functionally associated with RNA helicase DDX3X [22], apoptosis regulator BCL2 [23] and tumor suppressor BRCA1 [24]. BRCA1 in turn interacts itself with BCL2 [25] and transcription factor E2F1 [26]. The presented data support the regulatory role of identified miRNAs in response to exercise.

Dynamically regulated miRNA-mRNA networks

We monitored the transcriptome expression level before and following exercise and this allowed us to reveal dynamically regulated miRNA-mRNA networks. We used a two-step approach to identify the mRNA targets for the differentially expressed miRNAs. First, we looked for anti-correlating groups of miRNAs and mRNAs expression of which over time tended to have opposite profiles. Target mRNA degradation is one of the mechanisms of miRNA action when their perfect complementarity occurs [1,27]. Thus, the second step of our strategy was either analysis of published data and selection of experimentally validated target mRNAs for a given miRNA or theoretical prediction of miRNA targets based on their complementarity, using one of the most popular web resources TargetScan [28]. The expression profiles and biological function of selected miRNAs and mRNAs were analysed in more detail. Based on this analysis, our final

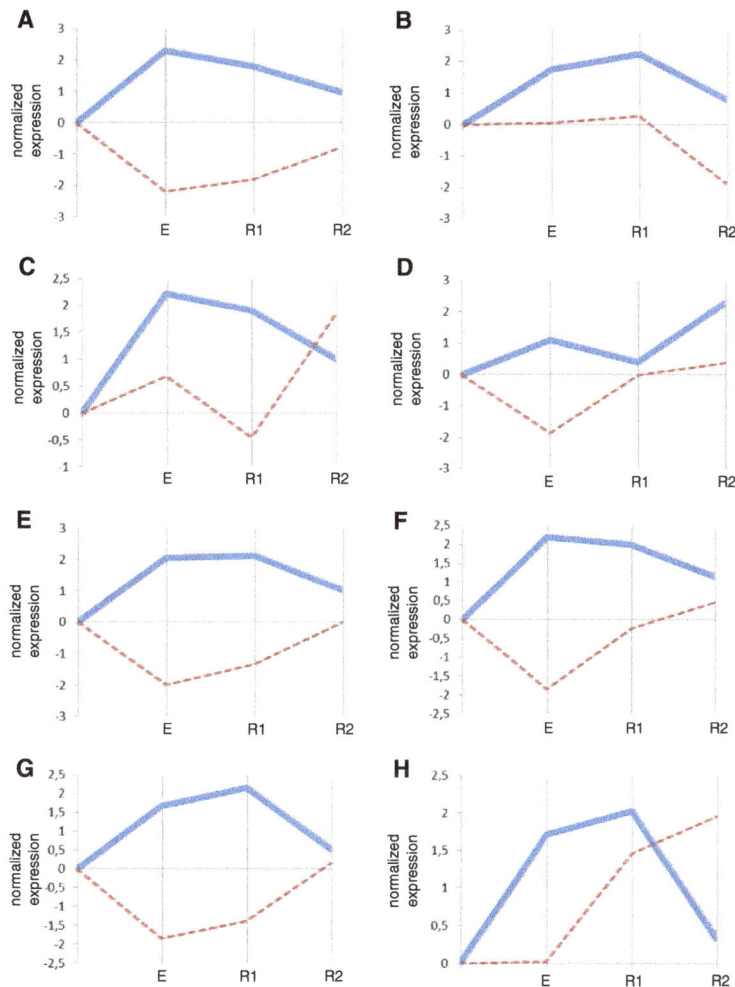

Figure 3 Expression profiles of hsa-miR-27a-5p and its target mRNA. (A-H) the tested athletes. E, after 30 min of exercise; R1, after 30 min relaxation; R2, after 60 min relaxation. Bold blue, hsa-miR-27a-5p; dashed brown, predicted potential target mRNA ST3GAL6.

identified miRNA-mRNA pairs have a high probability of being involved in the regulation of exercise-related physiological processes.

hsa-miR-21-5p

MiRNA hsa-miR-21-5p demonstrated different expression profiles over time (adjusted P-value 0.0039) however remarkably anti-correlating with experimentally validated target mRNAs TGFBR3 (adjusted P-value 1.079E-06), PDGFD (adjusted P-value 1.28E-06) and PPM1L (adjusted P-value 6.78E-07) (Figure 1). RHOBTB3 mRNA (adjusted P-value 0.002) predicted by TargetScan to be a potential target for hsa-miR-21-2-5p behaved similarly. We observed the up-regulation of hsa-miR-21-5p one hour after exercise. The differences in kinetics can be potentially explained by individualities of each athlete.

The expression level of hsa-miR-21-5p itself is known to be stress-responsive and play an important role in heart failure [29] and renal ischemia reperfusion injury [30].

Notably the up-regulation of circulating hsa-miR-21-5p was recently reported to occur in plasma upon exercise [6]. The overall action of hsa-miR-21-5p has been described by several authors to be strongly anti-inflammatory [6,31]. Note, that 60 min into relaxation, there was an up-regulation of hsa-miR-21-5p in all 8 subjects. This may reflect the self-protective anti-inflammatory reaction to exercise.

We identified four pairing targets for this miRNA namely TGFBR3, PDGFD, PPM1L, and RHOBTB3. TGFBR3 is a transforming growth factor (TGF)-beta type III receptor, mRNA of which is known to be up-regulated in the peripheral blood leukocytes in allograft rejection-prone recipients after intestinal transplantation thus mediating innate and adaptive inflammatory functions of leukocytes [32]. PDGFD encodes for platelet derived growth factor D [33], a member of the platelet-derived growth factor family which can regulate many cellular processes, including cell proliferation, apoptosis, transformation, migration,

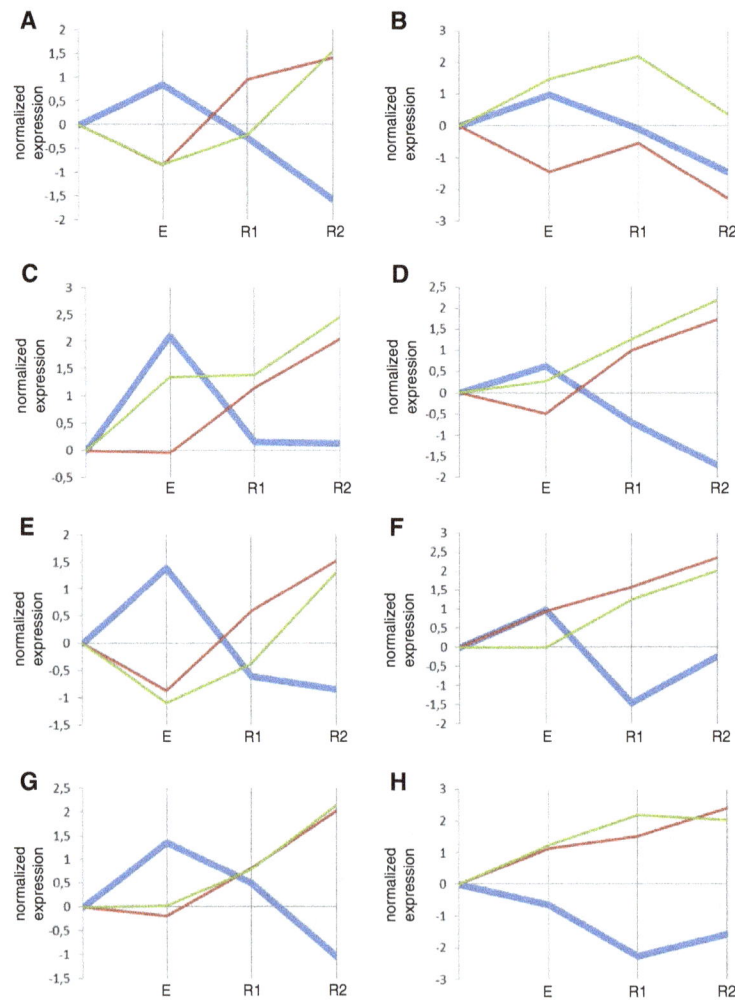

Figure 4 Expression profiles of hsa-miR-181a-5p and its validated target mRNAs. (A-H) the tested athletes. **E**, after 30 min of exercise; R1, after 30 min relaxation; R2, after 60 min relaxation. Bold blue, hsa-miR-181a-5p; brown, ROPN1L; green, SCL37A3.

invasion, angiogenesis and metastasis [34]. PPM1L encodes a protein phosphatase gene [35] responsible for the regulation of stress-activated protein kinase signaling cascade and apoptosis [36]. Finally, the fourth identified target for hsa-miR-21-5p is RHOBTB3 mRNA [33] which encodes for the Rho GTPase regulating the membrane traffic of proteins [37]. Interestingly, this mRNA proved to be a blood biomarker of psychosis and shows a decreased expression level in high hallucinations states [38].

hsa-miR-24-2-5p

MiRNA hsa-miR-24-2-5p (adjusted P-value 0.00017) was up-regulated immediately after exercise, then tended to decrease during the recovery period except athlete D (Figure 2). In our study for the first time we report the reaction to exercise of this miRNA which is known to have protective effects on myocytes against myocardial ischaemia/reperfusion-induced apoptosis [39].

MYC mRNA (adjusted P-value 0.00013) which is known to be the target for this miRNA from the literature, and KCNJ2 mRNA (adjusted P-value 0.00023) predicted by TargetScan to be a potential target essentially followed anti-profile of hsa-miR-24-2-5p. The protein encoded by the *MYC* gene is a multifunctional, nuclear phosphoprotein that plays a role in cell cycle progression, apoptosis and cellular transformation. It functions as a transcription factor that regulates transcription of specific target genes. Interestingly, hsa-miR-24-2-5p is known to be up-regulated during hematopoietic cell terminal differentiation suppressing MYC expression [40]. Thus the increase of this miRNA we observed (Figure 2) may reflect the regulation of hematopoiesis upon exercise. Remarkably, MYC mRNA is among those which are regulated by 2 differentially expressed miRNAs, namely hsa-miR-21-5p and hsa-miR-24-2-5p (Figure 5), however its expression profile is anti-correlated with only the profile of hsa-miR-24-2-5p (Figures 1 and 2).

Table 4 Pathway analysis of differentially expressed mRNAs

Pathway	Number of genes	Adjusted P-value
Glycoprotein	76	3.00E-09
Natural killer cell mediated cytotoxicity	22	1.80E-15
Immune response	13	3.10E-03
Response to wounding	7	8.70E-01
Inflammatory response	7	1.90E-01
Regulation of lymphocyte mediated immunity	5	1.40E-01
Leukocyte activation	5	8.90E-01
Response to mechanical stimulus	3	3.80E-02
Stress response	3	5.90E-02
Cytolysis	3	3.20E-02

KCNJ2 protein is an integral membrane protein and inward-rectifier type potassium channel participating in establishing the action potential waveform and excitability of neuronal and muscle tissues [41]. This mRNA expressed in peripheral blood lymphocytes is a biomarker for Parkinson's disease [42].

hsa-miR-27a-5p

MiRNA hsa-miR-27a-5p is clustered with hsa-miR-24-2-5p and behaved similarly to it increasing after exercise and decreasing during the recovery period except athlete D (Figure 3) with the adjusted P-value 0.00012. This miRNA was reported to promote myoblast proliferation by reducing the expression of myostatin [43].

The only mRNA target identified is predicted by TargetScan ST3GAL6. The encoded protein belongs to the sialyltransferase family and is responsible for the synthesis of selectin ligands [44].

hsa-miR-181a-5p

hsa-miR-181a-5p tended to increase after exercise and then to down-regulate during the first as well as the second period of the relaxation time (Figure 4) with an

Table 5 Pathway analysis of all validated mRNA targets of differentially expressed miRNAs

Pathway	Number of genes	Adjusted P-value
Transcription regulation	283	2.03E-13
Apoptotic process	157	2.59E-11
Cell cycle	148	5.95E-12
Regulation of kinase activity	76	1.08E-08
Regulation of cellular response to stress	34	1.63E-04
p53 signaling pathway	19	4.26E-08
E2F transcription factor network	19	1.51E-07
Validated targets of C-MYC transcriptional activation	14	1.08E-03

Table 6 Pathway analysis of mRNAs validated to be targets for 2 or 3 differentially expressed miRNAs

Pathway	Number of genes	Adjusted P-value
Cell death	17	7.64E-07
Regulation of cell proliferation	15	2.10E-07
Cellular response to stress	12	5.35E-05

adjusted P-value of 5.83E-05. The observed differential expression of hsa-miR-181a-5p in our athletes is consistent with previously published results [7,8]. This miRNA is characterized as a regulator of hematopoietic lineage differentiation [45] and a modulator of T cell sensitivity and selection [46]. Radom-Aizik showed up-regulation of this miRNA after 30 min interval exercise. They related it to increased T cell responsiveness and reduced susceptibility to infection due to physical activity. In our study 7 subjects showed up-regulation immediately after exercise (Figure 4).

The mRNAs ROPN1L (adjusted P-value 0.00024) and SLC37A3 (adjusted P-value 0.0019) were previously validated to be targets for hsa-miR-181a-5p and demonstrated pronounced anti-correlation with the miRNA expression profile. The *ROPN1L* gene encodes a member of the ropporin family. The encoded protein is involved in the targeting towards specific physiological substrates of Protein Kinase A, regulating glycogen, sugar, and lipid metabolism [47]. The SLC37A3 protein belongs to transmembrane sugar transporters and is responsible for sugar metabolism [48].

Conclusion

We have identified metabolic pathways enriched with differentially expressed mRNAs and with mRNA targets of differentially expressed miRNAs, including mRNAs known to be regulated by 2 or 3 miRNAs described here. The result supports previously published data. Moreover, we revealed four miRNA-mRNA networks dynamically regulated following exercise. These observations provide a novel insight into the potential regulatory role of miRNAs in the numerous physiological processes involved in stress adaptation.

Methods

Ethical approval and study participants

Eight national level ski athletes took part in this study. None of them suffered from acute or chronic diseases or reported intake of medication. Participants were informed about the nature, purpose, and potential risks of the experiments and signed an informed consent statement approved by the ethics committee of Scientific Research Center Bioclinicum (Moscow, Russia).

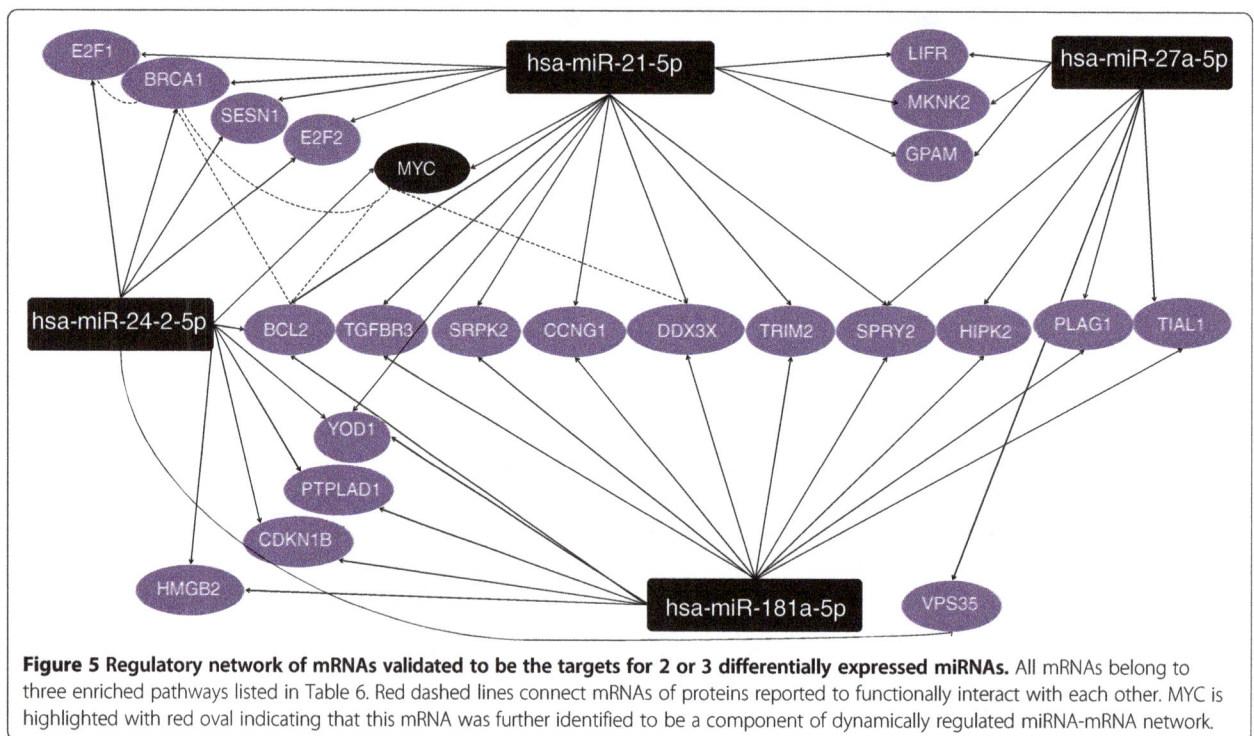

Figure 5 Regulatory network of mRNAs validated to be the targets for 2 or 3 differentially expressed miRNAs. All mRNAs belong to three enriched pathways listed in Table 6. Red dashed lines connect mRNAs of proteins reported to functionally interact with each other. MYC is highlighted with red oval indicating that this mRNA was further identified to be a component of dynamically regulated miRNA-mRNA network.

Anthropometric measurements

Height, weight, medical historical data and resting vital signs were recorded at the time of enrolment.

Exercise test protocol

In order to determine the VO_{2max} values, each subject performed a treadmill test with an incremental step protocol until exhaustion as described previously [47]. VO_{2max} was calculated as described [49]. The anaerobic threshold was calculated using the standard V-slope method [50].

Two weeks later, athletes participated in the main exercise, consisting of running at 80% VO_2 peak for 30 min on a treadmill. The exercise was performed during the morning hours (between 8 and 11 a.m.) keeping the exact test time for each participant constant.

Lactate concentration

Lactate concentration in capillary blood was measured electrochemically using the automated analyzer Biosen C_Line (EFK Diagnostic, Germany).

Analysis of aminoacids

Sera derived from the venous blood samples were analyzed for aminoacids in Genome Analysis Centre (Helmholtz Zentrum, Munich, Germany) using the BIOCRATES AbsoluteIDQ p150 Kit (Biocrates Life Sciences AG, Innsbruck, Austria) in a combined FIA-MS/MS and LC-MS/MS assay as recommended by the manufacturer and described previously [51].

Blood sampling

Venous blood was collected at four time points during the exercise. A 20-gauge intravenous catheter was placed antiseptically into a dorsal hand vein or a vein in the distal forearm as dictated by favourable anatomy using the Seldinger technique and then secured with tape. During ME 2.5 ml of blood was collected in PAXgene blood RNA tube, 7 ml in a Serum separator tube (BD, USA) and 4.5 ml in a tube containing buffered tri-sodium citrate (BD, USA) for flow cytometry analysis at baseline (prior to exercise testing) and immediately post-exercise (within 1 min of completion of exercise testing). After 30 min of rest and after 60 min of rest following exercise testing 2.5 ml of blood was collected in PAXgene blood RNA tubes.

RNA extraction

According to the Affymetrix Manual P/N 701880 Rev. 4 total RNA was extracted using the PAXgene Blood RNA kit as recommended by the manufacturer. RNA concentrations were determined by the Nanodrop photometer (NanoDrop, USA). RNA quality was checked using the Agilent Bioanalyser 2100 System (Agilent Technologies, USA). For all samples RNA integrity number (RIN) was greater than 7.

Flow cytometry analysis

Flow cytometry analysis of blood samples was performed using fluorescently labeled antibodies against B and T cell receptors and natural killer (NK) cell markers. Cells were labeled with antibodies against CD3 (FITC), CD4 (PE), CD8 (PE), CD16 (FITC), CD56 (PE), CD19 (FITC) (Sorbent, Russia), where NK cells were distinguished from the rest of the lymphocytes via positive expression of CD56 and negative expression of CD3.

The samples were analyzed on a FACScan Calibur flow cytometer (BD Biosciences, USA) and leukocytes were gated based on forward and side scatter properties. Events in the range of 40,000–200,000 were collected depending on the occurrence of the investigated leukocyte population, and analyzed with CELLQuest Pro analysis software (BD Biosciences, USA). To ensure flow cytometric standardization, the voltage settings were updated daily using 'Calibrate Beads' (BD Biosciences, USA).

Microarray analysis

RNA samples were prepared according to manufacturer's instructions (Affymetrix Manual P/N 701880 Rev. 4) as described elsewhere [52]. The samples were hybridized on GeneChip Human Gene 1.0 ST Arrays containing both miRNA and mRNA probes (Affymetrix, USA) for 16 h at 45°C. Arrays were washed to remove non-specifically bound nucleic acids and stained on Fluidics Station 450 (Affymetrix) using FS450_0007 protocol followed by scanning on a GeneChip Scanner 3000 7G system (Affymetrix). The microarray CEL files have been deposited in the GEO database (accession GSE46075).

Microarray data processing

Microarray data was processed using bioconductor [53] xps package implementation of RMA [54]. At the first step background correction was performed based on a global model for the distribution of probe intensities [54]. Then a quantile normalization algorithm [55] (so-called probe-level normalization) was applied to the preprocessed data. Finally, fitting a robust linear model using Tukey's median polish procedure [56] was done to convert probe intensities to the expression levels of probesets.

The statistical analysis of microarray data was performed using bioconductor [53] package limma [57]. The analysis was based on a generalized linear model [57,58] approach. In this approach one constructs a linear data model with a structure determined by the experiment layout, and then fits this model to the actual data. The linear model is defined in terms of a so-called design matrix. The number of rows in this matrix coincides with the number of experiment samples, and the number of columns coincides with the number of factors that have an essential influence on the measurable values. The value at the i-th row and j-th column of a design matrix specifies an effect of a factor j on a sample i. Each measurable value (i.e., each probeset) in this approach is analysed independently. For each probeset a vector of its expression values E is

represented in the form $E = D\beta + \varepsilon$, where D is a design matrix, β is a vector of coefficients indicating values of each factor's actual influence on the analyzed probeset, ε is a vector of error, and model fitting consists in the minimization of "error term" ε by finding optimal coefficients β. After the coefficients β are computed for each probeset, one can test various hypotheses on the structure of considered factors. For example, in order to find probesets that are affected by a factor i, one should search for the probesets with β_i statistically different from zero.

The general linear model was applied in the analysis of the studied transcriptome changes as follows. The model that takes into account both experiment time points and athletes individual features was used. Thus, the total number of factors was eleven: $c_1, ..., c_8$ correspond to an expression level of each athlete in a normal state (for all samples the effect of these factors is set to 1 if a sample and a factor correspond to the same athlete, and set to 0 otherwise), and d_1, d_2, d_3 correspond to the changes induces by the exercises, exercises and 30-minutes relaxation, and exercises and 60-minutes relaxation respectively (for all samples the effect of these factors is set to 1 if a sample and a factor correspond to the same experiment time point, and set to 0 otherwise). The total number of samples was 32: 4 samples for each athlete.

For each pair of experiment time points the detection of probesets with reliable difference between time points was performed. The probeset was considered to have a reliable difference between time points k, m if an adjusted p-value of an equality $\beta_k = \beta_m$ (where β_l was an actual influence of exercises at experiment time point for $l = 1,2,3$, and $\beta_0 = 0$) was less than 0.05, and a log-fold change was greater than 0.484 (this threshold corresponds to an intensity change by more than 40%). The Benjamini-Hochberg [59] algorithm was used for multiple testing adjustment. The minimum adjusted p-value for all pairs of time points is indicated for each differentially expressed probeset in the Table of differentially expressed mRNAs and miRNAs (Additional file 1) as a statistical significance value.

Pathway analysis

Bioinformatic analysis was performed using DAVID online tool (http://david.abcc.ncifcrf.gov) as described elsewhere [60]. So all the analyzed genes were classified into several functional groups, and the groups that may be potentially associated with physiological stress were considered and listed in the tabs of excel document. P-values on the tabs are modified Fisher Exact P-Values. When members of two independent groups can fall into one of two mutually exclusive categories, Fisher Exact test is used to determine whether the proportions of those falling into each category differs by group. In DAVID annotation system, Fisher Exact test is adopted to measure the gene-enrichment in annotation terms.

Abbreviations

miRNA: microRNA; mRNA: messenger RNA.

Competing interests

The authors declare that they have no competing interests.

Authors' contributions

Conception and design of the experiments: AGT, AIG. Collection, analysis and interpretation of data: DVM, DAS, MUS, AEL, VVG. Drafting the article and revising it critically TRS, AGT, AA, HN. All authors read and approved the final manuscript.

Acknowledgements

We thank Svetlana Vinogradova for the help with bioinformatic data analysis. This work was supported by BMBF grant RUS 10/040 and by Russian Ministry of Science Grants No. 16.522.12.2015 and 16.522.11.2004.

Author details

[1]Moscow State University, Leninskie Gory, Moscow 119991, Russia. [2]The Institute of General Pathology and Pathophysiology, Russian Academy of Medical Sciences, Baltiiskaya str. 8, Moscow 125315, Russia. [3]SRC Bioclinicum, Ugreshskaya str 2/85, Moscow 115088, Russia. [4]Institute of Clinical and Experimental Transfusion Medicine (IKET), University of Tübingen, Otfried-Müller-str. 4/1, Tübingen 72076, Germany. [5]Institute for Biomedical Problems, Russian Academy of Sciences, Khoroshevskoe road 76a, Moscow 123007, Russia.

References

1. Bartel DP: MicroRNAs: genomics, biogenesis, mechanism, and function. Cell 2004, 116:281–297.
2. Davidson-Moncada J, Papavasiliou FN, Tam W: MicroRNAs of the immune system: roles in inflammation and cancer. Ann N Y Acad Sci 2010, 1183:183–194.
3. Zhang C: MicroRNAs in vascular biology and vascular disease. J Cardiovasc Transl Res 2010, 3:235–240.
4. Dang CV: Rethinking the Warburg effect with Myc micromanaging glutamine metabolism. Cancer Res 2010, 70:859–862.
5. Davidsen PK, Gallagher IJ, Hartman JW, Tarnopolsky MA, Dela F, Helge JW, Timmons JA, Phillips SM: High responders to resistance exercise training demonstrate differential regulation of skeletal muscle microRNA expression. J Appl Physiol 2011, 110:309–317.
6. Baggish AL, Hale A, Weiner RB, Lewis GD, Systrom D, Wang F, Wang TJ, Chan SY: Dynamic regulation of circulating microRNA during acute exhaustive exercise and sustained aerobic exercise training. J Physiol 2011, 589:3983–3994.
7. Radom-Aizik S, Zaldivar F Jr, Oliver S, Galassetti P, Cooper DM: Evidence for microRNA involvement in exercise-associated neutrophil gene expression changes. J Appl Physiol 2010, 109:252–261.
8. Radom-Aizik S, Zaldivar F Jr, Leu SY, Adams GR, Oliver S, Cooper DM: Effects of exercise on microRNA expression in young males peripheral blood mononuclear cells. Clin Transl Sci 2012, 5:32–38.
9. Fernandes T, Magalhães FC, Roque FR, Phillips MI, Oliveira EM: Exercise training prevents the microvascular rarefaction in hypertension balancing angiogenic and apoptotic factors: role of microRNAs-16, -21, and −126. Hypertension 2012, 59:513–520.
10. Radom-Aizik S, Zaldivar FP, Haddad F, Cooper DM: Impact of brief exercise on peripheral blood NK cell gene and microRNA expression in young adults. J Appl Physiol 2013, 114:628–636.
11. Uhlemann M, Möbius-Winkler S, Fikenzer S, Adam J, Redlich M, Möhlenkamp S, Hilberg T, Schuler GC, Adams V: Circulating microRNA-126 increases after different forms of endurance exercise in healthy adults. Eur J Prev Cardiol 2012. doi:10.1177/2047487312467902.
12. Bye A, Røsjø H, Aspenes ST, Condorelli G, Omland T, Wisløff U: Circulating MicroRNAs and Aerobic Fitness - The HUNT-Study. PLoS One 2013, 8:e57496.
13. McKenzie S, Phillips SM, Carter SL, Lowther S, Gibala MJ, Tarnopolsky MA: Endurance exercise training attenuates leucine oxidation and BCOAD activation during exercise in humans. Am J Physiol Endocrinol Metab 2000, 278:E580–587.
14. Huang CC, Lin WT, Hsu FL, Tsai PW, Hou CC: Metabolomics investigation of exercise-modulated changes in metabolism in rat liver after exhaustive and endurance exercises. Eur J Appl Physiol 2010, 108:557–566.
15. Ribas GS, Sitta A, Wajner M, Vargas CR: Oxidative stress in phenylketonuria: what is the evidence? Cell Mol Neurobiol 2011, 31:653–662.
16. Mashima R, Nakanishi-Ueda T, Yamamoto Y: Simultaneous determination of methionine sulfoxide and methionine in blood plasma using gas chromatography–mass spectrometry. Anal Biochem 2003, 313:28–33.
17. Gibala MJ: Protein metabolism and endurance exercise. Sports Med 2007, 37:337–340.
18. Horn P, Kalz A, Lim CL, Pyne D, Saunders P, Mackinnon L, Peake J, Suzuki K: Exercise-recruited NK cells display exercise-associated eHSP-70. Exerc Immunol Rev 2007, 13:100–111.
19. Feezor RJ, Baker HV, Mindrinos M, Hayden D, Tannahill CL, Brownstein BH, Fay A, MacMillan S, Laramie J, Xiao W, Moldawer LL, Cobb JP, Laudanski K, Miller-Graziano CL, Maier RV, Schoenfeld D, Davis RW, Tompkins RG, Inflammation and Host Response to Injury, Large-Scale Collaborative Research Program: Whole blood and leukocyte RNA isolation for gene expression analyses. Physiol Genomics 2004, 19:247–254.
20. Broderick JA, Salomon WE, Ryder SP, Aronin N, Zamore PD: Argonaute protein identity and pairing geometry determine cooperativity in mammalian RNA silencing. RNA 2011, 17:1858–1869.
21. Takimoto K, Wakiyama M, Yokoyama S: Mammalian GW182 contains multiple Argonaute-binding sites and functions in microRNA-mediated translational repression. RNA 2009, 15:1078–1089.
22. Davidson ME, Kerepesi LA, Soto A, Chan VT: D-Serine exposure resulted in gene expression changes implicated in neurodegenerative disorders and neuronal dysfunction in male Fischer 344 rats. Arch Toxicol 2009, 83:747–762.
23. Jin Z, May WS, Gao F, Flagg T, Deng X: Bcl2 suppresses DNA repair by enhancing c-Myc transcriptional activity. J Biol Chem 2006, 281:14446–14456.
24. Chen Y, Olopade OI: MYC in breast tumor progression. Expert Rev Anticancer Ther 2008, 8:1689–1698.
25. Tonic I, Yu WN, Park Y, Chen CC, Hay N: Akt activation emulates Chk1 inhibition and Bcl2 overexpression and abrogates G2 cell cycle checkpoint by inhibiting BRCA1 foci. J Biol Chem 2010, 285:23790–23798.
26. De Siervi A, De Luca P, Byun JS, Di LJ, Fufa T, Haggerty CM, Vazquez E, Moiola C, Longo DL, Gardner K: Transcriptional autoregulation by BRCA1. Cancer Res 2010, 70:532–542.
27. Rhoades MW, Reinhart BJ, Lim LP, Burge CB, Bartel B, Bartel DP: Prediction of plant microRNA targets. Cell 2002, 110:513–520.
28. Lewis BP, Burge CB, Bartel DP: Conserved seed pairing, often flanked by adenosines, indicates that thousands of human genes are microRNA targets. Cell 2005, 120:15–20.
29. Thum T, Gross C, Fiedler J, Fischer T, Kissler S, Bussen M, Galuppo P, Just S, Rottbauer W, Frantz S, Castoldi M, Soutschek J, Koteliansky V, Rosenwald A, Basson MA, Licht JD, Pena JT, Rouhanifard SH, Muckenthaler MU, Tuschl T, Martin GR, Bauersachs J, Engelhardt S: MicroRNA-21 contributes to myocardial disease by stimulating MAP kinase signalling in fibroblasts. Nature 2008, 456:980–984.
30. Godwin JG, Ge X, Stephan K, Jurisch A, Tullius SG, Iacomini J: Identification of a microRNA signature of renal ischemia reperfusion injury. Proc Natl Acad Sci USA 2010, 107:14339–14344.
31. O'Neill LA, Sheedy FJ, McCoy CE: MicroRNAs: the fine-tuners of Toll-like receptor signalling. Nat Rev Immunol 2011, 11:163–175.
32. Ashokkumar C, Ningappa M, Ranganathan S, Higgs BW, Sun Q, Schmitt L, Snyder S, Dobberstein J, Branca M, Jaffe R, Zeevi A, Squires R, Alissa F, Shneider B, Soltys K, Bond G, Abu-Elmagd K, Humar A, Mazariegos G, Hakonarson H, Sindhi R: Increased expression of peripheral blood leukocyte genes implicate CD14+ tissue macrophages in cellular intestine allograft rejection. Am J Pathol 2011, 179:1929–1938.

33. Gabriely G, Wurdinger T, Kesari S, Esau CC, Burchard J, Linsley PS, Krichevsky AM: MicroRNA 21 promotes glioma invasion by targeting matrix metalloproteinase regulators. *Mol Cell Biol* 2008, **28**:5369–5380.

34. Wang Z, Ahmad A, Li Y, Kong D, Azmi AS, Banerjee S, Sarkar FH: Emerging roles of PDGF-D signaling pathway in tumor development and progression. *Biochim Biophys Acta* 1806, **2010**:122–130.

35. Hafner M, Landthaler M, Burger L, Khorshid M, Hausser J, Berninger P, Rothballer A, Ascano M Jr, Jungkamp AC, Munschauer M, Ulrich A, Wardle GS, Dewell S, Zavolan M, Tuschl T: Transcriptome-wide identification of RNA-binding protein and microRNA target sites by PAR-CLIP. *Cell* 2010, **141**:129–141.

36. Saito J, Toriumi S, Awano K, Ichijo H, Sasaki K, Kobayashi T, Tamura S: Regulation of apoptosis signal-regulating kinase 1 by protein phosphatase 2Cepsilon. *Biochem J* 2007, **405**:591–596.

37. Espinosa EJ, Calero M, Sridevi K, Pfeffer SR: RhoBTB3: a Rho GTPase-family ATPase required for endosome to Golgi transport. *Cell* 2009, **137**:938–948.

38. Kurian SM, Le-Niculescu H, Patel SD, Bertram D, Davis J, Dike C, Yehyawi N, Lysaker P, Dustin J, Caligiuri M, Lohr J, Lahiri DK, Nurnberger JI Jr, Faraone SV, Geyer MA, Tsuang MT, Schork NJ, Salomon DR, Niculescu AB: Identification of blood biomarkers for psychosis using convergent functional genomics. *Mol Psychiatry* 2011, **16**:37–58.

39. Zhu H, Fan GC: Role of microRNAs in the reperfused myocardium towards post-infarct remodelling. *Cardiovasc Res* 2012, **94**:284–292.

40. Lal A, Navarro F, Maher CA, Maliszewski LE, Yan N, O'Day E, Chowdhury D, Dykxhoorn DM, Tsai P, Hofmann O, Becker KG, Gorospe M, Hide W, Lieberman J: miR-24 Inhibits cell proliferation by targeting E2F2, MYC, and other cell-cycle genes via binding to "seedless" 3′UTR microRNA recognition elements. *Mol Cell* 2009, **35**:610–625.

41. Burge JA, Hanna MG: Novel insights into the pathomechanisms of skeletal muscle channelopathies. *Curr Neurol Neurosci Rep* 2012, **12**:62–69.

42. Gui YX, Wan Y, Xiao Q, Wang Y, Wang G, Chen SD: Verification of expressions of Kir2 as potential peripheral biomarkers in lymphocytes from patients with Parkinson's disease. *Neurosci Lett* 2011, **505**:104–108.

43. Huang Z, Chen X, Yu B, He J, Chen D: MicroRNA-27a promotes myoblast proliferation by targeting myostatin. *Biochem Biophys Res Commun* 2012, **423**:265–269.

44. Yang WH, Nussbaum C, Grewal PK, Marth JD, Sperandio M: Coordinated roles of ST3Gal-VI and ST3Gal-IV sialyltransferases in the synthesis of selectin ligands. *Blood* 2012, **120**:1015–1026.

45. Chen CZ, Li L, Lodish HF, Bartel DP: MicroRNAs modulate hematopoietic lineage differentiation. *Science* 2004, **303**:83–86.

46. Li QJ, Chau J, Ebert PJ, Sylvester G, Min H, Liu G, Braich R, Manoharan M, Soutschek J, Skare P, Klein LO, Davis MM, Chen CZ: miR-181a is an intrinsic modulator of T cell sensitivity and selection. *Cell* 2007, **129**:147–161.

47. Chen L, Kass RS: A-kinase anchoring proteins: different partners, different dance. *Nat Cell Biol* 2005, **7**:1050–1051.

48. Bartoloni L, Antonarakis SE: The human sugar-phosphate/phosphate exchanger family SLC37. *Pflugers Arch* 2004, **447**:780–783.

49. Cooper DM, Weiler-Ravell D, Whipp BJ, Wasserman K: Aerobic parameters of exercise as a function of body size during growth in children. *J Appl Physiol* 1984, **56**:628–634.

50. Beaver WL, Wasserman K, Whipp BJ: A new method for detecting anaerobic threshold by gas exchange. *J Appl Physiol* 1986, **60**:2020–2027.

51. Floegel A, Stefan N, Yu Z, Mühlenbruch K, Drogan D, Joost HG, Fritsche A, Häring HU, Hrabe de Angelis M, Peters A, Roden M, Prehn C, Wang-Sattler R, Illig T, Schulze MB, Adamski J, Boeing H, Pischon T: Identification of serum metabolites associated with risk of type 2 diabetes using a targeted metabolomic approach. *Diabetes* 2013, **62**:639–648.

52. Sakharov DA, Maltseva DV, Riabenko EA, Shkurnikov MU, Northoff H, Tonevitsky AG, Grigoriev AI: Passing the anaerobic threshold is associated with substantial changes in the gene expression profile in white blood cells. *Eur J Appl Physiol* 2012, **112**:963–972.

53. Gentleman RC, Carey VJ, Bates DM, Bolstad B, Dettling M, Dudoit S, Ellis B, Gautier L, Ge Y, Gentry J, Hornik K, Hothorn T, Huber W, Iacus S, Irizarry R, Leisch F, Li C, Maechler M, Rossini AJ, Sawitzki G, Smith C, Smyth G, Tierney L, Yang JY, Zhang J: Bioconductor: open software development for computational biology and bioinformatics. *Genome Biol* 2004, **5**:R80.

54. Irizarry RA, Hobbs B, Collin F, Beazer-Barclay YD, Antonellis KJ, Scherf U, Speed TP: Exploration, normalization, and summaries of high density oligonucleotide array probe level data. *Biostatistics* 2003, **4**:249–264.

55. Bolstad BM, Irizarry RA, Astrand M, Speed TP: A comparison of normalization methods for high density oligonucleotide array data based on variance and bias. *Bioinformatics* 2003, **19**:185–193.

56. Tukey JW: *Exploratory data analysis*. Reading: Addison-Wesley; 1977.

57. Smyth GK: Limma: linear models for microarray data. In *Bioinformatics and computational biology solutions using R and bioconductor*. Edited by Gentleman R, Carey V, Dudoit S, Irizarry R, Huber W. New York: Springer; 2005:397–420.

58. Yang YH, Speed TP: *Design and analysis of comparative microarray experiments*. In: Statistical analysis of gene expression microarray data. Edited by Speed TP. Chapman and Hall/CRC Press; 2003:35–93.

59. Benjamini Y, Hochberg Y: Controlling the false discovery rate: a practical and powerful approach to multiple testing. *J R Statist Soc B (Methodological)* 1995, **57**:289–300.

60. da Huang W, Sherman BT, Lempicki RA: Systematic and integrative analysis of large gene lists using DAVID bioinformatics resources. *Nat Protoc* 2009, **4**:44–57.

14

Localization of lipoprotein lipase and GPIHBP1 in mouse pancreas: effects of diet and leptin deficiency

Rakel Nyrén[1], Chuchun L Chang[2], Per Lindström[3], Anastasia Barmina[3], Evelina Vorrsjö[1], Yusuf Ali[4], Lisa Juntti-Berggren[4], André Bensadoun[5], Stephen G Young[6], Thomas Olivecrona[1] and Gunilla Olivecrona[1*]

Abstract

Background: Lipoprotein lipase (LPL) hydrolyzes triglycerides in plasma lipoproteins and enables uptake of lipolysis products for energy production or storage in tissues. Our aim was to study the localization of LPL and its endothelial anchoring protein glycosylphosphatidylinositol-anchored high density lipoprotein-binding protein 1 (GPIHBP1) in mouse pancreas, and effects of diet and leptin deficiency on their expression patterns. For this, immunofluorescence microscopy was used on pancreatic tissue from C57BL/6 mouse embryos (E18), adult mice on normal or high-fat diet, and adult *ob/ob*-mice treated or not with leptin. The distribution of LPL and GPIHBP1 was compared to insulin, glucagon and CD31. Heparin injections were used to discriminate between intracellular and extracellular LPL.

Results: In the exocrine pancreas LPL was found in capillaries, and was mostly co-localized with GPIHBP1. LPL was releasable by heparin, indicating localization on cell surfaces. Within the islets, most of the LPL was associated with beta cells and could not be released by heparin, indicating that the enzyme remained mostly within cells. Staining for LPL was found also in the glucagon-producing alpha cells, both in embryos (E18) and in adult mice. Only small amounts of LPL were found together with GPIHBP1 within the capillaries of islets. Neither a high fat diet nor fasting/re-feeding markedly altered the distribution pattern of LPL or GPIHBP1 in mouse pancreas. Islets from *ob/ob* mice appeared completely deficient of LPL in the beta cells, while LPL-staining was normal in alpha cells and in the exocrine pancreas. Leptin treatment of *ob/ob* mice for 12 days reversed this pattern, so that most of the islets expressed LPL in beta cells.

Conclusions: We conclude that both LPL and GPIHBP1 are present in mouse pancreas, and that LPL expression in beta cells is dependent on leptin.

Keywords: Lipoprotein lipase, Diabetes mellitus, Islet cells, Exocrine pancreas, Endothelium, *Ob/ob* mice, High fat diet, Heparin, qPCR, Immunofluorescence

Background

Lipoprotein lipase (LPL) is responsible for the hydrolysis of triglycerides in plasma lipoproteins, generating fatty acids and monoglycerides for uptake in tissues and use in metabolic processes [1,2]. LPL is synthesized and secreted by parenchymal cells such as adipocytes and myocytes, but the enzyme acts at the luminal face of endothelial cells in capillaries where it is anchored to the plasma membrane in a heparin-releasable manner. The mechanism by which LPL is transported from the interstitial spaces surrounding parenchymal cells into capillaries involves an endothelial cell protein, glycosylphosphatidylinositol-anchored high density lipoprotein binding protein 1 (GPIHBP1), that binds LPL at the basolateral surface of capillaries and transports it into the capillary lumen [3]. In the absence of GPIHBP1, LPL is mislocalized to the subendothelial spaces, resulting in severe hypertriglyceridemia [4]. Two structural motifs

* Correspondence: Gunilla.Olivecrona@medbio.umu.se
[1]Department of Medical Biosciences/Physiological Chemistry, Umeå University, Umeå, Sweden
Full list of author information is available at the end of the article

within GPIHBP1 are important for its ability to bind LPL. Mutations within one of the motifs have been identified in patients with severe chylomicronemia [5-8]. Recently it was demonstrated that the transendothelial transport of LPL is bidirectional [9].

LPL is found in large amounts in heart, skeletal muscle, and adipose tissue, but it is also present in kidneys, lungs, fetal liver, lactating mammary gland and macrophages, as well as in scattered cells of the brain [1]. In addition, LPL is found in the islets of Langerhans [10,11]. In INS-1 cells (clonal cells from a rat insulinoma cell line), high glucose levels stimulate the activity of LPL both in total cell extracts and in the heparin-releasable fractions of LPL that is secreted and associated to the cell surfaces [12]. The function of beta cell-derived LPL is unknown, but the stimulation by glucose of LPL activity suggests that it may contribute to beta cell function (or dysfunction) by increasing delivery of lipids to the islets. Acute exposure of islets to fatty acids potentiates glucose-stimulated insulin secretion [13], but chronic exposure causes impaired insulin responses and beta cell death [14]. In other tissues the expression and activity of LPL is regulated by nutritional and hormonal factors [1,2]. LPL activity is usually affected by insulin resistance, diabetes and obesity, although the mechanisms are not fully resolved. The aim here was to study the relative distribution of LPL and its endothelial transport protein GPIHBP1 in mouse pancreas, and to study effects on LPL and GPIHBP1 expression in pancreas by changes in nutritional state (fed compared to fasted), diet composition (normal chow compared to high-fat diet) and by obesity due to leptin deficiency.

Methods

Reagents and buffers

Phosphate buffered saline (PBS) was 0.15 M NaCl containing 0.1 M Na2HPO4 and 0.1 M NaH2PO4 (pH 7.5). TBST buffer consisted of 50 mM Tris–HCl, pH 7.4, 0.15 M NaCl, and 0.1% (w/v) Triton X-100. Paraformaldehyde (PFA) (Sigma-Aldrich, P6148) was diluted in 0.1 M PBS pH 7.5 to a final concentration of 4%. Sucrose for fixation of tissues was from BDH (AnalaR, 10274 7E), and the tissue mounting media Tissue Tek 4583 was from Sakura Finetek. The antibodies were diluted in 10% (v/v) heat-inactivated fetal calf serum (FCS) from Invitrogen. TBST was also used for washing of the slides. The sections were mounted in Vectasheild Mounting medium for Fluorescence (Vector Laboratories, CA 94010). Dalteparin sodium (Fragmin®) 2500 IE/KY anti-Xa/ml, a low molecular weight heparin, was from Pharmacia. Glass slides (Super Frost plus) and cover slips were from Menzel-Gläser (J1800AM).

Animals and procedures

Wild-type (WT) male mice (C57BL/6), six weeks of age, were fed a chow diet (CRM (E) 801730, SDS). C57BL/6 embryos were harvested at eighteen days of gestation (E18), and the pancreas was removed for immunofluorescence. Some mice were treated with Fragmin® 2500 IE (diluted 1:10 in 0.15 M NaCl), administered intraperitoneally (i.p. 1 ml/mouse), and sacrificed 20 minutes later. The animals were on a 12-hours light/dark cycle with free access to water, unless otherwise stated. All animal procedures were approved by the regional ethical committee on studies involving animal experiments, Umeå, Sweden and the corresponding Columbia University's Institutional Animal Care and Use Committee.

Mice on high fat diet, fasted and re-fed

Two groups of three-month-old C57BL/6 male mice, 9 in each group, were included in the experiment. One group was given regular pellets (Research Diets D12450B, 10% kcal% fat and high in carbohydrates) and the other group was given a high fat diet (HFD) for 10 days (Research Diets D12492, 60% kcal% fat). Food was then removed at 4 p.m. and the animals were fasted overnight. In the morning food was given back to five animals in the HFD-group and 5 animals in the control group and they were re-fed for 3 hours before sacrifice. The remaining 4 animals in each group stayed fasted during the corresponding time.

Mice fed a diet rich in saturated fatty acids (SAT) for 12 weeks

Four-weeks old male C57BL/6 mice were fed a HFD containing predominantly saturated fat (SAT, 21% fat) or a control, low fat, diet (chow, 4.5% fat) with compositions as detailed previously for 12 weeks [15]. In this experiment the animals were fasted for 2hours before fixation by perfusion of the whole body. Then the pancreases were taken out and treated as described for the other animals. We examined 5 pancreases from the SAT-group and 5 from the chow group.

Ob/ob mice

Ob/ob mice lack leptin [16]. They were taken from a local colony (Umeå ob/ob, Histology and Cell Biology, IMB, Umeå University, Sweden). The ob/ob genotype was identified by rapid increase in body weight and rise in blood glucose levels compared to the healthy siblings. All mice (female) were fed standard pellets high in carbohydrates (R3, Lactamin, Sweden). The youngest mice were 5.2 and 5.7 weeks old when sacrificed (in total two animals). In addition we examined 6 pancreases each from three and nine months old ob/ob mice obtained at two different experimental occasions. Ob/ob mice from The Rolf Luft Research Center for Diabetes and

Endocrinology, Karolinska Institutet, Stockholm, Sweden (same original strain as the Umeå colony) were used for qPCR on age related LPL expression (1–4, 8 and 11 months old).

Treatment of ob/ob mice with leptin

Ob/ob mice used for the leptin experiment were six months of age, and all were females. In one set of experiments, 4 animals were given leptin for 12 days, while 4 were given 0.15 M NaCl. In another set, 6 animals were treated with leptin and 6 used as controls. Leptin or vehicle was injected i.p. twice every day for 12 days. The starting concentration was 0.4 µg leptin/g body weight. After 2 days the concentration was reduced to 0.2 µg leptin/g for 2 days and finally 0.1 µg/g was given for the remaining 7 days. Body weight and food intake were measured on a daily basis. Blood glucose (Ascensia Elite, Bayer) was measured during leptin treatment. The mice had free access to water and food, standard pellets (R3, Lactamin, Sweden).

Isolation of islets

Ob/ob mice were sacrificed after anesthesia and the pancreas was dissected out. Six *ob/ob* mice were leptin treated and 6 were used as controls. Age and sex-matched (female) C57BL/6 (n=10) was used for comparison. The pancreas was placed in collagenase solution (1.5 mg/ml Collagenase P, Roche Inc.) and shaken for 18 minutes at 37°C. A Krebs - Ringer medium buffer was used with the following composition in mM: 130 NaCl, 4.7 KCl, 1.2 KH2PO4, 1.2 MgSO4 and 2.56 CaCl2 and supplemented with 1 mg/ml BSA and 3 mM D-glucose. The medium was buffered with 20 mM HEPES and NaOH to reach pH 7.4. Islets were picked, counted, placed in buffer RLT from Qiagen and frozen at –80°C.

Real-time PCR

RNA was extracted from isolated islets and DNAse treated using an RNeasy Micro Kit from Qiagen (Cat. No. 74004). cDNA was prepared from 20 ng total RNA using Moloney Murine Leukemia Virus Reverse Transcriptase, RNase H Minus (M-MLV RT [H–]) (Fermentas) and pd (N)6 Random Hexamer (Fermentas) in total volume of 20 µl. The expression of LPL was quantified by real time PCR as previously described using Maxima probe/ROX qPCR Master Mix (Fermentas) and the ABI Prism 7000 Sequence Detection System (Applied Biosystems, Foster City, CA, USA), using the same primers and probes [17]. Expression levels were normalized to 18S mRNA using the Eukaryotic18S rRNA Endogenous Control Reagent Set supplied from Applied Biosystems. In the experiment with leptin treatment, one pancreas from a leptin treated *ob/ob* mouse gave low islet count for technical reasons and was discarded. Another mouse in the leptin-treated

group died, leaving 4 mice for the leptin–treated group and 6 mice for the untreated group.

Analyses of LPL expression on isolated islets from untreated *ob/ob* mice were done using SYBR-Green with beta actin as reference gene. Four mice were used in each age group, except at three months where 3 mice were used.

Tissue preparation

For sectioning, the organs were dissected free from contaminating tissue in cold PBS and fixed in 4% PFA (paraformaldehyde), at 4°C for 1–2 hours. The tissue pieces were then placed in 30% sucrose in 0.1 M PBS, pH 7.5, at 4°C overnight. The pieces were mounted in Tissue Tek and quickly frozen on dry ice for storage at –80°C or for direct cryosectioning (8-µm sections, put on Super Frost glass).

Immunofluorescence microscopy

Tissue sections were first blocked with 10% (v/v) FCS in TBST for 1 hour at room temperature. Then they were incubated overnight at 4°C with primary antibodies diluted in the blocking solution. After washing three times with TBST, secondary antibodies diluted in blocking solution were added and incubated for 1 hour at room temperature. Slides were mounted in Vectasheild Mounting Media for Fluorescence (Vector Labs). Visualization of the stained sections was made with a Nikon confocal microscope Eclipse E800, Japan, with the software EZ-C1 Digital Eclipse and Nikon ACT-1. The pictures were taken with magnification 10x, 40x and 60x.

Antibodies

The anti-LPL antibody was raised by immunizing chickens with bovine LPL; affinity-purified IgY was obtained as described [18]. The batch used was diluted 1:400 and was the same as the one previously thoroughly investigated for specificity [3]. Control IgY (purified from a non-immunized chicken) was diluted to the same protein concentration. AlexaFluor 488– or AlexaFluor 594–labeled goat-anti-chicken antibodies from Molecular Probes (A-11039, A-11042) were diluted 1:1000. The endothelium was identified by staining with rat anti-PECAM (CD31) antibodies from BP Pharmagen (553371) diluted 1:250, and Alexa Fluor 594 goat-anti-rat (A-11007). Islet cells were visualized with antibodies against glucagon (alpha cells), insulin (beta cells), somatostatin (delta cells) and PP-cells. Rabbit anti-glucagon from Linco (403101F) was diluted 1:1000, and visualized with Alexa Fluor 488 or 594 goat-anti-rabbit from Molecular Probes (A-11034,   A-11076). Guinea pig-anti-insulin (from Dako, A0564) was diluted 1:500 and visualized with Alexa Fluor 488 or 594 goat-anti-guinea pig antibodies from Molecular Probes (A-11073, A-11076). Rat-anti-somatostatin from Biogenesis (83300009) was diluted 1:500 and visualized with Alexa Fluor 594 goat-anti-rat. Guinea pig-anti-pancreatic polypeptide from Linco (404101) was diluted 1:500 and visualized with Alexa Fluor 594 goat-anti-guinea pig. Nuclei were stained by DAPI from Sigma (D9542). The GPIHBP1 antibody was raised in a rabbit against recombinant mouse GPIHBP1 (amino acids 23–205 in pQE-30 (QIA-GEN) expressed in *E. coli* [4]. An immunoglobulin fraction was purified on a 6His-GPIHBP1-Sepharose column, used at 5 µg/ml and visualized with Alexa Fluor goat-anti-rabbit 488 or 594. Monoclonal rat-anti-mouse GPIHBP1, (11A12 concentration 2.67 mg/ml) diluted 1:1500 was visualized with Alexa Fluor 594 goat-anti-rat.

Statistics

Data was normalized and presented as mean ± SEM (Kruskal-Wallis). Statistical analysis was performed using Graph Pad Prism 5.

Results

LPL in endocrine pancreas

Most of the cells in the islets of Langerhans were stained by the anti LPL antibody, but some cells were more fluorescent than others (Figure 1A and D). With antibodies to insulin, co-localization with LPL was evident in most cells in the center of the islets (Figure 1B-C), while cells in the periphery stained only for LPL. With antibodies to glucagon, co-localization with LPL was seen in cells with the peripheral distribution pattern typical for alpha cells (Figure 1D-F). No staining for LPL was seen in the less abundant delta or PP cells (data not shown).

LPL in embryonic mice at stage E18 and antibody specificity

It is known that alpha cells tend to show autofluorescence due to their high content of granulae. To investigate whether LPL is really expressed in alpha cells we studied staining for LPL, insulin and glucagon in embryonic pancreases at stage E18 when the alpha cells have not yet developed secretory granules. Immunofluorescence for LPL was seen connected to both beta and alpha cells (Figure 2). The staining for glucagon was weaker than for insulin, but co-staining was visible between glucagon and LPL also at this early stage. This finding supported the results from the adult mice indicating that LPL is expressed both in alpha and beta cells.

LPL and GPIHBP1 in exocrine pancreas

Next we wanted to exclude the possibility that the staining for LPL was non-specific. Therefore control experiments were made with pre-immune IgY (data not shown), with only secondary antibodies, or with adsorption of the anti-LPL IgY with purified bovine LPL. Compared to the results with anti-LPL IgY, there was little or no fluorescence in either islets or the exocrine pancreas with any of the tested antibodies (Figure 3). In contrast,

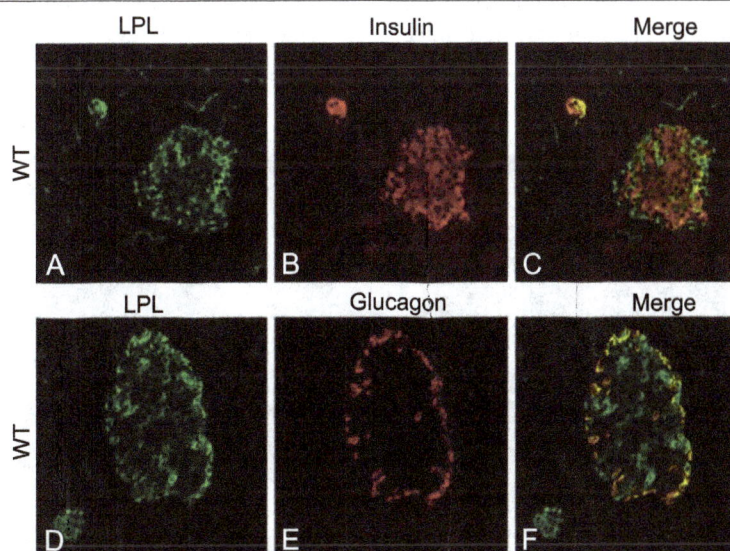

Figure 1 LPL immune-reactivity in mouse islets. Islets of Langerhans in pancreas from normal mice (WT) stained with antibodies against LPL and insulin or glucagon. (**A**) Section containing one large and one small islet stained with anti-LPL (green), (**B**) same section stained with anti-insulin to visualize beta cells (red) and (**C**) a merge between A and B demonstrating co-localization between LPL and beta cells. (**D**) Section containing one large and one small islet stained with anti-LPL, (**E**) same section stained with anti-glucagon to visualize alpha cells and (**F**) a merge between D and E demonstrating co-localization between LPL and alpha cells.

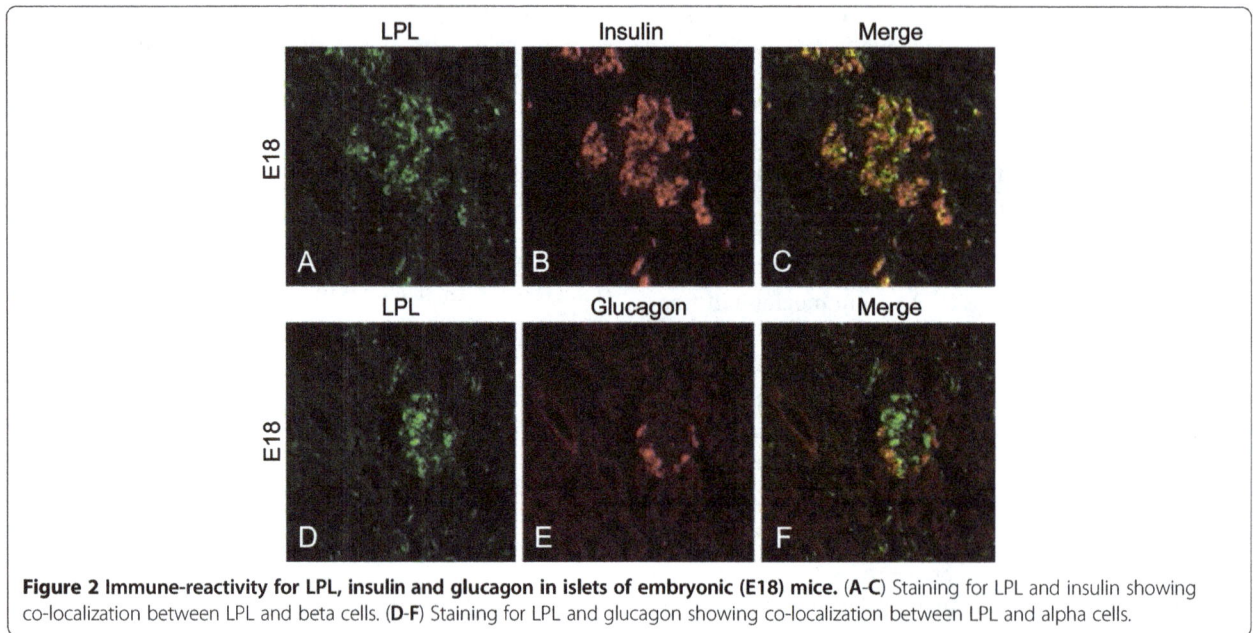

Figure 2 Immune-reactivity for LPL, insulin and glucagon in islets of embryonic (E18) mice. (A-C) Staining for LPL and insulin showing co-localization between LPL and beta cells. **(D-F)** Staining for LPL and glucagon showing co-localization between LPL and alpha cells.

the positive staining for LPL in exocrine pancreatic tissue with anti-LPL IgY was localized to capillaries, as evidenced by co-localization with the endothelial marker CD31 (Figure 4A-C).

To investigate whether the immune-reactive LPL was heparin-releasable, mice were first injected with low molecular weight heparin (Fragmin®) [19], and were then sacrificed 20 minutes later for studies of LPL in pancreas. Compared to mice that had not been given Fragmin®, much of the LPL immune-reactivity had disappeared from capillaries and small blood vessels of the exocrine pancreas in the Fragmin®-treated mice (Figure 4D), while the staining for CD31 remained

associated with the endothelium, as expected (Figure 4E-F). A lower magnification (Figure 4G-H) demonstrated that in the islets the staining for LPL was not much changed in Fragmin®-treated animals compared to non-treated animals. The resistance to Fragmin® indicated that LPL was mostly localized within islets cells. This is in contrast to LPL in exocrine pancreas that was heparin-releasable and therefore presumably exposed on endothelial cell surfaces.

Immunostaining for GPIHBP1 (the LPL-binding protein) was associated with capillaries and small vessels in exocrine pancreas (Figure 5B) in a pattern similar to that seen with the anti LPL antibodies (Figure 5A). The

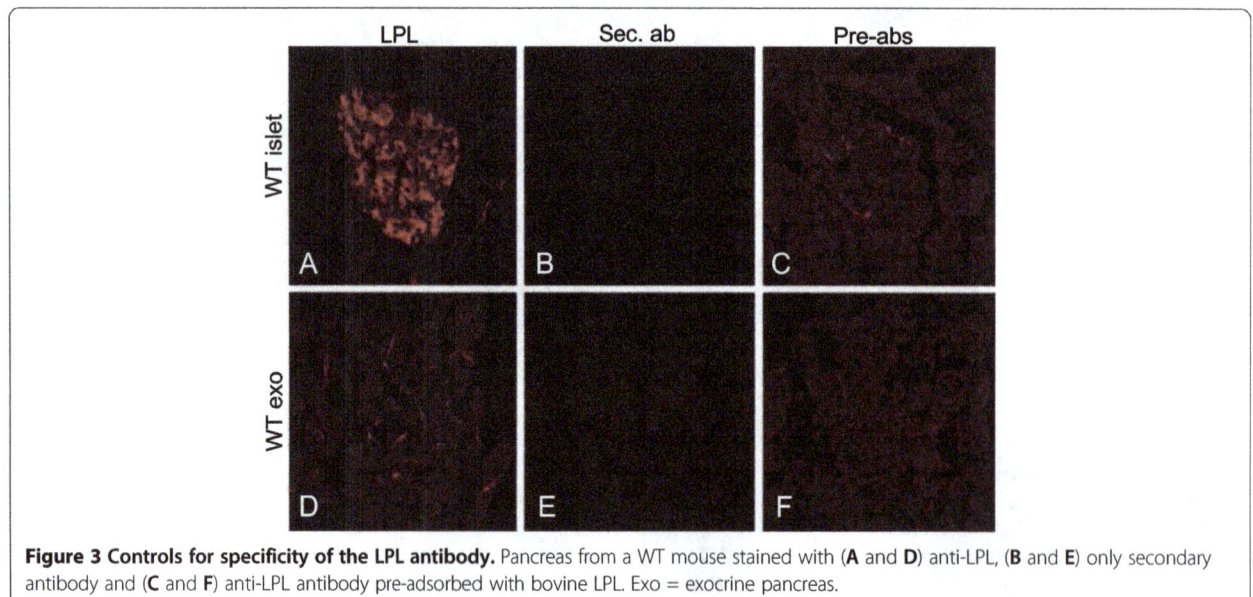

Figure 3 Controls for specificity of the LPL antibody. Pancreas from a WT mouse stained with **(A and D)** anti-LPL, **(B and E)** only secondary antibody and **(C and F)** anti-LPL antibody pre-adsorbed with bovine LPL. Exo = exocrine pancreas.

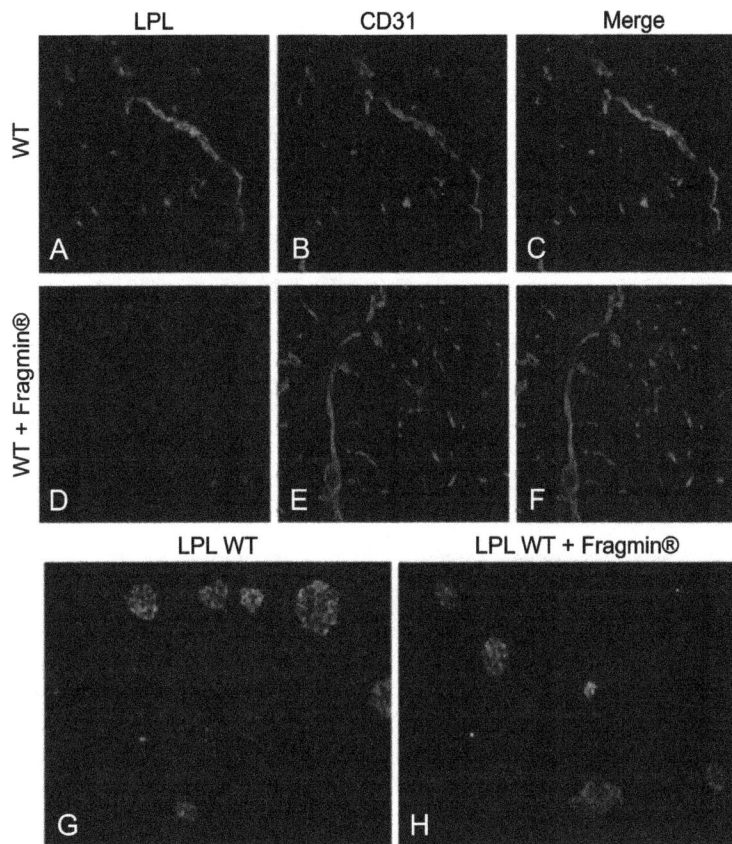

Figure 4 Release of LPL from blood vessels in exocrine pancreas by heparin injection. LPL in exocrine pancreas from normal and heparinized (Fragmin®) mice. (**A**) Staining for LPL (green) in a non-treated, WT mouse, (**B**) staining for endothelium of small vessels with anti-CD31 (red) in the same section as A, and (**C**) a merge between A and B. (**D**) Staining for LPL in a Fragmin®-treated mouse. (**E**) Staining with anti-CD31 of the same section as D, (**F**) a merge between D and E. (**G**) Pancreas from a non-treated WT mouse in lower magnification stained for LPL (green) and (**H**) pancreas from a Fragmin®-treated WT mouse stained for LPL.

staining for GPIHBP1 co-localized with the staining for CD31 (Figure 5G-I). In accord with previous findings in other tissues [4] GPIHBP1 was mostly seen within the smallest blood vessels, but was not present in larger ones. As expected, mice treated with Fragmin® showed the same staining pattern for GPIHBP1 in exocrine pancreas as untreated animals (data not shown). Co-localization between LPL and GPIHBP1 was seen in many of the small blood vessels in the exocrine pancreas and also in the islets vessels (Figure 5A-F).

LPL in pancreas of *ob/ob* mice and leptin-treated *ob/ob* mice

Islets in leptin-deficient *ob/ob* mice are known to be enlarged and to produce increased amounts of insulin [16]. We studied LPL in pancreas of *ob/ob* mice at five weeks and at three, six or nine months of age. In contrast to what was seen in control mice, there were almost no LPL-positive cells in the center of the islets and only scattered LPL-positive cells in the periphery of the islets (Figure 6A and G) at three, six and nine months.

Most of the scattered cells stained positively also for glucagon (Figure 6G-I) and hence were presumably alpha cells. The beta cells in *ob/ob* mice stained for insulin, but not for LPL (Figure 6A-C). In five weeks old *ob/ob* mice the islets were smaller than at the older ages, but the pattern for LPL distribution was similar to that in three, six and nine months old animals (data not shown). To study if LPL in the islets was intracellular, or associated with endothelial cells in capillaries, islets from WT and *ob/ob* mice were stained with antibodies to CD31 and LPL (Figure 7). Co-localization was seen between LPL and CD31, but in WT mice the majority of LPL was intracellular in alpha and beta cells. In *ob/ob* mice islets there was very little LPL staining. Some of the immune-reactivity co-localized with extracellular CD31 and the rest with intracellular glucagon.

To investigate whether it was possible to reverse the aberrant pattern for LPL reactivity in islets of *ob/ob* mice towards the pattern seen in WT mice, *ob/ob* mice were treated with daily injections of leptin for 12 days. During this time the treated animals ate less, probably due to

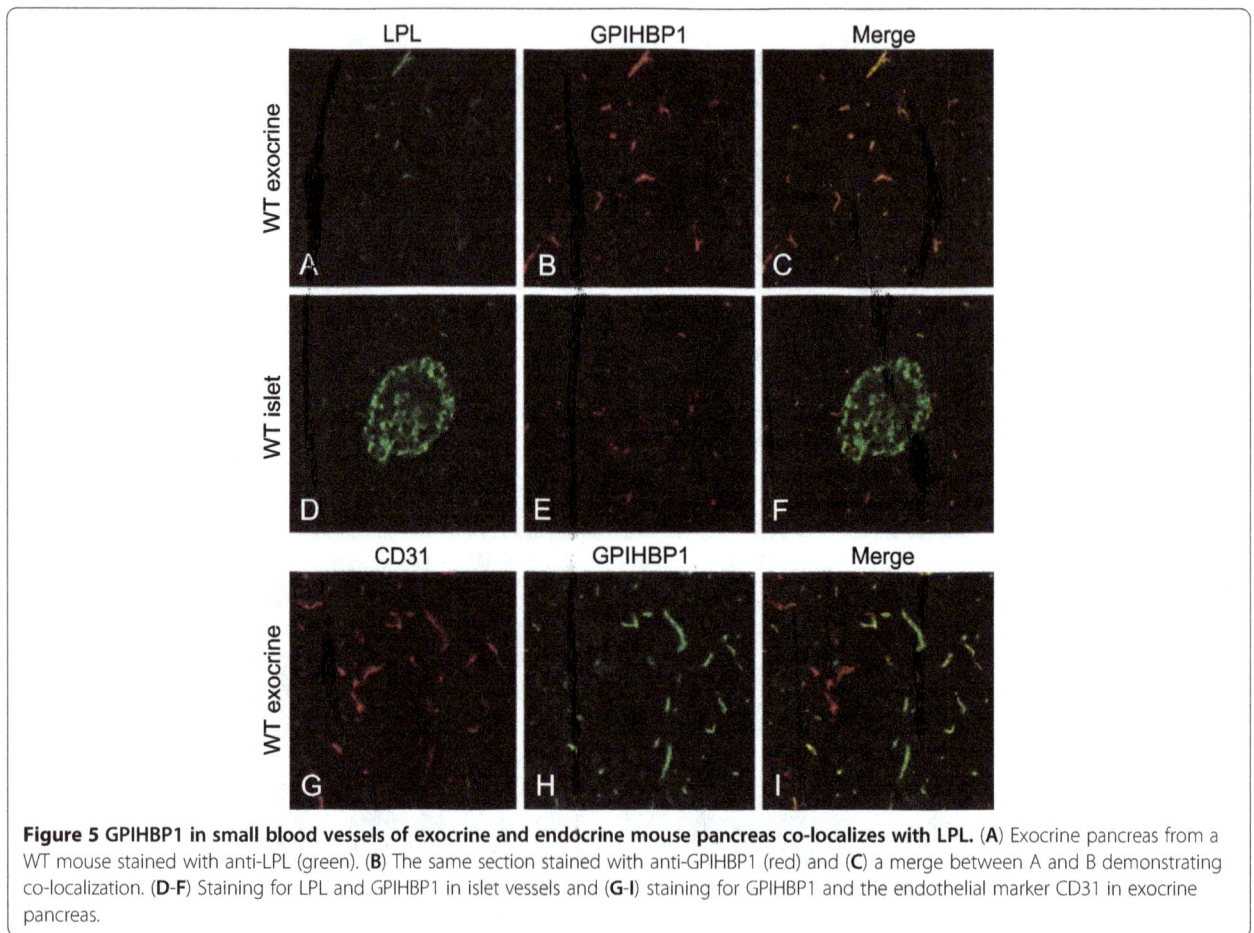

Figure 5 GPIHBP1 in small blood vessels of exocrine and endocrine mouse pancreas co-localizes with LPL. (A) Exocrine pancreas from a WT mouse stained with anti-LPL (green). **(B)** The same section stained with anti-GPIHBP1 (red) and **(C)** a merge between A and B demonstrating co-localization. **(D-F)** Staining for LPL and GPIHBP1 in islet vessels and **(G-I)** staining for GPIHBP1 and the endothelial marker CD31 in exocrine pancreas.

the anorectic effect of leptin, and their body weight and plasma glucose levels decreased (Table 1). After treatment with leptin for 12 days, immunofluorescence for LPL was again found in islet beta cells (Figure 6D-F and J). The expression pattern differed from islet to islet. Some islets had recovered almost completely, while others stained for LPL mostly in alpha cells and only in a few beta cells. *Ob/ob* mice in the control group ate more than the leptin-treated group, but still lost some weight, probably due to that they were somewhat disturbed by the daily i.p. injections of saline (Table 1). They did not show any LPL expression in their beta cells. Immune-reaction for LPL was visible in alpha cells in the saline-injected group (Figure 6A and G), just like in *ob/ob* mice at all ages studied. Exocrine tissue of *ob/ob* mice stained for LPL in the same way as that of WT mice, showing co-localization of LPL and CD31 (data not shown). Lean control mice, from the same colony, had a mean weight of 24.8 ± 3.9 g and blood glucose levels of 7.9 ± 0.7 mmol/L (n=4).

In another comparable experiment mRNA expression analyses were performed on isolated islets. Values from leptin-treated and untreated *ob/ob* mice, compared to WT mice, for blood glucose, weight and food intake are presented in Table 2. LPL mRNA expression was found in both WT and *ob/ob* islets; however, the level of LPL mRNA was significantly lower in islets of saline-injected *ob/ob* mice than in islets from WT mice (p=0.044, Figure 6M). This was consistent with the low or absent immunofluorescence found for LPL in beta cells in *ob/ob* mice. Leptin treatment for 12 days tended to increase the mRNA level for LPL in the islets, but the increase did not reach statistical significance (Figure 6M). There was no significant difference (p>0.05) in the mRNA-levels for LPL in islets from young *ob/ob* mice compared to older *ob/ob* mice (mice were analyzed at 1–4, 8 and 11 months, Figure 6N). The largest difference was seen between three and eleven months with a p-value of 0.057. The mean glucose level in control WT mice was 6.9 ± 0.7 mmol/L (n=10).

Effects of high fat diet for 10 days and 12 weeks in WT mice

In other tissues than pancreas, both LPL and GPIHBP1 are known to be affected by nutritional and/or hormonal factors [20]. To investigate possible nutritional effects on

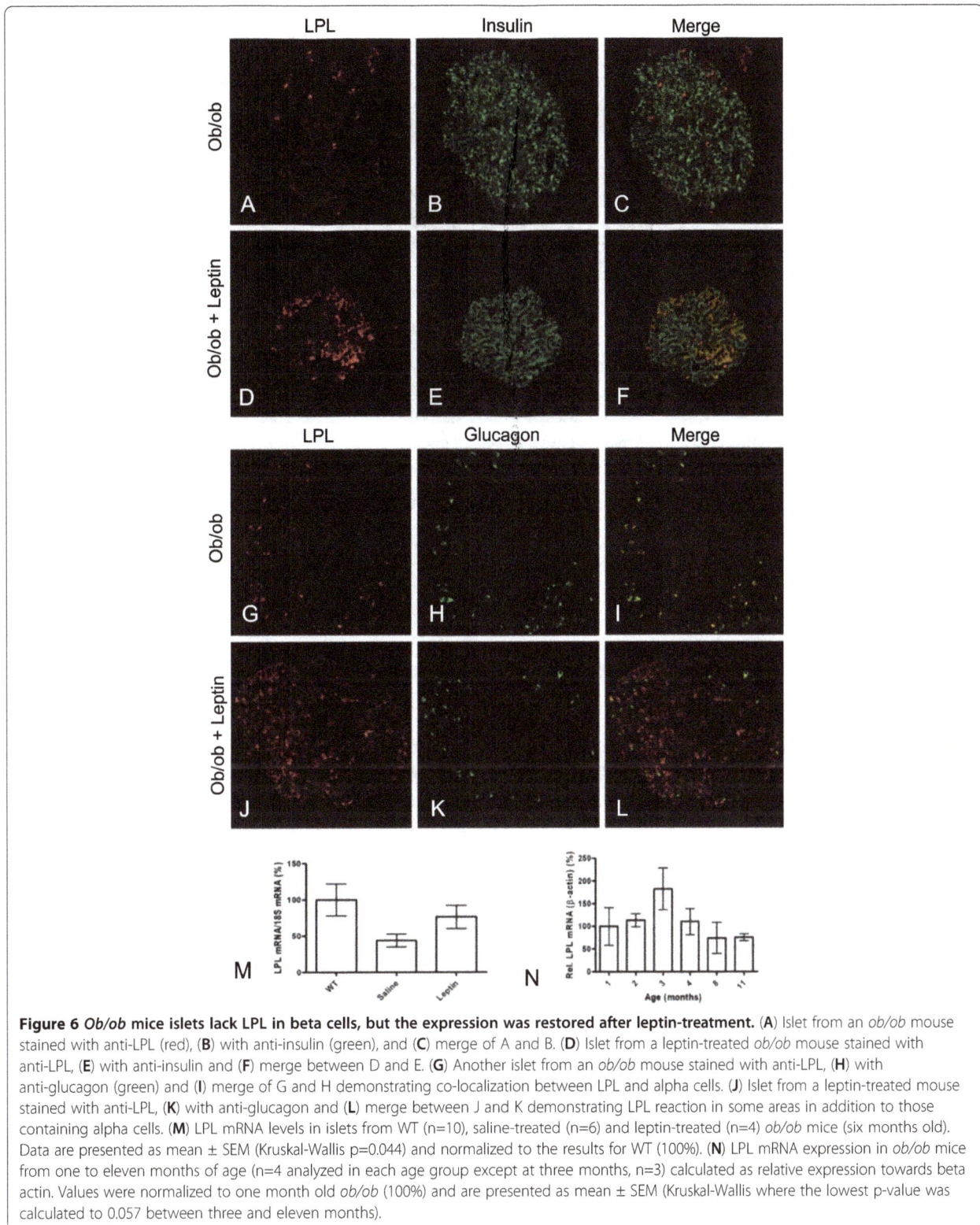

Figure 6 *Ob/ob* **mice islets lack LPL in beta cells, but the expression was restored after leptin-treatment.** (**A**) Islet from an *ob/ob* mouse stained with anti-LPL (red), (**B**) with anti-insulin (green), and (**C**) merge of A and B. (**D**) Islet from a leptin-treated *ob/ob* mouse stained with anti-LPL, (**E**) with anti-insulin and (**F**) merge between D and E. (**G**) Another islet from an *ob/ob* mouse stained with anti-LPL, (**H**) with anti-glucagon (green) and (**I**) merge of G and H demonstrating co-localization between LPL and alpha cells. (**J**) Islet from a leptin-treated mouse stained with anti-LPL, (**K**) with anti-glucagon and (**L**) merge between J and K demonstrating LPL reaction in some areas in addition to those containing alpha cells. (**M**) LPL mRNA levels in islets from WT (n=10), saline-treated (n=6) and leptin-treated (n=4) *ob/ob* mice (six months old). Data are presented as mean ± SEM (Kruskal-Wallis p=0.044) and normalized to the results for WT (100%). (**N**) LPL mRNA expression in *ob/ob* mice from one to eleven months of age (n=4 analyzed in each age group except at three months, n=3) calculated as relative expression towards beta actin. Values were normalized to one month old *ob/ob* (100%) and are presented as mean ± SEM (Kruskal-Wallis where the lowest p-value was calculated to 0.057 between three and eleven months).

the distribution of LPL and GPIHBP1 in pancreas we studied WT mice that had been on high fat diet (HFD) for 10 days and compared them to mice on normal chow. Half of the total number of animals in each group (n=10) was sacrificed after overnight fasting, and the other half was re-fed for 3 hours before they were sacrificed. After the different diets there was no difference in blood glucose levels between the ones on HFD for

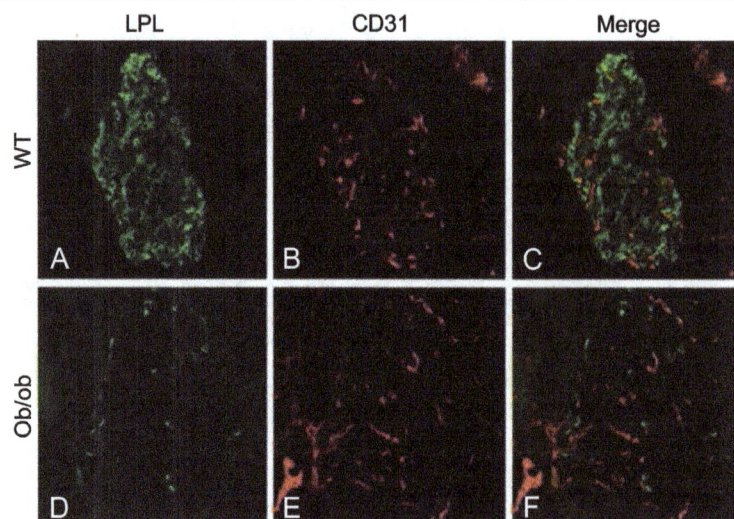

Figure 7 Islet LPL was mainly intracellular in WT mice but absent in *ob/ob* mice. Islets from WT and *ob/ob* mice stained for LPL and endothelium (with anti-CD31). (**A**) LPL in an islet from a WT mouse. (**B**) Staining for CD31 and (**C**) a merge showing co-localization between LPL and CD31. (**D**) Pancreatic tissue from an *ob/ob* mouse, LPL staining was only visible in the periphery of the islet (similar to the pattern for alpha cells). (**E**) Anti-CD31 demonstrates small vessels in the islet and (**F**) a merge between D and E showing that most of the LPL reaction was separate from the staining of vessels.

10 days and the ones on chow diet, but the HFD group weighed 2 g more than the chow group (median, 28 g compared to 26 g). Investigation of their pancreas showed no obvious difference in LPL between the re-fed and the fasted animals or between the ones on HFD for 10 days compared to those on chow diet (Figure 8C-F). Next we investigated pancreases from mice fed a diet high in saturated fatty acids (SAT) for 12 weeks, rendering them hyperlipidemic with regard to plasma triglycerides and non-esterified fatty acids (NEFA) [15], and slightly hyperglycemic (glucose levels were 1.3-fold elevated) compared to mice on normal chow for the same time. A somewhat weaker signal for LPL was seen in the islets from animals on SAT diet compared to animals fed chow diet for 12 weeks, but the differences were not clear enough to be conclusive (Figure 8A-B). The staining for LPL was still mostly in beta cells, both in the SAT-fed mice and in the control mice on chow (data not shown). In both groups the staining for LPL and CD31 in the exocrine parts appeared comparable.

The immune-reaction for GPIHBP1 was similar in islets from the fasted and re-fed mice fed a regular diet (Figure 9A-B), and also in those fed a high fat diet for 10 days (Figure 9C-D). The distribution of the immune-reactivity for GPIHBP1 was comparable to the staining for vessels by anti-CD31 (Figure 5). There was no obvious effect on this pattern or intensity after 12 weeks on a diet high in saturated fats (Figure 9E-F). In *ob/ob* mice treated with or without leptin the fluorescence intensity for

Table 1 Weight, food intake and blood glucose levels of *ob/ob* mice before and after treatment with leptin for immunofluorescence

Ob/ob mice leptin or saline	Weight before (g)	Weight after (g)	Total food intake after injections (g)	Glucose measure day 2 (mmol/L)	Glucose measure day 11 (mmol/L)
Leptin 1	56.9	46.3	40.8	5.5	4.8
Leptin 2	67.7	59.2	45.9	11.1	3.8
Leptin 3	64.3	52	28.5	7.4	3.7
Leptin 4	62.7	54.5	41.8	5.1	4.5
Control 1	64	56.7	57.9	24.1	31.4
Control 2	58.9	55	74	27.8	23
Control 3	66.9	62.7	84.5	8.8	23.1
Control 4	69.4	68.1	70.5	23.8	25.2

The table demonstrates weight, food intake and glucose levels in ob/ob mice treated with leptin or saline for 12 days. The mice were used for immunofluorescence (IF). All glucose values are from non-fasted animals.

Table 2 Weight, food intake and blood glucose levels of *ob/ob* mice before and after treatment with leptin for qPCR

Ob/ob mice leptin or saline	Weight before (g)	Weight after (g)	Total food intake after injections (g)	Glucose measure day 0 (mmol/L)	Glucose measure day 13 (mmol/L)
Leptin 1	53.7	43.9	54.2	8.2	6.2
Leptin 2	53.7	43.5	41.3	9.6	4.7
Leptin 3	52.5	45.6	50.8	9.3	5.4
Leptin 4	52	42.5	37.6	7.1	5.6
Control 1	64.6	68.3	89.1	10.2	17.7
Control 2	53.4	55.2	66.9	7.2	6.6
Control 3	49.9	54.1	76.3	10.3	11.1
Control 4	58	60.9	75.1	7.5	10.8
Control 5	52	56	84.1	11.1	14.3
Control 6	48.3	51.5	89.5	6.7	12

The table demonstrates weight, food intake and glucose levels in ob/ob mice treated with leptin or saline for 12 days. The mice were used for determination of mRNA levels by qPCR. All glucose values are from non-fasted animals.

GPIHBP1 was somewhat increased in the islets (Figure 9G-H). The capillaries and small vessels containing GPIHBP1 appeared wider than in WT mice and this was similar to what was seen with anti-CD31 in islets of *ob/ob* mice (Figure 7E compared to B). In exocrine pancreatic tissue, no effects were seen on the distribution or intensity of GPIHBP1 immune-reactivity by nutritional status, diet or leptin deficiency (Figure 10A-H).

Discussion

A major new finding in this study is that the expression of LPL in pancreatic beta cells is suppressed in *ob/ob* mice. While there was strong immunostaining for LPL in beta cells from normal mice, there was virtually no staining in beta cells from obese and leptin deficient *ob/ob* mice. This suggests that leptin has an important role for the expression of LPL in beta cells. *Ob/ob* mice eat constantly and become obese, insulin resistant and hyperglycemic. To cope with this they develop islet hyperplasia, and in addition the *ob/ob* mice have a higher proportion of beta cells in their islets than WT mice (>90%) [16]. In contrast to humans with diabetes type 2 due to insufficient insulin secretion [21], the beta cells of *ob/ob* mice have normal glucose-stimulated insulin secretion and produce large amounts of insulin [16]. We found that supplementation of *ob/ob* mice for 12 days with leptin reduced food intake, body weight and blood glucose levels, and restored LPL-expression in the beta cells. Some islets were almost completely restored, while others had only started to recover LPL expression at this time. LPL mRNA levels responded in a similar way. They were lower in *ob/ob* compared to WT mice, and tended to increase in *ob/ob* mice after leptin treatment. The lack of LPL in beta cells of *ob/ob* mice could be due to the lack of leptin *per se*, or could be a consequence of obesity and/or the high levels of glucose, fatty acids and insulin in the blood. A similar response to leptin had been described for hormone sensitive lipase (HSL) in *ob/ob* mice. After 7 days with leptin injections there was increased immunostaining for HSL in islets [22]. Leptin is known to affect LPL in other tissues. In skeletal muscle, but not in adipose tissue, an increase

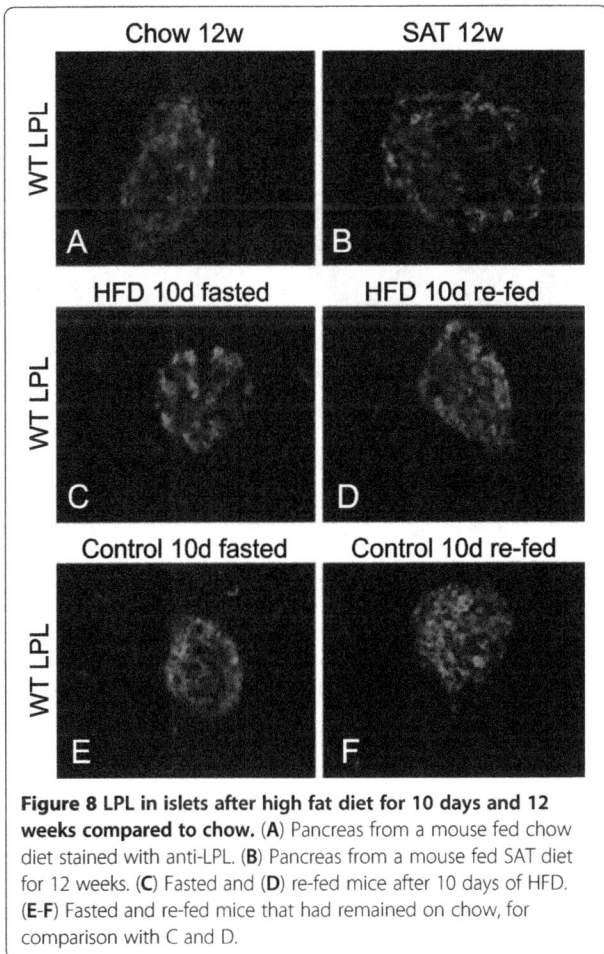

Figure 8 LPL in islets after high fat diet for 10 days and 12 weeks compared to chow. (A) Pancreas from a mouse fed chow diet stained with anti-LPL. **(B)** Pancreas from a mouse fed SAT diet for 12 weeks. **(C)** Fasted and **(D)** re-fed mice after 10 days of HFD. **(E-F)** Fasted and re-fed mice that had remained on chow, for comparison with C and D.

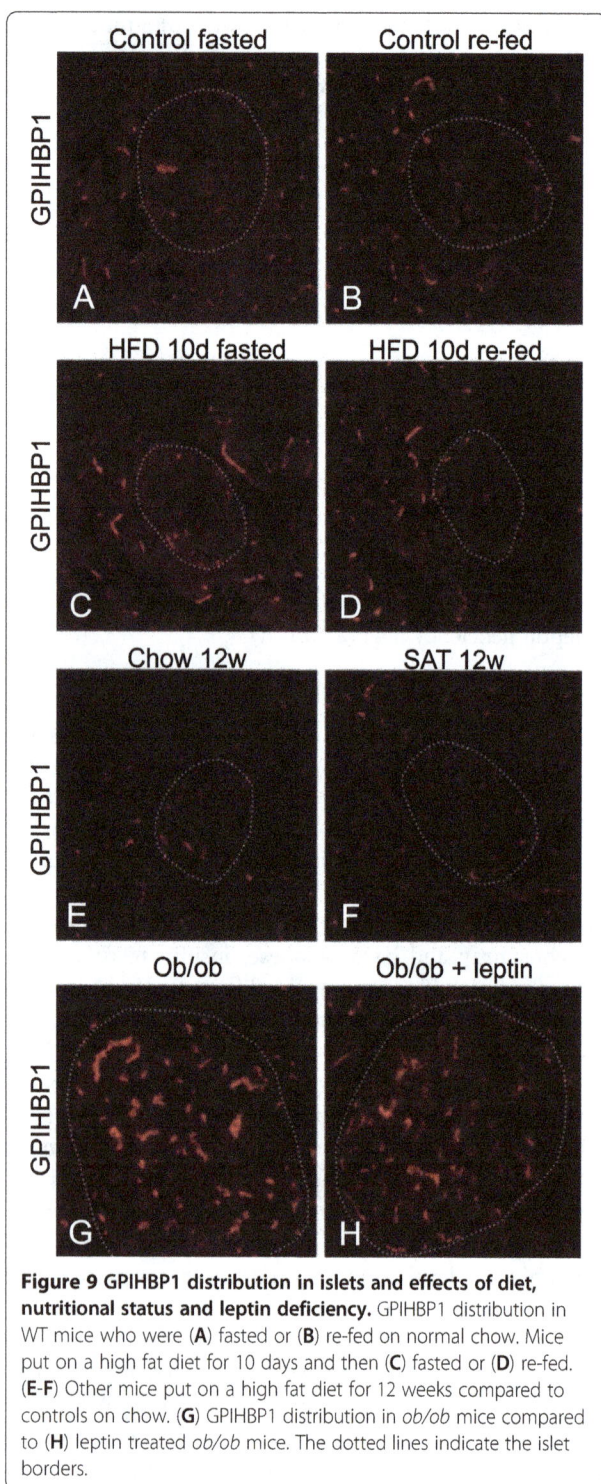

Figure 9 GPIHBP1 distribution in islets and effects of diet, nutritional status and leptin deficiency. GPIHBP1 distribution in WT mice who were (**A**) fasted or (**B**) re-fed on normal chow. Mice put on a high fat diet for 10 days and then (**C**) fasted or (**D**) re-fed. (**E-F**) Other mice put on a high fat diet for 12 weeks compared to controls on chow. (**G**) GPIHBP1 distribution in *ob/ob* mice compared to (**H**) leptin treated *ob/ob* mice. The dotted lines indicate the islet borders.

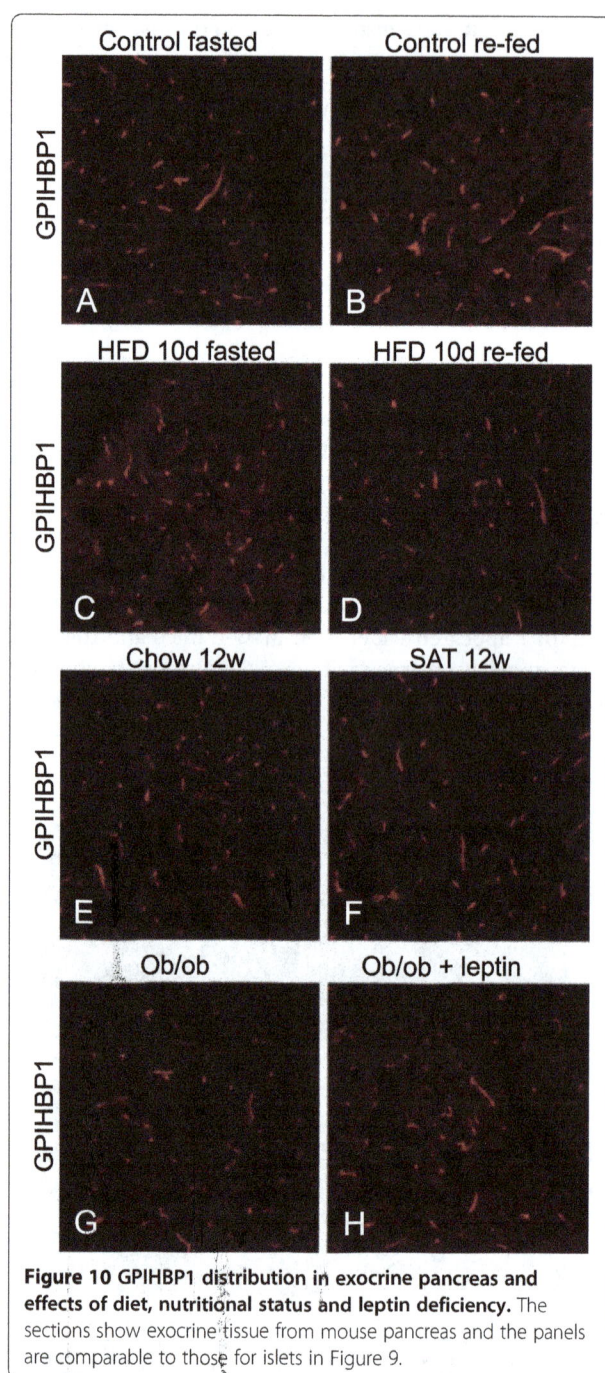

Figure 10 GPIHBP1 distribution in exocrine pancreas and effects of diet, nutritional status and leptin deficiency. The sections show exocrine tissue from mouse pancreas and the panels are comparable to those for islets in Figure 9.

in LPL activity is seen both in WT and *ob/ob* mice after leptin injections [23]. Leptin also affects expression of LPL in J774 macrophages [24]. Taken together, these observations imply an important role for leptin in modulation of the LPL system, and hence in lipoprotein metabolism.

It is known that leptin affects alpha and beta cells through the leptin receptor ObR and that this leads to inhibited insulin and glucagon secretion [25,26]. Pancreas-specific ObR −/− mice show no difference in body weight, food intake or percentage of body fat compared to control mice, while differences are seen in blood insulin concentrations and response to glucose [27]. Like *ob/ob* mice, the pancreas-specific ObR −/− mice develop islet hyperplasia due to increased beta-cell mass. This animal model could be used to investigate whether islet LPL, and HSL, are affected by the local lack of leptin signaling, or by the general metabolic disturbances seen in the *ob/ob* mice.

LPL has previously been shown to be expressed in beta cells and to be closely linked to the function of these cells [11]. Both beta cell-specific overexpression of LPL, and deletion of LPL in beta cells, resulted in a diabetic phenotype [11]. Overexpression of LPL in beta cells decreased islet glucose metabolism, while beta cell-specific knock-out of LPL increased islet glucose metabolism. It is therefore likely that optimal beta cell function requires a delicate balance between metabolism of glucose and fatty acids. In the normal situation, some of the fatty acids may be provided by the LPL system, in addition to the fatty acids that arrive from adipose tissue as albumin-bound NEFAs and fatty acids released from intracellular islet stores by adipose tissue triglyceride lipase (ATGL) and HSL [28]. The intracellular localization of LPL within alpha and beta cells, rather than on the capillary endothelium in the islets, demonstrate that only a minor fraction of the synthesized LPL is secreted from these cells and argues against a function of LPL in lipid uptake by the islet cells. LPL is present in vesicles separate from the insulin-containing granulae in INS1 cells and it was proposed that glucose stimulates LPL translocation to the cell surface [12]. The expression of LPL in INS1 cells has been shown to be up-regulated by agonists to the peroxisome proliferator-activated receptor delta and by cytokines that induce expression of this receptor [29]. We thought that the predominant intracellular localization of LPL in islets could be due to a relative lack of the endothelial LPL-binding protein GPIHBP1. This was not the case. GPIHBP1 was found to be associated with capillaries and smaller vessels both in exocrine pancreas, and in islets. As expected, immune-reaction for GPIHBP1 was co-localized with the endothelial marker CD31 and also with LPL. In islets from *ob/ob* mice the immune-reaction for GPIHBP1 appeared somewhat stronger and the capillaries somewhat wider than in WT mice. After leptin treatment for 12 days, LPL expression was restored in beta cells, but the expression pattern for GPIHBP1 remained the same as in untreated mice, possibly due to that the islets were still enlarged.

An important argument against an involvement of LPL in insulin secretion is that insulin-dependent diabetes is not a commonly reported problem in animal models of LPL deficiency [30,31], or in patients with either total LPL deficiency or with non-functional LPL protein [32]. In one study on human LPL-deficient subjects, enhanced glucose-stimulated insulin secretion after an oral glucose tolerance test was found, compared to other groups of non-diabetic patients with hypertriglyceridemia [33]. Islets from LPL-deficient mice were re-ported to secrete more insulin than islets from normal mice, and the LPL-deficient mice had lower fasting blood glucose levels and no signs of abnormal insulin responsiveness [10]. With age, LPL-deficient mice were found to display glucose intolerance and decreased first-phase insulin secretion [34]. Thus, a direct effect of LPL on insulin secretion is unlikely, but secondary effects of LPL deficiency on insulin secretion, showing up when the metabolism is in some way challenged, cannot be excluded.

It is well known that the expression of both LPL and GPIHBP1 is regulated by nutritional and hormonal factors. For LPL the adaptation to feeding or fasting occurs mostly by posttranslational mechanism [1,2], while the transcription of GPIHBP1 is upregulated on fasting through activation of peroxisome proliferator-activated receptor-gamma [20]. We studied the response of LPL and GPIHBP1 expression in pancreas of mice exposed to a high fat diet for 10 days or 12 weeks, respectively. The latter group showed increased plasma NEFA and hypertriglyceridemia, indicating insulin resistance [15], while such changes were not yet evident after 10 days on HFD. There were no obvious differences in the LPL distribution pattern in islets of these two groups of diet-treated mice compared to littermates on normal chow. In the 10 day experiment we looked for rapid nutritional effects by comparing LPL distribution in pancreas from fasted mice to those re-fed for 3 hours after fasting. Neither the HFD nor the control groups showed any significant changes in LPL distribution pattern in response to fasting. This was also the case for mice fed a diet containing a high proportion of saturated fat (SAT) for 12 weeks. We conclude that expression and distribution of LPL in mouse pancreatic tissue appears relatively robust with respect to nutritional state and to metabolic disturbances connected to obesity and insulin resistance. A similar conclusion was reached for the expression and distribution of GPIHBP1, but in *ob/ob* mice with or without leptin treatment there is an increase in islet vessel GPIHBP1. This followed the vessel structure in the *ob/ob* islets, which was larger than in islets of WT mice. After leptin treatment for 12 days LPL expression returned in beta cells, but the GPIHBP1 pattern remained the same as in un-treated mice.

In the exocrine pancreatic tissue LPL appeared to co-localize with the endothelial marker CD31 and with GPIHBP1. The function of LPL in exocrine pancreas is not known, but the enzyme is likely to provide the acinar cells with lipolysis products for energy production to support synthesis and secretion of digestive enzymes. In contrast to LPL in islet cells, LPL in exocrine pancreas disappeared after injection of Fragmin®, demonstrating that most of the LPL in exocrine pancreas is localized on cell surfaces in a heparin-releasable manner. This supports the view that the main function of LPL in exocrine pancreas is to act on the triglyceride-rich plasma lipoproteins to release fatty acids and monoglycerides for uptake in the tissue. As expected, GPIHBP1, which is linked to plasma membranes of endothelial cell via a glycosylphosphatidylinositol (GPI) anchor [4], remained at the endothelium after Fragmin® treatment. The source of LPL in pancreatic exocrine tissue is presently not known. We did not see much immunoreaction for LPL over the acinar cells, indicating that they, in contrast to islets cells, secrete most of the newly synthesized LPL. If the acinar cells are not the origin of LPL, endocrine cells might provide exocrine vessels with LPL [35]. In *ob/ob* mice LPL in exocrine pancreas was not affected by the leptin deficiency in beta cells. This argues against the hypothesis that LPL in the exocrine pancreas originates from the islets, unless most of the exocrine LPL comes from alpha cells.

Conclusions

We have shown that LPL and GPIHBP1 are present on capillaries both in exocrine and endocrine parts of pancreas and that expression of GPIHBP1 is not markedly dependent on either leptin or metabolic status. In islets, LPL is mostly intracellular and LPL expression in beta cells, but not in alpha cells, is dependent on leptin and can be restored after leptin-treatment of *ob/ob* mice. Taken together with earlier studies it is clear that LPL is present within insulin-producing cells, but further studies will be needed to understand its regulation and function.

Abbreviations
ATGL: Adipose tissue triglyceride lipase; GPIHBP1: Glycosylphosphatidylinositol-anchored HDL-binding protein 1; HSL: hormone sensitive lipase; LPL: Lipoprotein lipase.

Competing interest
The authors declare that they have no competing interest.

Authors' contributions
RN and GO did the conception and design of the research. CLC, PL, AB, YA, LJ-B and TO conducted the animal experiments. RN, EV and YA performed the analytical work and AB and S.G.Y. provided necessary knowledge and tools for studies of GPIHBP1. All authors contributed to analyses of data and to interpretation of the results. RN prepared the figures and RN and GO drafted the manuscript. All authors contributed to edition and revision of the manuscript. All authors read and approved the final manuscript.

Acknowledgements
We thank P. Steneberg and H. Edlund (Umeå University) for valuable technical and scientific advice, and for providing us with antibodies and mouse embryos. We also thank Dr. R.J. Deckelbaum (Columbia University, New York) for supporting the diet studies. This work was financed by grants from the Swedish Science Council (grant no 12203), the Swedish Heart and Lung foundation and the Biotechnology fund at Umeå University.

Author details
[1]Department of Medical Biosciences/Physiological Chemistry, Umeå University, Umeå, Sweden. [2]Institute of Human Nutrition, College of Physicians and Surgeons, Columbia University, New York, NY, USA. [3]Department of Integrative Medical Biology (IMB), Umeå University, Umeå, Sweden. [4]The Rolf Luft Research Center for Diabetes and Endocrinology, Karolinska Institutet, Stockholm, Sweden. [5]Division of Nutritional Science, Cornell University, Ithaca, NY, USA. [6]Department of Medicine, David Geffen School of Medicine, University of California, Los Angeles, CA, USA.

References
1. Wang H, Eckel RH: **Lipoprotein lipase: from gene to obesity.** *Am J Physiol Endocrinol Metab* 2009, 297:E271–E288.
2. Olivecrona T, Olivecrona G: **The ins and outs of adipose tissue.** In *Cellular lipid metabolism.* Edited by Ehnholm C. Heidelberg: Springer; 2009:315–369.
3. Davies BS, Beigneux AP, Barnes RH 2nd, Tu Y, Gin P, Weinstein MM, Nobumori C, Nyren R, Goldberg I, Olivecrona G, et al: **GPIHBP1 is responsible for the entry of lipoprotein lipase into capillaries.** *Cell Metab* 2010, 12:42–52.
4. Beigneux AP, Davies BS, Gin P, Weinstein MM, Farber E, Qiao X, Peale F, Bunting S, Walzem RL, Wong JS, et al: **Glycosylphosphatidylinositol-anchored high-density lipoprotein-binding protein 1 plays a critical role in the lipolytic processing of chylomicrons.** *Cell Metab* 2007, 5:279–291.
5. Beigneux AP, Franssen R, Bensadoun A, Gin P, Melford K, Peter J, Walzem RL, Weinstein MM, Davies BS, Kuivenhoven JA, et al: **Chylomicronemia with a mutant GPIHBP1 (Q115P) that cannot bind lipoprotein lipase.** *Arterioscler Thromb Vasc Biol* 2009, 29:956–962.
6. Olivecrona G, Ehrenborg E, Semb H, Makoveichuk E, Lindberg A, Hayden MR, Gin P, Davies BS, Weinstein MM, Fong LG, et al: **Mutation of conserved cysteines in the Ly6 domain of GPIHBP1 in familial chylomicronemia.** *J Lipid Res* 2010, 51:1535–1545.
7. Franssen R, Young SG, Peelman F, Hertecant J, Sierts JA, Schimmel AW, Bensadoun A, Kastelein JJ, Fong LG, Dallinga-Thie GM, Beigneux AP: **Chylomicronemia with low postheparin lipoprotein lipase levels in the setting of GPIHBP1 defects.** *Circ Cardiovasc Genet* 2010, 3:169–178.
8. Coca-Prieto I, Kroupa O, Gonzalez-Santos P, Magne J, Olivecrona G, Ehrenborg E, Valdivielso P: **Childhood-onset chylomicronaemia with reduced plasma lipoprotein lipase activity and mass: identification of a novel GPIHBP1 mutation.** *J Intern Med* 2011, 270:224–228.
9. Davies BS, Goulbourne CN, Barnes RH 2nd, Turlo KA, Gin P, Vaughan S, Vaux DJ, Bensadoun A, Beigneux AP, Fong LG, Young SG: **Assessing mechanisms of GPIHBP1 and lipoprotein lipase movement across endothelial cells.** *J Lipid Res* 2012, 53:2690–2697.
10. Marshall BA, Tordjman K, Host HH, Ensor NJ, Kwon G, Marshall CA, Coleman T, McDaniel ML, Semenkovich CF: **Relative hypoglycemia and hyperinsulinemia in mice with heterozygous lipoprotein lipase (LPL) deficiency. Islet LPL regulates insulin secretion.** *J Biol Chem* 1999, 274:27426–27432.
11. Pappan KL, Pan Z, Kwon G, Marshall CA, Coleman T, Goldberg IJ, McDaniel ML, Semenkovich CF: **Pancreatic beta-cell lipoprotein lipase independently regulates islet glucose metabolism and normal insulin secretion.** *J Biol Chem* 2005, 280:9023–9029.
12. Cruz WS, Kwon G, Marshall CA, McDaniel ML, Semenkovich CF: **Glucose and insulin stimulate heparin-releasable lipoprotein lipase activity in mouse islets and INS-1 cells. A potential link between insulin resistance and beta-cell dysfunction.** *J Biol Chem* 2001, 276:12162–12168.
13. Yaney GC, Corkey BE: **Fatty acid metabolism and insulin secretion in pancreatic beta cells.** *Diabetologia* 2003, 46:1297–1312.
14. Newsholme P, Keane D, Welters HJ, Morgan NG: **Life and death decisions of the pancreatic beta-cell: the role of fatty acids.** *Clin Sci (Lond)* 2007, 112:27–42.
15. Chang CL, Seo T, Matsuzaki M, Worgall TS, Deckelbaum RJ: **n-3 fatty acids reduce arterial LDL-cholesterol delivery and arterial lipoprotein lipase levels and lipase distribution.** *Arterioscler Thromb Vasc Biol* 2009, 29:555–561.
16. Lindstrom P: **beta-cell function in obese-hyperglycemic mice [ob/ob Mice].** *Adv Exp Med Biol* 2010, 654:463–477.
17. Ruge T, Sukonina V, Myrnas T, Lundgren M, Eriksson JW, Olivecrona G: **Lipoprotein lipase activity/mass ratio is higher in omental than in subcutaneous adipose tissue.** *Eur J Clin Invest* 2006, 36:16–21.

18. Olivecrona T, Bengtsson G: **Immunochemical properties of lipoprotein lipase. Development of an immunoassay applicable to several mammalian species.** *Biochim Biophys Acta* 1983, **752**:38–45.

19. Chevreuil O, Hultin M, Ostergaard P, Olivecrona T: **Biphasic effects of low-molecular-weight and conventional heparins on chylomicron clearance in rats.** *Arterioscler Thromb* 1993, **13**:1397–1403.

20. Davies BS, Waki H, Beigneux AP, Farber E, Weinstein MM, Wilpitz DC, Tai LJ, Evans RM, Fong LG, Tontonoz P, Young SG: **The expression of GPIHBP1, an endothelial cell binding site for lipoprotein lipase and chylomicrons, is induced by peroxisome proliferator-activated receptor-gamma.** *Mol Endocrinol* 2008, **22**:2496–2504.

21. Weir GC, Bonner-Weir S: **Five stages of evolving beta-cell dysfunction during progression to diabetes.** *Diabetes* 2004, **53**(Suppl 3):S16–S21.

22. Khan A, Narangoda S, Ahren B, Holm C, Sundler F, Efendic S: **Long-term leptin treatment of ob/ob mice improves glucose-induced insulin secretion.** *Int J Obes Relat Metab Disord* 2001, **25**:816–821.

23. Donahoo WT, Stob NR, Ammon S, Levin N, Eckel RH: **Leptin increases skeletal muscle lipoprotein lipase and postprandial lipid metabolism in mice.** *Metabolism* 2011, **60**:438–443.

24. Maingrette F, Renier G: **Leptin increases lipoprotein lipase secretion by macrophages: involvement of oxidative stress and protein kinase C.** *Diabetes* 2003, **52**:2121–2128.

25. Kieffer TJ, Habener JF: **The adipoinsular axis: effects of leptin on pancreatic beta-cells.** *Am J Physiol Endocrinol Metab* 2000, **278**:E1–E14.

26. Tuduri E, Marroqui L, Soriano S, Ropero AB, Batista TM, Piquer S, Lopez-Boado MA, Carneiro EM, Gomis R, Nadal A, Quesada I: **Inhibitory effects of leptin on pancreatic alpha-cell function.** *Diabetes* 2009, **58**:1616–1624.

27. Morioka T, Asilmaz E, Hu J, Dishinger JF, Kurpad AJ, Elias CF, Li H, Elmquist JK, Kennedy RT, Kulkarni RN: **Disruption of leptin receptor expression in the pancreas directly affects beta cell growth and function in mice.** *J Clin Invest* 2007, **117**:2860–2868.

28. Mulder H, Sorhede-Winzell M, Contreras JA, Fex M, Strom K, Ploug T, Galbo H, Arner P, Lundberg C, Sundler F, *et al*: **Hormone-sensitive lipase null mice exhibit signs of impaired insulin sensitivity whereas insulin secretion is intact.** *J Biol Chem* 2003, **278**:36380–36388.

29. Kharroubi I, Lee CH, Hekerman P, Darville MI, Evans RM, Eizirik DL, Cnop M: **BCL-6: a possible missing link for anti-inflammatory PPAR-delta signalling in pancreatic beta cells.** *Diabetologia* 2006, **49**:2350–2358.

30. Liu G, Ashbourne Excoffon KJ, Wilson JE, McManus BM, Rogers QR, Miao L, Kastelein JJ, Lewis ME, Hayden MR: **Phenotypic correction of feline lipoprotein lipase deficiency by adenoviral gene transfer.** *Hum Gene Ther* 2000, **11**:21–32.

31. Christophersen B, Nordstoga K, Shen Y, Olivecrona T, Olivecrona G: **Lipoprotein lipase deficiency with pancreatitis in mink: biochemical characterization and pathology.** *J Lipid Res* 1997, **38**:837–846.

32. Brunzell JD, Deeb SS: **Familial lipoprotein lipase deficiency, apoC-II deficiency, and hepatic lipase deficiency.** In *The Metabolic and molecular bases of inherited disease.* Edited by Scriver CR B, Beaudet AL, Sly WS, Valle D, Childs B, Kinzler K, Vogelstein B. New York: McGraw-Hill; 2001:2789–2816.

33. Tamasawa N, Matsui J, Murakami H, Tanabe J, Matsuki K, Ogawa Y, Ikeda Y, Takagi A, Suda T: **Glucose-stimulated insulin response in non-diabetic patients with lipoprotein lipase deficiency and hypertriglyceridemia.** *Diabetes Res Clin Pract* 2006, **72**:6–11.

34. Ding YL, Wang YH, Huang W, Liu G, Ross C, Hayden MR, Yang JK: **Glucose intolerance and decreased early insulin response in mice with severe hypertriglyceridemia.** *Exp Biol Med (Maywood)* 2010, **235**:40–46.

35. Henderson JR, Moss MC: **A morphometric study of the endocrine and exocrine capillaries of the pancreas.** *Q J Exp Physiol* 1985, **70**:347–356.

15

MAPK-activated protein kinase 2-deficiency causes hyperacute tumor necrosis factor-induced inflammatory shock

Benjamin Vandendriessche[1,2], An Goethals[1,2†], Alba Simats[1,2†], Evelien Van Hamme[3], Peter Brouckaert[1,2†] and Anje Cauwels[1,2,4*†]

Abstract

Background: MAPK-activated protein kinase 2 (MK2) plays a pivotal role in the cell response to (inflammatory) stress. Among others, MK2 is known to be involved in the regulation of cytokine mRNA metabolism and regulation of actin cytoskeleton dynamics. Previously, MK2-deficient mice were shown to be highly resistant to LPS/D-Galactosamine-induced hepatitis. Additionally, research in various disease models has indicated the kinase as an interesting inhibitory drug target for various acute or chronic inflammatory diseases.

Results: We show that in striking contrast to the known resistance of MK2-deficient mice to a challenge with LPS/D-Gal, a low dose of tumor necrosis factor (TNF) causes hyperacute mortality via an oxidative stress driven mechanism. We identified *in vivo* defects in the stress fiber response in endothelial cells, which could have resulted in reduced resistance of the endothelial barrier to deal with exposure to oxidative stress. In addition, MK2-deficient mice were found to be more sensitive to cecal ligation and puncture-induced sepsis.

Conclusions: The capacity of the endothelial barrier to deal with inflammatory and oxidative stress is imperative to allow a regulated immune response and maintain endothelial barrier integrity. Our results indicate that, considering the central role of TNF in pro-inflammatory signaling, therapeutic strategies examining pharmacological inhibition of MK2 should take potentially dangerous side effects at the level of endothelial barrier integrity into account.

Keywords: MK2, Inflammatory shock, Tumor necrosis factor, Reactive oxygen species, Actin cytoskeleton, Endothelial permeability, Cecal ligation and puncture

Background

MAP kinase (MAPK)-activated protein kinase 2 (MK2) is involved in very diverse cellular processes ranging from cell migration, to reorganization of the cytoskeleton, inflammation and apoptosis. MK2 is located downstream from p38 MAPK, a major transducer of cell stress responses, such as heat shock, bacterial lipopolysaccharide (LPS), tumor necrosis factor (TNF) and IL-1β (reviewed in [1,2]). In response to an inflammatory stressor such as LPS, p38 will phosphorylate and activate a number of effectors, including MK2. The resulting p38-MK2 complex will translocate from the nucleus to the cytoplasm, followed by MK2-mediated phosphorylation of target proteins (reviewed in [3]). Because of this requirement for co-translocation of p38 and MK2, MK2-deficient mice are also partially p38 MAPK-deficient [4].

One of the better characterized MK2-mediated processes is the post-transcriptional regulation of pro-inflammatory cytokine production [5], including but not limited to TNF [6], IL-6 [7,8], IFN-γ [9], and possibly IL-1β [10]. Tristetra-prolin (TTP), an mRNA-binding zinc-finger protein, destabilizes many mRNAs by binding to AU-rich elements (AREs) in their 3' untranslated region [11], and subsequently targeting them to exosomes or proteasomes [12,13]. MK2 can phosphorylate TTP, thereby reducing its affinity for the ARE [14,15] and allowing other mRNA-binding protein complexes to form that alter the dynamics of pro-

---

* Correspondence: anje.cauwels@vib-ugent.be
†Equal contributors
[1]Inflammation Research Center, VIB, 9052 Ghent, Belgium
[2]Department of Biomedical Molecular Biology, Ghent University, 9000 Ghent, Belgium
Full list of author information is available at the end of the article

inflammatory mRNA metabolism. For instance, in the case of TNF mRNA translation, human antigen R (HuR) can replace phosphorylated TTP, thereby stabilizing the mRNA and initiating translation of TNF [16]. In addition, the expression and post-translational regulation of TTP itself is also regulated by p38-MK2-dependent signal transduction, which allows intrinsic feedback control of the inflammatory response [15,16]. As a result of the dependency of many pro-inflammatory mRNAs on MK2-mediated stabilization, the expression of these cytokines in response to many inflammatory challenges is severely altered in MK2-deficient mice. This was first shown for TNF biosynthesis in response to a combined LPS/D-Galactosamine (D-Gal) challenge, a model of acute hepatitis [6]. Another target of p38 MAPK is MK3. The documented functions and expression patterns of MK2 and MK3 overlap, but MK2 is expressed at significantly higher levels, and assumed to be the dominant isoform. Consistently, TNF production in MK3-deficient mice is comparable to wild type, while expression in MK2/MK3 double-knockout mice was reduced further compared to MK2-deficient mice [17].

A second major p38/MK2-mediated function is the regulation of actin cytoskeleton dynamics through phosphorylation of the small heat shock protein (sHSP) 25 (mouse equivalent to human sHSP27) [1,18]. The actin cytoskeleton plays essential roles in many cellular processes, including regulation of cell shape, endocytosis, anchorage to cells and substrates, and signal transduction. Because of the ability of sHSPs to exist in various states of oligomerization, depending on their phosphorylation status, they can be involved in highly diverse cellular functions, including molecular chaperoning [19], modulation of the glutathione redox status [20], and regulation of actin polymerization dynamics [21].

The endothelial cell layer plays a pivotal role in the inflammatory response by regulating the passage of leukocytes and various signaling molecules, and is an important signal transduction interface. Put differently, its main function is to maintain a highly specialized and selective barrier between the blood and other tissues. During systemic inflammatory conditions, endothelial cells can become exposed to extremely high levels of inflammatory mediators, such as reactive oxygen species (ROS). When ROS-induced damage reaches critical levels or cannot be dealt with appropriately, the barrier function can become severely impaired, resulting in uncontrolled fluid leak, a dysregulated immune response, cell death, and tissue damage. Therefore, endothelial cells have evolved mechanisms to quickly reorganize their actin cytoskeleton into stress fibers that serve both as a contraction scaffold to allow a controlled increase in endothelial permeability and extravasation of leukocytes [22,23], as well as firmly anchor the cells to their neighbors and the matrix to preserve overall barrier integrity [24-26].

In the current study, we examined MK2-deficiency in a model of TNF or LPS-induced systemic inflammation, as well as cecal ligation and puncture (CLP)-induced sepsis. We identified profound and hyperacute TNF-induced mortality, in sharp contrast to the previously described resistance of MK2-deficient mice to LPS/D-Gal-induced hepatitis [6] and similar results we obtained here in an endotoxic shock model. This hyperacute phenotype appeared to be caused by the inability of MK2-deficient endothelial cells to mount a proper stress fiber response, resulting in excessive fluid leak, tissue damage and mortality. Additionally, MK2-deficient mice were also sensitized to CLP-induced mortality.

Results

The effect of MK2-deficiency on mortality induced by systemic inflammation or sepsis

MK2-deficient mice were originally shown to be resistant to LPS/D-Gal [6]. However, LPS/D-Gal causes apoptosis-dependent hepatitis and not endotoxic shock [27], as often mentioned. In order to determine the response of MK2-deficient animals to endotoxic shock, we administered a high i.v. dose of LPS and found that MK2-deficiency also confers extreme protection to LPS-induced hypothermia and mortality (Figure 1A-B). In sharp contrast to these results, MK2-deficient mice were hypersensitive to TNF-induced inflammatory shock (Figure 1C-D). Low to very low doses of TNF (10 – 250 µg/kg), which in wild type (WT) mice only induced a small and temporary drop in body temperature, caused a very fast drop in body temperature in MK2-deficient animals, followed by acute mortality 2–8 h after challenge. In addition, we examined the response of MK2-deficient animals to cecal ligation and puncture (CLP)-induced sepsis. Similarly to TNF, MK2-deficient mice were also sensitized to CLP-induced sepsis (Figure 1E).

Acute TNF-induced inflammatory mediators and cell damage parameters

IL-1β and IL-6 levels were significantly increased in MK2-deficient mice 2.5 h after TNF challenge compared to their WT counterparts (Figure 2A-B). Of note, a high dose of TNF (450 µg/kg) was used to also evoke a clear inflammatory response in WT mice. Intracellular proteins such as hexosaminidase, a lysosomal enzyme, and lactate dehydrogenase (LDH) are indicative for cellular damage and (necrotic) disintegration when detected systemically. Plasma hexosaminidase was significantly increased above baseline in MK2-deficient mice only, 2.5 h after challenge (Figure 2C). Similarly, LDH was only significantly increased for MK2-deficient animals (Figure 2D).

The hypersensitivity of MK2-deficient mice for TNF can be prevented by antioxidant treatment

Circulating peroxide equivalents, a measure for total oxidative stress exposure, were significantly higher in plasma

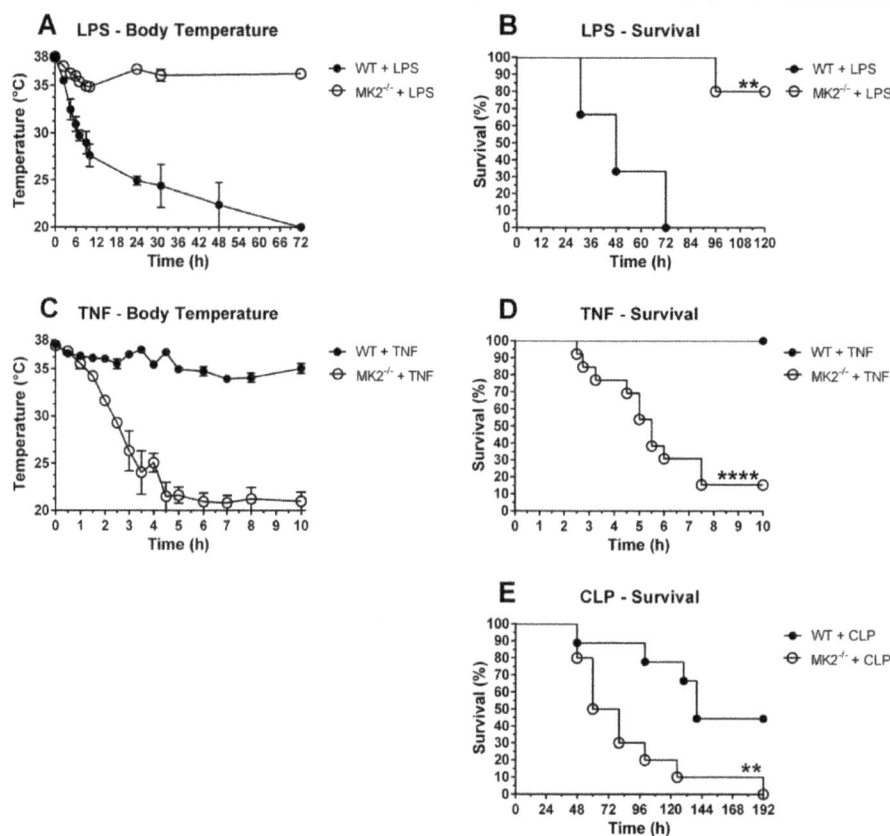

Figure 1 Effect of MK2-deficiency on morbidity and mortality in systemic inflammation and sepsis. (A-B) Body temperature and mortality for WT (n = 3) and MK2$^{-/-}$ (n = 5) mice after i.v. injection of 10 mg/kg LPS. **(C)** Body temperature for WT (n = 5) and MK2$^{-/-}$ (n = 9) mice after i.v. injection of 50 or 125 µg/kg TNF. Dose groups were pooled together because statistical comparison within one genotype revealed no differences. **(D)** Mortality for WT (n = 10) and MK2$^{-/-}$ (n = 13) mice after i.v. injection of 10, 50, 125 or 250 µg/kg TNF. Dose groups were pooled together because statistical comparison within one genotype revealed no differences. **(E)** Mortality for WT (n = 9) and MK2$^{-/-}$ (n = 10) mice after CLP surgery. Survival curves of different genotypes were compared via log-rank test. ****, p $\leq$ 0.0001; **, p $\leq$ 0.01.

of MK2-deficient animals compared to WT mice, already 2.5 h after injection of TNF (Figure 3A), while NO$_x^-$ levels, a measure for total nitric oxide (NO) production, were similarly increased from baseline for both genotypes (Figure 3B). We treated MK2-deficient animals with antioxidants to verify the influence of oxidative stress in the pathophysiology of the hyperacute response. The membrane-permeable superoxide dismutase (SOD) mimetic and radical scavenger tempol could significantly protect against TNF-induced mortality as a combined pre- and post-treatment, while the non-membrane permeable SOD had no effect (Figure 3C).

TNF challenged MK2-deficient animals have a defective stress fiber response

Liver sections were stained for F-actin and 3 small vessels per section were imaged. Representative examples are shown in Figure 4A1-3. Part of the endothelial cell sheet was manually defined as a region of interest (ROI), followed by segmentation of the ROI in discrete actin structures. Next, a number of parameters were calculated: (1) the

percentage of F-actin positive voxels in the ROI, as a measure for the density of the actin network (Figure 4B); (2) the number of discrete actin structures per 100 000 voxels (Figure 4C); and (3) the total number of F-actin positive voxels per actin structure normalized over the number of discrete actin structures, as an estimator of the size of the actin structures (Figure 4D). F-actin density and the number of F-actin structures were not increased from baseline in MK2-deficient mice, in contrast to WT controls, indicating a failure of the endothelial cells to mount a proper stress fiber response (Figure 4B-C). In addition, the size of the F-actin structures was lower in the TNF challenged MK2-deficient animals compared to WT but this difference was not significant (Figure 4D).

TNF-induced vascular leak is much more pronounced in MK2-deficient mice

Vascular permeability was quantified by examining extravasation of FITC-dextran (4 kDa) and Evans Blue. The latter binds albumin with high affinity, resulting in an approximate molecular weight of 70 kDa. No significant

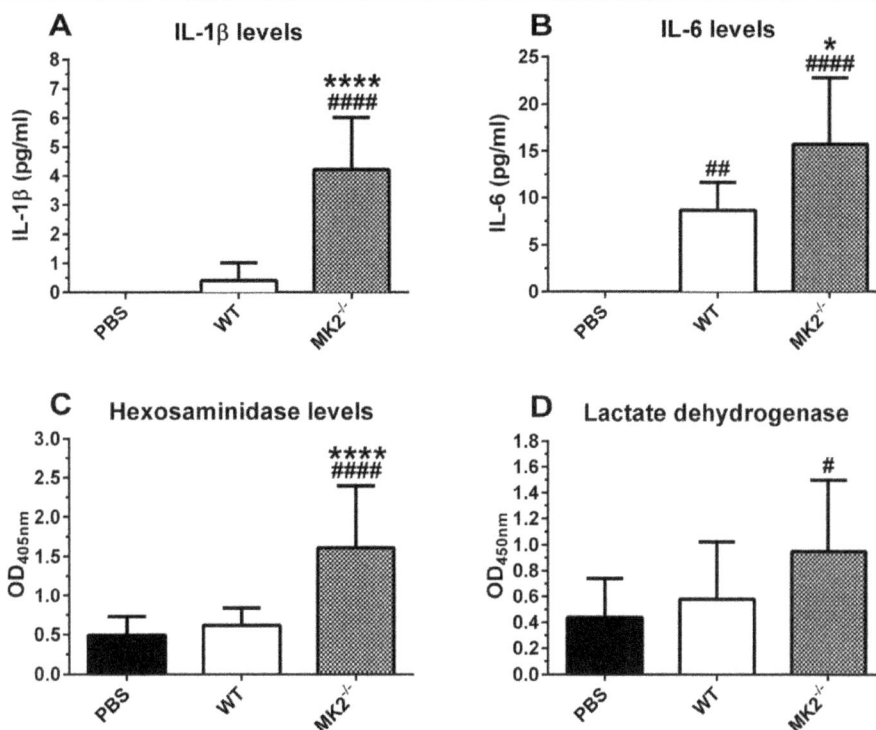

Figure 2 IL-1β, IL-6, hexosaminidase and lactate dehydrogenase levels. (A-B) Plasma IL-1β and IL-6 levels for WT and MK2$^{-/-}$ mice, 2.5 h after i.v. injection of 450 μg/kg TNF (n^{PBS} (WT and MK2$^{-/-}$) = 10, n^{TNF} (WT) = 5, n^{TNF} (MK2$^{-/-}$) = 5). **(C-D)** Plasma hexosaminidase and lactate dehydrogenase plasma levels for WT and MK2$^{-/-}$ mice, 2.5 h after i.v. injection of 450 μg/kg TNF. Pooled data from 2 separate experiments is shown (n^{PBS} (WT and MK2$^{-/-}$) = 17, n^{TNF} (WT) = 10, n^{TNF} (MK2$^{-/-}$) = 8). Comparisons were made between baseline (PBS) and TNF challenged animals (#), and between genotypes (*) via one-way ANOVA with Sidak's multiple comparisons test. Error bars indicate SD. ****, p ≤ 0.0001; **, p ≤ 0.01; *, p ≤ 0.05.

differences in Evans blue extravasation were observed (data not shown). However, the smaller molecular weight FITC-dextran was significantly increased from baseline in liver, kidney and spleen of MK2-deficient mice, in contrast to WT controls (Figure 5A-B and E). Also in the lungs, a small increase in permeability was observed, albeit non-significant, while no effect was observed in the heart (Figure 5C-D).

Discussion

Our results show that TNF induces a hyperacute inflammatory shock phenotype in MK2-deficient mice. A lethal TNF challenge in WT mice will cause mortality between roughly 16–24 h post-challenge (data not shown), while a low dose of TNF normally causes only mild and transient morbidity in healthy WT mice. However, in MK2-deficient mice, very low doses of TNF caused hyperacute mortality already 2–8 h post-challenge. In addition, we corroborated earlier results that demonstrated the resistance of MK2-deficient mice to LPS/D-Gal induced hepatitis [6,27], by showing that MK2-deficient mice are also resistant to endotoxic shock. The resistance of MK2-deficient mice to LPS/D-Gal has been clearly linked to reduced stability of TNF and other mRNAs encoding

pro-inflammatory cytokines, via p38 MAPK/MK2/TTP-mediated signaling [7,8,14]. However, in our TNF model, IL-6 and IL-1β levels in circulation were increased more in MK2-deficient animals after the challenge, compared to WT controls. This could indicate that the hyperacute phenotype is caused by such a severe inflammatory response that, despite decreased mRNA stability of pro-inflammatory cytokines, high levels of these cytokines could still be detected in circulation. To corroborate this further, parameters indicative for (necrotic) cellular disintegration were highly increased early after TNF challenge in MK2-deficient mice, while they were not increased from baseline for WT controls that received a high dose of TNF.

We previously observed a similar hyperacute phenotype in WT mice after a combined challenge with TNF and the pan-caspase inhibitor zVAD-fmk [28]. In that case and others, ROS were found to play an important role in the pathophysiology [28,29]. Also in the current study, highly increased levels of radicals were detected after challenge with TNF in the MK2-deficient animals. Therefore, we treated these animals with the antioxidants tempol or SOD. Tempol is a membrane permeable antioxidant that dismutates superoxide catalytically and limits Fenton-mediated hydroxyl radical formation [30].

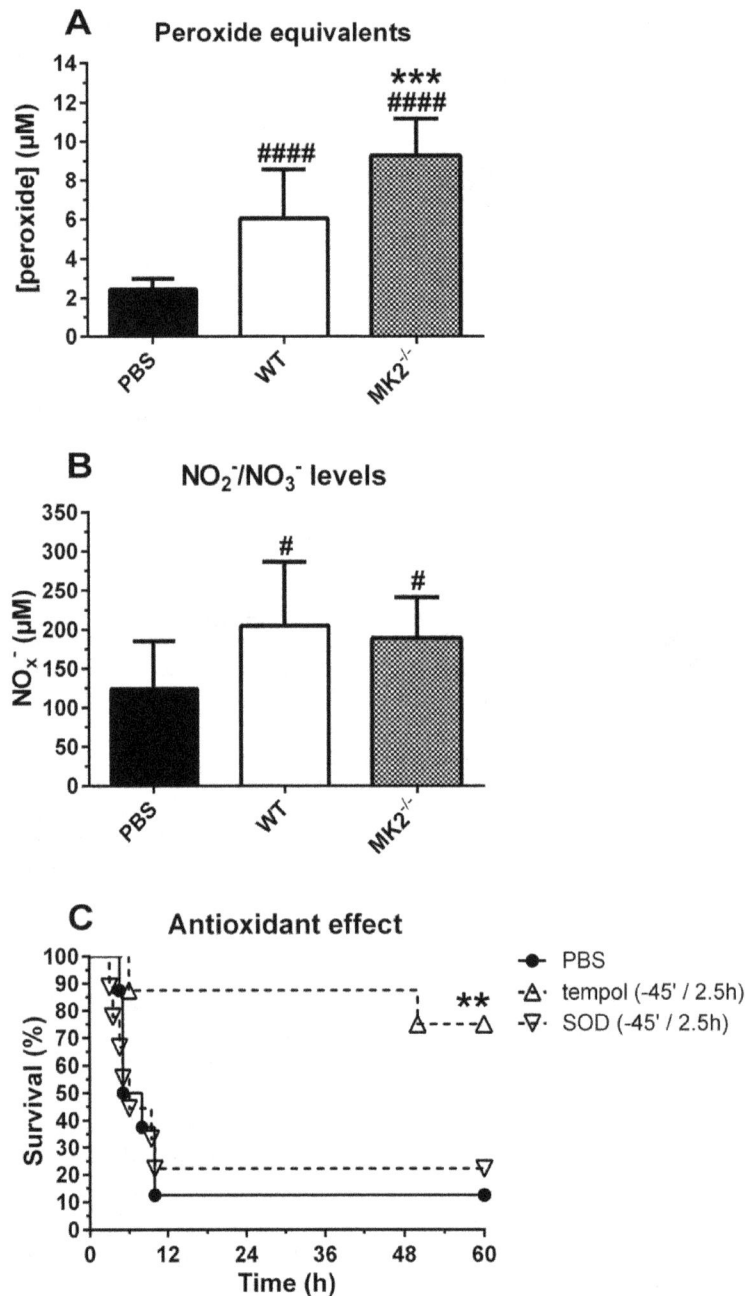

Figure 3 Peroxide equivalents, NO$_x^-$ levels, and effect of antioxidant treatment on mortality. (A) Plasma peroxide equivalents for WT and MK2$^{-/-}$ mice, 2.5 h after i.v. injection of 125 µg/kg TNF. Pooled data from 2 separate experiments is shown (n^{PBS} (WT and MK2$^{-/-}$) = 13, n^{TNF} (WT) = 11, n^{TNF} (MK2$^{-/-}$) = 12). **(B)** Plasma NO$_x^-$ levels for WT and MK2$^{-/-}$ mice, 2.5 h after i.v. injection of 125 µg/kg TNF. Pooled data from 2 separate experiments is shown (n^{PBS} (WT and MK2$^{-/-}$) = 12, n^{TNF} (WT) = 7, n^{TNF} (MK2$^{-/-}$) = 9). Comparisons were made between baseline (PBS) and TNF challenged animals (#), and between genotypes (*) via one-way ANOVA with Sidak's multiple comparisons test. **(C)** Mortality for TNF challenged MK2$^{-/-}$ mice after pre- and post-treatment with tempol or SOD. Survival curves of different treatment groups were compared to controls via log-rank test (*). Error bars indicate SD. ****, $p \leq 0.0001$; ***, $p \leq 0.001$; **, $p \leq 0.01$; *, $p \leq 0.05$.

Contrary, the action of SOD is limited to the dismutation of superoxide and it is not membrane permeable. Thus, the observed difference in response could indicate that the ability of tempol to diffuse into cells and/or its broader spectrum antioxidant activity are key factors for preventing the acute TNF-induced toxicity. In any case, it indicates that ROS are an important driver of the TNF-induced pathophysiology in the absence of MK2. The small heat shock protein 25 (sHSP25) can form large oligomers that are known to be involved in the

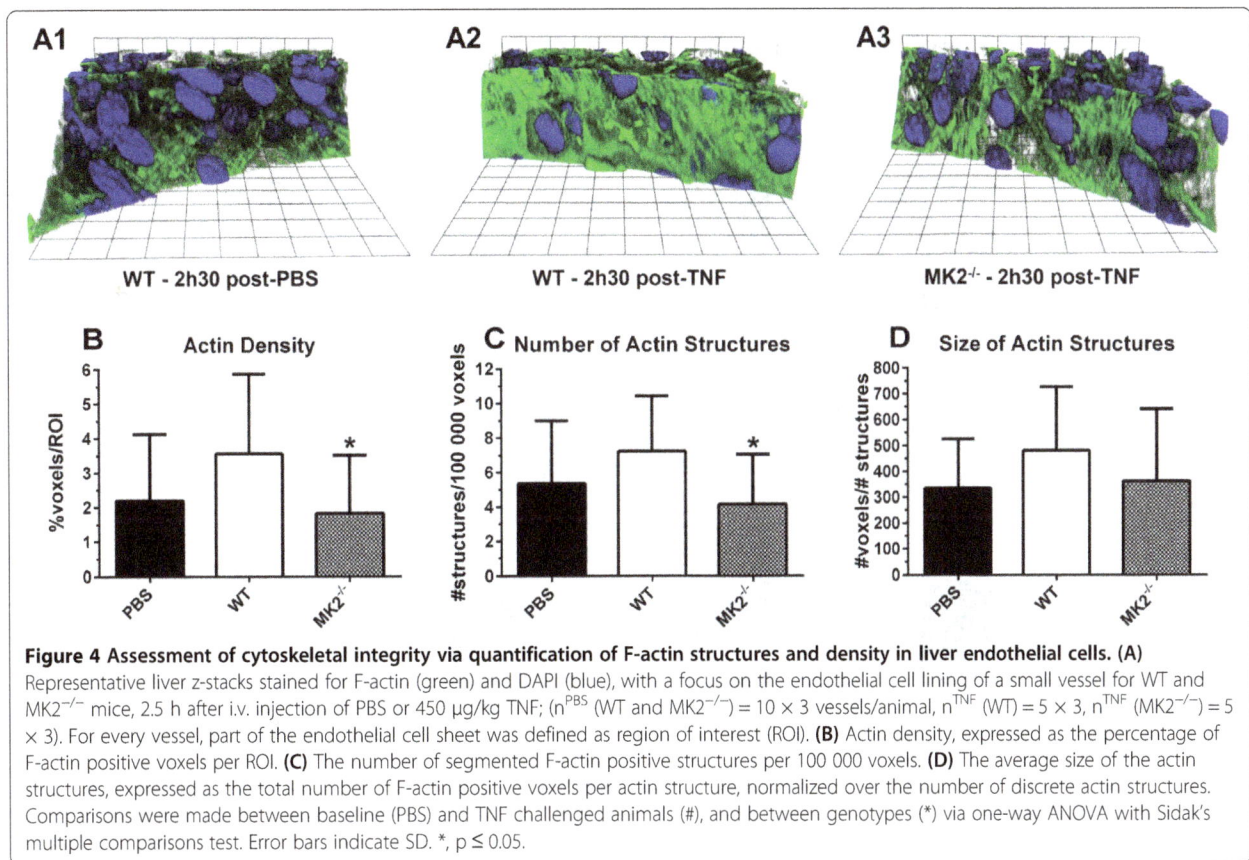

Figure 4 Assessment of cytoskeletal integrity via quantification of F-actin structures and density in liver endothelial cells. (A) Representative liver z-stacks stained for F-actin (green) and DAPI (blue), with a focus on the endothelial cell lining of a small vessel for WT and MK2$^{-/-}$ mice, 2.5 h after i.v. injection of PBS or 450 μg/kg TNF; (n^{PBS} (WT and MK2$^{-/-}$) = 10 × 3 vessels/animal, n^{TNF} (WT) = 5 × 3, n^{TNF} (MK2$^{-/-}$) = 5 × 3). For every vessel, part of the endothelial cell sheet was defined as region of interest (ROI). **(B)** Actin density, expressed as the percentage of F-actin positive voxels per ROI. **(C)** The number of segmented F-actin positive structures per 100 000 voxels. **(D)** The average size of the actin structures, expressed as the total number of F-actin positive voxels per actin structure, normalized over the number of discrete actin structures. Comparisons were made between baseline (PBS) and TNF challenged animals (#), and between genotypes (*) via one-way ANOVA with Sidak's multiple comparisons test. Error bars indicate SD. *, p ≤ 0.05.

maintenance of intracellular glutathione (GSH) levels and help keep GSH in its reduced form under conditions of oxidative stress [20,31], in addition to their well-known protein chaperoning functions [32]. It is therefore tempting to speculate that the absence of MK2, which can modulate the function of sHSP25 via phosphorylation, could be the cause of the high ROS levels, resulting in tissue damage and the observed acute mortality. However, upon MK2-mediated phosphorylation the large sHSP25 oligomers dissociate into smaller oligomers and monomers [33,34], and the antioxidant capacity of sHSP25 has been clearly linked to its unphosphorylated oligomerized form [31]. Decreased sHSP25-mediated antioxidant capacity is therefore unlikely to be a dominant mechanism in the current model.

Next, we examined actin cytoskeleton dynamics, another target of MK2 via phosphorylation of sHSP25. As mentioned earlier, large sHSP25 oligomers will dissociate into smaller oligomers and monomers [33,34]. Considering that signal transduction occurs through the stress-activated p38 MAPK/MK2 pathway, phosphorylation of sHSP25 will be induced by exposure to inflammatory mediators such as TNF and ROS. The resulting small phosphorylated sHSP25 oligomers can bind to F-actin filaments, thereby promoting increased F-actin dynamics and stress fiber formation [21], manifested by rapid reorganization of cortically localized F-actin into long transcytoplasmic fibers [35-37]. In HUVEC cells, this process was shown to be severely impaired after pharmacological inhibition of p38 MAPK [38]. Because of its unique location, the endothelial actin cytoskeleton is one of the earliest targets of ROS-mediated toxicity during an inflammatory response. In fact, it has been suggested that endothelial barrier function, which hinges on the integrity of the cytoskeleton, could be the limiting factor determining the capacity of endothelial cells to deal with oxidative stress [35]. The change in F-actin dynamics serves two main functions in the endothelium: (1) modulation of intercellular contacts [39], as well as providing a scaffold for actomyosin-based contractility to allow cell rounding and inter-endothelial gap formation [40], required for the regulated extravasation of leukocytes in response to inflammatory mediators; and (2) firmly anchor the cells to their neighbors by connecting intracellular stress fiber networks together through so-called discontinuous adherens junctions to preserve barrier function in response to stress [25,26]. Our *in vivo* results confirmed that the endothelial cell barrier in MK2-deficient liver vessels appeared to be unable to mount a proper stress fiber response, as evidenced by the absence of increased actin density and changes in the observable actin structures after TNF challenge. The failure of endothelial cells to respond appropriately to inflammatory mediators, such as TNF and

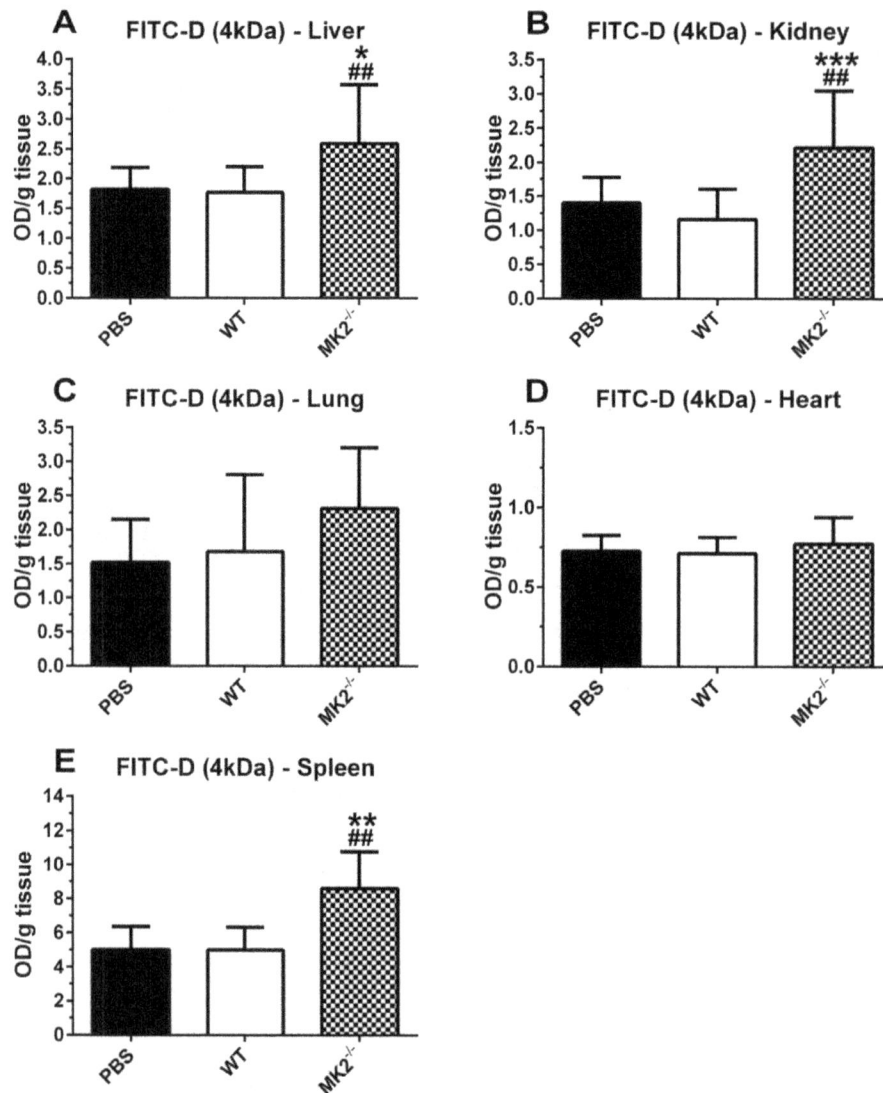

Figure 5 Vascular permeability assessed by extravasation of FITC-Dextran (4 kDa). FITC-Dextran quantification for WT and MK2$^{-/-}$ mice, 2.5 h after i.v. injection of 450 µg/kg TNF for liver **(A)**, kidney **(B)**, lung **(C)**, heart **(D)**, and spleen **(E)**; (n = 5 × 2 for liver, kidney and lungs; n = 5 for heart and spleen). Comparisons were made between baseline (PBS) and TNF challenged animals (#), and between genotypes (*) via one-way ANOVA with Sidak's multiple comparisons test. Error bars indicate SD. ***, p ≤ 0.001; **, p ≤ 0.01; *, p ≤ 0.05.

TNF-induced ROS, may then result in loss of barrier integrity because of cellular damage, and excessive fluid leak, which we observed in the liver, kidneys and spleen, culminating into end-organ failure and hyperacute mortality. The speed of these events was further emphasized by the pronounced drop in body temperature, starting as early as 90–120 min after TNF challenge, indicative for microcirculatory failure of end-organs. Curiously, we only observed increased permeability for a 4 kDa tracer, while no increased albumin (70 kDa) permeability was observed. This suggests that the failure of endothelial cells to reorganize their actin cytoskeleton appeared to result mainly in increased permeability for fluid and small solutes, while uncontrolled passage of larger molecules did not occur.

Contrary to our results, an earlier study reported decreased lung endothelial permeability for Evans Blue in an ovalbumin-induced asthma model [41], indicating that the response of stress-induced regulation of the cytoskeleton is highly dependent on the initial stressor and the dynamics of the model.

In order to extend our results to a more clinically relevant model of sepsis, MK2-deficient mice were subjected to CLP surgery. Also CLP-induced mortality was exacerbated in MK2-deficient mice. The reason for this increased sensitivity remains to be determined, but similar mechanisms as described for the TNF model could be involved. In addition, blocking TNF in CLP is known to actually exacerbate mortality [42]. Thus, reduced TNF levels in MK2-deficient animals because of increased instability of pro-inflammatory cytokine mRNAs could also have contributed to increased mortality.

Conclusions

In summary, we showed that MK2-deficient mice are highly sensitized to even very low doses of TNF, leading to hyperacute mortality. ROS play an important role in this pathophysiology since the phenotype could be rescued by antioxidant treatment with tempol. In addition, the failure of endothelial cells to respond to ROS-induced toxicity with an appropriate stress fiber response, required to preserve barrier function and efficiently regulate the immune response, appeared to be involved in the phenotype. In turn, this could have led to massive edema formation, increased cellular and tissue damage, and mortality. Our results thus corroborate the dependency of actin cytoskeletal dynamics on the stress-induced p38 MAPK/ MK2 pathway in an *in vivo* setting, and emphasize the importance of this pathway for stabilizing the endothelial barrier under conditions of oxidative stress. Multiple studies have highlighted the inflammation-driving role of MK2 and MK3 (reviewed in [43]) by showing that mice deficient for one or more of these kinases are protected against diverse inflammatory conditions, including arthritis, pancreatitis, skin inflammation, acute proliferative glomerulonephritis, colitis, cardiac ischemia-reperfusion injury [44], and asthma [41] or ventilator-induced [45] lung injury. Consequently, pharmacological inhibition of MK proteins has been proposed as a potential therapeutic strategy. However, our results warrant caution for the unbridled pharmacological targeting of MK2. Considering the pivotal role of TNF in many acute and chronic inflammatory conditions, systemic inhibition of MK2 could have potentially dangerous side effects at the level of endothelial barrier integrity.

Methods

Mice

MK2-deficient mice were generated on a C57BL/6J background, as described previously [6], and bred homozygously in our SPF facility. All mice were housed in temperature-controlled, individually ventilated cages in an SPF facility with 14/10 h light/dark cycles, food and water *ad libitum*, and used at 10–20 weeks of age. All experiments were approved by the animal ethics committee of the Faculty of Sciences of Ghent University (Belgium), performed according to its guidelines, and comply with Directive 2010/63/EU. For each experiment, mice were monitored every 30 min for the first 6 h, followed by several times daily until recovery. Moribund or surviving animals were euthanized by CO_2 asphyxiation, followed by cervical dislocation.

Reagents and injections

All reagents were dissolved in sterile phosphate buffered saline (PBS) and 200 µl was injected intravenously (i.v.), unless stated otherwise. Recombinant mouse TNF was produced in and purified from *Escherichia coli*, LPS content was <0.02 ng/mg (chromogenic *Limulus amebocyte* lysate assay), and was administered at various sublethal doses (10, 50, 125 or 250 µg/kg) or a lethal dose (450 µg/kg) for wild type (WT) mice. Phenol extracted *E. coli* LPS (serotype O111:B4) was purchased from Sigma (St. Louis, MO) and injected i.v. at 10 mg/kg. Tempol (Sigma) was injected intraperitoneally (i.p.) at 285 mg/kg (−45 min) and 125 mg/kg (+2.5 h). Superoxide dismutase (SOD, ICN, Aurora, OH) was injected i.p. at 3500 U/animal (−45 min) and 1800 U/animal (+2.5 h). 0.2% Evans blue (Sigma) and 50 mg/ml FITC-dextran (4 kDa, Sigma) were used to examine vascular permeability.

Cecal ligation and puncture surgery

The CLP procedure was performed as described earlier [46]. Briefly, the mice were anesthetized using 2% isoflurane in oxygen. After shaving and disinfecting the abdomen, a 10 mm midline laparotomy was performed, followed by exposure of the cecum. Using 5–0 Ethicon suture, the cecum was ligated immediately under the ileocecal valve and subsequently perforated by a single through-and-through puncture with a 22G needle. Next, the cecum was slightly compressed until a small drop of feces appeared. The abdomen was closed in two layers, using 5–0 suture for the peritoneum and abdominal musculature, and wound clips for the skin. Following surgery, the animals were resuscitated with 1 ml 0.9% saline subcutaneously. All animals were given pre- and postoperative analgesia (Ibuprofen, 200 µg/ml in drinking water), starting 24 h before until 48 h after surgery. Mice were randomized with regard to age and genotype.

Body temperature

Rectal body temperatures were recorded on an electronic thermometer (C28K, Comark Electronics; Littlehampton, UK).

Vascular permeability

Animals were injected with Evans blue and FITC-dextran 30 min before dissection, followed by terminal anesthesia with ketamine/xylazine and perfusion with 50 ml heparin (Sigma) in sterile saline (5 mg/ml). Liver, kidneys, lungs, heart and spleen were dissected, minced and incubated for 24 h at 37°C in formamide (Sigma) to extract the tracers. After clearance by centrifugation, Evans blue and FITC-dextran levels were determined at 620 nm and 520 nm, respectively.

Plasma NO$_x^-$, peroxide, and cytokine levels

EDTA plasma was prepared from blood collected via cardiac puncture after terminal anesthesia with ketamine/xylazine and immediately flash frozen in liquid nitrogen. Plasma concentrations of NO$_2^-$ and NO$_3^-$ (collectively NO$_x^-$) were determined via the Griess method as previously described [29]. Plasma peroxide equivalents were determined with a QuantiChrom Peroxide assay (DIOX-250, BioAssay Systems, CA) as per the manufacturer's instructions. IL-1β and IL-6 levels were determined with a Bio-Plex Pro cytokine kit (Bio-Rad, Hercules, CA), as per the manufacturer's instructions.

Plasma hexosaminidase and lactate dehydrogenase levels

Hexosaminidase levels were determined using p-nitrophenol-N-acetyl-β-D-glucosamine substrate as described previously [47]. Lactate dehydrogenase levels were determined with a CytoTox 96 assay (Promega, Madison, WI), as per the manufacturer's instructions.

Immunohistochemical detection of F-actin

Livers and kidneys were dissected and fixed in 4% PFA, followed by embedding in 5% low-melting point agarose (type VIIa, Sigma). Tissue sections of 60 μm were cut on a vibratome, stained with phalloidin Alexa Fluor 488 (1/25, Invitrogen, Paisley, UK) for 20 min at RT, and counterstained with DAPI nuclear staining (1/1000, Invitrogen). Images were taken on a Zeiss LSM780 confocal microscope (Carl Zeiss Microscopy, Jena, Germany) with a 100× Plan-Apochromat/1.46 oil objective. Pixel size was 0.083 μm at an image resolution of 1024 × 1024 pixels. DAPI was excited with a Ti:Sa Laser Mai Tai (Spectra-Physics) at 790 nm and detected with a spectral bandwidth of 415–494 nm by the PMT. Alexa fluor 488 was excited using the 488 line of a Multi-Argon laser and detected with a spectral bandwidth of 499–587 nm by the Quasar detection unit. The pinhole was set at 1 Airy Unit. 80 z-sections were made with 0.34 μm z-spacing. 3D segmentation was performed using Volocity™ software, version 6.1.5 (PerkinElmer Inc., Waltham, MA). Objects were identified in a manually defined region of interest. Intensity threshold was set at 38.5% and objects smaller than 0.01 μm^3 were discarded. For each region of interest the total number and volume of phalloidin-positive structures were determined. The number of objects per unit of volume was derived from these data, and the average size of the detected objects was calculated.

Statistical analysis

Statistical analysis was performed with GraphPad Prism 6.03 (GraphPad Software, La Jolla, CA (USA)). Survival results were compared to each other using a log-rank (Mantel-Cox) test. For *ex vivo* analysis, WT were compared to MK2-deficient animals via one-way ANOVA with Sidak's multiple comparisons test. Control (PBS) groups for both genetic backgrounds were pooled because they were statistically similar. Values are means ± SD.

Abbreviations

ARE: AU-rich element; CLP: Cecal ligation and puncture; D-Gal: D-Galactosamine; FITC: Fluorescein isothiocyanate; GSH: Glutathione; HuR: Human antigen R; HUVEC: Human umbilical vein endothelial cell; IFN: Interferon; IL: Interleukin; LDH: Lactate dehydrogenase; LPS: Lipopolysaccharide; MAPK: Mitogen-activated protein kinase; MK2: MAPK-activated protein kinase 2; NO: Nitric oxide; PMT: Photomultiplier tube; ROI: Region of interest; ROS: Reactive oxygen species; sHSP: Small heat shock protein; SOD: Superoxide dismutase; SPF: Specific pathogen free; TNF: Tumor necrosis factor; TTP: Tristetraprolin; WT: Wild type.

Competing interests

The authors declare that they have no competing interests.

Authors' contributions

BV designed experiments, acquired and analyzed data, and drafted the manuscript. AG designed experiments, acquired and analyzed data. AS acquired and analyzed data. EV acquired and analyzed the microscopy data. PB participated in project coordination and revised the manuscript. AC designed experiments, participated in project coordination and helped draft the manuscript. All authors read and approved the final manuscript.

Authors' information

An Goethals and Alba Simats share second authorship.
Peter Brouckaert and Anje Cauwels share senior authorship.

Acknowledgments

The authors thank Prof. Matthias Gaestel for kindly providing the MK2-deficient mice, Elke Rogge for technical assistance with experiments, and all animal caretakers of the Inflammation Research Center at VIB – Ghent University. Research was supported by the agency for Innovation by Science and Technology (IWT); Research Foundation Flanders (FWO); and Ghent University: Concerted Research Actions (GOA).

Author details

[1]Inflammation Research Center, VIB, 9052 Ghent, Belgium. [2]Department of Biomedical Molecular Biology, Ghent University, 9000 Ghent, Belgium. [3]Bio Imaging Core, Inflammation Research Center, VIB, 9052 Ghent, Belgium. [4]Cytokine Receptor Lab - Department of Medical Protein Research, VIB, 9000 Ghent, Belgium.

References

1. Ronkina N, Kotlyarov A, Gaestel M: MK2 and MK3–a pair of isoenzymes? *Front Biosci* 2008, **13**:5511–5521.
2. Cuadrado A, Nebreda AR: Mechanisms and functions of p38 MAPK signalling. *Biochem J* 2010, **429**:403–417.
3. Kotlyarov A, Gaestel M: Is MK2 (mitogen-activated protein kinase-activated protein kinase 2) the key for understanding post-transcriptional regulation of gene expression? *Biochem Soc Trans* 2002, **30**(Pt 6):959–963.
4. Ben-Levy R, Hooper S, Wilson R, Paterson HF, Marshall CJ: Nuclear export of the stress-activated protein kinase p38 mediated by its substrate MAPKAP kinase-2. *Curr Biol* 1998, **8**:1049–1057.
5. Anderson P: Post-transcriptional control of cytokine production. *Nat Immunol* 2008, **9**:353–359.
6. Kotlyarov A, Neininger A, Schubert C, Eckert R, Birchmeier C, Volk HD, Gaestel M: MAPKAP kinase 2 is essential for LPS-induced TNF-alpha biosynthesis. *Nat Cell Biol* 1999, **1**:94–97.
7. Neininger A, Kontoyiannis D, Kotlyarov A, Winzen R, Eckert R, Volk H-D, Holtmann H, Kollias G, Gaestel M: MK2 targets AU-rich elements and regulates biosynthesis of tumor necrosis factor and interleukin-6 independently at different post-transcriptional levels. *J Biol Chem* 2002, **277**:3065–3068.

MAPK-activated protein kinase 2-deficiency causes hyperacute tumor necrosis factor-induced...

191

8. Zhao W, Liu M, D'Silva NJ, Kirkwood KL: **Tristetraprolin regulates interleukin-6 expression through p38 MAPK-dependent affinity changes with mRNA 3′ untranslated region.** *J Interf Cytokine Res* 2011, **31:**629–637.

9. Ogilvie RL, Sternjohn JR, Rattenbacher B, Vlasova IA, Williams DA, Hau HH, Blackshear PJ, Bohjanen PR: **Tristetraprolin mediates interferon-gamma mRNA decay.** *J Biol Chem* 2009, **284:**11216–11223.

10. Wang X-Y, Tang Q-Q, Zhang J-L, Fang M-Y, Li Y-X: **Effect of SB203580 on pathologic change of pancreatic tissue and expression of TNF-α and IL-1β in rats with severe acute pancreatitis.** *Eur Rev Med Pharmacol Sci* 2014, **18:**338–343.

11. Carballo E, Lai WS, Blackshear PJ: **Feedback inhibition of macrophage tumor necrosis factor-alpha production by tristetraprolin.** *Science* 1998, **281:**1001–1005.

12. Chen CY, Gherzi R, Ong SE, Chan EL, Raijmakers R, Pruijn GJ, Stoecklin G, Moroni C, Mann M, Karin M: **AU binding proteins recruit the exosome to degrade ARE-containing mRNAs.** *Cell* 2001, **107:**451–464.

13. Deleault KM, Skinner SJ, Brooks SA: **Tristetraprolin regulates TNF TNF-alpha mRNA stability via a proteasome dependent mechanism involving the combined action of the ERK and p38 pathways.** *Mol Immunol* 2008, **45:**13–24.

14. Hitti E, Iakovleva T, Brook M, Deppenmeier S, Gruber AD, Radzioch D, Clark AR, Blackshear PJ, Kotlyarov A, Gaestel M: **Mitogen-activated protein kinase-activated protein kinase 2 regulates tumor necrosis factor mRNA stability and translation mainly by altering tristetraprolin expression, stability, and binding to adenine/uridine-rich element.** *Mol Cell Biol* 2006, **26:**2399–2407.

15. Mahtani KR, Brook M, Dean JL, Sully G, Saklatvala J, Clark AR: **Mitogen-activated protein kinase p38 controls the expression and posttranslational modification of tristetraprolin, a regulator of tumor necrosis factor alpha mRNA stability.** *Mol Cell Biol* 2001, **21:**6461–6469.

16. Tiedje C, Ronkina N, Tehrani M, Dhamija S, Laass K, Holtmann H, Kotlyarov A, Gaestel M: **The p38/MK2-driven exchange between tristetraprolin and HuR regulates AU-rich element-dependent translation.** *PLoS Genet* 2012, **8:**e1002977.

17. Ronkina N, Kotlyarov A, Dittrich-Breiholz O, Kracht M, Hitti E, Milarski K, Askew R, Marusic S, Lin L-L, Gaestel M, Telliez J-B: **The mitogen-activated protein kinase (MAPK)-activated protein kinases MK2 and MK3 cooperate in stimulation of tumor necrosis factor biosynthesis and stabilization of p38 MAPK.** *Mol Cell Biol* 2007, **27:**170–181.

18. Lavoie JN, Hickey E, Weber LA, Landry J: **Modulation of actin microfilament dynamics and fluid phase pinocytosis by phosphorylation of heat shock protein 27.** *J Biol Chem* 1993, **268:**24210–24214.

19. Haslbeck M, Franzmann T, Weinfurtner D, Buchner J: **Some like it hot: the structure and function of small heat-shock proteins.** *Nat Struct Mol Biol* 2005, **12:**842–846.

20. Arrigo A-P, Virot S, Chaufour S, Firdaus W, Kretz-Remy C, Diaz-Latoud C: **Hsp27 consolidates intracellular redox homeostasis by upholding glutathione in its reduced form and by decreasing iron intracellular levels.** *Antioxid Redox Signal* 2005, **7:**414–422.

21. Mounier N, Arrigo A-P: **Actin cytoskeleton and small heat shock proteins: how do they interact?** *Cell Stress Chaperon* 2002, **7:**167–176.

22. Vandenbroucke E, Mehta D, Minshall R, Malik AB: **Regulation of endothelial junctional permeability.** *Ann N Y Acad Sci* 2008, **1123:**134–145.

23. Bogatcheva NV, Verin AD: **Reprint of "The role of cytoskeleton in the regulation of vascular endothelial barrier function" [Microvascular Research 76 (2008) 202–207].** *Microvasc Res* 2009, **77:**64–69.

24. Nehls V, Drenckhahn D: **Demonstration of actin filament stress fibers in microvascular endothelial cells in situ.** *Microvasc Res* 1991, **42:**103–112.

25. Millán J, Cain RJ, Reglero-Real N, Bigarella C, Marcos-Ramiro B, Fernández-Martín L, Correas I, Ridley AJ: **Adherens junctions connect stress fibres between adjacent endothelial cells.** *BMC Biol* 2010, **8:**11.

26. Lampugnani MG: **Endothelial adherens junctions and the actin cytoskeleton: an "infinity net"?** *J Biol* 2010, **9:**16.

27. Mignon A, Rouquet N, Fabre M, Martin S, Pagès JC, Dhainaut JF, Kahn A, Briand P, Joulin V: **LPS challenge in D-galactosamine-sensitized mice accounts for caspase-dependent fulminant hepatitis, not for septic shock.** *Am J Respir Crit Care Med* 1999, **159:**1308–1315.

28. Cauwels A, Janssen B, Waeytens A, Cuvelier C, Brouckaert P: **Caspase inhibition causes hyperacute tumor necrosis factor-induced shock via oxidative stress and phospholipase A2.** *Nat Immunol* 2003, **4:**387–393.

29. Cauwels A, Rogge E, Janssen B, Brouckaert P: **Reactive oxygen species and small-conductance calcium-dependent potassium channels are key mediators of inflammation-induced hypotension and shock.** *J Mol Med* 2010, **88:**921–930.

30. Wilcox CS, Pearlman A: **Chemistry and antihypertensive effects of tempol and other nitroxides.** *Pharmacol Rev* 2008, **60:**418–469.

31. Mehlen P, Hickey E, Weber LA, Arrigo AP: **Large unphosphorylated aggregates as the active form of hsp27 which controls intracellular reactive oxygen species and glutathione levels and generates a protection against TNFalpha in NIH-3 T3-ras cells.** *Biochem Biophys Res Commun* 1997, **241:**187–192.

32. Ehrnsperger M, Gräber S, Gaestel M, Buchner J: **Binding of non-native protein to Hsp25 during heat shock creates a reservoir of folding intermediates for reactivation.** *EMBO J* 1997, **16:**221–229.

33. Rogalla T, Ehrnsperger M, Preville X, Kotlyarov A, Lutsch G, Ducasse C, Paul C, Wieske M, Arrigo AP, Buchner J, Gaestel M: **Regulation of Hsp27 oligomerization, chaperone function, and protective activity against oxidative stress/tumor necrosis factor alpha by phosphorylation.** *J Biol Chem* 1999, **274:**18947–18956.

34. Benndorf R, Hayess K, Ryazantsev S, Wieske M, Behlke J, Lutsch G: **Phosphorylation and supramolecular organization of murine small heat shock protein HSP25 abolish its actin polymerization-inhibiting activity.** *J Biol Chem* 1994, **269:**20780–20784.

35. Huot J, Houle F, Marceau F, Landry J: **Oxidative stress-induced actin reorganization mediated by the p38 mitogen-activated protein kinase/heat shock protein 27 pathway in vascular endothelial cells.** *Circ Res* 1997, **80:**383–392.

36. Goldblum SE, Ding X, Campbell-Washington J: **TNF-alpha induces endothelial cell F-actin depolymerization, new actin synthesis, and barrier dysfunction.** *Am J Physiol* 1993, **264**(4 Pt 1):C894–C905.

37. Mehlen P, Mehlen A, Guillet D, Preville X, Arrigo AP: **Tumor necrosis factor-alpha induces changes in the phosphorylation, cellular localization, and oligomerization of human hsp27, a stress protein that confers cellular resistance to this cytokine.** *J Cell Biochem* 1995, **58:**248–259.

38. Kiemer AK, Weber NC, Fürst R, Bildner N, Kulhanek-Heinze S, Vollmar AM: **Inhibition of p38 MAPK Activation via Induction of MKP-1: Atrial Natriuretic Peptide Reduces TNF-alpha-Induced Actin Polymerization and Endothelial Permeability.** *Circ Res* 2002, **90:**874–881.

39. McKenzie JAG, Ridley AJ: **Roles of Rho/ROCK and MLCK in TNF-alpha-induced changes in endothelial morphology and permeability.** *J Cell Physiol* 2007, **213:**221–228.

40. Bogatcheva NV, Garcia JGN, Verin AD: **Molecular mechanisms of thrombin-induced endothelial cell permeability.** *Biochemistry* 2002, **67:**75–84.

41. Gorska MM, Liang Q, Stafford SJ, Goplen N, Dharajiya N, Guo L, Sur S, Gaestel M, Alam R: **MK2 controls the level of negative feedback in the NF-kappaB pathway and is essential for vascular permeability and airway inflammation.** *J Exp Med* 2007, **204:**1637–1652.

42. Eskandari MK, Bolgos G, Miller C, Nguyen DT, DeForge LE, Remick DG: **Anti-tumor necrosis factor antibody therapy fails to prevent lethality after cecal ligation and puncture or endotoxemia.** *J Immunol* 1992, **148:**2724–2730.

43. Gaestel M: **What goes up must come down: molecular basis of MAPKAP kinase 2/3-dependent regulation of the inflammatory response and its inhibition.** *Biol Chem* 2013, **394:**1301–1315.

44. Shiroto K, Otani H, Yamamoto F, Huang C-K, Maulik N, Das DK: **MK2−/− gene knockout mouse hearts carry anti-apoptotic signal and are resistant to ischemia reperfusion injury.** *J Mol Cell Cardiol* 2005, **38:**93–97.

45. Damarla M, Hasan E, Boueiz A, Le A, Pae HH, Montouchet C, Kolb T, Simms T, Myers A, Kayyali US, Gaestel M, Peng X, Reddy SP, Damico R, Hassoun PM: **Mitogen activated protein kinase activated protein kinase 2 regulates actin polymerization and vascular leak in ventilator associated lung injury.** *PLoS One* 2009, **4:**e4600.

46. Rittirsch D, Huber-Lang MS, Flierl MA, Ward PA: **Immunodesign of experimental sepsis by cecal ligation and puncture.** *Nat Protoc* 2009, **4:**31–36.

47. Wendeler M, Sandhoff K: **Hexosaminidase assays.** *Glycoconj J* 2009, **26:**945–952.

16

VEGF induces sensory and motor peripheral plasticity, alters bladder function, and promotes visceral sensitivity

Anna P Malykhina[1], Qi Lei[1], Chris S Erickson[2], Miles L Epstein[2], Marcia R Saban[3], Carole A Davis[3] and Ricardo Saban[3*]

Abstract

Background: This work tests the hypothesis that bladder instillation with vascular endothelial growth factor (VEGF) modulates sensory and motor nerve plasticity, and, consequently, bladder function and visceral sensitivity. In addition to C57BL/6J, ChAT-cre mice were used for visualization of bladder cholinergic nerves. The direct effect of VEGF on the density of sensory nerves expressing the transient receptor potential vanilloid subfamily 1 (TRPV1) and cholinergic nerves (ChAT) was studied one week after one or two intravesical instillations of the growth factor. To study the effects of VEGF on bladder function, mice were intravesically instilled with VEGF and urodynamic evaluation was assessed. VEGF-induced alteration in bladder dorsal root ganglion (DRG) neurons was performed on retrogradly labeled urinary bladder afferents by patch-clamp recording of voltage gated Na+ currents. Determination of VEGF-induced changes in sensitivity to abdominal mechanostimulation was performed by application of von Frey filaments.

Results: In addition to an overwhelming increase in TRPV1 immunoreactivity, VEGF instillation resulted in an increase in ChAT-directed expression of a fluorescent protein in several layers of the urinary bladder. Intravesical VEGF caused a profound change in the function of the urinary bladder: acute VEGF (1 week post VEGF treatment) reduced micturition pressure and longer treatment (2 weeks post-VEGF instillation) caused a substantial reduction in inter-micturition interval. In addition, intravesical VEGF resulted in an up-regulation of voltage gated Na$^+$ channels (VGSC) in bladder DRG neurons and enhanced abdominal sensitivity to mechanical stimulation.

Conclusions: For the first time, evidence is presented indicating that VEGF instillation into the mouse bladder promotes a significant increase in peripheral nerve density together with alterations in bladder function and visceral sensitivity. The VEGF pathway is being proposed as a key modulator of neural plasticity in the pelvis and enhanced VEGF content may be associated with visceral hyperalgesia, abdominal discomfort, and/or pelvic pain.

Background

It is highly likely that neurogenic dysfunction of the urinary bladder is involved in various disorders of the lower urinary tract (LUT) including neurogenic bladder, outflow obstruction, idiopathic detrusor instability, overactive bladder, painful bladder syndrome, and diabetic neuropathy. In addition, chronic pathological conditions that cause tissue irritation or inflammation can alter the properties of sensory pathways, leading to a reduction in pain threshold and/or an amplification of painful sensation (hyperalgesia) [1].

Depending on the pathology, several mediators and their respective receptors have been proposed to modulate peripheral nerve plasticity in the LUT, including but not limited to: purinergic receptors in general [2] or P2X receptor in particular [3], TRPV1 [1,4], substance P acting on NK1 receptors [5], protease activated receptors [6], and nerve growth factor and its receptors [7].

* Correspondence: ricardo-saban@ouhsc.edu
[3]Department of Physiology, College of Medicine, Urinary Tract Physiological Genomics Laboratory, University of Oklahoma Health Sciences Center (OUHSC), 800 Research Parkway, Room 410, Oklahoma City, OK 73104, USA
Full list of author information is available at the end of the article

In this context, the development of cross-sensitization in the pelvis is one of the suggested mechanisms underlying co-morbidity of pelvic disorders which is frequently observed in the clinical setting [8]. Recently, evidence indicated that acute colonic inflammation triggers the occurrence of urinary bladder detrusor instability via activation of the transient receptor potential vanilloid subfamily 1 (TRPV1) related pathways [4]. Moreover, colonic inflammation-induced activation of TRPV1 receptors at the peripheral sensory terminals results in an up-regulation of voltage gated Na^+ channels on the cell soma of bladder sensory neurons [9]. This increase in channels may underlie the occurrence of peripheral cross-sensitization in the pelvis and functional chronic pelvic pain [9].

The new hypothesis being tested in this manuscript is that increased levels of VEGF observed during bladder inflammation provoke nerve plasticity. This hypothesis is based on evidence indicating that nerves and blood vessels are anatomically associated, follow a common molecular pathway during development, and their maturation in adulthood may be controlled by the same key molecules responsible for their development [10,11]. The finding that mutant mice (neurogenin1/neurogenin2 double knockout embryos) lacking sensory nerves also show disorganized blood vessel branching [12], suggests that local signals such as VEGF supplied by nerve fibers, may provide a cue that determines blood vessel patterning.

Evidence has been presented supporting the hypothesis that many proteins that were originally discovered to be required for axon guidance are implicated in the development of the vascular [11] and lymphatic systems [13]. But perhaps the most striking observation linking the nervous and vascular systems is the finding that angiogenic factors, when deregulated, contribute to various neurological disorders, such as neurodegeneration. The prototypic example of this cross-talk between nerves and vessels is the vascular endothelial growth factor, VEGF [14]. Although originally described as a key angiogenic and permeability factor, it is now well established that VEGF also plays a crucial role in the development of the nervous system [14].

Recently, we provided evidence that chronic inflammation increases the density of bladder sensory nerves that express: a) the transient receptor potential vanilloid subfamily 1 (TRPV1) [15], b) protein gene product (PGP9.5) [16], c) substance P, and d) calcitonin gene-related peptide (CGRP) [17]. We also determined that B20, a VEGF neutralizing antibody, prevented inflammation-induced increase in sensory nerves [17]. Furthermore, instillation of VEGF into the bladder recapitulated the effect of inflammation on sensory nerve plasticity [17], and represents direct evidence of VEGF action on the peripheral nervous system.

The scope of the present work was to determine whether VEGF, in addition to increased sensory nerve density, also alters the density of cholinergic nerves, and, consequently, bladder function and visceral sensitivity.

Results

Instillation of VEGF into the mouse bladder results in an increase in sensory nerve density

It was reported that VEGF is expressed at relatively higher amounts in nerves than in the surrounding mesenchymal tissue [12]. This finding led to a new appreciation of the role of VEGF in neuronal development [14,18] and stimulated us to review a possible link between VEGF-induced inflammation and bladder nerve plasticity. To provide direct evidence that VEGF induces bladder neuronal plasticity, VEGF was instilled into the C57BL/6 mouse bladder. Previous results from our laboratory indicated that acute or chronic instillation of VEGF into the mouse bladder caused inflammation, characterized predominantly by the accumulation of macrophages [17], and an increase in sensory nerve density as indicated by image analysis of nerve fibers positive for the nociceptive transducer vanilloid type 1 transient receptor potential receptor (TRPV1) [17]. In the present manuscript, we expanded the time course of VEGF exposure by including a group that received two weekly instillations of VEGF. Female C57BL/6 mice were instilled weekly for two weeks with VEGF (6.41 nM in 100 µl). Mice were euthanized one week after the second VEGF instillation and the bladder was removed for image analysis of TRPV1-positive fibers. One VEGF instillation promotes a substantial increase in TRPV1-positive fibers in the urothelium and lamina propria (Figure 1A) and in the detrusor and adventitia (Figure 1B). Two VEGF instillations resulted in the most pronounced alteration in sensory nerve plasticity, as indicated by a peak increase in TRPV1-positive fibers. After the 4th weekly treatment with VEGF, the response was reduced. Similar results were obtained with ChAT mice indicating that 1 and 2 weekly VEGF instillations provoked similar increases in TRPV1 immune reactivity (data not shown). These results provide direct evidence that VEGF participates in the plasticity of bladder sensory nerves and that two weekly instillations of VEGF produced the largest increase in sensory nerve density.

A mouse model for the study of bladder cholinergic innervation

We sought to extend our studies by investigating whether VEGF also alters the plasticity of bladder cholinergic nerves. The rationale for the use of the ChAT-cre mouse model was based on reports that staining

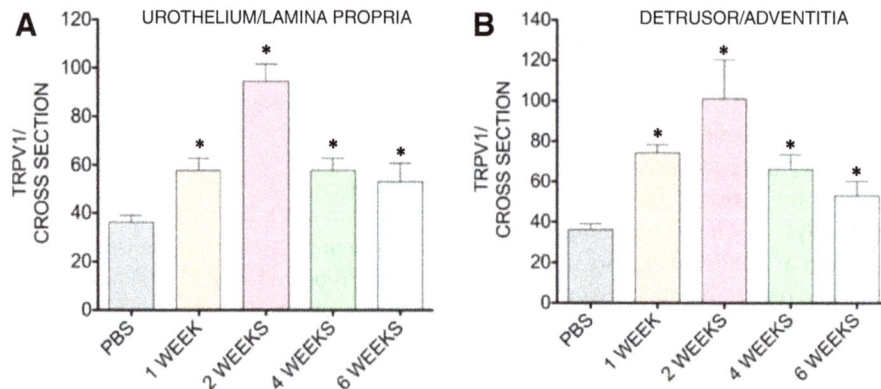

Figure 1 Intravesical instillation of VEGF induces a time-dependent alteration in the density of TRPV1-positive sensory fibers in the urothelium and lamina propria (A) and detrusor and and adventitia (B) layers. Quantification of TRPV1-IR in the C57BL/6 urinary bladder isolated 1 week after: 1, 2, 4, and 6 weekly instillations of VEGF of PBS (N=8 per group). Asterisks indicate a statistically significant difference (p values < 0.05) when compared to the PBS group.

peripheric nerves with antibodies targeting the synthe-sizing enzyme choline acetyltransferase (ChAT) is not consistent and often fails to detect these neurons. In contrast, cholinergic neurons and fibers of the urinary bladder and surrounding tissues are readily visualized in whole mount preparations isolated from adult ChAT mice (Figure 2A and 2B). High quality photomicro-graphs were used to detailed the disctribution of ChAT-positive nerves (Figure 2C, 2D, and 2E). However, using these high quality micrographs, we found the pelvic gan-glia to be so intensely fluorescent that the signals from the surrounding tissues were not readily apparent (Figure 2C, red circle). When the fluorescence of the PG region was electronically reduced, it was possible to image the innervation of the colon, uterus, and urinary bladder (Figure 2D). Both preparations also allow the

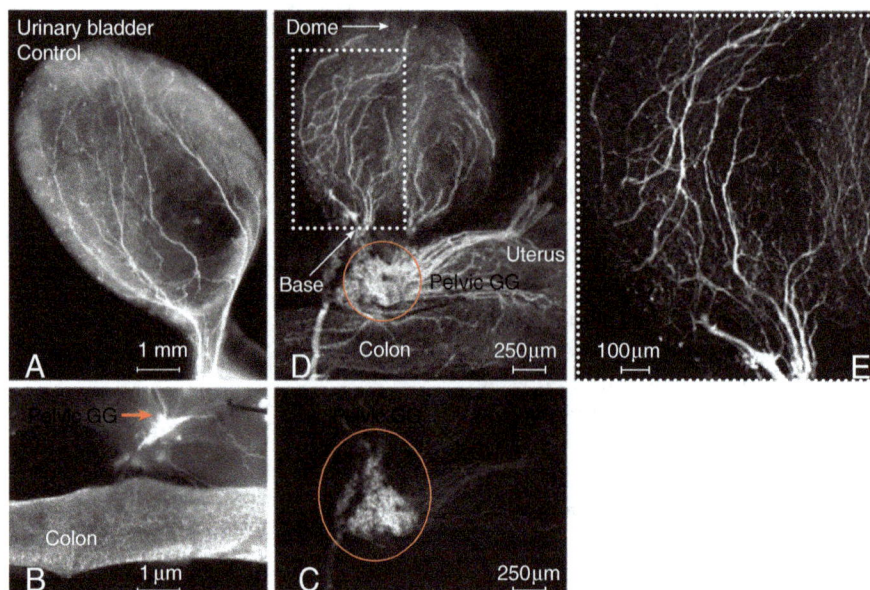

Figure 2 A ChAT transgenic mouse permits the visualization of cholinergic cells and fibers in a pelvic ganglion and cholinergic fibers in the urinary bladder, gastrointestinal tract, and uterus. Representative photomicrographs of whole mount preparations of the urinary bladder removed from ChAT mice instilled with PBS (**A**). The pelvic ganglion and colon are also illustrated. (**B**). ChAT nerves appeared intact confirming previous results that intravesical instillation does not cause damage to the bladder wall. **C**, **D**, and **E** are confocal photomicrographs of whole mount preparations isolated from another control ChAT mouse. An intense fluorescence was observed in the pelvic ganglion region (**C**). In order to permit visualization of the ChAT-positive fibers in the bladder, uterus, and colon, the intensity of the pelvic ganglion (red circle) was reduced. **E** is a high magnification of the area delimited by the white dotted rectangle in figure **D** and permits the visualization of large and small cholinergic fibers innervating the urinary bladder.

visualization of the pelvic ganglia and its relationship with cholinergic nerves innervating the urinary bladder and other pelvic organs (Figure 2B and 2C), which will permit the capture of these cells for future patch clamp studies. Figure 2E is a high magnification image of the dotted square region of Figure 2D and shows the large superficial nerve trunks innervating the adventitial coat. As described in cross-sections presented below, these fibers penetrate deep into the lamina propria and ramify in the urothelium.

In order to confirm that ChAT positive fibers crossing the urinary bladder were indeed nerve fibers, we stained with an antibody targeting the class III β-tubulin, a specific neuronal marker [19]. Both β-III tubulin- and ChAT-positive fibers are distributed within the urothelium and detrusor smooth muscle (Figure 3A-D). Areas highlighted by dotted squares in Figure 3D were photographed at higher magnification to discriminate the overlap of the green and red fluorescence in the urothelium

(Figure 3E-H) and detrusor smooth muscle (Figure 3I-L). These images indicate substantial overlap between the cholinergic and tubulin markers and thus show that the cholinergic fibers are indeed neuronal.

An analysis of images from sections shows the relative density of ChAT fluorescent fibers in the urothelium, lamina propria (sub-urothelium), detrusor muscle, and adventitia in comparison with areas immunostained by a pan-neuronal marker (PGP9.5), sensory nerves (TRPV1), and substance P containing fibers (Figure 4). It has to be noted that PGP9.5 antibodies resulted in a non-specific labeling of the urothelial layer. A reasonable explanation for this artifact is that the methods recommended for permeabilization of the tissues caused such labeling. These findings precluded the use of the urothelium for quantification purposes of PGP9.5 but not for TRPV1 and SP. PGP9.5 image analysis was performed in two layers: the detrusor smooth muscle and the sub-urothelium that extended from the basal layer of the

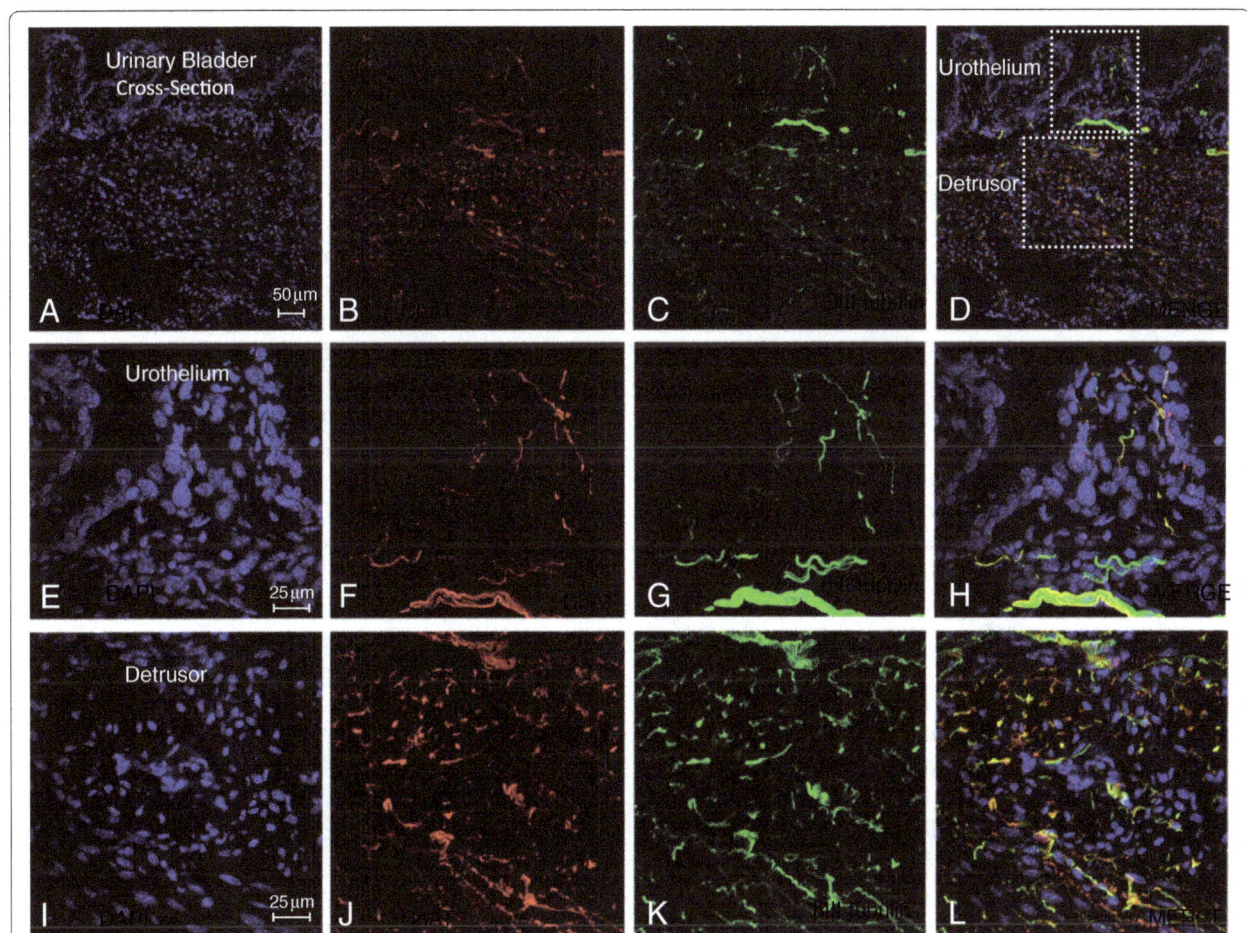

Figure 3 ChAT–positive fibers are nerve elements. Representative photomicrographs of 12 μm thick cross-sections of the urinary bladder isolated from ChAT mice. Sections were stained with DAPI (4′,6-diamidino-2-phenylindole) to highlight the cell nucleus and with class III β-tubulin antibody. **A-D** illustrates that both β-III tubulin- and ChAT-positive fibers are distributed within the urothelium and detrusor smooth muscle. Areas highlighted by dotted squares in **D** were photographed at higher magnification to show the overlap of beta-III tubulin(green)- and ChAT (red)- positive fibers fluorescence in the urothelium (**E-H**) and detrusor smooth muscle (**I-L**).

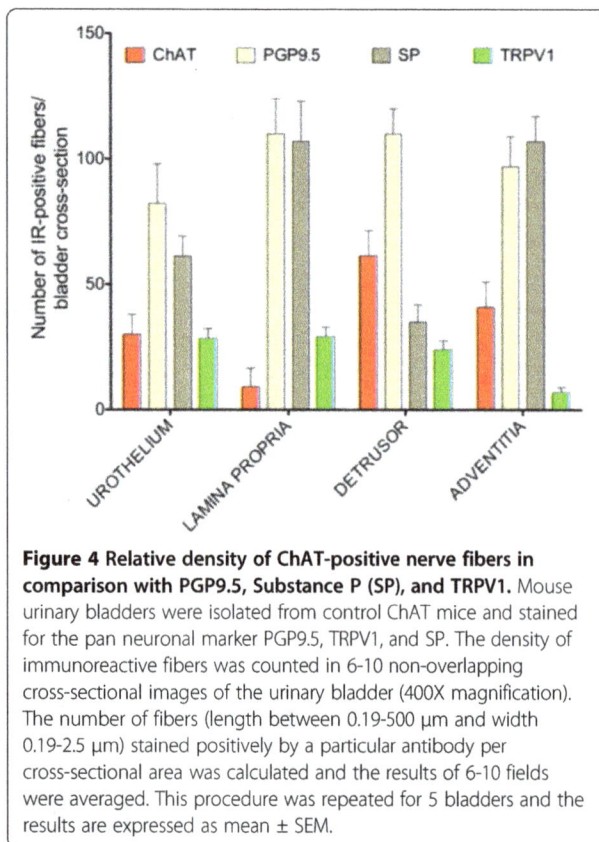

Figure 4 Relative density of ChAT-positive nerve fibers in comparison with PGP9.5, Substance P (SP), and TRPV1. Mouse urinary bladders were isolated from control ChAT mice and stained for the pan neuronal marker PGP9.5, TRPV1, and SP. The density of immunoreactive fibers was counted in 6-10 non-overlapping cross-sectional images of the urinary bladder (400X magnification). The number of fibers (length between 0.19-500 μm and width 0.19-2.5 μm) stained positively by a particular antibody per cross-sectional area was calculated and the results of 6-10 fields were averaged. This procedure was repeated for 5 bladders and the results are expressed as mean ± SEM.

urothelium to detrusor. Overall, these results indicate ChAT nerves are more prominent in the detrusor muscle when compared to TRPV1 nerves, whereas, TRPV1 nerves are more prominent than ChAT nerves in the lamina propria.

The finding that both sensory (TRPV1-positive) and cholinergic nerves are involved in urinary tract disorders such as overactive bladders [20] raises the question of whether these two systems are anatomically distinct. Therefore, we sought to determine whether sensory and motor nerves are co-localized in urinary bladder. Using bladder whole mounts that underwent blunt dissection to separate the lamina propria from the detrusor (Figure 5), we observed that TRPV1 and ChAT signals appear to overlap in the lamina propria (yellow arrow on Figure 5D) and to a lesser degree in the detrusor smooth muscle (Figure 5H). However, high magnification photomicrographs (Figures 5I-L) indicate that the two types of fibers are separate and run adjacent to each other, primarily around the blood vessels (Figure 5L). Photomicrographs of bladder cross-sections confirm the results obtained with whole mounts (Figure 6D). In addition, higher magnification images illustrate the separation of TRPV1 and ChAT fibers in intramural ganglia (Figure 6H) as well as in the lamina propria (Figure 6L). We conclude that the sensory and motor components do not overlap.

VEGF instillation increases the number of ChAT positive fibers

Figure 7 contains representative photomicrographs of urinary bladders isolated from control and VEGF-treated ChAT mice. These cross-sections suggest that VEGF treatment resulted in an increased density of ChAT- (Figure 7B and 7E) and TRPV1- positive fibers (Figure 7C and 7F). For better appreciation of sensory and cholinergic nerves, merged microphotographs were digitally amplified and are presented on Figure 7G and 7H (note the calibration bar on Figures 7G and H and compare with the bars on Figures 7A and D). Image analysis of nerve density indicates that single or repeated challenge of mouse bladders with VEGF resulted in a significant increase in ChAT density in the urothelium, lamina propria, and detrusor smooth muscle (Figure 8). Together these results indicate that in addition to alterations of peripheral sensory nerve plasticity (Figure 1), direct administration of VEGF also promotes an increase in bladder cholinergic nerve plasticity.

Urodynamic analysis of bladder function after intravesical VEGF instillation in awake (unrestrained) mice

To evaluate the effects of intravesical VEGF on urodynamic parameters and function of the urinary bladder *in vivo*, we performed cystometric assessment in conscious mice. Micturition cycles were first recorded under control conditions (N=5) and served as a baseline (internal control) followed by urodynamic evaluation at 1 and 2 weeks after beginning VEGF treatment. Figure 9 shows raw cystometric traces recorded in the same animal before (Figure 9A, baseline) and 2 weeks after intravesical VEGF (Figure 9B). Urodynamic parameters were first compared to the baseline for each mouse followed by further comparisons between the groups (before and after treatment). Intravesical VEGF caused significant changes in the function of the urinary bladder over the course of treatment (Figure 9B).

At 1 week post-VEGF, significant changes included a reduction in micturition pressure (19.75 ± 0.53 mmHg at baseline *vs* 14.4 ± 0.32 mmHg at 1 week, (Figure 10B, p≤0.005) and decreased micturition volume (by 26% in comparison to baseline, (p≤0.001, Figure 10C). These parameters were also significantly reduced 2 weeks after the initiation of VEGF treatment. Longer treatment (2 weeks) caused a substantial reduction in inter-micturition interval from 341.2 ± 25.6 s to 188.0 ± 20.8 s (p≤0.001, Figure 10A) and a decrease in bladder capacity from 57.1 ± 4.3 μl to 31.6 ± 3.5 μl (p≤0.001, Figure 10D). There was a tendency towards an increase in the number of non-micturition contractions (pointed by arrows in Figure 9B) after intravesical VEGF, although the difference did not reach statistical significance (Figure 10E). Other cystometric parameters such as intermicturition pressure interval,

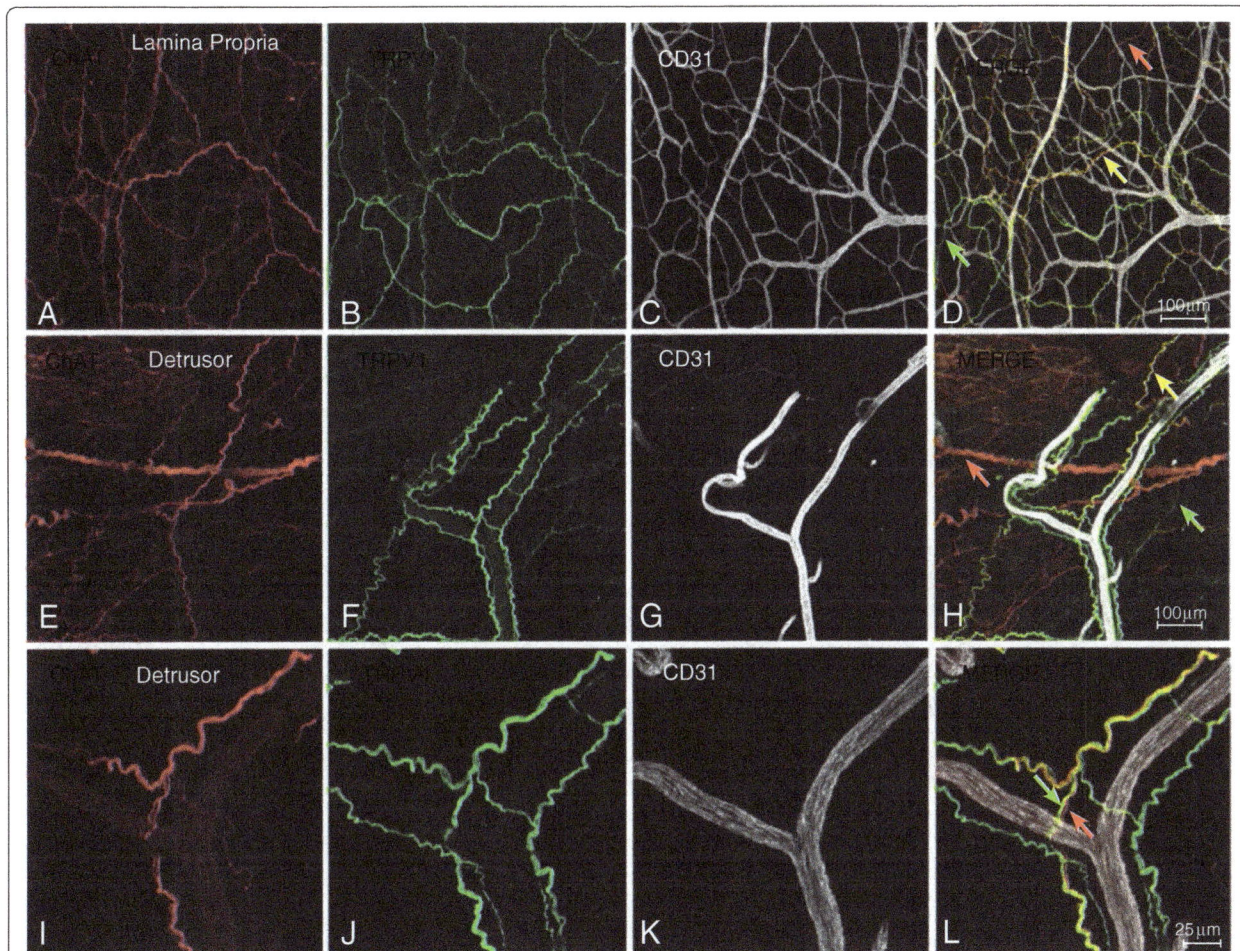

Figure 5 Representative photomicrographs of bladder whole mounts showing ChAT-positive nerve fibers, sensory nerves (TRPV1), and blood vessels (CD31). Representative photomicrographs taken from bladders isolated from ChAT mice and prepared as whole mounts that underwent blunt dissection to separate the lamina propria from the detrusor. In the lamina propria (**D**) the ChAT and TRPV1 fibers are usually associated (yellow arrow) but sometimes take separate paths (red and green arrows). In the detrusor (**H**) ChAT-positive fibers dominate although the ChAT and TRPV1 fibers around blood vessels are usually associated (yellow arrow). High magnification microphotographs (**I-L**) indicate that the two type of fibers run adjacent to each other (**L**).

threshold pressure and basal pressure were unaltered by VEGF treatment. Additional group of mice (N=5) underwent intravesical instillations with PBS and cystometric parameters were recorded at the same time points as in the VEGF group. Intravesical PBS did not significantly affect the function of the urinary bladder (Figure 10A-E). In addition, the baseline values did not differed between the PBS and VEGF groups and, therefore, baseline values were combined in Figure 10.

Intravesical VEGF caused an up-regulation of voltage gated Na$^+$ channels (VGSC) in bladder DRG neurons

It is well established that bladder inflammation causes an increase in VGSC expressed in sensory neurons receiving input from the urinary bladder [21]. In this set of experiments we aimed to determine if intravesical VEGF would cause any changes in VGSC, thereby, affecting neuronal excitability of bladder projecting afferents.

Retrograde labeling of lumbosacral sensory neurons with Fast Blue allowed identification of bladder projecting DRG cells used for electrophysiological recordings and data analysis. Bladder inflammation caused by intravesical VEGF triggered an increase in the amplitude of total Na$^+$ current recorded from bladder afferent neurons. Representative raw recordings of total Na$^+$ current obtained from the control (intravesical PBS) and experimental (intravesical VEGF) groups are presented in Figure 11A. The current–voltage (I-V) relationship of total Na$^+$ current normalized to the cell size shows that these neurons produced a large amplitude Na$^+$ current upon membrane depolarization, reaching maximal amplitude at -20 mV (Figure 11B). VEGF application increased the peak amplitude of total Na$^+$ current in bladder DRG

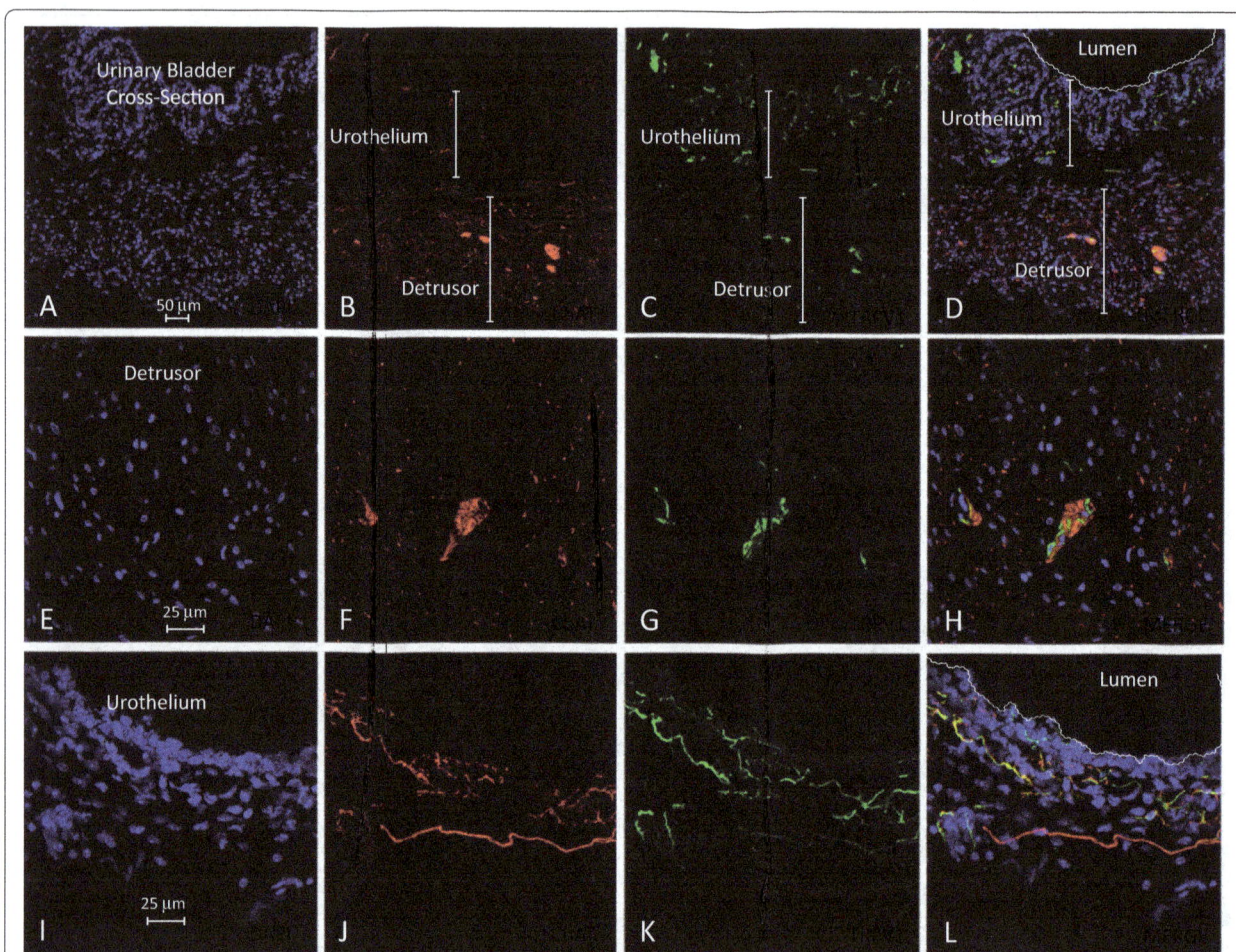

Figure 6 Photomicrographs of bladder cross-sections confirm the results obtained with whole mounts and indicate the predominance of TRPV1 fibers in the urothelium and the predominance of ChAT fibers in the detrusor smooth muscle. **A-D** are representative photomicrographs of the entire bladder cross section. **E-H** are representative photomicrographs of the detrusor smooth muscle taken at high magnification to show some areas of overlap between ChAT and TRPV1, primarily in intramural fascicles (**H**). **I- L** are representative photomicrographs of bladder urothelium taken at high magnification to show some areas of overlap between ChAT and TRPV1, primarily in the lamina propria (sub urothelium), as illustrate (**L**).

neurons at -10 mV from -152.1 ± 16.8 pA/pF (n=11) in the control group to -253.5 ± 43.5 pA/pF (n=9) in the VEGF group (p≤0.05). Significant enhancement of total Na^+ current was observed at all voltages from -30 mV to +20 mV (Figure 11B).

We next assessed the kinetic parameters of total Na^+ currents after the induction of neurogenic bladder inflammation caused by VEGF. The steady-state activation was studied by using a three-pulse protocol with a negative pre-pulse to -110 mV and a series of short depolarizing pulses (10 ms duration) to activate Na^+ currents (Figure 12A, top panel). The amplitude of steady-state activation was measured at the peak of tail current upon the voltage step to -70 mV, normalized and plotted as I/I_{max} against the voltage (Figure 12A, lower panel). Intravesical VEGF led to the leftward shift in the steady-state activation of total Na^+ current by 8 mV ($V_{1/2}$=-19.9

± 2.6 mV in the control group *vs* -27.6± 2.0 mV at 2 weeks of treatment, Figure 12B, p≤0.05). The amplitude of steady-state inactivation was measured at a series of membrane depolarizing steps ranging from -100 mV to +70 mV (Figure 12C). Bladder inflammation did not affect the parameters of steady-state inactivation of total Na^+ current in bladder sensory neurons (Figure 12D).

VEGF triggered an enhanced abdominal sensitivity to mechanical stimulation with von Frey filaments

Abdominal sensitivity was tested in a separate group of mice (N=7) before and after bladder treatments with VEGF. Figure 13 summarizes the frequency of responses to von Frey filament testing in the lower abdominal area before, and 1 week and 2 weeks after intravesical instillations of VEGF in the same group of mice. The response frequency correlated with the applied force, reaching a

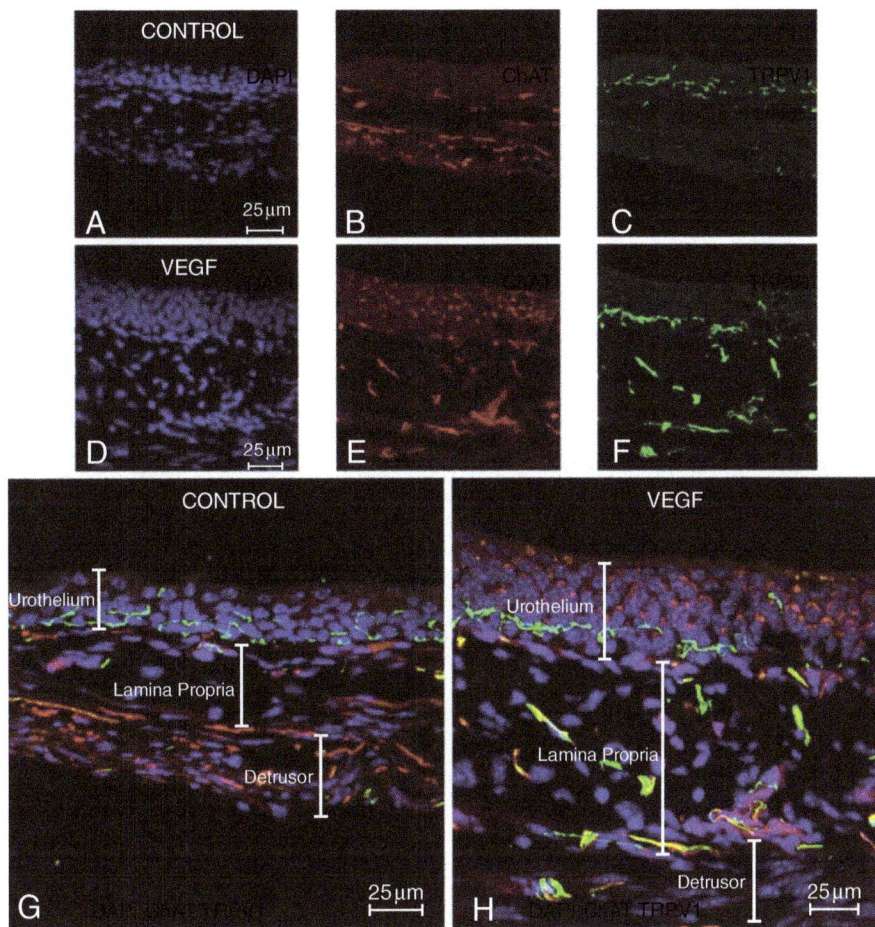

Figure 7 Representative photomicrographs of ChAT mouse bladder cross-sections isolated from control and a single VEGF instillation (Table 1). Flattened images from 10 μm thick cross-sections from control and VEGF treated are presented side by side to permit comparison. DAPI staining highlighted the cell nuclei (**A** and **D**), ChAT was visualized by the fluorescent protein (td tomato; **B** and **E**), and sensory nerves were identified by TRPV1 immunoreactivity (**C** and **F**). Enlarged and merged microphotographs are presented to permit a better appreciation of the differences between control (**G**) and VEGF-treated bladders (**H**).

plateau of 20% at the maximal tested force of 4 g (Figure 13). One week after VEGF treatment, mice became more sensitive to the filament testing and responses reached more than 40% at lower forces of 0.16 g and 0.4 g (Figure 13, p≤0.05 to baseline). Two weeks after the treatment the frequency response showed significant differences with stimuli of 1 and 4 g filaments in comparison to 1 week (Figure 13, p≤0.05 to baseline).

These results provide evidence that intravesical VEGF leads to an increased viscerosomatic response to cutaneous stimulation in the pelvic region. Such a response is usually associated with abdominal discomfort and/or pelvic pain.

Discussion

The major findings of the present manuscript are: 1) the instillation of VEGF produces an increase in sensory nerve density, presumably by nerve sprouting, that reaches a maximum at 2 weeks and declines by 4 weeks; 2) in addition to significant increase in sensory nerve fibers, VEGF increases the density of bladder cholinergic nerve fibers; and 3) the increase in nerve density produced by VEGF results in altered bladder function and visceral sensitivity. The unique feature of our findings is that VEGF produces an increase in nerve density via urothelium.

The nervous and vascular systems share several anatomical parallels. Both systems utilize a complex branching network of neuronal cells or blood vessels reaching all regions of the body. The anatomical similarity of the nervous and vascular systems suggests that axons might guide blood vessels and vice-versa [22]. Indeed, signal molecules produced by peripheral neuronal cells, such as VEGF [12], guide blood vessels [14] and signals from vessels, such as the neurotrophins NGF and NT-3, are required for, and orchestrate extension of neurons adjacent to vessels [23]. In this manner, the neuronal and

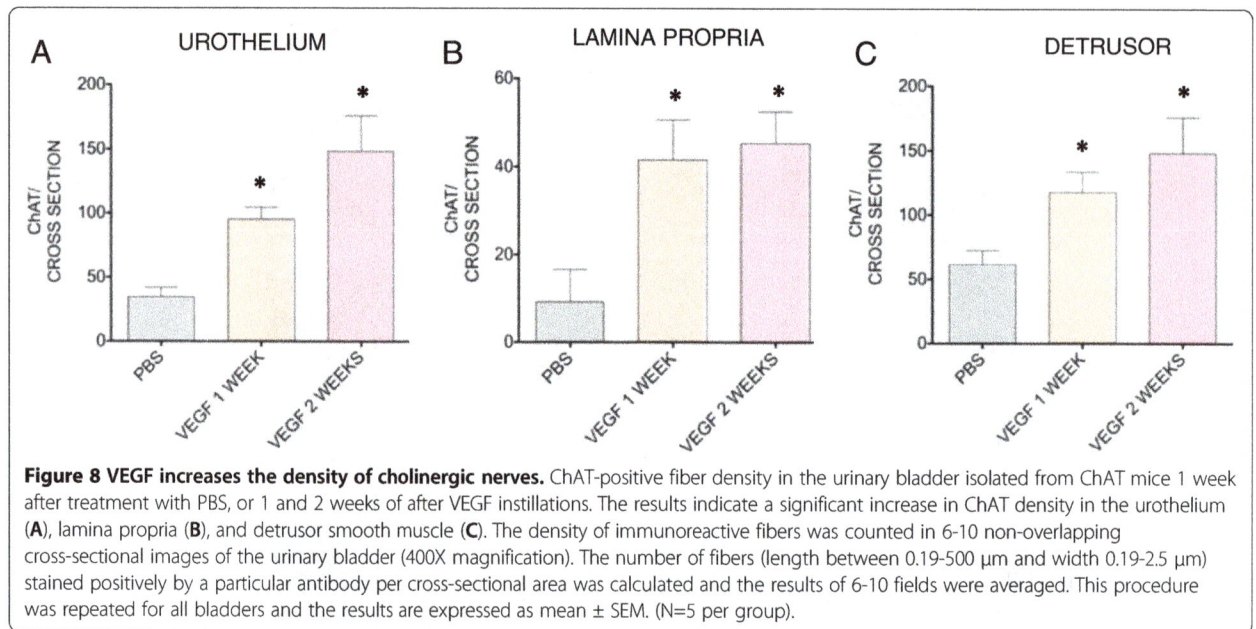

Figure 8 VEGF increases the density of cholinergic nerves. ChAT-positive fiber density in the urinary bladder isolated from ChAT mice 1 week after treatment with PBS, or 1 and 2 weeks of after VEGF instillations. The results indicate a significant increase in ChAT density in the urothelium (**A**), lamina propria (**B**), and detrusor smooth muscle (**C**). The density of immunoreactive fibers was counted in 6-10 non-overlapping cross-sectional images of the urinary bladder (400X magnification). The number of fibers (length between 0.19-500 μm and width 0.19-2.5 μm) stained positively by a particular antibody per cross-sectional area was calculated and the results of 6-10 fields were averaged. This procedure was repeated for all bladders and the results are expressed as mean ± SEM. (N=5 per group).

vascular systems are well organized and coordinated in normal adult tissues. However, in chronic inflammatory states particularly in the LUT, little is known about how the nerve-vessel relationship functions and whether it could underlie the chronic pain syndrome observed in patients with disorders of the lower urinary tract. In this context, this manuscript presents a body of evidence implicating VEGF signaling in the enhanced innervation of the urinary bladders in mice and the consequent alteration in mechanical responses and visceral sensitivity.

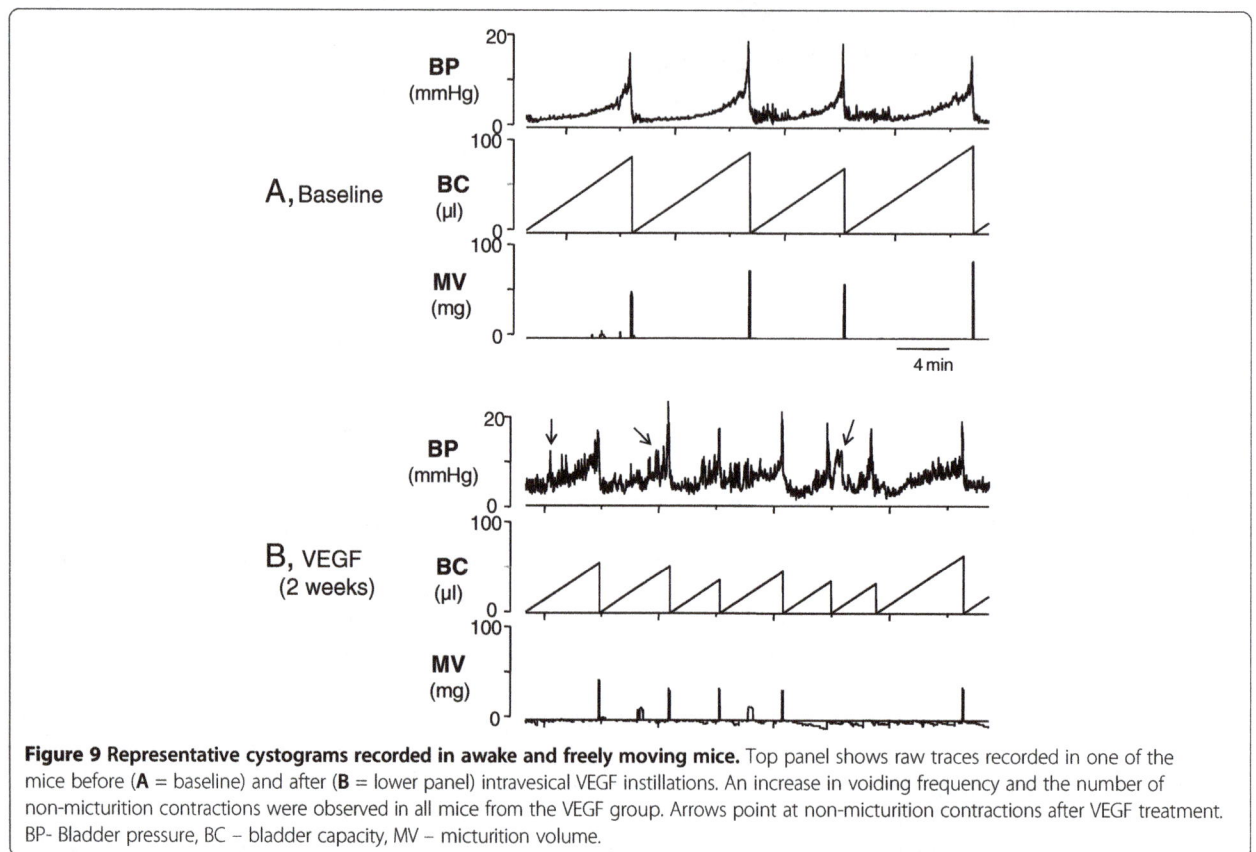

Figure 9 Representative cystograms recorded in awake and freely moving mice. Top panel shows raw traces recorded in one of the mice before (**A** = baseline) and after (**B** = lower panel) intravesical VEGF instillations. An increase in voiding frequency and the number of non-micturition contractions were observed in all mice from the VEGF group. Arrows point at non-micturition contractions after VEGF treatment. BP- Bladder pressure, BC – bladder capacity, MV – micturition volume.

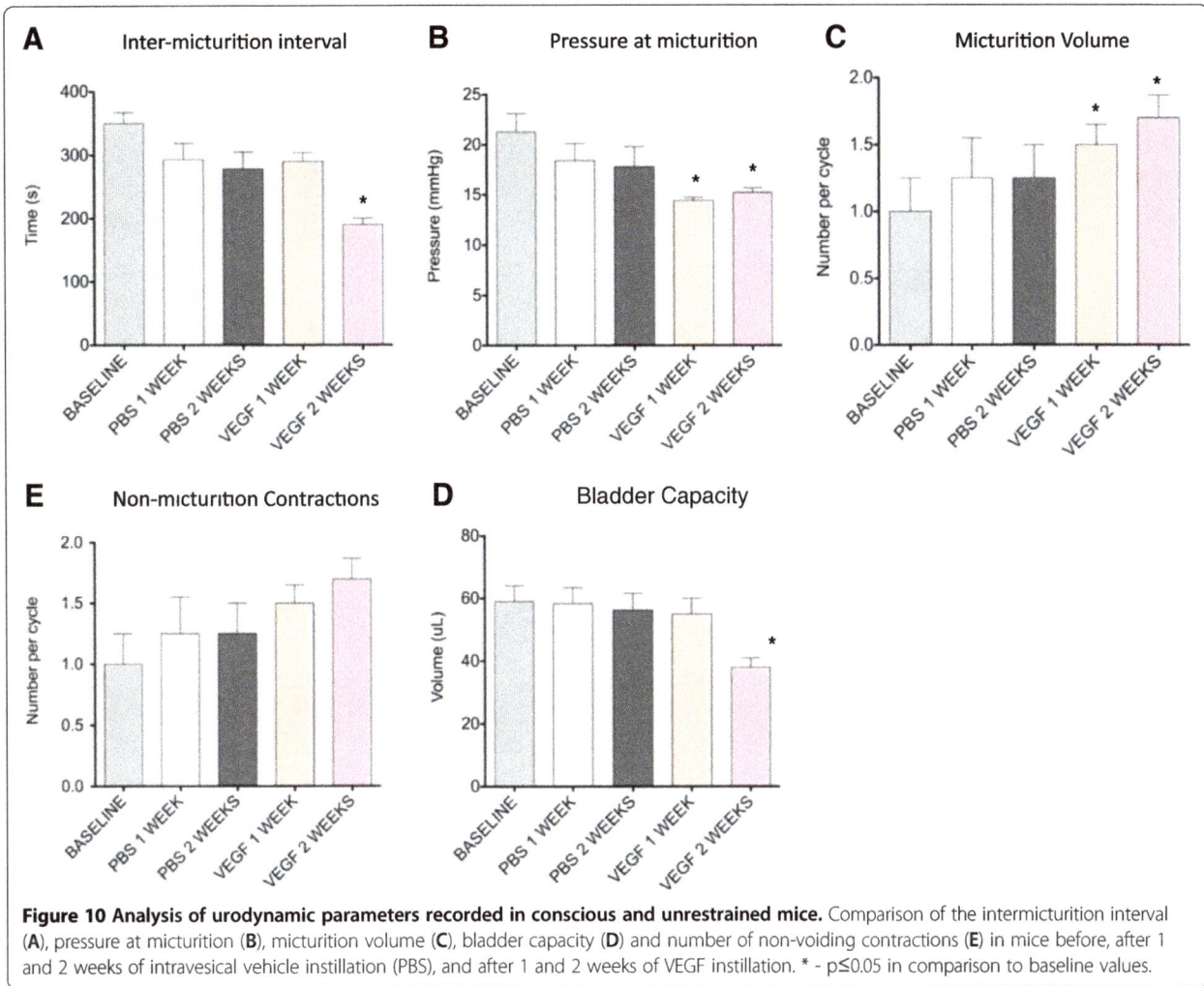

Figure 10 Analysis of urodynamic parameters recorded in conscious and unrestrained mice. Comparison of the intermicturition interval (**A**), pressure at micturition (**B**), micturition volume (**C**), bladder capacity (**D**) and number of non-voiding contractions (**E**) in mice before, after 1 and 2 weeks of intravesical vehicle instillation (PBS), and after 1 and 2 weeks of VEGF instillation. * - $p \leq 0.05$ in comparison to baseline values.

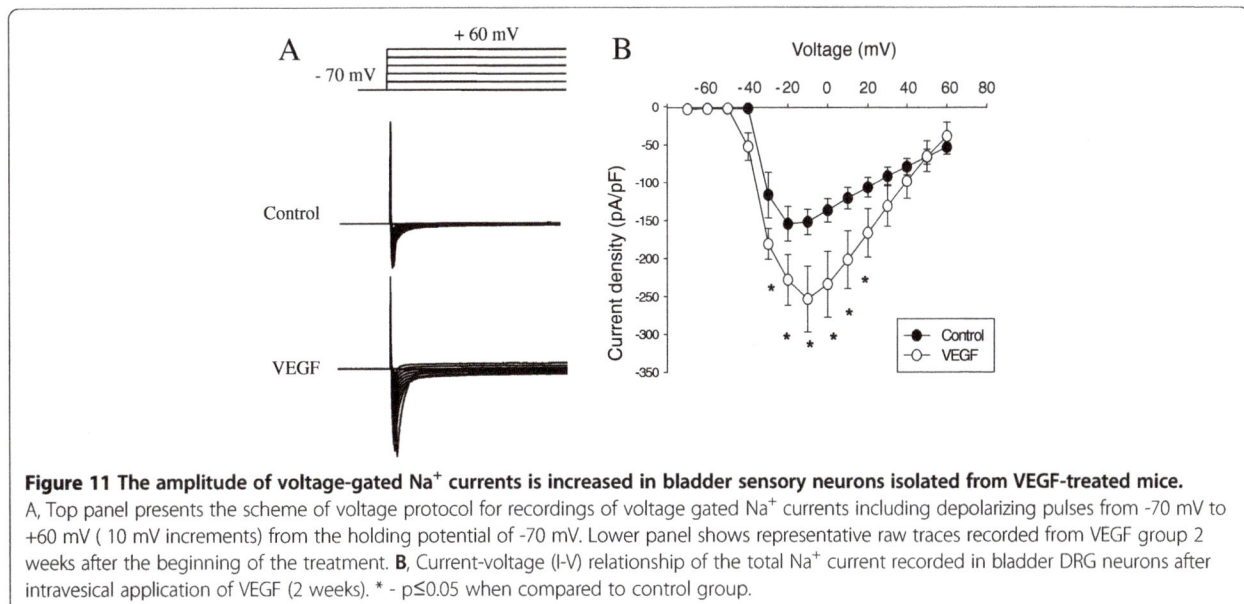

Figure 11 The amplitude of voltage-gated Na$^+$ currents is increased in bladder sensory neurons isolated from VEGF-treated mice.
A, Top panel presents the scheme of voltage protocol for recordings of voltage gated Na$^+$ currents including depolarizing pulses from -70 mV to +60 mV (10 mV increments) from the holding potential of -70 mV. Lower panel shows representative raw traces recorded from VEGF group 2 weeks after the beginning of the treatment. **B**, Current-voltage (I-V) relationship of the total Na$^+$ current recorded in bladder DRG neurons after intravesical application of VEGF (2 weeks). * - $p \leq 0.05$ when compared to control group.

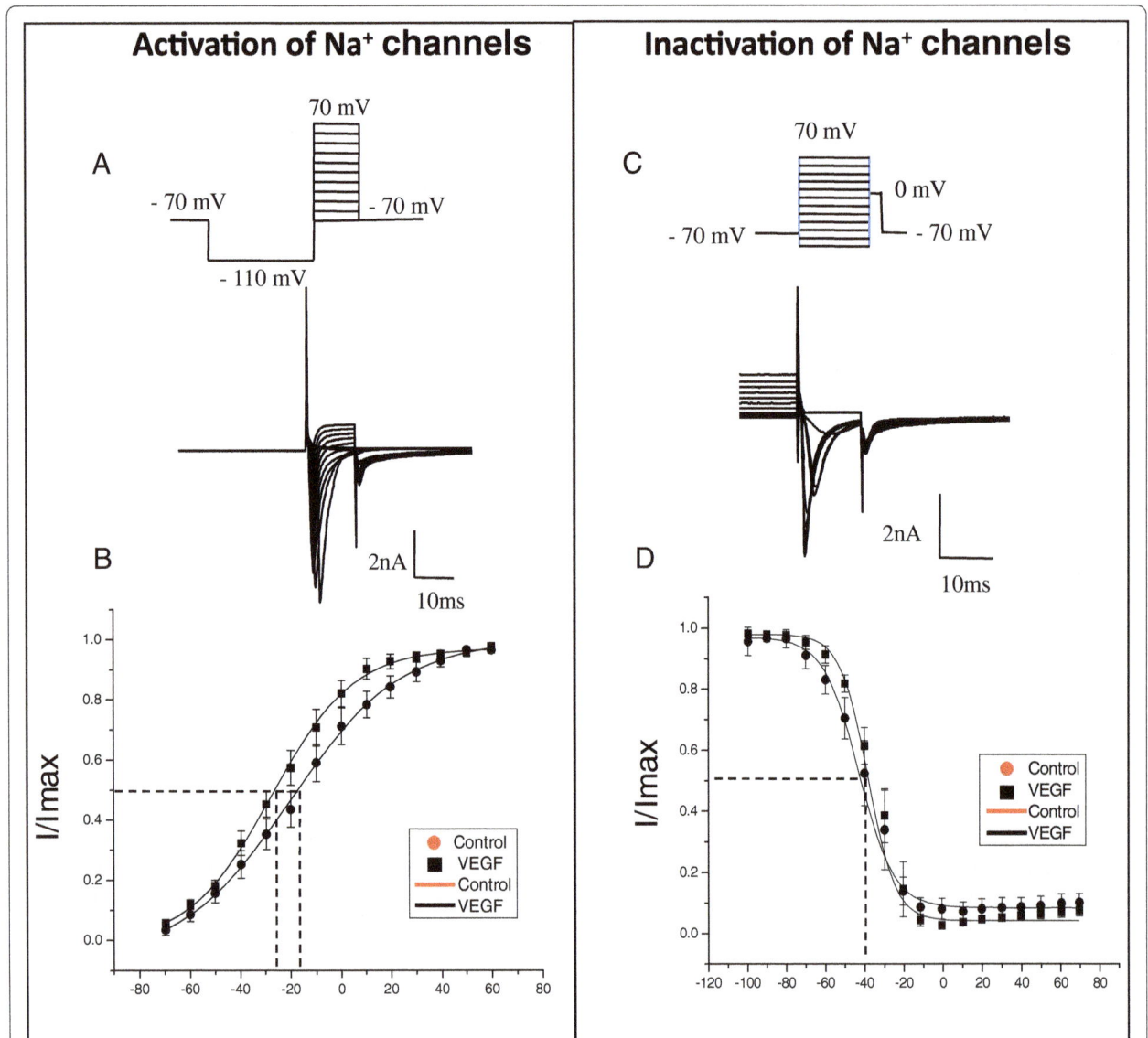

Figure 12 Kinetics of voltage gated Na⁺ channels recorded in bladder DRG neurons. A: The protocol (top panel) of steady-state activation and raw traces (bottom panel) of total Na⁺ current. The steady-state activation of VGSC was assessed by using a three-pulse protocol with a negative pre-pulse to -110 mV and a series of short pulses of 10 ms duration from -110 mV to +70 mV to activate Na+ currents. **B**: Voltage dependence of steady-state activation in bladder neurons from control and VEGF treated animals. Please note a leftward shift in the group with VEGF instillations suggestive of channel opening at more negative potentials. **C**: The protocol of steady-state inactivation (top panel) and raw traces of the recorded Na⁺ current (bottom panel). The amplitude of steady-state inactivation was measured at 0 mV after 150 ms depolarizing pulses ranging from -100 mV to 70 mV. **D**: Voltage dependence of steady-state inactivation of Na⁺ channels in lumbosacral bladder DRG neurons was not different in the control group and VEGF-treated mice.

Interest in guidance molecules, and particularly VEGF, modulating both vascular and neuronal pathology is emerging [14]. Changes in VEGF levels are associated with alterations in the vascular system of the urinary bladder [17]. VEGF is increased in bladders of patients with painful bladder syndrome, and this increase is associated with glomerulations on hydrodistension [24]. However, increased bladder VEGF is not observed in patients who do not show petechial bleeding or in controls [24], suggesting that VEGF levels are associated

with those PBS patients exhibiting alterations in the bladder microvascular system.

At this moment, it is not readily apparent which of the VEGF receptor subtypes mediates the bladder neuroplasticity in the mouse model. Both VEGFR1 and VEGFR2 as well as NRP1 and NRP2 are highly expressed in urothelium and intramural ganglia [25]. We also reported that control human bladders urothelium present a predominance of VEGFR1 and NRP2 over VEGFR2 and NRP1 immunoreactivity and that PBS

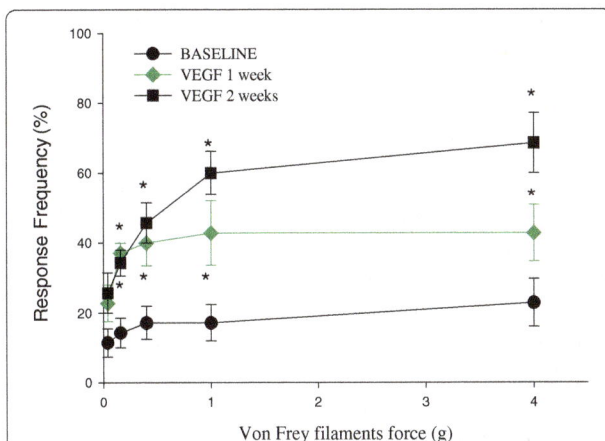

Figure 13 VEGF triggered an enhanced abdominal sensitivity in response to mechanical stimulation with von Frey filaments. Effects of intravesical VEGF on the development of viscerosomatic hyperalgesia as measured by the response to mechanical stimulation of the lower abdominal area using von Frey filaments. * - p≤0.05 when compared to the control group. This data suggests that intravesical VEGF induced the development of abdominal hypersensitivity in pelvic area which could be a reflection of abdominal discomfort/pain.

patients present a decrease in VEGFR1 and NRP2 expression [26]. Nevertheless, our results strongly suggest a new and blossoming VEGF-driven processes in the bladder that may be a putative target in neuronal plasticity. However, the role of VEGF pathway in bladder neuroplasticity is in its infancy. In contrast, the roles of NGF and BNDF in neuroplasticity are well established in bladder pathology (e.g., due to spinal cord injury) and have resulted in the testing of NGF-/BNDF-antibodies (or siRNA knockdown) as possible therapeutic options. Therefore, it is tempting to propose that VEGF neutralizing antibodies, such as avastin, or VEGF receptor antagonists may be of benefit to reduce inflammation-induced bladder neuronal plasticity. However, it has to be kept in mind that this growth factor is necessary not only for developing vessels and angiogenesis but also VEGF signaling is required for vascular homeostasis [27] and the consequences of reduced levels of VEGF can impact the kidney vasculature as seen in pre- eclampsia [28]. A promising alternative for neutralization of VEGF seems to be the blockade of neuropilins by engineered antibodies [29]. However, it is too early to predict whether neutralization of neuropilins will have any deleterious effect on the established vasculature.

The rationale for the methodology employed here is based upon our previous observations that VEGF is taken up by the intact urothelium. We showed that following intravesical instillation of a fluorescent VEGF tracer (scVEGF/Cy5.5) which only internalizes in cells expressing active VEGF receptors [30], results in accumulation of this growth factor in suburothelial layers

[31,32]. After binding these receptors, VEGF may be transcytosed by the urothelial cells into deeper suburothelial layers. Alternatively, VEGF could affect the permeability of the urothelium through mechanisms reminiscent of VEGF's effects on vascular permeability, which results in paracellular transport of VEGF. Indeed, the protein constituents comprising this highly effective urothelial barrier (tight junctions), occludins [33], claudins [34], and zonula occludens-1 [35] have been recently studied in detail [36] and are known targets of VEGF-mediated effects on vascular permeability. After the uptake, VEGF produces both bladder inflammation and changes in neuronal plasticity [17]. The hypothesis that VEGF is taken up by the urothelium was substantiated by the following findings: 1- VEGF receptors are expressed in the mouse [32] and human bladders [31]; 2-VEGF neutralizing antibodies significantly reduced inflammation and neuronal plasticity induced by intravesical Bacillus Calmette-Guérin (BCG) stimulation [17]; 3- An antibody targeting neuropilins (VEGF co-receptors) reduces bladder inflammation [37]; 4- VEGF itself reproduced the findings obtained with BCG by causing bladder inflammation and sensory nerve plasticity [17].

Increase in cholinergic fibers
Although an increase in sensory nerve density, particularly those expressing TRPV1-IR, has been proposed to underlie pain sensation and neurogenic detrusor overactivity [38], our past work did not explore whether the increased nerve density also resulted in altered function [17]. In order to investigate motor nerves, we used a unique mouse model expressing a fluorescent protein under the endogenous *Chat* gene promoter, we present evidence that direct application of VEGF into the mouse bladder increases the density of peripheral cholinergic nerves. To the best of our knowledge this increase in cholinergic nerve fibers represents a new finding that was only possible by the use this ChAT transgenic mouse, a model which will open a new area of research on the role of VEGF and its receptors in bladder motor function.

How does VEGF produce its effects?
VEGF and its receptors are known neuronal guidance molecules and, therefore, it is expected that they affect nerves. However, the inflammation induced by VEGF may be another possible mechanism leading to an increase in neuronal density. Indeed, VEGF mediates inflammation in the bladder as shown by the findings that instillation of VEGF causes vasodilation, edema, and macrophage recruitment, hallmarks of inflammation [17], while application of neutralizing VEGF antibodies significantly reduce bladder inflammation [37]. At this time, there is no definitive evidence suggesting a specific

inflammatory cell regulating bladder nerve plasticity. However, given the known trophic effects of VEGF on neurite growth prolonged survival of neurons [39,40], and reinnervation following local nerve damage [41,42], it is reasonable to propose that inflammatory cells producing VEGF may mediate these growth effects on neurons. This new appreciation of VEGF signaling in bladder inflammation is supported by emerging evidence that VEGF is increased at the site of inflammation, and that infiltrating lymphocytes and other inflammatory cells may represent additional sources of VEGF [43]. The involvement of cholinergic nerves on bladder inflammatory responses to VEGF suggests a cross-talk between the autonomic and immune systems. Whether the immune system is functionally and anatomically connected to the bladder nervous system remains to be determined. However, a recent investigation proposes that afferent and efferent signals transmitted in the vagus nerve modulate innate immune responses and are components of an inflammatory reflex [44,45]. Therefore, it is fair to propose that VEGF increases the cross-talk between the immune and autonomic systems.

VEGF alters bladder function
We showed for the first time that VEGF affects bladder function and modulates micturition reflex pathways.

Analysis of urodynamic parameters recorded in conscious mice confirmed the suggested role of VEGF in modulation of micturition reflex pathways. It is known that exogenous VEGF (or hypoxia induced upregulation of the growth factor) can lead to detrusor and urothelial hypertrophy and hyperplasia [46]. In addition, previous immunohistochemical analyses of human specimens detected increased innervation in the suburothelial and detrusor layers of the urinary bladder in PBS patients [47,48]. In our mouse model, we established that intravesical VEGF treatment resulted in an increase in the density of ChAT fibers in both the detrusor smooth muscle and urothelial layers. This increase in nerve density was associated with altered bladder function as indicated by a decrease in the duration of intermicturition interval, reduced voiding pressure, micturition volume and bladder capacity during continuous filling cystometry. At this time, the individual contributions of sensory and motor nerves to the VEGF-induced increased bladder motility are not clear. Blockade of TRPV1 with capsazepine may shed some light in this respect.

Our results are consistent with other studies which established similar urodynamic changes in animal models of bladder irritation/inflammation [49-51]. For instance, overexpression of neurotrophic nerve growth factor (NGF), a well-known modulator of neural plasticity, in the urinary bladder of mice caused bladder hyperreflexia associated with increased voiding frequency [7,52]. These

changes were accompanied by an increased density of calcitonin gene-related peptide, SP and neurofilament (NF) 100 positive fibers, as well as tyrosine hydroxylase-positive sympathetic nerve fibers within the suburothelial nerve plexus of the urinary bladder [7]. Additionally, expression of several TRP channels, including TRPA1, TRPV1, and TRPV4, was increased in the urinary bladder of mice over-expressing NGF [53]. Interestingly, the urinary bladder phenotype observed in mice with urothelial overexpression of NGF was associated predominantly with the afferent limb of the micturition reflex, whereas our results provide evidence that VEGF affects both afferent and efferent neural pathways. Our data confirmed the suggestion that VEGF may be a potent modulator of neural plasticity in the LUT. Other investigators also suggested that VEGF is a more potent stimulator of neuronal plasticity compared to a number of different neurothrophic factors [54-56]. However, a cross-talk between VEGF and neurotrophins cannot be discarded. On one hand administration of VEGF can support and enhance the growth of regenerating nerve fibers, probably through a combination of angiogenic, neurotrophic, and neuroprotective effects [57] and conversely, neurotrophins, such as NGF have been described as pro-angiogenic factors [58]. On the other hand VEGF had neurotrophic effects comparable with BDNF, NT3, or NT4 on the rat isolated pelvic ganglia in culture, [54]. In addition, VEGF was found to be more potent than BDNF in inducing ChAT-expressing fibers [54,55]. Moreover, the synergistic biological activity of VEGF and NGF [59] is supported by the finding that mechanical stretch of sympathetic neurons seems to induce VEGF expression via a NGF and CNTF signaling pathway [60]. An intriguing recent hypothesis explaining the cross-talk between VEGF and neurotrophins proposes the convergence of putative signaling downstream of receptor tyrosine kinases [61]. In this work, Kidins220 /ARMS (Ankyrin repeat-rich membrane spanning) was identified as a main player in the modulation of neurotrophin and VEGF signaling *in vivo*, and a primary determinant for neuronal and cardiovascular development [61]. In support of this hypothesis, it was demonstrated that Kidins220 interacts with neurotrophin, VEGF, ephrin, and glutamate receptors, and is a common downstream target of several trophic stimuli [61,62]. Adding to the cross-talk between neurotrophins and VEGF on neuronal plasticity, the present results go one step further by indicating that VEGF alters both sensory (TRPV1) as well as motor (ChAT) nerves. Our present results suggest the idea that across-talk between VEGF and neurotropins controls bladder motor (ChAT) nerve plasticity.

Electrophysiological recordings *in vitro* and *in vivo* revealed several distinct classes of afferent fibers that participate in transmission of sensory signaling upon physiological bladder filling, noxious distension, chemical irritation and inflammation [63]. Sensory neurons located within DRG are the first cells to receive afferent input from the pelvic viscera and, therefore, play a substantial role in the development of visceral sensitivity and pelvic discomfort during pathophysiological conditions. DRG neurons express several types of ion channels including TRPV1 and voltage-gated sodium channels (VGSC), both of which are well known transducers of nociceptive processing in pain pathways [64,65]. Experiments utilizing animal models of acute and chronic inflammation in the genitourinary tract showed an increased excitability of DRG neurons receiving direct input from the affected organs [49,66,67]. In this study, we determined that instillations of intravesical VEGF caused an up-regulation of VGSC in bladder sensory neurons identified by retrograde labeling. Overexpression of VGSC in bladder DRG cells is associated with increased neuronal excitability and enhanced firing rate [21]. Our results also support the data from human studies which suggested that abdominal pain and altered bladder and pelvic hypersensitivity in patients with OAB and PBS may involve organizational and/or functional changes in visceral afferent pathways when bladder sensory neurons become sensitized and hyper-responsive to normally innocuous stimuli such as bladder filling [68,69].

Multiple sodium channel isoforms are expressed in DRG neurons [70]. Sodium channels play a central role in neuronal electrogenesis, therefore, variations in the level of expression of any one of the sodium channel isoforms could, in principle, alter their level of excitability [71]. However, a number of modulatory factors such as neuronal functional status, homeostatic regulation of ion channel expression, post-translational modifications, and interactions with regulating molecules and trophic factors can also significantly affect neuronal excitability [70]. For instance, brief exposure to NGF, interferon gamma, epidermal growth factor or basic fibroblast growth factor can induce an up-regulation of expression of $Na_V1.7$ channel [72]. Interactions of Na^+ channels with partner molecules including NGF [73,74], GDNF [73], contactin [75,76], annexin [77], gabapentin [78], and other modulators [79] were established to regulate expression of multiple sodium channel isoforms. Based on these observations, we suggest that the effects of VEGF treatment on Na^+ channels in our study could be associated either with the changes in the expression ratio between different Na^+ channel isoforms in bladder sensory neurons or modulation of Na^+ channel function by regulatory molecules as outlined above [70]. Additional studies are warranted to identify the exact mechanisms of VEGF action on specific Na^+ channels isoforms and electrical activity of bladder sensory neurons.

The results of behavioral experiments revealed, for the first time, that intravesical VEGF induced the development of abdominal hypersensitivity detected by mechanical stimulation of the lower pelvic region. These effects may be explained, in part, by the ability of VEGF to increase the density of SP and TRPV1 positive fibers [17]. This suggestion correlates with the previously published studies, which confirmed participation of TRPV1 in the development of abdominal hyperalgesia and neuropathic pain [80]. Results with TRPV1 knockout mice support the role of TRPV1 in mediating changes in sensitivity. Wang et al. determined that abdominal hyperreactivity and cutaneous allodynia were significantly diminished in these genetically modified animals although the lack of functional TRPV1 receptors did not improve the histological changes in the inflamed bladder induced by either cyclophosphamide (CYP) or acrolein [51]. In addition to the involvement of TRPV1 afferents in pelvic sensitivity, other receptors and molecules can also contribute to abdominal hyperalgesia depending on the model and nature of chosen inflammatory agents [81]. Thus, increased peripheral sensitivity in mice with bacterial cystitis was related to activation of toll-like receptor 4 [82]. In the acrolein model of bladder inflammation in rats, increased mechanical sensitivity was conveyed, in part, via NGF and trk receptors [83]. Likewise, inflammatory events experienced earlier in life were established to trigger long lasting changes in sensory pathways leading to altered pelvic sensations during the adulthood [84,85]. Altogether, our data provide direct evidence that VEGF-induced neurogenic inflammation in the urinary bladder is associated with significant structural and functional changes that may play a key role in the development of neurogenic bladder dysfunctions in humans.

Conclusion

The discovery that neuronal guidance molecules such as neuropilins function as co-receptors for VEGF has opened up a new field of VEGF research and has even revealed potentially new roles for VEGF in axonal growth [86]. In other words, sprouting of neuronal axons and vessels appear to use common molecular mechanisms for navigation based upon NRP-VEGF interactions [87].

We previously provided strong evidence indicating that the mouse [25] and human urothelium [31] express an extraordinary level of VEGF receptors and that the expression of these receptors is fundamentally altered in bladder biopsies of PBS patients [31]. Additional results supported the hypothesis that the mouse bladder urothelium actively internalizes VEGF [31].

Nevertheless, the function exerted by VEGF in the LUT is not clear. In both neuronal and vascular cells VEGF is known to increase permeability, prevent apoptosis [88], and promote cell survival [89] and proliferation [90]. Whether VEGF exhibits the same functions on urothelial cells remains to be determined. The results presented in this manuscript indicate that VEGF also participates in bladder neuronal plasticity and that the increased nerve density is accompanied by alterations in bladder function and visceral sensitivity.

Methods
Animals and experimental groups
All animal experimentation conformed to the APS's Guiding Principles in the Care and Use of Animals and was approved by the OUHSC Animal Care & Use Committee (protocol #08-105), University of Wisconsin-Madison (protocol M02497), and University of Pennsylvania School of Medicine (protocol # 802979)

For the visualization of cholinergic neurons we used genetically engineered mice with an "IRES-Cre" sequence inserted downstream of the stop codon such that *cre* expression is controlled by the endogenous *Chat* gene promoter (B6;129S6-$Chat^{tm1(cre)Lowl}$/J.; Jackson Laboratories stock # 006410). We mated the ChAT-cre mice with Rosa stop *td* tomato mice. The resulting offspring express the fluorescent protein (td tomato) in all cholinergic cells and fibers, as the cre deletes the stop signals flanking the td tomato sequence. In these mice, *Chat* gene expression, however, is unaffected. For simplicity, this mouse strain will be referred as ChAT mice.

Adult C57BL/6J and ChAT female mice (10-12 wks old, Jackson Laboratory) were used in this study and maintained on a 12-hour light/dark cycle with *ad libitum* access to water and food.

Intravesical instillation was described in [91]. Briefly, 2-4 month-old female mice were anesthetized with isoflurane (between 1 and 2.5% titrated to effect) and transurethrally catheterized with a polypropylene catheter (24 gauge; ¾ in.; 19 mm long, inside diameter 0.47 mm, outside diameter 0.67 mm; Angiocath, Becton-Dickinson, Sandy, UT). Test compounds were instilled via a syringe attached to the catheter at a slow rate to avoid trauma and vesicoureteral reflux. 100 µl of one of the following substances were instilled: pyrogen-free saline (PBS; controls) or mouse recombinant VEGF, also known as VEGF-A or $VEGF_{165}$ (6.41 nM in 100 µl; ProSpec-Tany TechnoGene Ltd [Rehovot 76124, Israel; catalog # MGC70609]). To ensure consistent contact of substances with the bladder and to avoid reflux or leakage, the catheter was occluded and left in place for 30 minutes. Mice received one or twice weekly innstillation of VEGF, as described in the particular figure legend. The groups of mice were euthanized one week post-instillation, and the urinary bladders were removed and examined as whole mounts. Subsequently, the urinary bladders were sectioned and visualized as cross-sections and immunofluorescence was used for image analysis of cholinergic and sensory nerves.

Functional Studies
C57BL/6J female mice were randomly divided into three experimental groups: 1 – cystometry studies (N=5); 2 - control group for electrophysiological experiments (intravesical PBS, N=5); 3 – VEGF group (intravesical VEGF, N=5). Animals in all groups first underwent survival surgeries as described below followed by 3 intravesical instillations of either PBS or vascular endothelial growth factor (VEGF, 100 µL, 6.41 nM in 100 µl, groups 1 and 3) within a 2-week period (every 4th day), see Table 1.

Bladder whole mounts
Urinary bladders were isolated from ChAT mice, the urine was drained, and tissues were fixed in 4% paraformaldehyde for 4-6 hours at room temperature or overnight at 4°C. After fixation, the tissue was washed in PBS twice and placed in 1% triton X-100 for 4-6 hours at room temperature or overnight at 4°C. After the tissue was washed in PBS, the primary antibodies were added for 4-6 hours at room temperature or overnight at 4°C, washed off in PBS, and the secondary antibodies were added for 4-6 hours at room temperature or overnight at 4°C. Whole mounts were visualized and photographed with a dissecting fluorescence microscope (Nikon SMZ 1500 microscope equipped with high-resolution Plan 1.6 WD24 objective lenses). For detailed visualization of ChAT and TRPV1 nerves along with blood vessels, some of the whole mounts were blunt dissected to separate the urothelium together with the suburothelium/lamina propria [92] from the detrusor smooth muscle. Photomicrographs were taken with the lamina propria facing upward and the urothelium downward or the detrusor smooth muscle facing upward and the adventitia downward. Subsequently, tissues were frozen in 1:1 tissue freezing media (TFM, Triangle Biomed Sciences) and OCT (Tissue Tek®) and sectioned with a cryostat. Cross-sections were examined by immunofluorescence, as described below.

Immunofluorescence (IF) of mouse tissues
Urinary bladders were processed for IF according to published methods [93]. For all tissues, appropriate cross-sectional morphology was confirmed by H&E staining and examination by light microscopy prior to preparing slides for IF labeling. Frozen sections (10, 15, or 40 µm thick, as indicated in the figure legend) were post-fixed in 1% MeOH-free formaldehyde for all stains. Briefly, slides were blocked for 35 minutes with 5% normal donkey serum (NDS; Jackson Immunolabs), then co-incubated with primary antibodies in 0.5% NDS for 90 minutes in a humidified chamber or overnight at 4°C. When double IF was used, following brief rinses with PBS, slides were co-incubated with both secondary antibodies at the same time. Controls included slides labeled only with individual primary or secondary antibodies.

Table 1 Experimental scheme for functional studies

DAYS	0	1	5	7	9	14
PROCEDURES						
		1st instillation of VEGF	2nd instillation of VEGF		3rd instillation of VEGF	
	Cystometry (Baseline)			Cystometry (1 week)		Cystometry (2 weeks)
				Von Frey Testing (1 week)		Von Frey testing (2 weeks)
						Electrophysiology (2 weeks)

Primary antibodies

TRPV1 antibody (1:10,000) was raised in rabbits against the 15 C-terminal amino acids of the rat TRPV1 sequence [94]. Commercially available antibodies included: rabbit anti-human protein gene product 9.5 [PGP9.5] (Neuromics; catalog # RB12103, 1:1500 dilution), rabbit anti-mouse substance P (Millipore; catalog AB1566; 1:250 dilution), guinea pig anti-rat substance P (Millipore; catalog AB15810; 1:1000 dilution), rat anti-mouse-derived endothelioma cell line [CD31] (BD Pharmingen; #550274; 1:200), rabbit anti-β III tubulin [TuJ1] (Gift from Dr. Anthony Frankfurter; 1:250).

Secondary antibodies

All secondary antibodies were used at a 1:500 dilution and included donkey anti-rabbit IgG Alexafluor 488 and 546 conjugate (Molecular Probes), donkey anti-goat IgG Alexafluor 546, donkey anti-rat IgG Alexafluor 488, goat anti-guinea pig 546 ,donkey anti-rat Cy5 (Jackson ImmunoResearch), donkey anti-rabbit Dylight 488), donkey anti-rabbit Cy5. Slides were washed, counter-stained with 4, 6-diamidino-2-phenylindole (DAPI), and coverslipped.

Image analysis

A Nikon A1R scanning confocal microscope (Melville, NY) controlled by NIS-Elements C (Nikon) was used to image whole mounts and cross sections at UW-Madison. For image analysis, all tissue cross-sections were viewed with a Nikon Eclipse TE 2000-S inverted fluorescent microscope at OUHSC and imaged at room temperature using a digital CCD camera (Roper Scientific; Sarasota, Florida 34240) driven by NIS-Elements AR 3.0 Imaging software. A control slide stained only with secondary antibody was used to determine exposure time and to set minimum background fluorescence levels for each fluorophore imaged. Once set, exposure times were not changed during acquisition of each respective fluorophore in the staining series. Staining was considered positive only when the acquired signal exceeded the established background. Absence of signal bleed-through was determined using previously optimized multi-acquisition settings on single fluorophore stained slides. DAPI staining was viewed using a DAPI filter set (340-380nm ex, 435-485nm em). Imaging of Alexafluor 488 utilized an excitation filter of 465-495nm and an emission filter of 515-555nm. Alexafluor 546 was imaged with an excitation of 528-553nm and 590-650nm emission range.

Quantification of nerve fibers

Histologically nerve fibers undulate in and out of the plane of the section, sometimes appearing as linear structures, and sometimes as punctate staining, indicating presumed nerves in cross-section. Therefore, the following parameters were used in order to exclude structures above or below a certain size as being potentially non-neuronal and to exclude inflammatory cells since monocytes and macrophages have been reported to express TRPV1 [95]. In this context, for image analysis of nerves, the NIS-Elements AR 3.0 Imaging software was set to count only structures with length between 0.19-500 μm and width 0.19-2.5 μm. [Length is a derived feature appropriate for elongated or thin structures. Length = (Perimeter + sqrt (Perimeter^2 - 16*Area))/4]; and Width is a derived feature appropriate for elongated or thin structures. It is based on the rod model and is calculated according to the following formula: Width = Area/Length].

To meet the independent randomized sampling assumption required for our statistical test(s), the following measures were taken: blinding the reader to treatment groups and picking a random starting position and proceeding clockwise with 6-10 non-overlapping images. As 12-20 fields are necessary to view the whole bladder cross-section at 400X magnification, the sampling of 6-10 non-overlapping images represented half of the entire bladder cross-section. The area occupied by cells stained positively with td tomato or TRPV1 antibody was calculated as percent of the total area of the region of interest (ROI), as indicated in the individual figure legend and the results of 6-10 fields were averaged. This procedure was repeated for all bladders used per treatment group and the results are expressed as mean ± SEM of cross-sections. The data were examined to determine if the distributions were homoscedastic and Gaussian. As these conditions were met, groups were compared through a two-sample Student's t test. An alpha of 0.05 was considered statistically significant. P-values were adjusted for multiple comparisons through a Bonferroni correction.

Surgical procedure to catheterize the urinary bladder in mice

Mice included in the group for urodynamic evaluation of the urinary bladder function (awake cystometry) underwent the following survival surgical procedure to insert bladder catheters. An animal was anesthetized with isoflurane (VEDCO, St. Joseph, MO), and a PTF catheter with a blunted end (Catamount Research, St. Albans, VT) was sutured in place at the bladder dome and tunneled out the abdomen to the nape of the neck where it was then inserted into the end of a 22-gauge angiocath iv catheter. Upon determination of the optimal length, the PTF catheter was affixed to the angiocath with super glue. The angiocath was first tested with a gentle saline infusion to reveal no leak at the bladder, and then capped and the abdomen was closed in layers. The angiocath was anchored to the fascia and skin of the neck using two to three 3–0 Vicryl sutures. Animals were kept in individual cages to avoid possible damage to the catheters by their cage mates. Mice were allowed to recover from surgery for 4 days followed by cystometric evaluation of bladder function under normal conditions (baseline cystometry). After initial urodynamic evaluation mice received 3 intravesical instillations of VEGF as described above.

Surgical procedure for labeling urinary bladder DRG neurons

Mice were anaesthetized with 2% isoflurane and held on a warming pad inside a fume hood to minimize the investigator's exposure to the anesthetic. A midline laparotomy was performed under sterile conditions to gain access to the urinary bladder. Urinary bladder was exposed and Fast Blue (Polysciences Inc., Warrington, PA, USA; 1.5% w/v in water) was injected into the urinary bladder wall (detrusor at 6 – 10 sites) using a Hamilton syringe with 26-gauge needle. The total volume of dye injected into the bladder was 20–25 μl. Adjacent pelvic organs were isolated with gauze to soak up any spills and prevent the labeling of adjacent structures during injections. Additionally, the needle was kept in place for 30 minutes after each injection. Any leaked dye was removed with a cotton swab before placing the organ into the pelvic cavity. Incisions were sutured in layers under sterile conditions followed by subcutaneous injection of buprenorphine (0.5 mg/kg). Animals were allowed to recover on a warm blanket until they gained full consciousness and then were returned to their cages. Mice started treatments with intravesical VEGF (or PBS in the control group) 10 days after labeling of bladder sensory neurons.

Urodynamic evaluation of bladder function

Conscious mice were placed in cystometry cages (16 cm width, 12 cm height, and 24 cm length) without any restraint and allowed to acclimate for 30 min. The tip of the exteriorized bladder catheter located at the base of the mouse neck was connected to a pressure transducer and an infusion pump of the cystometry station (Small Animal Laboratory Cystometry, Catamount Research and Development, St. Albans, VT) using a T-shaped valve. Room temperature saline solution (0.9% NaCl) was infused into the bladder at a rate of 10 μl/min. Voided urine was collected in the tray connected to a force displacement transducer integrated into the data acquisition system. Each animal was observed for up to six-eight voiding cycles. Urodynamic values were recorded continuously using data acquisition software (Small Animal Laboratory Cystometry, Catamount Research and Development). The following cystometric parameters were recorded and analyzed in this study: bladder capacity, pressure at the start of micturition, micturition rate, continuous intravesicular pressure, intermicturition interval, and the number of non-micturition contractions. Non-micturition contractions were defined as increased values in detrusor pressure from the baseline that had amplitudes of at least a third of maximal pressure at the start of micturition. Each animal underwent baseline cystometric evaluation followed by intravesical instillations of VEGF. The second cystometric assessment was done after two VEGF instillations (1 week after the first dose) and the third cystometry was performed 3 days after completion of all three VEGF treatments at 2 weeks after the baseline measurement (day 0), Table 1.

Cystometric parameters were uploaded from the acquisition software into analysis software (SOF-552 Cystometry Data Analysis, Version 1.4, Catamount Research and Development Inc., St. Albans, Vermont). Maximum pressure at micturition, bladder capacity, micturition volume, number of non-micturition contractions, intermicturition interval and micturition rate indices were calculated. All data are expressed as the mean ± standard error of the mean (S.E.M). The results were statistically analyzed using one-way repeated measures ANOVA between baseline and 2 urodynamic assessments followed by Bonferroni's post test, as appropriate (Systat Software Inc., San Jose, CA). A difference in values between the baseline and treatments was considered statistically significant at $p \leq 0.05$.

Isolation of bladder DRG neurons for patch-clamp experiments

Animals were euthanized by overdose of sodium pentobarbital (130 mg/kg) 2 weeks after the beginning of VEGF treatments. Dorsal root ganglia were dissected and removed bilaterally at L6-S2 levels. The ganglia were treated with collagenase (Worthington, type 2, Biochemical Corp., Lakewood, NJ, USA) in F-12 medium (Invitrogen,

Carlsbad, CA, USA) for 90 min in an incubator with 95% O_2 and 5% CO_2 at 37° C. Isolated ganglia were then rinsed in phosphate-buffered saline (PBS) and incubated for 15 min in the presence of trypsin (Sigma, St Louis, MO, USA; 1 mg/ml) at room temperature. The enzymatic reaction was terminated in Dulbecco's Modified Eagle's Medium (DMEM) containing 10% of fetal bovine serum (FBS). Single neurons were obtained by gentle trituration using fire-polished Pasteur pipettes in DMEM with trypsin inhibitor (Sigma; 2 mg/ml) and deoxyribonuclease (Sigma; DNase 1 mg/ml). The cell suspension was centrifuged for 10 min at 700 rpm (4° C), and supernatant was discarded. The pellet, containing sensory neurons, was resuspended in 2 ml of DMEM containing 10% FBS. Neurons were plated on poly-L-ornithine coated 35 mm Petri dishes. Isolated cells were maintained overnight in an incubator at 37° C with 95% O_2/5% CO_2 and were used for electrophysiological experiments within 24 hours.

Electrophysiological recordings of voltage gated Na⁺ currents from bladder dorsal root ganglion neurons

Bladder labeled neurons were identified with an inverted fluorescent microscope (Ti E2000–5, Nikon containing a specific filter for Fast Blue (UV-2A, Nikon). Only neurons exhibiting bright blue fluorescence (Fast Blue labeled) were used for Na⁺ current recordings using the whole-cell patch clamp technique. For voltage clamp experiments the external solution contained (in mM): NaCl 45, TEA Chloride 30, Choline Chloride 60, KCl 5.4, $MgCl_2$ 1, $CaCl_2$ 1, HEPES 5, D-glucose 5.5, adjusted with NaOH to pH 7.4. Pipette solution for these experiments consisted of (in mM): L-aspartic acid 100, CsCl 30, $MgCl_2$ 2, Na-ATP 5, EGTA 5, HEPES 5 adjusted with CsOH to pH 7.2. CdCl (100 µM) was added to the external solution in order to block voltage gated calcium currents. Freshly made Amphotericin B (0.24 mg/ml, ACROS, NJ, USA) was added to the pipette solution for perforated whole cell recordings. Microelectrodes were fabricated from borosilicate capillary glass (Sutter instruments, Novato, CA) and had resistances of 2–5 MΩ when filled with internal solution. Recordings commenced 5 min after the establishment of whole cell access. Series resistance was compensated ≥80–85%, and the calculated junction potential was around 5 mV. Cells were excluded from analysis if uncompensated series resistance resulted in a maximum voltage error >5 mV or if the seal or access resistance were unstable. Recordings and analysis of kinetic parameters of voltage gated Na⁺ channels were performed using previously established protocols [9].

pCLAMP software (Axon Instruments, CA) was used for data acquisition and analysis. All data are expressed as means ± SEM. Statistical significance between the groups was assessed by one-way ANOVA followed by Bonferroni`s test. Data with p≤0.05 were considered statistically significant.

Assessment of visceral sensitivity using von Frey filaments

Mice were tested before and after intravesical instillations of VEGF. Irritation and/or inflammation in the pelvic viscera are associated with enhanced abdominal sensitivity due to convergence of visceral and somatic inputs on the second order neurons in the dorsal horn of the spinal cord [21]. This phenomenon is known as viscerosomatic (called hyperalgesia) and is measured by using mechanical stimulation with von Frey filaments on the lower abdominal/ pelvic area. Mice were tested in individual Plexiglas chambers (6 x 10 x 12 cm) with a stainless steel wire grid floor (mouse acclimation period was 30 min before testing). Frequency of withdrawal responses was tested using five individual fibers with forces of 0.04, 0.16, 0.4, 1, and 4 g (Stoelting). Each filament was applied for 1–2 s with an interstimulus interval of 5 s for a total of 10 times, and the hairs were tested in ascending order of force. Stimulation was confined to the lower abdominal area in the general vicinity of the bladder, and care was taken to stimulate different areas within this region to avoid desensitization or "wind up" effects. Three types of behavior were considered as positive responses to filament stimulation: *1)* sharp retraction of the abdomen, *2)* immediate licking or scratching of the area of filament stimulation, or *3)* jumping as previously described [96].

Authors' contributions
This manuscript reports the results of studies developed at the University of Pennsylvania (UP), UW-Madison, and OUHSC. At the UW-Madison, under the directions of MLE, MRS anesthetized and instilled the ChAT mice and CSE developed the analysis of bladder whole mounts and immunofluorescence of mouse tissues. At the OUHSC, under the direction of MRS, CAD developed image analysis and quantification of nerve fibers. At the UP, under the direction of APM, QL developed the functional studies, including urodynamic evaluation of bladder function, isolation of bladder DRG neurons for patch-clamp experiments, electrophysiological recordings of voltage gated Na⁺ currents from bladder dorsal root ganglion neurons, and assessment of visceral sensitivity using von Frey filaments. RS conceived the study, analyzed the results, and prepared the manuscript. All authors read and approved the final manuscript.

Acknowledgements
This research was supported by the Department of Defense Medical Research Program (PRMRP) under award number PR080981 (RS). Views and opinions of, and endorsements by the author(s) do not reflect those of the US Army or the Department of Defense. Studies at UW-Madison were supported by R01-DK081634 (MLE). Studies at UP were supported by DK077699 (APM).

Author details
[1]Department of Surgery, Division of Urology, University of Pennsylvania School of Medicine, Glenolden, PA 19036-2307, USA. [2]Department of Neurosciences, University of Wisconsin-Madison, Madison, WI 53706, USA. [3]Department of Physiology, College of Medicine, Urinary Tract Physiological Genomics Laboratory, University of Oklahoma Health Sciences Center (OUHSC), 800 Research Parkway, Room 410, Oklahoma City, OK 73104, USA.

References

1. Avelino A, Cruz F: TRPV1 (vanilloid receptor) in the urinary tract: expression, function and clinical applications. *Naunyn Schmiedebergs Arch Pharmacol* 2006, **373**(4):287–299.

2. Andersson KE, Hedlund P: Pharmacologic perspective on the physiology of the lower urinary tract. *Urology* 2002, **60**(5 Suppl 1):13–20. discussion 20-11.

3. Ford AP, Cockayne DA: ATP and P2X purinoceptors in urinary tract disorders. *Handb Exp Pharmacol* 2011, **202**:485–526.

4. Asfaw TS, Hypolite J, Northington GM, Arya LA, Wein AJ, Malykhina AP: Acute colonic inflammation triggers detrusor instability via activation of TRPV1 receptors in a rat model of pelvic organ cross-sensitization. *Am J Physiol Regul Integr Comp Physiol* 2011, **300**(6):R1392–R1400.

5. Saban R, Saban MR, Nguyen NB, Lu B, Gerard C, Gerard NP, Hammond TG: Neurokinin-1 (NK-1) receptor is required in antigen-induced cystitis. *Am J Pathol* 2000, **156**(3):775–780.

6. Saban R, D'Andrea MR, Andrade-Gordon P, Derian CK, Dozmorov I, Ihnat MA, Hurst RE, Davis CA, Simpson C, Saban MR: Mandatory role of proteinase-activated receptor 1 in experimental bladder inflammation. *BMC Physiol* 2007, **7**:4.

7. Schnegelsberg B, Sun TT, Cain G, Bhattacharya A, Nunn PA, Ford AP, Vizzard MA, Cockayne DA: Overexpression of NGF in mouse urothelium leads to neuronal hyperinnervation, pelvic sensitivity, and changes in urinary bladder function. *Am J Physiol Regul Integr Comp Physiol* 2010, **298**(3):R534–R547.

8. Alagiri M, Chottiner S, Ratner V, Slade D, Hanno PM: Interstitial cystitis: unexplained associations with other chronic disease and pain syndromes. *Urology* 1997, **49**(5A Suppl):52–57.

9. Lei Q, Malykhina AP: Colonic inflammation up-regulates voltage-gated sodium channels in bladder sensory neurons via activation of peripheral transient potential vanilloid 1 receptors. *Neurogastroenterol Motil* 2012, **24**(6):575–585. e257.

10. Martin P, Lewis J: Origins of the neurovascular bundle: interactions between developing nerves and blood vessels in embryonic chick skin. *Int J Dev Biol* 1989, **33**(3):379–387.

11. Carmeliet P, Tessier-Lavigne M: Common mechanisms of nerve and blood vessel wiring. *Nature* 2005, **436**(7048):193–200.

12. Mukouyama YS, Shin D, Britsch S, Taniguchi M, Anderson DJ: Sensory nerves determine the pattern of arterial differentiation and blood vessel branching in the skin. *Cell* 2002, **109**(6):693–705.

13. Yuan L, Moyon D, Pardanaud L, Breant C, Karkkainen MJ, Alitalo K, Eichmann A: Abnormal lymphatic vessel development in neuropilin 2 mutant mice. *Development* 2002, **129**(20):4797–4806.

14. de Almodovar Ruiz C, Lambrechts D, Mazzone M, Carmeliet P: Role and therapeutic potential of VEGF in the nervous system. *Physiol Rev* 2009, **89**(2):607–648.

15. Charrua A, Reguenga C, Cordeiro JM, Correiade-Sa P, Paule C, Nagy I, Cruz F, Avelino A: Functional transient receptor potential vanilloid 1 is expressed in human urothelial cells. *J Urol* 2009, **182**(6):2944–2950.

16. Doran JF, Jackson P, Kynoch PA, Thompson RJ: Isolation of PGP 9.5, a new human neurone-specific protein detected by high-resolution two-dimensional electrophoresis. *J Neurochem* 1983, **40**(6):1542–1547.

17. Saban MR, Davis CA, Avelino A, Cruz F, Maier J, Bjorling DE, Sferra TJ, Hurst RE, Saban R: VEGF signaling mediates bladder neuroplasticity and inflammation in response to BCG. *BMC Physiol* 2011, **11**:16.

18. Carmeliet P: Neuro-vascular link: from genetic insights to therapeutic perspectives. *Bull Mem Acad R Med Belg* 2008, **163**(10-12):445–451. discussion 451-442.

19. Avwenagha O, Campbell G, Bird MM: Distribution of GAP-43, beta-III tubulin and F-actin in developing and regenerating axons and their growth cones in vitro, following neurotrophin treatment. *J Neurocytol* 2003, **32**(9):1077–1089.

20. Birder LA, Wolf-Johnston AS, Sun Y, Chai TC: Alteration in TRPV1 and Muscarinic (M3) receptor expression and function in idiopathic overactive bladder urothelial cells. *Acta Physiol (Oxf)* 2013, **207**(1):123–129.

21. Ritter AM, Martin WJ, Thorneloe KS: The voltage-gated sodium channel Nav1.9 is required for inflammation-based urinary bladder dysfunction. *Neurosci Lett* 2009, **452**(1):28–32.

22. Carmeliet P: Blood vessels and nerves: common signals, pathways and diseases. *Nat Rev Genet* 2003, **4**(9):710–720.

23. Kuruvilla R, Zweifel LS, Glebova NO, Lonze BE, Valdez G, Ye H, Ginty DD: A neurotrophin signaling cascade coordinates sympathetic neuron development through differential control of TrkA trafficking and retrograde signaling. *Cell* 2004, **118**(2):243–255.

24. Tamaki M, Saito R, Ogawa O, Yoshimura N, Ueda T: Possible mechanisms inducing glomerulations in interstitial cystitis: relationship between endoscopic findings and expression of angiogenic growth factors. *J Urol* 2004, **172**(3):945–948.

25. Saban MR, Backer JM, Backer MV, Maier J, Fowler B, Davis CA, Simpson C, Wu X-R, Birder L, Freeman MR, Soker S, Saban R: VEGF receptors and neuropilins are expressed in the urothelial and neuronal cells in normal mouse urinary bladder and are up-regulated in inflammation. *Am J Physiol Renal* 2008, **295**. doi:10.1152/ajprenal.00618.02007.

26. Saban R, Saban MR, Maier J, Fowler B, Tengowski M, Davis CA, Wu XR, Culkin DJ, Hauser P, Backer J, Hurst RE: Urothelial expression of neuropilins and VEGF receptors in control and interstitial cystitis patients. *Am J Physiol Renal Physiol* 2008, **295**(6):F1613–F1623.

27. Lee S, Chen TT, Barber CL, Jordan MC, Murdock J, Desai S, Ferrara N, Nagy A, Roos KP, Iruela-Arispe ML: Autocrine VEGF signaling is required for vascular homeostasis. *Cell* 2007, **130**(4):691–703.

28. Sugimoto H, Hamano Y, Charytan D, Cosgrove D, Kieran M, Sudhakar A, Kalluri R: Neutralization of circulating vascular endothelial growth factor (VEGF) by anti-VEGF antibodies and soluble VEGF receptor 1 (sFlt-1) induces proteinuria. *J Biol Chem* 2003, **278**(15):12605–12608.

29. Saban MR, Sferra TJ, Davis CA, Simpson C, Allen A, Maier J, Fowler B, Knowlton N, Birder L, Wu XR, Saban R: Neuropilin-VEGF signaling pathway acts as a key modulator of vascular, lymphatic, and inflammatory cell responses of the bladder to intravesical BCG treatment. *Am J Physiol Renal Physiol* 2010, **299**(6):F1245–F1256.

30. Backer MV, Levashova Z, Patel V, Jehning BT, Claffey K, Blankenberg FG, Backer JM: Molecular imaging of VEGF receptors in angiogenic vasculature with single-chain VEGF based probes. *Nat Med* 2007, **13**(4):504–509.

31. Saban R, Saban MR, Maier J, Fowler B, Tengowski M, Davis CA, Wu XR, Culkin DJ, Hauser P, Backer J, Hurst RE: Urothelial expression of neuropilins and VEGF receptors in control and interstitial cystitis patients. PMID: 18815217 American journal of physiology. *Ren Physiol* 2008, **295**(6):F1613–F1623.

32. Saban MR, Backer JM, Backer MV, Maier J, Fowler B, Davis CA, Simpson C, Wu XR, Birder L, Freeman MR, Soker S, Hurst RE, Saban R: VEGF receptors and neuropilins are expressed in the urothelial and neuronal cells in normal mouse urinary bladder and are upregulated in inflammation. *Am J Physiol Renal Physiol* 2008, **295**(1):F60–F72.

33. Schmitt M, Horbach A, Kubitz R, Frilling A, Haussinger D: Disruption of hepatocellular tight junctions by vascular endothelial growth factor (VEGF): a novel mechanism for tumor invasion. *J Hepatol* 2004, **41**(2):274–283.

34. Rodewald M, Herr D, Fraser HM, Hack G, Kreienberg R, Wulff C: Regulation of tight junction proteins occludin and claudin 5 in the primate ovary during the ovulatory cycle and after inhibition of vascular endothelial growth factor. *Mol Hum Reprod* 2007, **13**(11):781–789.

35. Nico B, Mangieri D, Crivellato E, Longo V, De Giorgis M, Capobianco C, Corsi P, Benagiano V, Roncali L, Ribatti D: HIF activation and VEGF overexpression are coupled with ZO-1 up-phosphorylation in the brain of dystrophic mdx mouse. *Brain Pathol* 2007, **17**(4):399–406.

36. Acharya P, Beckel J, Ruiz WG, Wang E, Rojas R, Birder L, Apodaca G: Distribution of the tight junction proteins ZO-1, occludin, and claudin-4, -8, and -12 in bladder epithelium. *Am J Physiol Renal Physiol* 2004, **287**(2):F305–F318.

37. Saban MR, Sferra TJ, Davis CA, Simpson C, Allen A, Maier J, Fowler B, Knowlton N, Birder L, Wu XR, Saban R: Neuropilin-VEGF signaling pathway acts as a key modulator of vascular, lymphatic, and inflammatory cell responses of the bladder to intravesical BCG treatment. PMID: 20861073. *Am J Physiol Renal Physiol* 2010, **299**(6):F1245–F1256.

38. Silva C, Avelino A, Souto-Moura C, Cruz F: A light- and electron-microscopic histopathological study of human bladder mucosa after intravesical resiniferatoxin application. *BJU Int* 2001, **88**(4):355–360.

39. Brockington A, Wharton SB, Fernando M, Gelsthorpe CH, Baxter L, Ince PG, Lewis CE, Shaw PJ: Expression of vascular endothelial growth factor and

its receptors in the central nervous system in amyotrophic lateral sclerosis. *J Neuropathol Exp Neurol* 2006, **65**(1):26–36.

40. Ogunshola OO, Antic A, Donoghue MJ, Fan SY, Kim H, Stewart WB, Madri JA, Ment LR: **Paracrine and autocrine functions of neuronal vascular endothelial growth factor (VEGF) in the central nervous system.** *J Biol Chem* 2002, **277**(13):11410–11415.

41. Damon DH: **Vascular endothelial-derived semaphorin 3 inhibits sympathetic axon growth.** *Am J Physiol Heart Circ Physiol* 2006, **290**(3):H1220–H1225.

42. Marko SB, Damon DH: **VEGF promotes vascular sympathetic innervation.** *Am J Physiol Heart Circ Physiol* 2008, **294**(6):H2646–H2652.

43. Freeman MR, Schneck FX, Gagnon ML, Corless C, Soker S, Niknejad K, Peoples GE, Klagsbrun M: **Peripheral blood T lymphocytes and lymphocytes infiltrating human cancers express vascular endothelial growth factor: a potential role for T cells in angiogenesis.** *Cancer Res* 1995, **55**(18):4140–4145.

44. Tracey KJ: **The inflammatory reflex.** *Nature* 2002, **420**(6917):853–859.

45. Andersson U, Tracey KJ: **Neural reflexes in inflammation and immunity.** *J Exp Med* 2012, **209**:1057–1068.

46. Burgu B, Medina Ortiz WE, Pitera JE, Woolf AS, Wilcox DT: **Vascular endothelial growth factor mediates hypoxic stimulated embryonic bladder growth in organ culture.** *J Urol* 2007, **177**(4):1552–1557.

47. Christmas TJ, Rode J, Chapple CR, Milroy EJ, Turner-Warwick RT: **Nerve fibre proliferation in interstitial cystitis.** *Virchows Arch A Pathol Anat Histopathol* 1990, **416**(5):447–451.

48. Lundeberg T, Liedberg H, Nordling L, Theodorsson E, Owzarski A, Ekman P: **Interstitial cystitis: correlation with nerve fibres, mast cells and histamine.** *Br J Urol* 1993, **71**(4):427–429.

49. Charrua A, Cruz CD, Cruz F, Avelino A: **Transient receptor potential vanilloid subfamily 1 is essential for the generation of noxious bladder input and bladder overactivity in cystitis.** *J Urol* 2007, **177**(4):1537–1541.

50. Dinis P, Charrua A, Avelino A, Yaqoob M, Bevan S, Nagy I, Cruz F: **Anandamide-evoked activation of vanilloid receptor 1 contributes to the development of bladder hyperreflexia and nociceptive transmission to spinal dorsal horn neurons in cystitis.** *J Neurosci* 2004, **24**(50):11253–11263.

51. Wang ZY, Wang P, Merriam FV, Bjorling DE: **Lack of TRPV1 inhibits cystitis-induced increased mechanical sensitivity in mice.** *Pain* 2008, **139**(1):158–167.

52. Girard BM, Tompkins JD, Parsons RL, May V, Vizzard MA: **Effects of CYP-induced cystitis on PACAP/VIP and receptor expression in micturition pathways and bladder function in mice with overexpression of NGF in urothelium.** *J Mol Neurosci* 2012, **48**(3):730–743.

53. Merrill L, Girard BM, May V, Vizzard MA: **Transcriptional and translational plasticity in rodent urinary bladder TRP channels with urinary bladder inflammation, bladder dysfunction, or postnatal maturation.** *J Mol Neurosci* 2012, **48**(3):744–756.

54. Lin G, Chen KC, Hsieh PS, Yeh CH, Lue TF, Lin CS: **Neurotrophic effects of vascular endothelial growth factor and neurotrophins on cultured major pelvic ganglia.** *BJU Int* 2003, **92**(6):631–635.

55. Lin G, Shindel AW, Fandel TM, Bella AJ, Lin CS, Lue TF: **Neurotrophic effects of brain-derived neurotrophic factor and vascular endothelial growth factor in major pelvic ganglia of young and aged rats.** *BJU Int* 2010, **105**(1):114–120.

56. Stewart AL, Anderson RB, Kobayashi K, Young HM: **Effects of NGF, NT-3 and GDNF family members on neurite outgrowth and migration from pelvic ganglia from embryonic and newborn mice.** *BMC Dev Biol* 2008, **8**:73.

57. Pereira Lopes FR, Lisboa BC, Frattini F, Almeida FM, Tomaz MA, Matsumoto PK, Langone F, Lora S, Melo PA, Borojevic R, Han SW, Martinez AM: **Enhancement of sciatic nerve regeneration after vascular endothelial growth factor (VEGF) gene therapy.** *Neuropathol Appl Neurobiol* 2011, **37**(6):600–612.

58. Nico B, Mangieri D, Benagiano V, Crivellato E, Ribatti D: **Nerve growth factor as an angiogenic factor.** *Microvasc Res* 2008, **75**(2):135–141.

59. Fan BS, Lou JY: **Enhancement of angiogenic effect of co-transfection human NGF and VEGF genes in rat bone marrow mesenchymal stem cells.** *Gene* 2011, **485**(2):167–171.

60. Saygili E, Pekassa M, Saygili E, Rackauskas G, Hommes D, Noor-Ebad F, Gemein C, Zink MD, Schwinger RH, Weis J, Marx N, Schauerte P, Rana OR: **Mechanical stretch of sympathetic neurons induces VEGF expression via a NGF and CNTF signaling pathway.** *Biochem Biophys Res Commun* 2011, **410**(1):62–67.

61. Cesca F, Yabe A, Spencer-Dene B, Scholz-Starke J, Medrihan L, Maden CH, Gerhardt H, Orriss IR, Baldelli P, Al-Qatari M, Koltzenburg M, Adams RH, Benfenati F, Schiavo G: **Kidins220/ARMS mediates the integration of the neurotrophin and VEGF pathways in the vascular and nervous systems.** *Cell Death Differ* 2012, **19**(2):194–208.

62. Neubrand VE, Cesca F, Benfenati F, Schiavo G: **Kidins220/ARMS as a functional mediator of multiple receptor signalling pathways.** *J Cell Sci* 2012, **125**(Pt 8):1845–1854.

63. Sun B, Li Q, Dong L, Rong W: **Ion channel and receptor mechanisms of bladder afferent nerve sensitivity.** *Auton Neurosci* 2010, **153**(1–2):26–32.

64. Caterina MJ: **Vanilloid receptors take a TRP beyond the sensory afferent.** *Pain* 2003, **105**(1–2):5–9.

65. Dib-Hajj SD, Cummins TR, Black JA, Waxman SG: **Sodium channels in normal and pathological pain.** *Annu Rev Neurosci* 2010, **33**:325–347.

66. Cheng Y, Keast JR: **Effects of estrogens and bladder inflammation on mitogen-activated protein kinases in lumbosacral dorsal root ganglia from adult female rats.** *BMC Neurosci* 2009, **10**:156.

67. Yu SJ, Xia CM, Kay JC, Qiao LY: **Activation of extracellular signal-regulated protein kinase 5 is essential for cystitis- and nerve growth factor-induced calcitonin gene-related peptide expression in sensory neurons.** *Mol Pain* 2012, **8**(1):48.

68. Driscoll A, Teichman JM: **How do patients with interstitial cystitis present?** *J Urol* 2001, **166**(6):2118–2120.

69. Yamaguchi O, Honda K, Nomiya M, Shishido K, Kakizaki H, Tanaka H, Yamanishi T, Homma Y, Takeda M, Araki I, Obara K, Nishizawa O, Igawa Y, Goto M, Yokoyama O, Seki N, Takei M, Yoshida M: **Defining overactive bladder as hypersensitivity.** *Neurourol Urodyn* 2007, **26**(6 Suppl):904–907.

70. Rush AM, Cummins TR, Waxman SG: **Multiple sodium channels and their roles in electrogenesis within dorsal root ganglion neurons.** *J Physiol* 2007, **579**(Pt 1):1–14.

71. Waxman SG: **Sodium channels, the electrogenisome and the electrogenistat: lessons and questions from the clinic.** *J Physiol* 2012, **590**(Pt 11):2601–2612.

72. Toledo-Aral JJ, Brehm P, Halegoua S, Mandel G: **A single pulse of nerve growth factor triggers long-term neuronal excitability through sodium channel gene induction.** *Neuron* 1995, **14**(3):607–611.

73. Leffler A, Cummins TR, Dib-Hajj SD, Hormuzdiar WN, Black JA, Waxman SG: **GDNF and NGF reverse changes in repriming of TTX-sensitive Na(+) currents following axotomy of dorsal root ganglion neurons.** *J Neurophysiol* 2002, **88**(2):650–658.

74. Dib-Hajj SD, Black JA, Cummins TR, Kenney AM, Kocsis JD, Waxman SG: **Rescue of alpha-SNS sodium channel expression in small dorsal root ganglion neurons after axotomy by nerve growth factor in vivo.** *J Neurophysiol* 1998, **79**(5):2668–2676.

75. Liu CJ, Dib-Hajj SD, Black JA, Greenwood J, Lian Z, Waxman SG: **Direct interaction with contactin targets voltage-gated sodium channel Na(v) 1.9/NaN to the cell membrane.** *J Biol Chem* 2001, **276**(49):46553–46561.

76. Rush AM, Craner MJ, Kageyama T, Dib-Hajj SD, Waxman SG, Ranscht B: **Contactin regulates the current density and axonal expression of tetrodotoxin-resistant but not tetrodotoxin-sensitive sodium channels in DRG neurons.** *Eur J Neurosci* 2005, **22**(1):39–49.

77. Okuse K, Malik-Hall M, Baker MD, Poon WY, Kong H, Chao MV, Wood JN: **Annexin II light chain regulates sensory neuron-specific sodium channel expression.** *Nature* 2002, **417**(6889):653–656.

78. Yang RH, Wang WT, Chen JY, Xie RG, Hu SJ: **Gabapentin selectively reduces persistent sodium current in injured type-a dorsal root ganglion neurons.** *Pain* 2009, **143**(1–2):48–55.

79. Wang W, Gu J, Li YQ, Tao YX: **Are voltage-gated sodium channels on the dorsal root ganglion involved in the development of neuropathic pain?** *Mol Pain* 2011, **7**:16.

80. Toth DM, Szoke E, Bolcskei K, Kvell K, Bender B, Bosze Z, Szolcsanyi J, Sandor Z: **Nociception, neurogenic inflammation and thermoregulation in TRPV1 knockdown transgenic mice.** *Cell Mol Life Sci* 2011, **68**(15):2589–2601.

81. Dupont MC, Spitsbergen JM, Kim KB, Tuttle JB, Steers WD: **Histological and neurotrophic changes triggered by varying models of bladder inflammation.** *J Urol* 2001, **166**(3):1111–1118.

82. Bjorling DE, Wang ZY, Boldon K, Bushman W: **Bacterial cystitis is accompanied by increased peripheral thermal sensitivity in mice.** *J Urol* 2008, **179**(2):759–763.

83. Guerios SD, Wang ZY, Boldon K, Bushman W, Bjorling DE: **Blockade of NGF and trk receptors inhibits increased peripheral mechanical sensitivity accompanying cystitis in rats.** *Am J Physiol Regul Integr Comp Physiol* 2008, **295**(1):R111–R122.

84. DeBerry J, Randich A, Shaffer AD, Robbins MT, Ness TJ: **Neonatal bladder inflammation produces functional changes and alters neuropeptide content in bladders of adult female rats.** *J Pain* 2010, **11**(3):247–255.

85. Randich A, Uzzell T, DeBerry JJ, Ness TJ: **Neonatal urinary bladder inflammation produces adult bladder hypersensitivity.** *J Pain* 2006, **7**(7):469–479.

86. Robinson CJ, Stringer SE: **The splice variants of vascular endothelial growth factor (VEGF) and their receptors.** *J Cell Sci* 2001, **114**(Pt 5):853–865.

87. Eichmann A, Makinen T, Alitalo K: **Neural guidance molecules regulate vascular remodeling and vessel navigation.** *Genes Dev* 2005, **19**(9):1013–1021.

88. Tran J, Master Z, Yu JL, Rak J, Dumont DJ, Kerbel RS: **A role for survivin in chemoresistance of endothelial cells mediated by VEGF.** *Proc Natl Acad Sci U S A* 2002, **99**(7):4349–4354.

89. Segarra M, Ohnuki H, Maric D, Salvucci O, Hou X, Kumar A, Li X, Tosato G: **Semaphorin 6A regulates angiogenesis by modulating VEGF signaling.** *Blood* 2012, **120**(19):4104–4115.

90. Yang S, Wu X, Luo C, Pan C, Pu J: **Expression and clinical significance of hepaCAM and VEGF in urothelial carcinoma.** *World J Urol* 2010, **28**(4):473–478.

91. Saban MR, Nguyen NB, Hammond TG, Saban R: **Gene expression profiling of mouse bladder inflammatory responses to LPS, substance P, and antigen-stimulation.** *Am J Pathol* 2002, **160**(6):2095–2110.

92. Yu W, Hill WG: **Defining protein expression in the urothelium: a problem of more than transitional interest.** *Am J Physiol Renal Physiol* 2011, **301**(5):F932–942.

93. Haarala M, Kiiholma P, Nurmi M, Uksila J, Alanen A: **The role of Borrelia burgdorferi in interstitial cystitis.** *European urology* 2000, **37**(4):395–399.

94. Charrua A, Cruz CD, Narayanan S, Gharat L, Gullapalli S, Cruz F, Avelino A: **GRC-6211, a new oral specific TRPV1 antagonist, decreases bladder overactivity and noxious bladder input in cystitis animal models.** *J Urol* 2009, **181**(1):379–386.

95. Finney-Hayward TK, Popa MO, Bahra P, Li S, Poll CT, Gosling M, Nicholson AG, Russell RE, Kon OM, Jarai G, Westwick J, Barnes PJ, Donnelly LE: **Expression of transient receptor potential c6 channels in human lung macrophages.** *Am J Respir Cell Mol Biol* 2010, **43**(3):296–304.

96. Rudick CN, Chen MC, Mongiu AK, Klumpp DJ: **Organ cross talk modulates pelvic pain.** *Am J Physiol Regul Integr Comp Physiol* 2007, **293**(3):R1191–1198.

17

Subcellular dissemination of prothymosin alpha at normal physiology: immunohistochemical vis-a-vis western blotting perspective

Caroline Mwendwa Kijogi[1,3], Christopher Khayeka-Wandabwa[2,3*], Keita Sasaki[4], Yoshimasa Tanaka[4], Hiroshi Kurosu[4], Hayato Matsunaga[4] and Hiroshi Ueda[4]

Abstract

Background: The cell type, cell status and specific localization of Prothymosin α (PTMA) within cells seemingly determine its function. PTMA undergoes 2 types of protease proteolytic modifications that are useful in elucidating its interactions with other molecules; a factor that typifies its roles. Preferably a nuclear protein, PTMA has been shown to function in the cytoplasm and extracellularly with much evidence leaning on pathognomonic status. As such, determination of its cellular distribution under normal physiological context while utilizing varied techniques is key to illuminating prospective validation of its distinct functions in different tissues. Differential distribution insights at normal physiology would also portent better basis for further clarification of its interactions and proteolytic modifications under pathological conditions like numerous cancer, ischemic stroke and immunomodulation. We therefore raised an antibody against the C terminal of PTMA to use in tandem with available antibody against the N terminal in a murine model to explicate the differences in its distribution in brain cell types and major peripheral organs through western blotting and immunohistochemical approaches.

Results: The newly generated antibody was applied against the N-terminal antibody to distinguish truncated versions of PTMA or deduce possible masking of the protein by other interacting molecules. Western blot analysis indicated presence of a truncated form of the protein only in the thymus, while immunohistochemical analysis showed that in brain hippocampus the full-length PTMA was stained prominently in the nucleus whereas in the stomach full-length PTMA staining was not observed in the nucleus but in the cytoplasm.

Conclusion: Truncated PTMA could not be detected by western blotting when both antibodies were applied in all tissues examined except the thymus. However, immunohistochemistry revealed differential staining by these antibodies suggesting possible masking of epitopes by interacting molecules. The differential localization patterns observed in the context of nucleic versus cytoplasmic presence as well as punctate versus diffuse pattern in tissues and cell types, warrant further investigations as to the forms of PTMA interacting partners.

Keywords: Prothymosin α, Anti-C terminal antibody, Anti- N terminal antibody, Immunohistochemistry, Western blotting and localization

* Correspondence: khayekachris@yahoo.com
[2]African Population and Health Research Center (APHRC), P. O. Box 10787-00100, Nairobi, Kenya
[3]Institute of Tropical Medicine and Infectious Diseases-KEMRI (ITROMID-KEMRI), Nairobi, Kenya
Full list of author information is available at the end of the article

Background

Prothymosin α (PTMA) is an unstructured, extremely acidic protein (pI 3.5), expressed in a wide variety of cell types. Progressively, research has attested to it as a protein of clinical significance and potential medical use [1, 2]. It is considered a nuclear protein with a potent nuclear localization signal (NLS), albeit reports indicate cytoplasmic and extracellular presence as well, under specific physiological or pathological conditions [3, 4]. It has a highly conserved amino acid sequence among mammals and this together with its wide distribution affirm that it plays an essential role in an organism other than the traditionally attributed role of immune modulation.

Even so, the precise function is still not well understood. Accumulating data point towards both intracellular and extracellular biological functions of PTMA [5–11]. The major intracellular role is associated with cell proliferation. It has been reported that PTMA stimulates cell proliferation by sequestering a repressor of estrogen receptor activity in various cells [12]. Cancer cells are known to be highly proliferative and indeed high expression of intracellular PTMA has been correlated with progression of a number of cancer types including bladder cancer, liver cancer, breast cancer, head and neck cancer, lung cancer, colon cancer, rectal cancer, ovarian cancer, neuroblastoma, prostate cancer and gastric cancer [13–26]. Moreover, PTMA binds to histones, p300 histone acetyl transferase and cAMP response element binding protein (CREB)-binding protein to induce gene transcription [27, 28]. Recent studies have explored the role of intracellular PTMA in acetylation regulation [29].

Further intracellular roles of PTMA include its involvement in cell survival. Nuclear Factor erythroid 2 related factor (Nrf2), a transcription factor that regulates expression of defensive genes such as antioxidant proteins and detoxifying enzymes, is inhibited by Kelch-like ECH-associated protein 1(Keap1). On one hand, PTMA binds to Keap1 to dissociate Keap1-Nrf2 complex thus upregulating the expression of Nrf2 dependent antioxidative stress genes [30]. On the other hand, it has been reported in mediating nuclear import of Keap1 to degrade nuclear Nrf2 and thus switch off downstream gene expression suggesting that it is involved in on/off switch of Keap1-Nrf2 system [31]. Moreover, PTMA acts as an anti-apoptotic molecule in the cytoplasm by interacting with Apaf1 to inhibit apoptosome formation [32] and by binding to cytochrome c [33] thereby inhibiting caspase activation. Reports also show that it interacts with p8 (nuclear protein 1), a natively unstructured protein with anti-apoptotic activity much like PTMA, to form a heterodimer complex that could act in concert to regulate the apoptotic cascade [34]. Interestingly however, PTMA undergoes caspase mediated fragmentation in apoptotic cells at two amino-terminal sub-optimal

sites and one carboxy-terminal optimal site [35, 36]. Cleavage at the latter site disrupts its nuclear localization and subsequently its intranuclear functioning [37].

Extracellularly, PTMA plays a role in immunomodulation via a pleiotropic mode by stimulating a variety of immune cells including natural killer cells, T cells and lymphokine-activated killer cells-dendritic cells, monocytes and macrophages. The mechanism by which it regulates immune responses is proposed to be through binding to TLR4 on innate immune cells to trigger induction of pro-inflammatory cytokines. Reports also show that the C-terminus of PTMA holds the immunologically active site of the polypeptide [38]. Seemingly, different parts of the molecule are responsible for the different biological functions it exerts.

Reports from our laboratory also show that extracellular PTMA can confer protection to neurons upon ischemic stress by inhibiting necrosis [39]. Cell death that occurs as a consequence of obstructed blood flow in a brain region causes damage to tissues and results in ischemic stroke. Two modes of cell death occur during ischemic stroke: necrosis at the ischemic core and apoptosis several days later at the region that surrounds the core called the penumbra. Necrosis, a rapid and expanding process contributes largely to cell damage but to this end there are no known inhibitors of necrosis. Apoptosis on the other hand can be inhibited by growth factors. Importantly, PTMA was identified as a molecule that can initiate a switch from uncontrollable necrosis to tractable apoptosis in ischemic neurons [40]. Further findings on the neuroprotective role of PTMA revealed neuron-specific extracellular release of the polypeptide following ischemic stress. PTMA was released in a non-classical manner and this release was mediated by its interaction with the cargo protein, S100A13 [41]. The interaction was shown to require the C-terminal region of PTMA. Since astrocytes have intrinsic caspase 3 activity it was postulated that the non-release of PTMA in astrocytes in brain following ischemia was as a result of caspase cleavage of PTMA in its C-terminus thus depriving it the interaction with S100A13. In addition, caspase cleavage of PTMA disrupts its nuclear localization, resulting in redistribution of the polypeptide. PTMA is also capable of proteolytic lysis by asparaginyl endopeptidase in its N-terminus to yield thymosin alpha 1 (TA_1) but it still remains to be elucidated if this proteolysis is simply a step in the catabolism of PTMA or a more specific selective process in view of some biological function of TA_1 [42].

Depending on the proteins which it interacts with, PTMA exerts different effects; a feature that is determined by its subcellular localization. To individualize PTMA interactions and proteolytic modifications that occur in different tissues, it is a prerequisite to determine its cellular modelling in diverse tissues. The subcellular localization in tissues under normal physiological context has been under reported yet this is a core basis for further elucidation of its interactions and proteolytic modifications under pathological conditions like the various cancer forms, ischemic stroke and immunomodulation mechanisms where it exhibits extensively contrasting roles depending on the pathognomonic status and localization. In the present study, we implore western blotting and immunohistochemical techniques to explore the expression of PTMA and its specific cellular localization in different murine tissues using a set of monoclonal antibodies raised against different epitopes on the polypeptide; the brain being the predominant organ of investigation based on our earlier findings [39–41]. First, we generated a monoclonal antibody against the C-terminal region of PTMA (AntiCT) and employed it in conjunction with the anti N-terminal monoclonal antibody (2 F11) for a comparison. We therefore observe that, the preferential combination of the applied techniques and monoclonal antibodies would lay ground to prospective examinations for better understanding of factors that mediate biological function of PTMA across brain cells and other peripheral tissues not only during proteolytic modifications in pathological conditions but also under normal physiology context.

Methods

Experimental animals

Two female Wistar rats were used for the generation of monoclonal antibodies. Male MP-BL mice were used for the western blotting and immunohistochemistry experiments. The animals were kept in a room maintained at constant temperature (21 ± 2 °C) and relative humidity (55 ± 5 %) with an automatic 12 h light/dark cycle with free access to standard laboratory diet and water *ad libitum*.

Immunization of animals

Synthetic biotinylated carboxy-terminal peptide of PTMA, (bearing the sequence DDVDTKKQKTEEDD, -Cat.No 293211. GL Biochem Shanghai Ltd), was used as immunogen. Wistar rats were anesthetized and immunized with 200 μg avidin conjugated immunogen, injected on the foot pads as emulsions (1:1 v/v) in complete Freund's adjuvant (Cat No. 263810, DIFCO Laboratories Detroit, MI) Blood was collected from the immunized animals 2 weeks after the injection and the serum tested for immune reactivity with recombinant mouse PTMA. A week later the animals were sacrificed and the medial iliac lymph nodes aseptically harvested as previously reported [43, 44].

Characterization of the antibody

Hybridomas were prepared using the isolated medial iliac lymph node cells and SP2/0 myeloma cells as the fusion partner in the presence of polyethylene glycol (PEG) and cultured in Hypoxthanthine Aminopterin Thymidine (HAT) selective medium. Cell culture media was then assayed by standard Enzyme linked Immunosorbent Assay (ELISA) for the presence of PTMA-reactive antibodies and cells from the ELISA-positive wells cloned by limiting dilution. Screening of hybridoma cell line supernatants was performed via ELISA. Positively identified hybridoma clones were expanded and inspected for monoclonality then assayed by ELISA for immune-reactivity. Desired clones were subsequently re-expanded and adapted to RPMI1640 medium. The monoclonal antibody was then purified from the supernatant by Protein G affinity chromatography and the concentration of purified antibody was determined by Lowry method.

Application of antibody in western blot analysis

Mice were decapitated and the desired brain regions (Olfactory bulb, cortex, amygdala, hippocampus, striatum, cerebellum, thalamus, hypothalamus, mid brain pons and medulla) and tissues (peripheral tissues including spleen, thymus, lung, heart, kidney, liver, colon, stomach, duodenum, jejunum, ileum and cecum) were obtained and transferred into ice-cold homogenizing buffer (20 mM Tris-HCl, pH 7.4, 10 mM NaCl, 1 mM EDTA, 0.01 % SDS, 1 % Triton X-100 and 1X protease inhibitor cocktail) . Tissue lysis was performed using tissue homogenizer or sonication. The homogenate was centrifuged at 15,000 rpm for 30 min at 4 °C. An aliquot of the supernatant was taken for protein quantification, equivalent amounts of total protein mixed with 2 x SDS sample buffer and heated in a boiling water bath for 5 min. The boiled samples were either used immediately or frozen at −20 °C.

Protein quantification of recombinant PTMA and total protein concentration of tissue homogenates was determined by Lowry protein assay method. Samples were prepared for loading onto gel using 1×SDS loading buffer as previously described. Indicated quantities of recombinant Prothymosin α and the tissue samples containing 20 μg of total protein were electrophoresed on 15 % SDS-polyacrylamide gels, transferred onto a nitrocellulose membrane by electroblotting performed at 30 V, 100 mA for 90 min and subjected to immunoblotting with appropriate antibody. In the case of untagged recombinant and tissue PTMA, transfer onto a membrane was by electroblotting with acidic buffer (20 mM sodium acetate buffer, pH 5.2) followed by fixation with 0.5 % glutaraldehyde. Blotted membranes were blocked with 5 % skim milk and 2 % FBS in TBST or 5 % BSA.

Membranes were then probed with rat/mouse anti-PTMA (AntiCT and 2 F11 from Alexis Biochemicals respectively) and mouse anti-GAPDH (internal control) primary antibodies followed by Horseradish Peroxidase (HRP)-conjugated goat secondary antibodies. Visualization of immunoreactive bands was executed by enhanced chemiluminescent (ECL). Densitometry of the detected protein bands was determined using ImageJ software. The densitometry ratio of PTMA to GAPDH was calculated. For the purpose of comparison between tissues and between different sets of experiments, the densitometry ratio of each tissue was plotted.

Application of antibody in immunoprecipitation assay

10 µg Protein G sepharose fast flow slurry was incubated with 10 µg of indicated antibody at 4 °C overnight in agitating condition. The beads were then washed 3 times each with wash buffer and incubated with sample (tissue lysate or recombinant protein), at 4 °C for 4 h followed by 3 washes and eluted with 1X SDS loading buffer. Immunoprecipitated samples were then boiled for 5 min and analysed by western blot.

Application of antibody to immunohistochemistry

Mice peripheral tissues and specific brain regions were fixed by vascular perfusion with 30 mL of 4 % paraformaldehyde (PFA) after perfusion with PBS for about 20 min. Desired organs were isolated and washed with PBS then processed using a rapid microwave automatic histo-processor using a standard protocol and embedded into paraffin wax. Subsequent immunohistochemistry assays were then performed per standard protocols previously described [15]. Briefly, sectioned tissues were deparrafinized then permeabilized with methanol. The sections were then blocked with 3 % BSA for 1 h at room temperature and later incubated with primary antibody (1:300 mouse monoclonal IgG 2 F11; Enzo Life Sciences Int., PA, USA and AntiCT)) at 4 °C overnight, washed with PBST then with secondary antibody conjugated to AlexFluor (1:600) for 2 h at room temperature. Counterstaining with Hoechst 33342 (1:10,000) was effected. The slides were then mounted by pristine mount and left to dry overnight at 4 °C. Images were collected by BZ-8000 microscope (KEYENCE, Osaka, Japan) with a × 20 Plan APO lens (Nikon, Tokyo, Japan).

Application of antibody to immunocytochemistry

Primary cortical cells on an eight-well Lab Tek chamber were fixed in 4 % PFA in PBS at 4 °C overnight followed by 3 wash steps with PBS. Fixed cells were permeabilized with 50 and 100 % methanol for 10 min each then washed with PBS 3 times. The permeabilized cells were washed with 0.1 % Triton X-100 in PBS (PBST), incubated in blocking buffer (3 % BSA in PBST) for 3 h at 4 °C, and then incubated in primary antibody (1 : 300; mouse monoclonal IgG 2 F11; Enzo Life Sciences Int., PA, USA and AntiCT) overnight at 4 °C. The cells were then washed with PBST and thereafter incubated in a secondary antibody conjugated to AlexFluor. The nuclei were visualized with Hoechst 33342. Images were collected using a BZ-8000 microscope (KEYENCE, Osaka, Japan) with a × 20 Plan APO lens (Nikon, Tokyo, Japan).

Ethical clearance

All the procedures were formally approved by Nagasaki University Animal Care Committee. The guidelines were strictly adhered to during the research.

Results

Selection of hybridoma cell lines secreting monoclonal antibodies by indirect ELISA was performed using purified Glutathione S- transferase (GST) and Maltose binding protein (MBP) tagged recombinant PTMA as the antigen. From approximately 1500 primary hybridomas 16 yielded immune reactive signals 3-100-fold above background as indicated by optical density (OD) values (data not shown). The 16 hybridomas were all confirmed to react with recombinant PTMA in a second round of ELISA screening. To determine whether the secreted antibodies could specifically detect full-length PTMA, the 16 hybridoma candidates were tested for their reactivity against recombinant mouse PTMA by western blot analysis (Fig. 1). The C-terminal truncated PTMA was included to assay the specific detection of C-terminus region. Supernatant from the hybridoma cell culture was used for the analysis. The antibodies from the cultures could detect full-length PTMA but not the C-terminal truncated one.

To further investigate if the generated antibody could detect rat and human PTMA, western blot analysis was carried out using purified recombinant full-length mouse, rat and human Prothymosin α (Fig. 2). Supernatant from the hybridoma culture was used for this analysis. Clones 1, 5 and 7 showed somewhat similar signal intensities for the detection of PTMA across the species. On the other hand, clones 3, 4, 8, 13, 15 and 16 showed higher affinity for mouse PTMA whereas clones 9, 11 and 12 lost their ability to secret the antibodies. Clones 10 and 14 showed relatively very weak signal intensities. PTMA sequence is highly conserved across species (Fig. 3), coloured amino acids denote less conserved sections. While amino termini of all three species show precise homology, the carboxy termini show some differences between the species. Nevertheless, some antibodies from various hybridoma cell lines could recognize the c-terminus of PTMA across species.

Clone 7 (Figs. 1 and 2) was selected for further culture due to its consistency in PTMA detection after cloning.

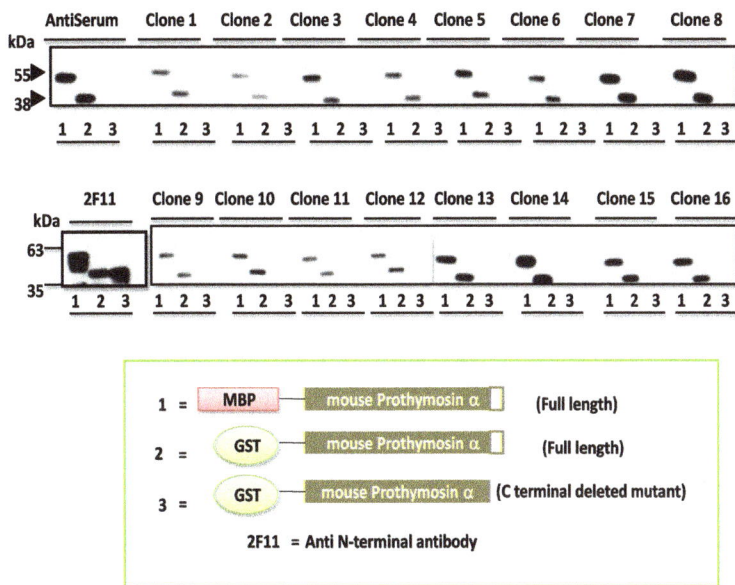

Fig. 1 Western blot analysis of hybridoma immune-reactivity MBP and GST tagged recombinant mouse PTMA (as shown in the inlet) were loaded onto gel for electrophoresis and thereafter blotted on to nitrocellulose membranes. Blotted membranes were incubated with supernatant from the hybridoma cultures from different clones as indicated. HRP conjugated anti-rat IgG secondary antibody and HRP substrate was used to develop the bands. Signals were detected by enhanced chemiluminescence. No band was detected on the C-terminal deleted mutant of PTMA (lane 3), while bands corresponding to full-length tagged recombinant PTMA were detected with different intensities across the clones

The selected clone was adapted to RPMI1640 medium and antibody immunoreactivity confirmed. The hybridoma clone was then grown in serum free GIT medium and the secreted antibodies were purified by protein G affinity chromatography, dialyzed with PBS and later antibody concentration was determined. Reactivity of the purified antibody was assayed by western blotting and antibody tested for capacity to immunoprecipitate PTMA from tissue and the recombinant PTMA. AntiCT antibody successfully immunoprecipitated PTMA from the cerebellum tissue lysate. Anti N-terminal PTMA (2 F11) was applied alongside AntiCT in the immunoprecipitation studies for a comparison. Detection of PTMA immunoprecipitated by both antibodies was carried out by 2 F11. Same amount of antibody was used for each antibody type. 2 F11 antibody showed greater capacity for immunoprecipitation than AntiCT.

The tissue-wide distribution of PTMA was assessed using the newly generated anti C-terminal PTMA (AntiCT) and the anti N-terminal PTMA (2 F11)

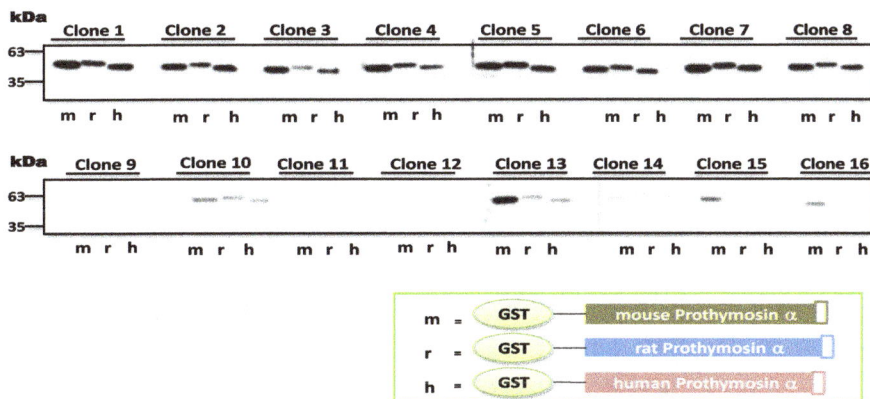

Fig. 2 Determination of cross reactivity of the antibodies with rat and human PTMA. GST tagged recombinant mouse, rat and human PTMA were loaded onto gel for electrophoresis and blotted on to nitrocellulose membranes thereafter. Blotted membranes were incubated with supernatant from the hybridoma cultures from different clones as indicated. Antibodies from most clones showed crossreactivity with rat and human PTMA. Some showed relatively similar or different signal intensities indicative of the affinity of the antibodies to the particular antigens. Clones 9, 11 and 12 lost their ability to secret antibodies

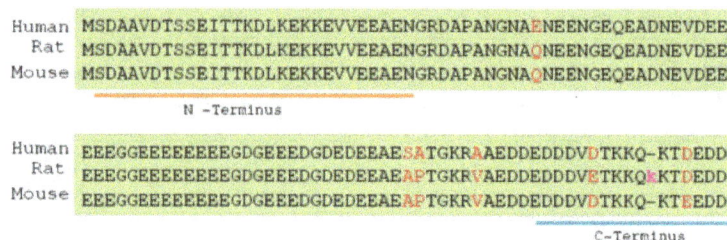

Fig. 3 Alignment of amino acid sequences of human, rat and mouse Prothymosin alpha

antibodies. To explore whether proteolytically modified forms of PTMA could be detected by the set of antibodies, the immunoblot assay was performed in brain regions and peripheral tissues. Immunoblot data revealed a single band detectable by both 2 F11 and AntiCT that corresponded to full-length PTMA in the brain regions (Fig. 4), no additional bands were detected indicative of proteolytic modification of PTMA. In peripheral tissues, a similar observation was made (Fig. 5), however an additional lower band was detectable by 2 F11 only in the thymus suggesting c-terminal truncated version o or several different variants of PTMA could be present. The relative levels of PTMA in different tissues were calculated according to densitometry measurements and the data are summarized. Densitometric quantification of the western blot bands of PTMA expression across peripheral tissues and selected brain regions [Additional files 1 and 2 correspondingly] corresponding to Figs. 4 and 5 respectively. In the brain, the highest levels of PTMA were detected in the olfactory bulb and cerebellum by both antibodies while in peripheral tissues, the thymus, spleen and lungs showed high PTMA levels by both antibodies. Relatively low PTMA levels were detected in the heart, kidney and liver.

PTMA localization was evaluated by immunohistochemistry in a spectrum of organs Multi-colour experiment was performed for PTMA visualization by co-staining with AntiCT and 2 F11 antibodies. Hoechst stain was used to visualize the nucleus. We observed a differential staining pattern among the tissues examined. Immunoreactivity of PTMA was mainly in the nucleus of most tissues, while other tissues indicated predominant cytoplasmic staining. In the hippocampus PTMA signals were intense in the nucleus (Fig. 6a iii) when detected by both Anti CT and 2 F11 (Fig. 6a i and ii) clearly indicated by the merge data (Fig. 6a iv). In the lungs, an intriguing observation was made in the pattern of distribution of PTMA expression. The AntiCT antibody stained both nucleus and cytoplasm (Fig. 6b i iii and iv) in majority of the cells while 2 F11 stained only the cytoplasm in most cells and the perinuclear space in few cells (Fig. 6b ii, iii and iv).

The heart presented weak PTMA immunostaining by both AntiCT and 2 F11 antibodies (Fig. 7a i, ii and iii) and clearly illustrated by the merge (Fig. 7a iv) in correlation with the western blot data that indicated weak PTMA expression. In the kidney, PTMA was primarily expressed in the nucleus (Fig. 7b iii) by both antibodies (Fig. 7b i and ii) with AntiCT showing more intense signal (Fig. 7b iv).

In the liver PTMA was demonstrated considerably in the nucleus (Fig. 8b iii) by both AntiCT ant 2 F11 (Fig. 8a i, ii and iv), this correlates with the western blot data that showed substantial expression of PTMA. In the stomach, PTMA immunoreactive cells of the mucosal

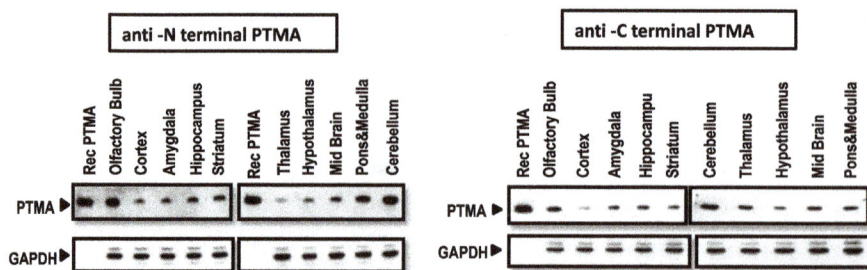

Fig. 4 Western blot analysis of the distribution of PTMA in selected brain regions. Immunoreactive PTMA from regions of the brain tissue shows single bands at apparent molecular weight of 12 kDa. Lysates from multiple sections of the brain were resolved in electrophoretic gel and transferred to nitrocellulose membranes. The western blot analysis was performed with monoclonal 2 F11 and monoclonal AntiCT. Untagged recombinant PTMA was used as positive control and GAPDH as internal control

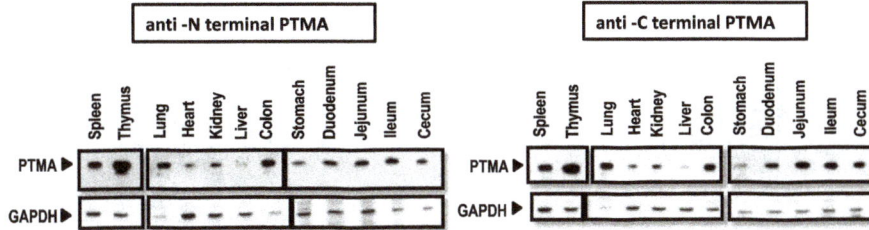

Fig. 5 Western blot analysis of the distribution of PTMA across peripheral tissues. Immunoreactive PTMA from various peripheral tissues shows single bands at apparent molecular weight of 12 kDa. Lysates from the peripheral tissues were resolved in electrophoretic gel and transferred to nitrocellulose membranes. The western blot analysis was performed with monoclonal 2 F11 and monoclonal AntiCT. GAPDH was used as internal control

layer demonstrated quite a unique distribution pattern. PTMA was not stained in the nucleus (Fig. 8b iii) of these cells by either of 2 F11 or AntiCT antibodies (Fig. 8b i and ii). Interestingly, only the cytoplasm was positively immunostained, clearly indicated by the merge data (Fig. 8b iv). Showing both antibodies exhibited strong cytoplasmic immunofluorescent intensity.

The duodenum showed PTMA immunoreactivity in the nucleus (Fig. 9a iii) and weakly in the cytoplasm but AntiCT (Fig. 9a i) demonstrated higher signal intensity than 2 F11 (Fig. 9a ii). Additionally, 2 F11 depicted perinuclear staining in some submucosal layer cells. The jejunum also presented an exceptional PTMA staining pattern in which the AntiCT shows immunoreactivity mainly in the nucleus (Fig. 9b i and iii) while 2 F11 depicts mainly a cytoplasmic immunostaining (Fig. 9b ii). Some cells show perinuclear staining with 2 F11 only,

while few show perinuclear staining with both antibodies (Merge, Fig. 9b iv).

Ileum, colon and cecum demonstrated a similar pattern of distribution of immunoreactive PTMA (Figs. 10a, b and 11 respectively). The AntiCT stained with much higher fluorescent intensity (Figs. 10a i, iii; b i, iii and Fig. 11 i, iii), depicting strong nucleus signal compared to cytoplasmic signal. 2 F11 showed moderate nucleus signal (Figs. 10a ii, iii; b ii, iii and Fig. 11 ii, iii). An overlay of PTMA and nuclear staining is shown in the merge data (Figs. 10a, b and 11iv).

Given that PTMA has previously been shown by 2 F11 to be exclusively located in the nuclei of neurons we explored cell-type specific distribution of PTMA: an immunocytochemical study, by immunostaining with newly generated anti C-terminus PTMA antibody whether a similar staining pattern would be observed. We used

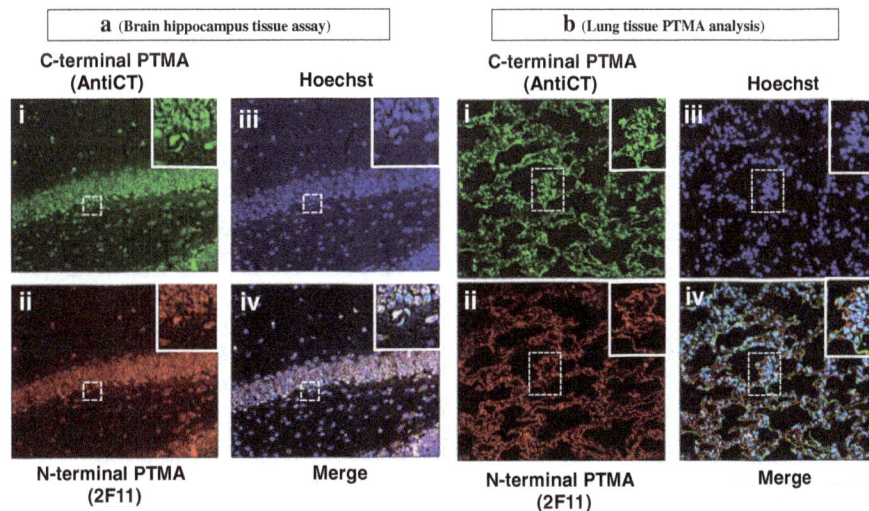

Fig. 6 Immunohistochemistry analysis of PTMA in (**a**) mouse brain hippocampus tissue and (**b**) Lung tissue. Whole animal vascular perfusion fixation was conducted with PFA and the required tissues were isolated. The brain hippocampus and lung were processed for immunohistochemistry by embedding to paraffin wax. Tissue sections were stained with AntiCT (a)i and (b)i and 2 F11 (a)ii and (b)ii together with relevant fluorescent tagged antibodies. Sections were then washed, counterstained with Hoechst (a)iii and (b)iii and processed for fluorescence microscopy. Both antibodies localized PTMA in the nucleus of the hippocampus (a)i and ii, while in the lung PTMA immunoreactivity was observed in the nucleus and cytoplasm by AntiCT (b)i but mainly in the cytoplasm by 2 F11 (b)ii

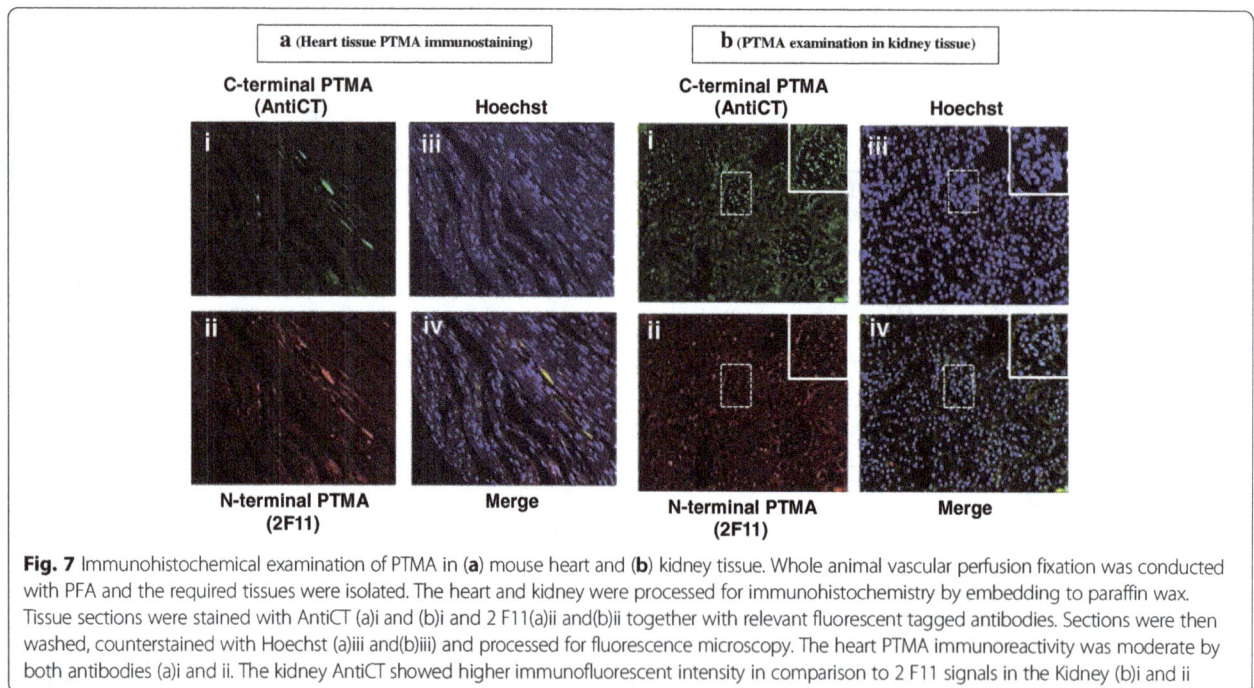

Fig. 7 Immunohistochemical examination of PTMA in (**a**) mouse heart and (**b**) kidney tissue. Whole animal vascular perfusion fixation was conducted with PFA and the required tissues were isolated. The heart and kidney were processed for immunohistochemistry by embedding to paraffin wax. Tissue sections were stained with AntiCT (a)i and (b)i and 2 F11(a)ii and(b)ii together with relevant fluorescent tagged antibodies. Sections were then washed, counterstained with Hoechst (a)iii and(b)iii and processed for fluorescence microscopy. The heart PTMA immunoreactivity was moderate by both antibodies (a)i and ii. The kidney AntiCT showed higher immunofluorescent intensity in comparison to 2 F11 signals in the Kidney (b)i and ii

primary cortical neurons cultured from 17 day-old embryonic rat brain. Anti C-terminal PTMA depicted a punctate signal that was widely distributed throughout the nucleus; weak signals were also detected in the cytoplasm as by the arrow heads shown (Fig. 12), eliciting contrast with the 2 F11 antibody.

Discussion

Prothymosin α (PTMA) generates a great deal of interest among investigators due to its robust involvement in a variety of biological processes ranging from cell proliferation as observed in several types of cancer [13–26] and apoptosis [34, 37, 39, 40, 45] to its association with cell-

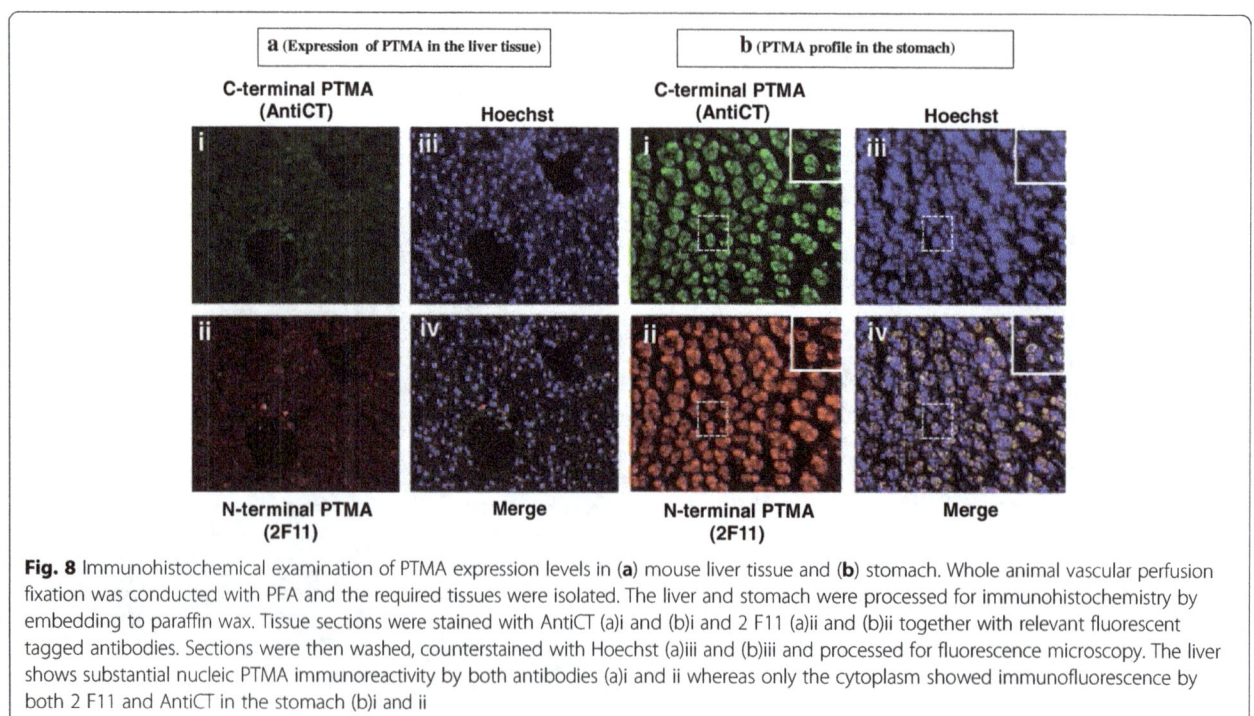

Fig. 8 Immunohistochemical examination of PTMA expression levels in (**a**) mouse liver tissue and (**b**) stomach. Whole animal vascular perfusion fixation was conducted with PFA and the required tissues were isolated. The liver and stomach were processed for immunohistochemistry by embedding to paraffin wax. Tissue sections were stained with AntiCT (a)i and (b)i and 2 F11 (a)ii and (b)ii together with relevant fluorescent tagged antibodies. Sections were then washed, counterstained with Hoechst (a)iii and (b)iii and processed for fluorescence microscopy. The liver shows substantial nucleic PTMA immunoreactivity by both antibodies (a)i and ii whereas only the cytoplasm showed immunofluorescence by both 2 F11 and AntiCT in the stomach (b)i and ii

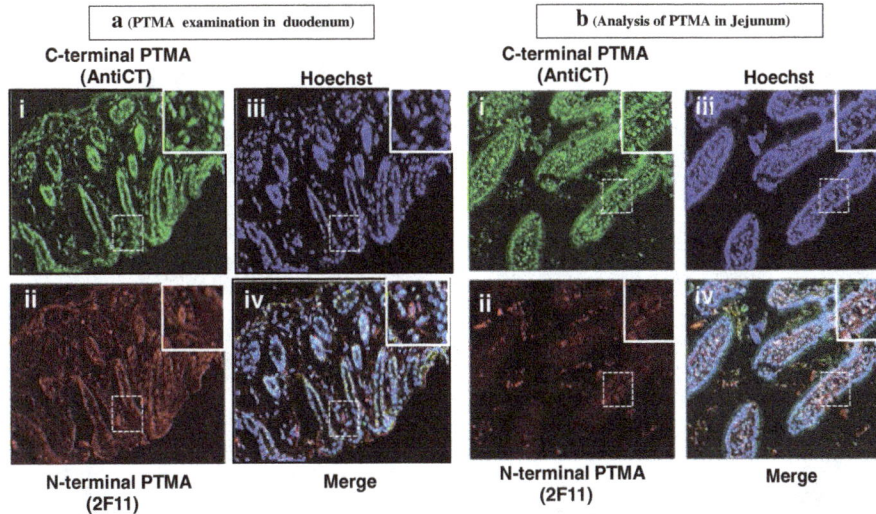

Fig. 9 Immunohistochemical analysis of PTMA in (**a**) mouse duodenum and (**b**) Jejunum. Whole animal vascular perfusion fixation was conducted with PFA and the required tissues were isolated. The duodenum and jejunum were processed for immunohistochemistry by embedding to paraffin wax. Tissue sections were stained with AntiCT (a)i and (b)i and 2 F11 (a)ii and (b)ii together with relevant fluorescent tagged antibodies. Sections were then washed, counterstained with Hoechst (a)iii and (b)iii and processed for fluorescence microscopy. In the duodenum, PTMA immunoreactivity revealed nucleic staining with AntiCT (b)i and cytoplasmic staining with 2 F11 (b)ii

mediated immunity [6, 8, 46]. Moreover, going by recent studies conducted to understand the role PTMA in non-mammalian vertebrates, insights into changes in PTMA functions and expression that have occurred with evolution is required. It has been shown that PTMA is involved in spermatogenesis in the frog [47, 48] and in the cartilaginous fish *Torpedo marmorata* [49]. In the zebrafish, the PTMA gene has been shown to be duplicated [50] and expressed differentially during embryonic development indicating that their function is more complex in fishes than in mammals.

As yet, its subcellular localization in tissues under normal physiological context has been underreported equally utilizing narrow range techniques. In the present study we demonstrated the tissue distribution and subcellular localization of PTMA in diverse murine organ

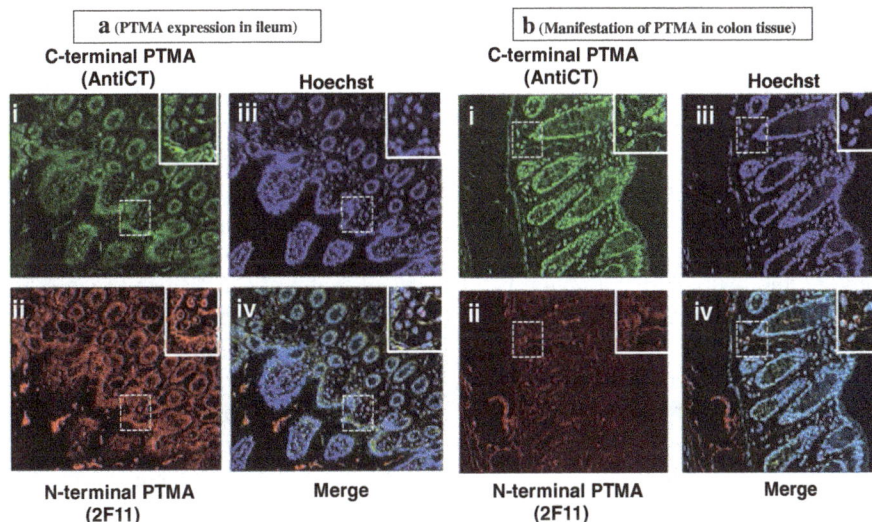

Fig. 10 Immuohistochemical analysis of PTMA in (**a**) mouse ileum tissue and (**b**) colon. Whole animal vascular perfusion fixation was conducted with PFA and the required tissues were isolated. The ileum and colon were processed for immunohistochemistry by embedding to paraffin wax. Tissue sections were stained with AntiCT (a)i and (b)i and 2 F11 (a)ii and(b)ii together with relevant fluorescent tagged antibodies. Sections were then washed, counterstained with Hoechst (a)iii and(b)iii and processed for fluorescence microscopy. The ileum and colon depict nucleic PTMA staining with AntiCT (a and b)i and cytoplasmic staining with 2 F11 (a and b)ii

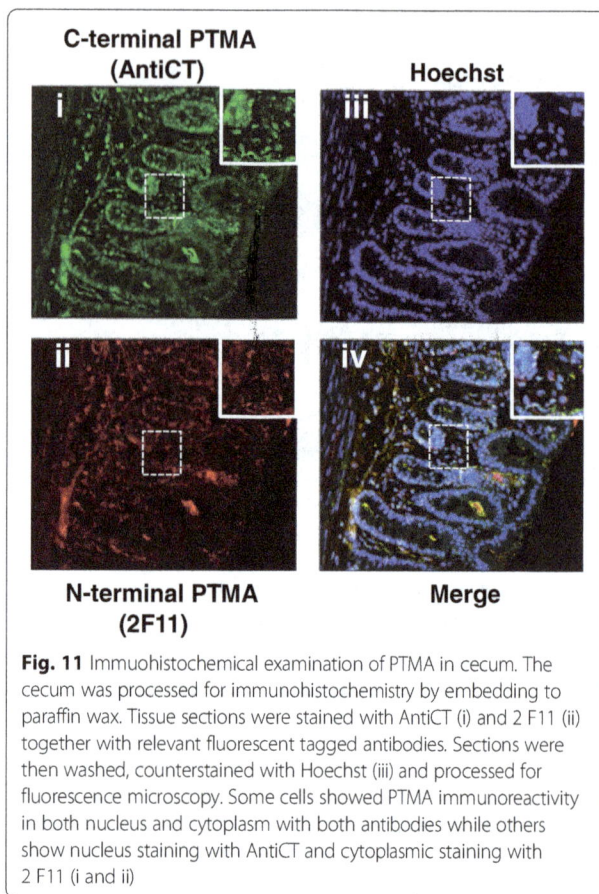

Fig. 11 Immuohistochemical examination of PTMA in cecum. The cecum was processed for immunohistochemistry by embedding to paraffin wax. Tissue sections were stained with AntiCT (i) and 2 F11 (ii) together with relevant fluorescent tagged antibodies. Sections were then washed, counterstained with Hoechst (iii) and processed for fluorescence microscopy. Some cells showed PTMA immunoreactivity in both nucleus and cytoplasm with both antibodies while others show nucleus staining with AntiCT and cytoplasmic staining with 2 F11 (i and ii)

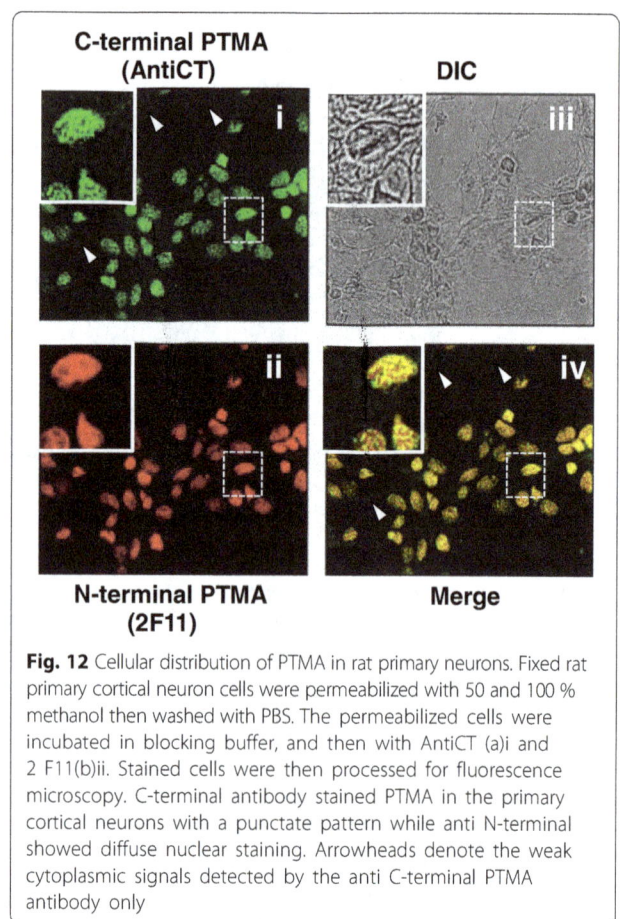

Fig. 12 Cellular distribution of PTMA in rat primary neurons. Fixed rat primary cortical neuron cells were permeabilized with 50 and 100 % methanol then washed with PBS. The permeabilized cells were incubated in blocking buffer, and then with AntiCT (a)i and 2 F11(b)ii. Stained cells were then processed for fluorescence microscopy. C-terminal antibody stained PTMA in the primary cortical neurons with a punctate pattern while anti N-terminal showed diffuse nuclear staining. Arrowheads denote the weak cytoplasmic signals detected by the anti C-terminal PTMA antibody only

tissues and cell types. The insights into its differential dissemination in brain cell types and major peripheral organs at normal physiology, would portent better basis for further elucidation of its interactions and proteolytic modifications under pathological conditions. This considers the fact that, it exhibits extensively contrasting roles depending on the pathognomonic status and localization as either intracellular or extracellular. To illuminate the differential distribution and localization of PTMA, with respect to different tissues and cell types, antibodies that discriminate the different epitopes on the polypeptide were useful tools. First we developed an antibody against the C-terminus of PTMA, a region that presents relatively high hydrophilicity and mobility indices and is therefore likely to have high antigenicity, according to a previous theoretical evaluation [51]. Additionally, antigenic determinants of polypeptides are usually located in their N and/or C termini therefore the C-terminus of PTMA is putatively immunogenic. The rat iliac lymph node method was utilized to produce the monoclonal antibodies instead of the conventional spleen method as it offers a number of benefits; (a) a single injection is sufficient for immunization, (b) lymph nodes are ready to use 2 weeks after injection and (c) increase in efficiency (10 times higher than conventional

method) due to higher yield of positive hybridomas. In this method, biotinylated C-terminal peptide of PTMA was used as antigen and emulsified with complete Freund's adjuvant. Rats were immunized once and 3 weeks later lymphocytes from the iliac lymph nodes of immunized rats were fused with SP2/0 myeloma cells. Antibody producing hybridomas were screened by ELISA and 16 positive clones were selected. On assaying reactivity of the purified antibody by western blotting and antibody testing for capacity to immunoprecipitate PTMA from tissue and the recombinant PTMA, it was evident that AntiCT antibody successfully immunoprecipitated PTMA from the cerebellum tissue lysate. When Anti N-terminal PTMA (2 F11) was applied alongside AntiCT for comparison and detection of PTMA immunoprecipitated by both antibodies carried out by 2 F11 using same amount of antibody for each antibody type; 2 F11 antibody showed greater capacity for immunoprecipitation than AntiCT. It is worth noting that the presence of variant proteins with the same N-terminal sequence generated from alternative splicing of the PTMA gene as recently reported [46] would possibly account for this difference. This observation needs to be verified in further prospective investigations.

The applied methodology revealed that the generated antibody was able to recognize full-length PTMA but could not detect the C-terminal truncated mutant as shown by the western blot results therefore, demonstrating the specificity of the antibodies to the C-terminal region of PTMA. Further characterization of the antibody by determining its cross reactivity with rat and human PTMA revealed clones with different species-specific affinities for PTMA while some clones lost the ability to secrete the antibodies possibly due to loss of chromosomes. Taken together, these results indicated successful generation of the C-terminal antibody. For subsequent experiments purified antibody from clone 7 (AntiCT) was used. A previous study by our laboratory showed that PTMA is a unique cell death regulatory molecule and therefore has neuroprotective roles in brain stroke [39, 45]. Additional studies demonstrated that PTMA exerts the neuroprotective function via its extracellular release upon interaction with S100A13 and that the C-terminal region of PTMA is required for this interaction [41]. However, PTMA cleavage by caspase in its C-terminus interferes with the interaction with S100A13 and disrupts its nuclear localization. Concurrently, PTMA undergoes asparaginyl endopeptidase-mediated cleavage in its N-terminus [42]. Such proteolytic modifications could present functional discontinuities of PTMA and aid to unearth other macromolecules that participate in PTMA functions. Therefore, we first investigated the presence of proteolytically modified variants of PTMA in mouse tissues by western blotting. When AntiCT was applied against 2 F11 in the immunoblot assay, a differential PTMA distribution pattern was observed in the brain regions and peripheral tissues. The tendency of PTMA expression pattern was similar by both antibodies, depicting a trend of high expression levels in brain regions associated with high neuron population (cerebellum) and regions in which neurogenesis is known to occur (olfactory bulb and hippocampus). Brain regions that showed the lowest levels include the thalamus and cortex. Only a single band signal was detectable, cleaved forms of PTMA were undetectable in brain region. In peripheral tissues PTMA expression was higher in lymphoid tissues such as thymus and spleen and lowest in the liver, only the thymus registered an additional lower band signal when detected by 2 F11 which was undetectable by AntiCT. It is plausible that this lower molecular weight band is indeed the C-terminal cleaved form of PTMA owing to the fact that the thymus is packed with apoptosing cells as a result of high cell turnover in this tissue. Further experiments will help to unequivocally determine the identity of the lower band. Overall, the expression level of cleaved forms of PTMA was undetectable in all tissues tested except the thymus under normal physiological context. It would be

interesting to explore this phenomenon after induction of some stress. Following the revelation of the PTMA expression trend in the various tissues, we explored the subcellular localization by use of immunohistochemistry techniques.

Immunohistochemical analysis was performed by co-staining with both antibodies (AntiCT and 2 F11). Immunostaining with AntiCT revealed that in most of the tissues analyzed, the expression of PTMA was localized in both the nucleus and cytoplasm while PTMA immunoreactivity was mostly detected in cytoplasm or perinuclear space by 2 F11. Specific cells of the mucosal layers of duodenum, jejunum, ileum, colon and cecum corroborated this observation. Some cells in the sub-mucosal layers of the duodenum and cecum showed PTMA immunoreactivity in the perinuclear space only by both antibodies. It is conceivable that this differential subcellular localization of PTMA is as a result of different PTMA interacting molecules in the different tissue and cell types or proteolytic modification of PTMA, however no PTMA cleaved forms were detected in these tissues. The brain hippocampus and stomach tissue sections revealed interesting staining patterns that differed from the aforementioned tissues. On one hand, exclusive nuclear staining of PTMA was observed in the hippocampus by both antibodies and on the other hand exclusive cytoplasmic staining was observed in the stomach when both antibodies were applied. As PTMA plays multiple cell robustness roles, this specified subcellular localization in the hippocampus and the stomach by both AntiCT and 2 F11 suggests cell type specific functioning of PTMA. The expression intensity in other tissues like the liver and the heart was relatively weak while the kidney showed comparatively higher signal intensity by immunohistochemistry where the signal was mainly localized in the nucleus. Interestingly the immunofluorescence detected in the lung tissues showed both nucleus and cytoplasmic staining by AntiCT but only cytoplasmic staining by 2 F11. This could be attributable to an interacting molecule involving the N-terminal of PTMA in the nucleus of lung cells. To determine the pattern of cellular distribution of PTMA in detail, immunocytochemistry analysis was carried out on primary neurons. As observed, AntiCT depicted a punctate distribution pattern in the nucleus of neurons and weakly stained the cytoplasm, features that differed from immunostaininng with 2 F11 which only stained the nucleus diffusely. We could consider the prospect that the punctate pattern detectable by AntiCT in primary neurons is a product of interacting molecules in the nucleus that mask C-terminal region and that the weak cytoplasmic signal detectable by AntiCT but not 2 F11, could indicate presence of interacting molecules in the cytoplasm that engage the N-terminal region of

PTMA therefore masking it from detection by 2 F11. All together these expression patterns seem to suggest functional differences of PTMA in diverse tissues and cellular compartments likely associated with different interacting proteins. Under apoptotic conditions intact intracellular PTMA can be processed by proteases leading to different fragments that may differ in biological functions as showed by PTMA-S100A13 binding studies, it would therefore be significant to examine subcellular localization of PTMA under such varying conditions. Moreover, we cannot rule out possibility of the presence of PTMA variants with similar N-terminal regions but differing C-terminal compartments resulting from alternative splicing. Further prospective studies are required to confirm such possible effect.

Conclusion

By analyzing how PTMA is distributed and localized in tissues and specific cell types under no pathological condition we have triggered prying into its precise role under such normal conditions given that in some tissues it was exclusively localized in the cytoplasm while in other tissues it was present predominantly in the nucleus. This will improve our understanding of mediators of PTMA biological function during disease. The next course of action would be to determine the particular cell types that express PTMA in the tissues that showed contrasting patterns of PTMA localization like the cells of the stomach, determine PTMA interacting partners and explore the biologic consequences of PTMA variants in same or different cells arising from alternative splicing.

Abbreviations

2 F11: antibody against the N-terminal region of prothymosin α; AntiCT: antibody against the C-terminal region of prothymosin α; CREB: cAMP response element binging protein; ECL: enhanced chemiluminescent; ELISA: Enzyme linked Immuno-sorbent Assay; HAT: Hypoxthanthine-Aminopterin-Thymidine; HRP: Horseradish Peroxidase; Keap1: Kelch-like ECH-associated protein 1; NLS: Nuclear Localization Signal; Nrf2: Nuclear Factor erythroid 2 related factor; OPD: O-phenylenediamine; PBS: Phosphate Buffered Saline; PEG: Polyethylene Glycol; PFA: Paraformaldehyde; PTMA: Prothymosin α; TA$_1$: Thymosin Alpha$_1$.

Authors' contributions

CMK and CKW conceptualized the paper and wrote the draft manuscript. CMK, KS, YT, HK, HM and HU were involved in the main study and gave substantial inputs to the plan for analysis and draft manuscript. All authors read and approved the final manuscript.

Acknowledgements

The authors thank Ms. Maeda Shiori and Mr. Takehiro Mukae of Nagasaki University for technical assistance during data analysis support in the different facets of this study. This study was partially supported by Grants-in-Aid for Scientific Research from the Ministry of Education, Culture, Sports, Science and Technology (MEXT).

Author details

[1]Department of Molecular Microbiology and Immunology, Division of Immunology, Graduate School of Biomedical Sciences, Nagasaki University, Nagasaki, Japan. [2]African Population and Health Research Center (APHRC), P. O. Box 10787-00100, Nairobi, Kenya. [3]Institute of Tropical Medicine and Infectious Diseases-KEMRI (ITROMID-KEMRI), Nairobi, Kenya. [4]Department of Pharmacology and Therapeutic Innovation, Graduate School of Biomedical Sciences, Nagasaki University, Nagasaki, Japan.

References

1.   Goldstein AL. History of the discovery of the thymosins. Ann N Y Acad Sci. 2007;1112:1–13.
2.   Haritos AA, Goodall GJ, Horecker BL. Prothymosin alpha: isolation and properties of the major immunoreactive form of thymosin alpha 1 in rat thymus. Proc Natl Acad Sci U S A. 1984;81(4):1008–11.
3.   Haritos AA, Tsolas O, Horecker BL. Distribution of prothymosin alpha in rat tissues. Proc Natl Acad Sci U S A. 1984;81(5):1391–3.
4.   Dosil M, Freire M, Gomez-Marquez J. Tissue-specific and differential expression of prothymosin alpha gene during rat development. FEBS Lett. 1990;269(2):373–6.
5.   Enkemann SA, Ward RD, Berger SL. Mobility within the nucleus and neighboring cytosol is a key feature of prothymosin-alpha. J Histochem Cytochem. 2000;48(10):1341–55.
6.   Salvin SB, Horecker BL, Pan LX, Rabin BS. The effect of dietary zinc and prothymosin alpha on cellular immune responses of RF/J mice. Clin Immunol Immunopathol. 1987;43(3):281–8.
7.   Barbini L, Gonzalez R, Dominguez F, Vega F. Apoptotic and proliferating hepatocytes differ in prothymosin alpha expression and cell localization. Mol Cell Biochem. 2006;291(1-2):83–91.
8.   Mosoian A, Teixeira A, Burns CS, Khitrov G, Zhang W, Gusella L, et al. Influence of prothymosin-alpha on HIV-1 target cells. Ann N Y Acad Sci. 2007;1112:269–85.
9.   Pineiro A, Cordero OJ, Nogueira M. Fifteen years of prothymosin alpha: contradictory past and new horizons. Peptides. 2000;21(9):1433–46.
10. Gomez-Marquez J, Rodriguez P. Prothymosin alpha is a chromatin-remodelling protein in mammalian cells. Biochem J. 1998;333(Pt 1):1–3.
11. Hannappel E, Huff T. The thymosins. Prothymosin alpha, parathymosin, and beta-thymosins: structure and function. Vitam Horm. 2003;66:257–96.
12. Martini PG, Delage-Mourroux R, Kraichely DM, Katzenellenbogen BS. Prothymosin alpha selectively enhances estrogen receptor transcriptional activity by interacting with a repressor of estrogen receptor activity. Mol Cell Biol. 2000;20(17):6224–32.
13. Tsai YS, Jou YC, Lee GF, Chen YC, Shiau AL, Tsai HT, et al. Aberrant prothymosin-alpha expression in human bladder cancer. Urology. 2009;73(1):188–92.
14. Tzai TS, Tsai YS, Shiau AL, Wu CL, Shieh GS, Tsai HT. Urine prothymosin-alpha as novel tumor marker for detection and follow-up of bladder cancer. Urology. 2006;67(2):294–9.
15. Tsitsiloni OE, Stiakakis J, Koutselinis A, Gogas J, Markopoulos C, Yialouris P, et al. Expression of alpha-thymosins in human tissues in normal and abnormal growth. Proc Natl Acad Sci U S A. 1993;90(20):9504–7.
16. Dominguez F, Magdalena C, Cancio E, Roson E, Paredes J, Loidi L, et al. Tissue concentrations of prothymosin alpha: a novel proliferation index of primary breast cancer. Eur J Cancer. 1993;29a(6):893–7.
17. Magdalena C, Dominguez F, Loidi L, Puente JL. Tumour prothymosin alpha content, a potential prognostic marker for primary breast cancer. Br J Cancer. 2000;82(3):584–90.
18. Suzuki S, Takahashi S, Takahashi S, Takeshita K, Hikosaka A, Wakita T, et al. Expression of prothymosin alpha is correlated with development and progression in human prostate cancers. Prostate. 2006;66(5):463–9.
19. Klimentzou P, Drougou A, Fehrenbacher B, Schaller M, Voelter W, Barbatis C, et al. Immunocytological and preliminary immunohistochemical studies of prothymosin alpha, a human cancer-associated polypeptide, with a well-characterized polyclonal antibody. J Histochem Cytochem. 2008;56(11):1023–31.
20. Wu CG, Habib NA, Mitry RR, Reitsma PH, van Deventer SJ, Chamuleau RA. Overexpression of hepatic prothymosin alpha, a novel marker for human hepatocellular carcinoma. Br J Cancer. 1997;76(9):1199–204.
21. Tripathi SC, Matta A, Kaur J, Grigull J, Chauhan SS, Thakar A, et al. Overexpression of prothymosin alpha predicts poor disease outcome in head and neck cancer. PLoS One. 2011;6(5), e19213.

22. Leys CM, Nomura S, LaFleur BJ, Ferrone S, Kaminishi M, Montgomery E, et al. Expression and prognostic significance of prothymosin-alpha and ERp57 in human gastric cancer. Surgery. 2007;141(1):41–50.

23. Sasaki H, Fujii Y, Masaoka A, Yamakawa Y, Fukai I, Kiriyama M, et al. Elevated plasma thymosin-alpha1 levels in lung cancer patients. Eur J Cardiothorac Surg. 1997;12(6):885–91.

24. Sasaki H, Nonaka M, Fujii Y, Yamakawa Y, Fukai I, Kiriyama M, et al. Expression of the prothymosin-a gene as a prognostic factor in lung cancer. Surg Today. 2001;31(10):936–8.

25. Sasaki H, Sato Y, Kondo S, Fukai I, Kiriyama M, Yamakawa Y, et al. Expression of the prothymosin alpha mRNA correlated with that of N-myc in neuroblastoma. Cancer Lett. 2001;168(2):191–5.

26. Ojima E, Inoue Y, Miki C, Mori M, Kusunoki M. Effectiveness of gene expression profiling for response prediction of rectal cancer to preoperative radiotherapy. J Gastroenterol. 2007;42(9):730–6.

27. Karetsou Z, Sandaltzopoulos R, Frangou-Lazaridis M, Lai CY, Tsolas O, Becker PB, et al. Prothymosin alpha modulates the interaction of histone H1 with chromatin. Nucleic Acids Res. 1998;26(13):3111–8.

28. Karetsou Z, Kretsovali A, Murphy C, Tsolas O, Papamarcaki T. Prothymosin alpha interacts with the CREB-binding protein and potentiates transcription. EMBO Rep. 2002;3(4):361–6.

29. Su BH, Tseng YL, Shieh GS, Chen YC, Shiang YC, Wu P, et al. Prothymosin alpha overexpression contributes to the development of pulmonary emphysema. Nat Commun. 2013;4:1906.

30. Karapetian RN, Evstafieva AG, Abaeva IS, Chichkova NV, Filonov GS, Rubtsov YP, et al. Nuclear oncoprotein prothymosin alpha is a partner of Keap1: implications for expression of oxidative stress-protecting genes. Mol Cell Biol. 2005;25(3):1089–99.

31. Niture SK, Jaiswal AK. Prothymosin-alpha mediates nuclear import of the INrf2/Cul3 Rbx1 complex to degrade nuclear Nrf2. J Biol Chem. 2009; 284(20):13856–68.

32. Jiang X, Kim HE, Shu H, Zhao Y, Zhang H, Kofron J, et al. Distinctive roles of PHAP proteins and prothymosin-alpha in a death regulatory pathway. Science. 2003;299(5604):223–6.

33. Markova OV, Evstafieva AG, Mansurova SE, Moussine SS, Palamarchuk LA, Pereverzev MO, et al. Cytochrome c is transformed from anti- to pro-oxidant when interacting with truncated oncoprotein prothymosin alpha. Biochim Biophys Acta. 2003;1557(1-3):109–17.

34. Malicet C, Giroux V, Vasseur S, Dagorn JC, Neira JL, Iovanna JL. Regulation of apoptosis by the p8/prothymosin alpha complex. Proc Natl Acad Sci U S A. 2006;103(8):2671–6.

35. Evstafieva AG, Belov GA, Kalkum M, Chichkova NV, Bogdanov AA, Agol VI, et al. Prothymosin alpha fragmentation in apoptosis. FEBS Lett. 2000;467(2-3):150–4.

36. Evstafieva AG, Belov GA, Rubtsov YP, Kalkum M, Joseph B, Chichkova NV, et al. Apoptosis-related fragmentation, translocation, and properties of human prothymosin alpha. Exp Cell Res. 2003;284(2):211–23.

37. Enkemann SA, Wang RH, Trumbore MW, Berger SL. Functional discontinuities in prothymosin alpha caused by caspase cleavage in apoptotic cells. J Cell Physiol. 2000;182(2):256–68.

38. Skopeliti M, Iconomidou VA, Derhovanessian E, Pawelec G, Voelter W, Kalbacher H, et al. Prothymosin alpha immunoactive carboxyl-terminal peptide TKKQKTDEDD stimulates lymphocyte reactions, induces dendritic

39. Ueda H, Fujita R, Yoshida A, Matsunaga H, Ueda M. Identification of prothymosin-alpha1, the necrosis-apoptosis switch molecule in cortical neuronal cultures. J Cell Biol. 2007;176(6):853–62.

40. Fujita R, Ueda H. Prothymosin-alpha1 prevents necrosis and apoptosis following stroke. Cell Death Differ. 2007;14(10):1839–42.

41. Matsunaga H, Ueda H. Stress-induced non-vesicular release of prothymosin-alpha initiated by an interaction with S100A13, and its blockade by caspase-3 cleavage. Cell Death Differ. 2010;17(11):1760–72.

42. Sarandeses CS, Covelo G, Diaz-Jullien C, Freire M. Prothymosin alpha is processed to thymosin alpha 1 and thymosin alpha 11 by a lysosomal asparaginyl endopeptidase. J Biol Chem. 2003;278(15):13286–93.

43. Kishiro Y, Kagawa M, Naito I, Sado Y. A novel method of preparing rat-monoclonal antibody-producing hybridomas by using rat medial iliac lymph node cells. Cell Struct Funct. 1995;20(2):151–6.

44. Sado Y, Inoue S, Tomono Y, Omori H. Lymphocytes from enlarged iliac lymph nodes as fusion partners for the production of monoclonal antibodies after a single tail base immunization attempt. Acta Histochemica Cytochemica. 2006;39(3):89–94.

45. Ueda H, Matsunaga H, Halder SK. Prothymosin alpha plays multifunctional cell robustness roles in genomic, epigenetic, and nongenomic mechanisms. Ann N Y Acad Sci. 2012;1269:34–43.

46. Teixeira A, Yen B, Gusella GL, Thomas AG, Mullen MP, Aberg J, et al. Prothymosin alpha variants isolated from CD8+ T cells and cervicovaginal fluid suppress HIV-1 replication through type I interferon induction. J Infect Dis. 2015;211(9):1467–75.

47. Aniello F, Branno M, De Rienzo G, Ferrara D, Palmiero C, Minucci S. First evidence of prothymosin alpha in a non-mammalian vertebrate and its involvement in the spermatogenesis of the frog Rana esculenta. Mech Dev. 2002;110(1-2):213–7.

48. Paolo Pariante, Raffaele Dotolo, Massimo Venditti, Diana Ferrara, Aldo Donizetti, Francesco Aniello and Sergio Minucci. Prothymosin alpha expression and localization during the spermatogenesis of Danio rerio. Zygote, available on CJO2015. doi:10.1017/S0967199415000568

49. Prisco M, Donizetti A, Aniello F, Locascio A, Del Giudice G, Agnese M, et al. Expression of Prothymosin alpha during the spermatogenesis of the spotted ray Torpedo marmorata. Gen Comp Endocrinol. 2009;164(1):70–6.

50. Donizetti A, Liccardo D, Esposito D, Del Gaudio R, Locascio A, Ferrara D, et al. Differential expression of duplicated genes for prothymosin alpha during zebrafish development. Dev Dyn. 2008;237(4):1112–8.

51. Costopoulou D, Leondiadis L, Czarnecki J, Ferderigos N, Ithakissios DS, Livaniou E, et al. Direct ELISA method for the specific determination of prothymosin alpha in human specimens. J Immunoass. 1998;19(4):295–316.

18

Deficiency of the BMP Type I receptor ALK3 partly protects mice from anemia of inflammation

Inka Gallitz[1], Niklas Lofruthe[1], Lisa Traeger[1], Nicole Bäumer[2], Verena Hoerr[3,4], Cornelius Faber[4], Tanja Kuhlmann[5], Carsten Müller-Tidow[2,6] and Andrea U. Steinbicker[1*]

Abstract

Background: Inflammatory stimuli induce the hepatic iron regulatory hormone hepcidin, which contributes to anaemia of inflammation (AI). Hepcidin expression is regulated by the bone morphogenetic protein (BMP) and the interleukin-6 (IL-6) signalling pathways. Prior results indicate that the BMP type I receptor ALK3 is mainly involved in the acute inflammatory hepcidin induction four and 72 h after IL-6 administration. In this study, the role of ALK3 in a chronic model of inflammation was investigated. The intact, heat-killed bacterium *Brucella abortus* (BA) was used to analyse its effect on the development of inflammation and hypoferremia in mice with hepatocyte-specific *Alk3*-deficiency (*Alk3*[fl/fl]; *Alb-Cre*) compared to control (*Alk3*[fl/fl]) mice.

Results: An iron restricted diet prevented development of the iron overload phenotype in mice with hepatocyte-specific *Alk3* deficiency. Regular diet leads to iron overload and increased haemoglobin levels in these mice, which protects from the development of AI per se. Fourteen days after BA injection *Alk3*[fl/fl]; *Alb-Cre* mice presented milder anaemia (Hb 16.7 g/dl to 11.6 g/dl) compared to *Alk3*[fl/fl] control mice (Hb 14.9 g/dl to 8.6 g/dl). BA injection led to an intact inflammatory response in all groups of mice. In *Alk3*[fl/fl]; *Alb-Cre* mice, SMAD1/5/8 phosphorylation was reduced after BA as well as after infection with *Staphylococcus aureus*. The reduction of the SMAD1/5/8 signalling pathway due to hepatocyte-specific *Alk3* deficiency partly suppressed the induction of STAT3 signalling.

Conclusion: The results reveal in vivo, that 1) hepatocyte-specific *Alk3* deficiency partly protects from AI, 2) the development of hypoferremia is partly dependent on ALK3, and 3) the ALK3/BMP/hepcidin axis may serve as a possible therapeutic target to attenuate AI.

Keywords: Bone Morphogenetic Protein (BMP) type I receptor, Inflammation, Iron, Hepcidin, Liver

Background

Patients with acute or chronic inflammatory diseases or malignancies often develop anaemia of inflammation (AI). More than a quarter of the world's population is anaemic. As the second most common form of anaemia, AI contributes substantially to the burden of disease [1, 2]. Patients with AI present with hypoferremia, as iron is trapped within the iron stores and iron bioavailability for erythropoiesis is therefore decreased [3]. The hepatic hormone hepcidin plays a major role in the maintenance of iron homeostasis. Hepcidin induces internalization and degradation of the sole known iron exporter ferroportin [4]. Induction of hepcidin decreases the bioavailability of iron and can lead to an iron-restricted erythropoiesis [5]. During inflammation, cytokines such as the pro-inflammatory cytokine interleukin 6 (IL-6) are induced [6]. IL-6 acts via the Janus kinase-signal transducer (JAK) and activator of transcription (STAT3) pathway. Hepcidin transcription is induced by binding of phosphorylated STAT3 to the STAT3-responsive element in the hepcidin promoter [7]. In addition, transcriptional regulation of hepcidin requires BMP signalling [8]. Upon ligand binding, the BMP type II receptor is phosphorylated and thereby activates the BMP type I

* Correspondence: andrea.steinbicker@ukmuenster.de
[1]Department of Anaesthesiology, Intensive Care and Pain Medicine, University Hospital Muenster, Albert-Schweitzer Campus 1, Building A1, 48149 Muenster, Germany
Full list of author information is available at the end of the article

receptor. Activation of the kinase domain of the BMP type I receptor phosphorylates SMAD (P-SMAD 1, 5, and 8) proteins, which translocate with SMAD4 to the nucleus. Hepcidin expression is induced after binding of the P-SMAD complex to the BMP-responsive element in the hepcidin promoter [9, 10]. Specific inhibitors of the BMP signalling pathway present novel therapeutic opportunities in different diseases such as pulmonary arterial hypertension, vascular calcification or AI [11, 12]. The hepatocyte-specific disruption of SMAD4, or hepatocyte-specific deficiency of the BMP type I receptors ALK2 or ALK3, cause moderate and severe iron overload and hepcidin suppression, respectively [9, 13]. Mice with hepatocyte-specific *Smad4* deficiency display not only attenuated baseline hepcidin expression, but also lack IL-6 mediated hepcidin expression [9]. In mice with hepatocyte-specific *Alk3* deficiency, neither iron nor BMP agonists were able to stimulate hepcidin [13]. In a model of acute inflammation, Mayeur et al. demonstrated, that IL-6 induced hepatic hepcidin mRNA expression after four (or 72) hours was dependent on the BMP type I receptor ALK3 [14]. In mice with hepatocyte-specific *Alk3* deficiency STAT3 was phosphorylated by IL-6, but the hepcidin induction was impeded and hepcidin levels remained at about 1–5% compared to control mice in short term experiments [13, 14]. The susceptibility of these mice to develop AI had yet to be investigated. The intraperitoneal application of a single dose of heat-killed *Brucella abortus* (BA) particles was utilized in this study to induce chronic inflammation and the development of AI in mice. This well described murine model of AI features the following hallmarks of the disease: i) early hepcidin induction, ii) cytokine release and, iii) impaired erythropoiesis [15–17].

We hypothesized that suppressed hepcidin levels and iron overload in hepatocyte-specific *Alk3* deficiency protect from AI development per se. Prior to BA or saline injection and throughout the experiment, nutritional iron was therefore restricted in all groups of mice in order to maintain similar baseline iron levels in mice with and without hepatocyte-specific *Alk3* deficiency. In a previous study, nutritional iron restriction did not alter the early BA mediated induction of hepatic hepcidin mRNA levels or BA mediated serum IL-6 induction in control mice [18]. As anaemia suppresses hepcidin expression per se, and Kim et al. reported decreased hepcidin expression 14 days after BA administration in WT mice due to anaemia, STAT3 and SMAD1/5/8 phosphorylation were investigated in a second model [16] : *S. aureus* was applied to control and hepatocyte-specific *Alk3* deficient mice on a standard rodent chow and proteins were analysed 24 h later. Upon *S. aureus* administration SMAD1/5/8 phosphorylation was detectable in control mice, but not in mice with hepatocyte-specific *Alk3* deficiency.

To conclude, various factors contribute to anaemia. The presented data indicate that ALK3 and subsequently hepcidin are involved in the cross-talk between iron and inflammation, and contribute to at least 30% of the AI development in this model. Therefore, ALK3 inhibition could be an approach to ameliorate AI.

Methods

Animal research

Mice with homozygous loxP-flanked ("floxed") Alk3 alleles ($Alk3^{fl/fl}$) on a C57BL/6 background were bred with B6.Cg-Tg$^{(Alb-Cre)21Mgn}$/J mice (Jackson Laboratory) to obtain homozygous animals ($Alk3^{fl/fl}$) with or without the hepatocyte-specific *Cre* recombinase driven by an albumin promotor [19]. Mice with hepatocyte-specific deficiency of *Alk3* ($Alk3^{fl/fl}$; *Alb-Cre*) were compared to $Alk3^{fl/fl}$ mice without expression of the *Alb-Cre* as described previously (on regular iron chow) [13]. In this study, all mice were fed an iron-deficient diet since weaning and throughout the experiment (5 ppm iron, Altromin C1038, Lage, Germany).

Murine heat-killed *Brucella abortus* model and injection with *Staphylococcus aureus*

All mouse experiments were carried out in accordance with the recommendations and approval of the institutional ethics committee for "Animal Care of North Rhine-Westphalia, the Landesamt fuer Natur, Umwelt und Verbraucherschutz (LANUV), North Rhine-Westphalia, Germany" permit numbers LANUV Az.84–02.04.2013. A281 and 87–51.04.2011.A003. *Brucella abortus* (BA, Strain 99, *Brucella abortus* MRT AG PA 0048) was prepared as described by Sasu et al. [17]. Mice were maintained according to institutional guidelines in individually ventilated cages and were given food and water ad libitum. 12-week-old female mice were injected once with BA (5×10^8 particles per mouse) or PBS intraperitoneally (Additional file 1a). Fourteen days after BA administration, mice had an average weight of 24 g ± 2,9. At that day blood withdrawal and organ collection were performed, when Hb levels reach nadir values [16]. Mice were sacrificed by cervical dislocation in deep anaesthesia.

Staphylococcus aureus (*S. aureus*) strain 6850 (ATCC 53657, Manassas, VA) was cultivated overnight in brain-heart infusion medium under shaking conditions at 37 °C [20]. The bacteria were washed twice with sterile PBS and the bacterial suspension was adjusted to optical density at 600 nm (OD600 = 1), and stored at − 80 °C until use. Mice were inoculated with 1×10^6 colony forming units (CFUs) of *S. aureus* microorganisms in 150 μL of PBS or with PBS alone as vehicle via a lateral tail vein. After 24 h, blood was collected in deep anaesthesia (Additional file 1b). Then mice were sacrificed by cervical dislocation and organs were collected. All animals were monitored daily. No sudden deaths occurred.

Erythroid progenitor cells

Bone marrow (BM) was collected and processed as described previously [21]. Cells were stained with APC-conjugated rat-anti-mouse CD44 (BD Pharmingen, Heidelberg, Germany) and PE-conjugated rat-anti-mouse TER119 (BD Pharmingen, Heidelberg, Germany) in 2% FBS/PBS for 30 min at RT protected from light. Analysis was performed using the BD FACSDiva™ software on a FACSCalibur™ (Becton Dickinson, Heidelberg, Germany). Unstained cells were used as negative controls. Mean fluorescence intensity (FLI) from 20.000 cell counts was used as a measure of protein surface expression of Ter119 and CD44 [22–24].

Reticulocytes

Reticulocytes were counted by flow cytometry (FACSCalibur™, Becton Dickinson, Heidelberg, Germany). Blood (5 µl) was added to 1 ml of thiazole orange reagent (Retic-COUNT™, BD Bioscience; San Jose, CA) and incubated at room temperature for 1 h. Unstained controls were used to establish a gate to exclude background fluorescence. The results are expressed as the reticulocyte production index: RPI = Retic% x Hb/14.46, with 14.46 g/dL as the mean baseline haemoglobin (Hb) level of healthy WT mice [18].

Hematologic and iron parameters

Blood samples were collected by retro-orbital puncture and serum iron parameters were determined as previously described [13]. Complete blood counts were obtained with the scil Vet abc Plus™ (Viernheim, Germany). Non-haem tissue iron levels were determined as previously described [25].

Hepatic mRNA levels

RNA was extracted from tissue using Trizol® (Sigma, Hamburg, Germany) and homogenized with an ultrasound dissector. cDNA was created by MMLV-reverse transcriptase (Sigma, Hamburg, Germany).

Quantitative RT-PCR was performed on an Applied Biosystems 7500 Fast Real-Time-PCR system with LuminoCt® SYBR® Green qPCR ReadyMix™ (Sigma, Hamburg, Germany). The relative CT method was used to normalize the levels of target transcripts to 18S rRNA levels (Additional file 2).

Protein analysis

Liver tissue samples were prepared with RIPA buffer supplemented with protease and phosphatase inhibitors (Sigma-Aldrich, Heidelberg, Germany). Extracted proteins (40 µg/lane) were separated by electrophoresis using 4%–10% bis-tris gels and nitrocellulose membranes (GE

Healthcare, Freiburg, Germany). Membranes were incubated with antibodies directed against phosphorylated STAT3 (at tyrosine705 (P-STAT3, Cat. No. 9145 L, Cell Signalling Technology)), STAT3 (Cat. No. 4904, Cell Signalling Technology), phosphorylated SMAD 1/5/8 (P-SMAD 1/5, Cat. No. 9516S, Cell Signalling Technology), SMAD1 (Cat. No. 6944, Cell Signalling Technology), Ferroportin (Cat. No. MTP11-A, Alpha Diagnostics) and α-tubulin (Cat. No. T6074, Sigma-Aldrich). Washed membranes were incubated with horseradish peroxidase–linked anti-rabbit or anti-mouse IgG (New England Biolabs, Frankfurt, Germany). Membranes were incubated with ECL-Plus (Bio-Rad, Munich, Germany), and chemiluminescence was detected with a ChemiDoc™ XRS+ (Bio-Rad, Munich, Germany). Densitometrical analysis was performed with Image Lab™ (Bio-Rad, Munich Germany).

Statistical analysis

All values are expressed as mean ± SD. Data were analysed using nonparametric Mann-Whitney U test with two tailed P values. Differences were considered statistically significant with $P \leq 0.05$ (*).

Results

Hepatocyte-specific deficiency of *Alk3* attenuated AI development

Mice with hepatocyte-specific *Alk3* deficiency fed a standard rodent diet develop iron overload. Iron overload could protect these mice from anaemia. In order to avoid development of the iron overload phenotype, mice were fed an iron–deficient diet since weaning and throughout the experiment. At the age of 12 weeks mice were exposed to the heat-killed *BA* model of AI. Alk3 mRNA levels were suppressed in $Alk3^{fl/fl}$; *Alb-Cre* mice injected either with saline or with BA, and compared to $Alk3^{fl/fl}$ control mice (Additional file 4). Fed an iron-deficient diet, $Alk3^{fl/fl}$; *Alb-Cre* and $Alk3^{fl/fl}$ control mice injected with PBS expressed comparable Hb levels, reticulocyte production index (RPI), serum iron levels and transferrin saturation (Fig. 1a-d). Tissue iron content in liver and spleen (Additional file 5) was comparable between control and hepatocyte-specific *Alk3* deficient mice. BA administration led to a slight increase in LIC of hepatocyte-specific *Alk3* deficient mice compared to saline application in these mice. The results indicate that development of the iron overload phenotype in $Alk3^{fl/fl}$; *Alb-Cre* compared to $Alk3^{fl/fl}$ mice was prevented by the iron-deficient diet. Fourteen days after the intraperitoneal injection of BA, $Alk3^{fl/fl}$ control mice developed anaemia indicated by a decrease of the mean Hb levels

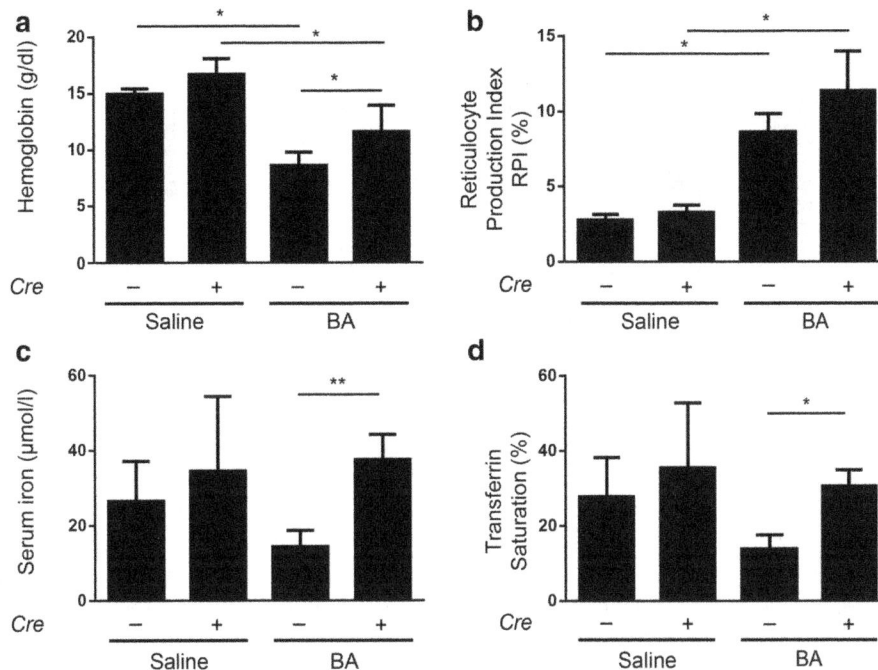

Fig. 1 Milder Anaemia of inflammation in *Alk3*^{fl/fl}; *Alb-Cre* mice compared to *Alk3*^{fl/fl} mice. **a** Haemoglobin values from *Alk3*^{fl/fl} and *Alk3*^{fl/fl}; *Alb-Cre* mice 14 days after heat-killed *Brucella abortus* (BA) or saline injection (*$P = 0.01$: *Alk3*^{fl/fl} injected with saline [$n = 4$] vs *Alk3*^{fl/fl} injected with BA [$n = 6$]; *$P = 0.01$: *Alk3*^{fl/fl}; *Alb-Cre* injected with saline [$n = 4$] vs *Alk3*^{fl/fl}; *Alb-Cre* injected with BA [$n = 6$]; *$P = 0.04$: *Alk3*^{fl/fl} injected with BA [$n = 6$] vs *Alk3*^{fl/fl}; *Alb-Cre* injected with BA [$n = 6$]). **b** Reticulocyte Production Index (*$P = 0.03$: *Alk3*^{fl/fl} injected with saline vs *Alk3*^{fl/fl} injected with BA; *$P = 0.01$: *Alk3*^{fl/fl}; *Alb-Cre* injected with saline vs *Alk3*^{fl/fl}; *Alb-Cre* injected with BA). **c** Serum iron from *Alk3*^{fl/fl} and *Alk3*^{fl/fl}; *Alb-Cre* mice 14 days after BA administration (**$P = 0.004$: *Alk3*^{fl/fl} injected with BA vs *Alk3*^{fl/fl}; *Alb-Cre* injected with BA). **d** Transferrin saturation (**$P = 0.01$: *Alk3*^{fl/fl} injected with BA vs *Alk3*^{fl/fl}; *Alb-Cre* injected with BA [$n = 5$])

from 14.9 g/dl to 8.6 g/dl (Fig. 1a). In contrast, *Alk3*^{fl/fl}; *Alb-Cre* mice presented moderate anaemia with a decrease in Hb levels from 16.7 g/dl to 11.6 g/dl. As a description of the relative reduction, Hb levels in control mice after BA administration were about one third lower compared to *Alk3* deficient mice after BA administration. The data indicate that mice with hepatocyte-specific *Alk3* deficiency were partially protected from the development of AI and hypoferremia.

The RPI was increased in both groups after BA administration (Fig. 1b) due to anaemia. Fed an iron-deficient diet and injected with PBS, *Alk3*^{fl/fl}; *Alb-Cre* mice and *Alk3*^{fl/fl} mice presented comparable serum iron levels and transferrin saturation (Fig. 1c-d). Fourteen days after BA injection *Alk3*^{fl/fl}; *Alb-Cre* mice showed higher serum iron levels and higher transferrin saturation compared to BA treated *Alk3*^{fl/fl} mice (Fig. 1c-d). In particular, the mean corpuscular volume (MCV) and the mean corpuscular haemoglobin (MCH) values were higher in *Alk3*^{fl/fl}; *Alb-Cre* mice injected with BA than in *Alk3*^{fl/fl} after BA injection (Fig. 2a-b). While *Alk3*^{fl/fl} mice fed an iron deficient diet and injected with BA developed a microcytic, hypochromic AI, the *Alk3*^{fl/fl}; *Alb-Cre* mice treated equally, developed a normocytic, normochromic AI with normal MCV and MCH values (Fig. 2a-b).

In mice with hepatocyte-specific *Alk3* deficiency BA induced hepatic ferroportin mRNA levels. Protein levels remained similarly high due to the hepcidin reduction caused by hepatocyte-specific *Alk3* deficiency (Fig. 3a-c). Hepatic ferritin expression was induced after BA application in control and in mice with hepatocyte-specific *Alk3* deficiency (Additional file 6). Hepatic TfR1 expression was elevated in hepatocyte-specific *Alk3* deficient mice after BA application. In control mice, a similar trend was observed (Fig. 4a-b). Splenic ferroportin mRNA levels were induced by BA in both, control and mice with hepatocyte-specific *Alk3* deficiency (Additional file 7). Splenic TfR1 mRNA levels were only elevated in control mice after BA administration (Additional file 7).

These data indicate that the BA-mediated decrease in serum iron levels led to an elevated extramedullary erythropoiesis as indicated by increased hepatic TfR1 protein and splenic TfR1 mRNA levels in *Alk3*^{fl/fl}; *Alb-Cre* and *Alk3*^{fl/fl} mice, respectively. Ferritin is not only an iron storage marker, but also an acute phase protein. Therefore, hepatic ferritin expression was induced after BA application in control and in mice with hepatocyte-specific *Alk3* deficiency as part of the acute phase reaction. LICs were slightly increased (Additional files 5 and 6).

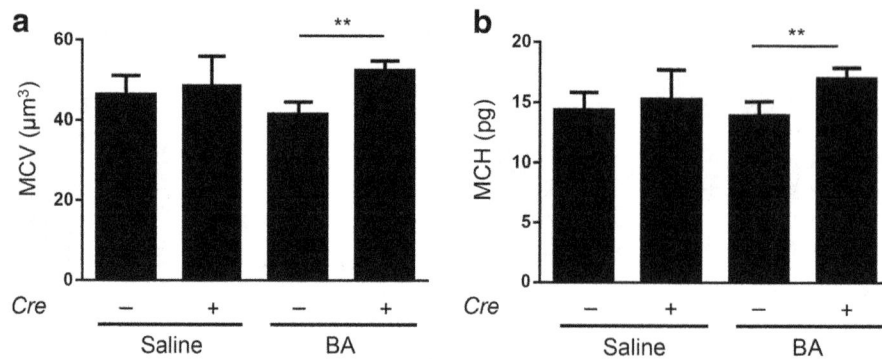

Fig. 2 MCV and MCH levels in $Alk3^{fl/fl}$; Alb-Cre mice compared to $Alk3^{fl/fl}$ mice. **a** Mean corpuscular volume (MCV) (**$P = 0.002$: $Alk3^{fl/fl}$ injected with BA vs $Alk3^{fl/fl}$; Alb-Cre injected with BA), and **b** Mean corpuscular haemoglobin (MCH) (**$P = 0.002$: $Alk3^{fl/fl}$ injected with BA vs $Alk3^{fl/fl}$; Alb-Cre injected with BA)

There were no discernible differences detectable in mRNA levels of ferroportin in the duodenum (Additional file 7). However, immunofluorescence staining of duodenal ferroportin of untreated mice with and without hepatocyte-specific $Alk3$ deficiency indicated a stronger ferroportin expression on the luminal surface of the mucosa in mice with hepatocyte-specific $Alk3$ deficiency compared to control mice (Additional files 8 and 9). These data suggest that a regional difference in ferroportin expression may result in the better iron mobilization in mice with hepatocyte-specific $Alk3$ deficiency.

Taken together, the data indicate that mice with hepatocyte-specific deficiency of $Alk3$ under iron-restricted conditions still developed AI after BA administration, but to a milder extent than control mice. Due to the relative

reduction in haemoglobin levels, the contribution of the ALK3/hepcidin/ferroportin circuitry to BA-mediated AI was estimated with about 30%. Hepatocyte-specific $Alk3$ deficiency partly prevented the development of hypoferremia and led to normocytic, normochromic erythrocytes.

The inflammatory response to BA administration was intact in mice with hepatocyte-specific $Alk3$ deficiency

In order to determine the inflammatory response to BA, mice with and without hepatocyte-specific $Alk3$ deficiency were analysed 14d after BA injection. AI was accompanied by an induction of granulocytes within comparable ranges after BA application in $Alk3^{fl/fl}$ and $Alk3^{fl/fl}$; Alb-Cre mice (Fig. 5a), which

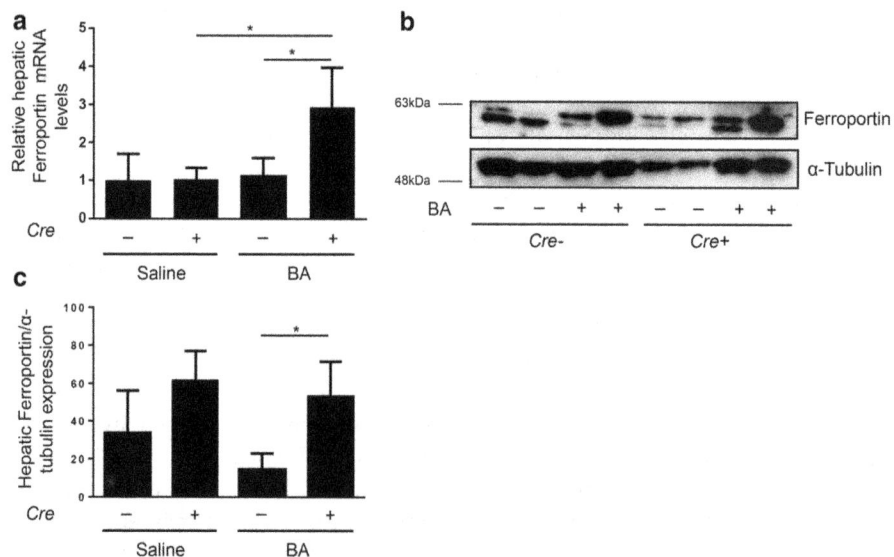

Fig. 3 Hepatocyte-specific $Alk3$ deficiency resulted in elevated liver ferroportin expression 14 days after BA injection. **a** Relative hepatic ferroportin mRNA levels (*$P = 0.01$: $Alk3^{fl/fl}$; Alb-Cre injected with saline [$n = 4$] vs $Alk3^{fl/fl}$; Alb-Cre injected with BA [$n = 6$]; *$P = 0.01$: $Alk3^{fl/fl}$ injected with BA [$n = 5$] vs $Alk3^{fl/fl}$; Alb-Cre injected with BA [$n = 6$]). Representative Western blots (**b**) and quantitative analyses (**c**) of hepatic ferroportin protein levels with α-tubulin as loading control

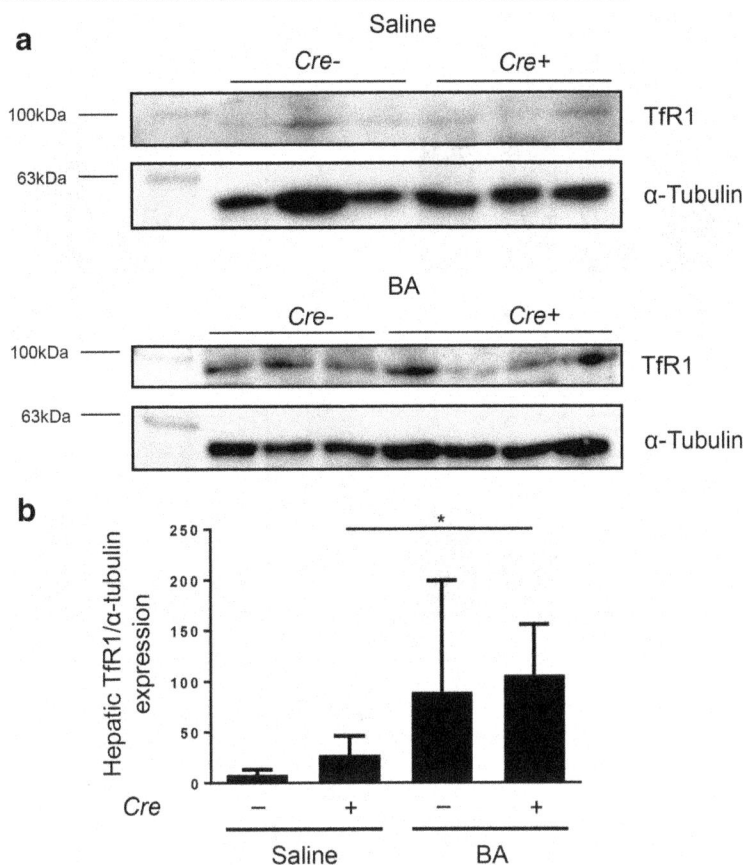

Fig. 4 Hepatic protein levels of transferrin receptor 1. **a** Representative Western blots and quantitative analyses (**b**) of hepatic TfR1 protein levels in $Alk3^{fl/fl}$ and $Alk3^{fl/fl}$; Alb-Cre mice 14 days after heat-killed $Brucella$ $abortus$ (BA) injection. As loading control α-tubulin expression is depicted. (*$P = 0.03$: $Alk3^{fl/fl}$; Alb-Cre injected with saline vs $Alk3^{fl/fl}$; Alb-Cre injected with BA)

indicate comparable grades of chronic inflammation in both groups. IL-6 and TNF-α mRNA levels were induced in both, $Alk3^{fl/fl}$; Alb-Cre and $Alk3^{fl/fl}$ mice, to a similar extent (Fig. 5b-c). HO-1 mRNA expression levels, a marker of oxidative stress, which is upregulated by the IL-6/STAT3 signalling pathway, were elevated in the liver of both, $Alk3^{fl/fl}$ and $Alk3^{fl/fl}$; Alb-Cre mice, after BA administration (Fig. 5d). IL-6 induces SAA-1 mRNA levels. Therefore, BA administration led to an increase in SAA-1 mRNA in $Alk3^{fl/fl}$; Alb-Cre and $Alk3^{fl/fl}$ mice (Fig. 6). Interestingly, SAA-1 mRNA levels were markedly higher in $Alk3^{fl/fl}$; Alb-Cre mice compared to $Alk3^{fl/fl}$ mice injected with BA. Hepcidin mRNA levels were suppressed 14d after BA-injection in all four groups of mice (Additional file 10). These data were expected, as the BA injection causes a hepcidin increase after 6 h, which decreases in chronic, prolonged inflammation and iron deficiency after 14d. To conclude, the BA-mediated inflammatory response was not altered in mice with hepatocyte-specific $Alk3$ deficiency. The elevated SAA-1 levels in mice with hepatocyte-specific $Alk3$ deficiency might reflect the

failure of early hepcidin induction upon inflammation and its anti-inflammatory properties.

Erythropoiesis was similar in $Alk3^{fl/fl}$ and $Alk3^{fl/fl}$; Alb-Cre mice after BA administration

To investigate whether an impaired erythropoiesis contributed to AI, total BM cells were selected for Ter119 cell surface expression via fluorescence-activated cell sorter to identify the amount of erythroid precursor cells. Cells from $Alk3^{fl/fl}$ and $Alk3^{fl/fl}$; Alb-Cre mice exhibited a similar reduction in their total erythroid cell population (43% decrease in $Alk3^{fl/fl}$ mice compared with 39% decrease in $Alk3^{fl/fl}$; Alb-Cre mice. Ter119$^+$ cells, Fig. 7a). To further distinguish the erythroid subpopulations, cells were sorted by CD44 expression and cell size (forward scatter). In later, further differentiated stages of erythroblasts, the CD44 surface expression declines (from proerythroblast to reticulocyte).

Gating for the Terr119$^+$ cell population, the subpopulations were analysed. BA administration led to an upregulation in basophilic erythroblasts in $Alk3^{fl/fl}$ mice only (population II, Fig. 7b). Polychromatic

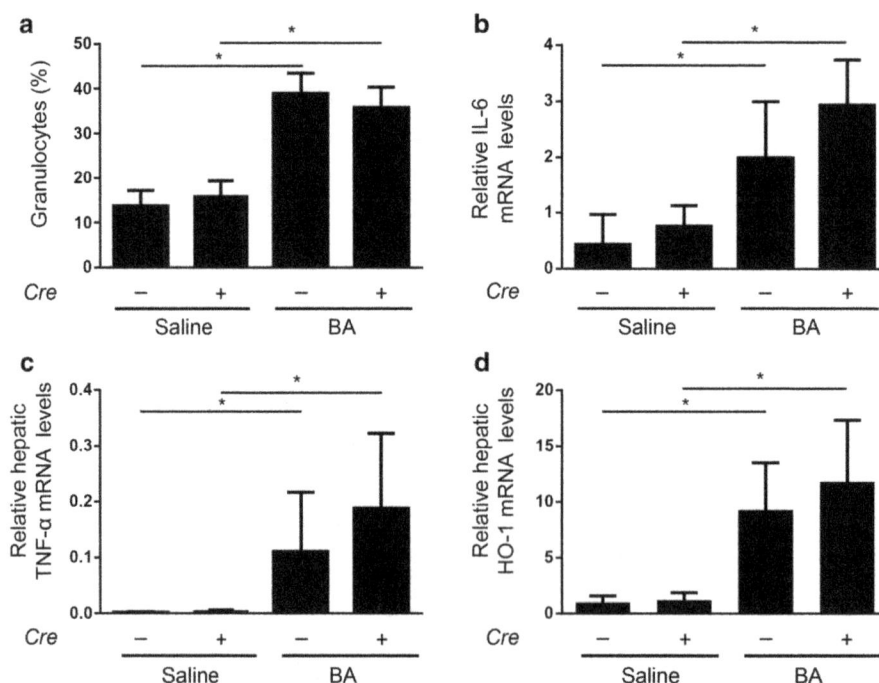

Fig. 5 Comparable BA-induced inflammation in *Alk3*^fl/fl^; *Alb-Cre* mice and *Alk3*^fl/fl^; mice. **a** Granulocytes from *Alk3*^fl/fl^ and *Alk3*^fl/fl^; *Alb-Cre* mice 14 days after heat-killed *Brucella abortus* (BA) or saline injection (*P = 0.01: *Alk3*^fl/fl^ injected with saline [n = 4] vs *Alk3*^fl/fl^ injected with BA [n = 4]; *P = 0.01: *Alk3*^fl/fl^; *Alb-Cre* injected with saline [n = 4] vs *Alk3*^fl/fl^; *Alb-Cre* injected with BA [n = 6]), and (**b**) Relative hepatic IL-6 mRNA levels from *Alk3*^fl/fl^ and *Alk3*^fl/fl^; *Alb-Cre* mice 14 days after BA administration (*P = 0.03: *Alk3*^fl/fl^ injected with saline [n = 3] vs *Alk3*^fl/fl^ injected with BA [n = 5]; **P = 0.01: *Alk3*^fl/fl^; *Alb-Cre* injected with saline [n = 4] vs *Alk3*^fl/fl^; *Alb-Cre* injected with BA [n = 6]). **c** Relative hepatic TNF-α mRNA levels (*P = 0.04: *Alk3*^fl/fl^ injected with saline [n = 3] vs *Alk3*^fl/fl^ injected with BA [n = 4]; *P = 0.01: *Alk3*^fl/fl^; *Alb-Cre* injected with saline [n = 5] vs *Alk3*^fl/fl^; *Alb-Cre* injected with BA [n = 6]). **d** Relative hepatic HO-1 mRNA levels (*P = 0.01: *Alk3*^fl/fl^ injected with saline [n = 4] vs *Alk3*^fl/fl^ injected with BA [n = 6]; *P = 0.01: *Alk3*^fl/fl^; *Alb-Cre* injected with saline [n = 4] vs *Alk3*^fl/fl^; *Alb-Cre* injected with BA [n = 6])

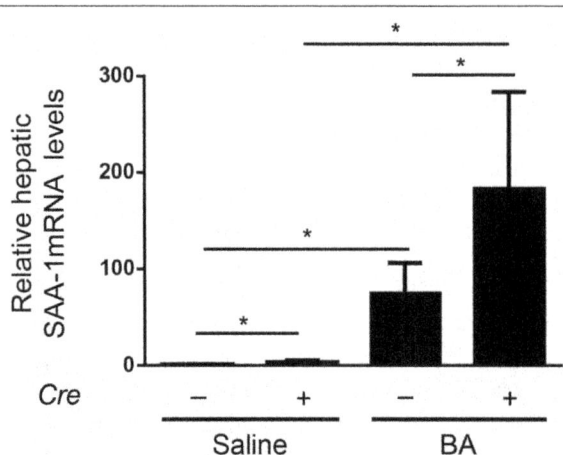

Fig. 6 BA-induced SAA-1 mRNA levels in *Alk3*^fl/fl^; *Alb-Cre* mice and *Alk3*^fl/fl^ mice. Relative hepatic SAA-1 mRNA levels (*P = 0,01: *Alk3*^fl/fl^ injected with saline [n = 4] vs *Alk3*^fl/fl^ injected with BA [n = 4]; *P = 0,01: *Alk3*^fl/fl^; *Alb-Cre* injected with saline [n = 6] vs *Alk3*^fl/fl^; *Alb-Cre* injected with BA [n = 6]; *P = 0.03: *Alk3*^fl/fl^ injected with saline vs *Alk3*^fl/fl^; *Alb-Cre* injected with saline; *P = 0.03: *Alk3*^fl/fl^ injected with BA vs *Alk3*^fl/fl^; *Alb-Cre* injected with BA). The relative CT method was used to normalize the levels of target transcripts to 18S rRNA levels

erythroblasts (population III) were upregulated in both groups, but more pronounced in *Alk3*^fl/fl^; *Alb-Cre* mice. BA administration resulted in a comparable decrease of terminal differentiated red cells from the BM in both groups (terminal differentiated red cells, population V, Fig. 7b). However, despite the differences in erythroid precursor cell distribution between both groups, BA administration led to an arrest in the maturation of erythroid cells before they differentiated into orthochromatic erythroblasts. This resulted in equally suppressed numbers of terminal differentiated red cells (population V) and the total of erythroid cells (Ter119+) from the BM in both, *Alk3*^fl/fl^ mice and *Alk3*^fl/fl^; *Alb-Cre* mice. Additionally, the number of red blood cells (RBCs) was equally decreased in both groups after BA administration (Additional file 10). The data reflect that BM erythropoiesis did not contribute to the protection of BA-mediated AI in *Alk3*^fl/fl^; *Alb-Cre* mice compared to controls. BA administration resulted in an impaired erythropoiesis of the BM in both, *Alk3*^fl/fl^ and *Alk3*^fl/fl^; *Alb-Cre* mice, with an arrest in maturation prior to differentiation into orthochromatic erythroblasts. The ratio of splenic weight/body weight was comparable and indicate that both

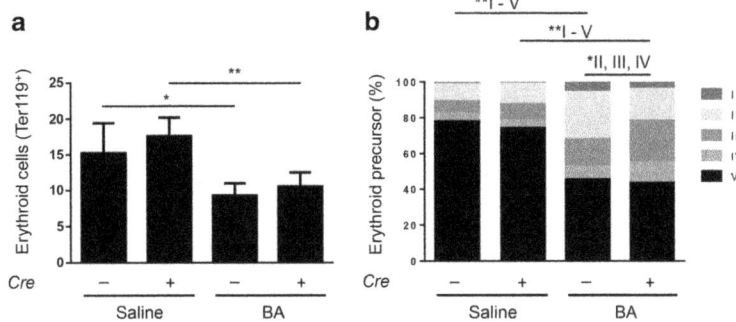

Fig. 7 Bone marrow erythropoiesis depicted through total erythroid cells and distribution of erythroid precursor cell populations. **a** Total erythroid cells (Ter119+) in the bone marrow 14 days after heat-killed *Brucella abortus* (BA) or saline injection (*$P = 0.03$: $Alk3^{fl/fl}$ injected with saline [$n = 4$] vs $Alk3^{fl/fl}$ injected with BA [$n = 6$]; **$P = 0.009$: $Alk3^{fl/fl}$; *Alb-Cre* injected with saline [$n = 4$] vs $Alk3^{fl/fl}$; *Alb-Cre* injected with BA [$n = 6$]). **b** Erythroid subpopulations in the bone marrow of $Alk3^{fl/fl}$ and $Alk3^{fl/fl}$; *Alb-Cre* mice 14d after BA administration (V and II: *$P = 0.01$: $Alk3^{fl/fl}$ injected with saline vs $Alk3^{fl/fl}$ injected with BA; III: *$P = 0.01$: $Alk3^{fl/fl}$ injected with saline vs $Alk3^{fl/fl}$ injected with BA; III and V: *$P = 0.01$: $Alk3^{fl/fl}$; *Alb-Cre* injected with saline vs $Alk3^{fl/fl}$; *Alb-Cre* injected with BA, II: $P = 0.01$: $Alk3^{fl/fl}$ injected with BA vs $Alk3^{fl/fl}$; *Alb-Cre* injected with BA; III: $P = 0.01$: $Alk3^{fl/fl}$ injected with BA vs $Alk3^{fl/fl}$; *Alb-Cre* injected with BA). [Subpopulation V = terminal differentiated red cells, IV = orthochromatic erythroblast, III = polychromatic erythroblast, II = basophilic erythroblast, I = proerythroblast]

groups compensated for the impaired erythropoiesis of the BM after BA administration with an enhanced erythropoiesis in the spleen (Additional file 10). The suppression of hepcidin develops due to the secretion of erythroid factors, such as erythroferrone, by the bone marrow. The way these erythroid factors repress hepcidin expression is partly known: Wang et al. showed that SMAD1/5 was required for erythropoietin and erythroferrone mediated hepcidin suppression [26]. As erythroferrone is proximal of BMP/SMAD signalling, there was no difference in erythroferrone mRNA

in liver and spleen of mice with and without hepatocyte-specific *Alk3* deficiency (Additional file 10).

Inhibition of BMP signalling did affect SMAD1/5/8 phosphorylation

In order to determine, if STAT3 phosphorylation was intact in mice with and without hepatocyte-specific *Alk3* deficiency, STAT3 phosphorylation was determined via immunoblotting. BA-injection induces IL-6 and thereby STAT3 phosphorylation. STAT3 phosphorylation was present in $Alk3^{fl/fl}$ and $Alk3^{fl/fl}$; *Alb-Cre* mice injected

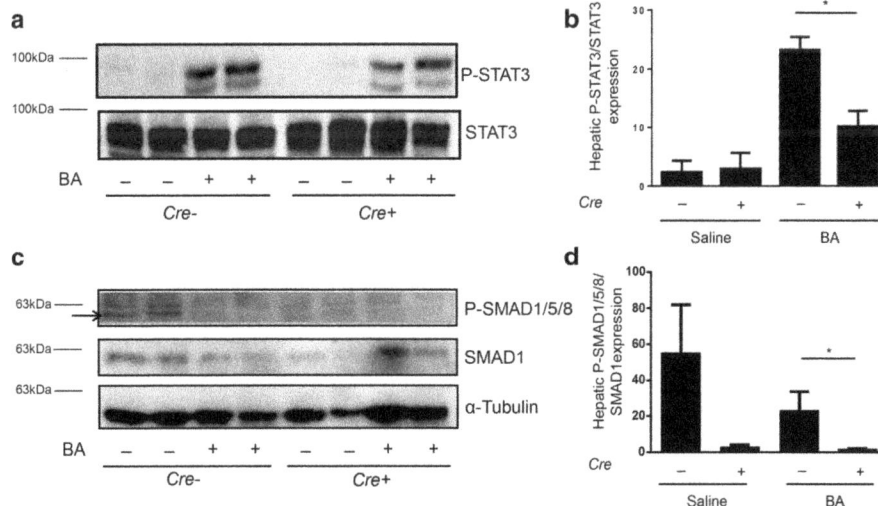

Fig. 8 Hepatic STAT3 and SMAD1/5/8 protein expression in $Alk3^{fl/fl}$; *Alb-Cre* and $Alk3^{fl/fl}$ mice. Representative western blots (**a**) and quantitative analyses (**b**) of phospho-STAT3 and total-STAT3 from $Alk3^{fl/fl}$ and $Alk3^{fl/fl}$; *Alb-Cre* mice 14 days after heat-killed *Brucella abortus* (BA) or saline injection. Two isoforms of phospho-STAT3 α and β (79/86 kDa) exist. Loading control is indicated by total STAT3 protein levels. **c** SMAD1/5/8 activation 14d after BA administration in $Alk3^{fl/fl}$ (*Cre-*) and hepatocyte-specific *Alk3* deficient ($Alk3^{fl/fl}$; *Alb-Cre*) (*Cre+*) mice fed an iron deficient diet. Western blots from liver proteins analysed with phosphorylated SMAD1/5/8, total SMAD1, and α-tubulin antibodies. Arrows indicate specific pSMAD signal. **d** Densitometric analyses of the ratio of SMAD1/5/8 to SMAD1

with BA, but weaker in the latter (Fig. 8a-b). SMAD1/5/8 baseline phosphorylation was detectable in control, but not in *Alk3* deficient mice. Fourteen days after BA administration SMAD1/5/8 phosphorylation seems reduced in control mice and still absent in *Alk3* deficient mice (Fig. 8c-d). These results indicate that BMP signalling is abrogated in mice with hepatocyte-specific *Alk3* deficiency, so that ALK3 is the critical receptor for intact BMP/SMAD signalling and that SMAD activation is required for the STAT3 pathway.

As SMAD1/5/8 phosphorylation, due to iron restriction and anaemia, was not induced 14 days after heat-killed BA administration, we administered the vital bacterium *S. aureus* in another set of experiments to mice with and without hepatocyte-specific *Alk3* deficiency and analysed the protein phosphorylation 24 h later. In mice with and without hepatocyte-specific *Alk3* deficiency, STAT3 phosphorylation was detectable 24 h after the *S. aureus* injection (Fig. 9a-b). SMAD1/5/8 phosphorylation was only detectable in control mice 24 h after *S. aureus* administration (Fig. 9c).

To conclude, the inhibition of the SMAD1/5/8 signalling pathway due to *Alk3* deficiency partly suppressed the induction of the STAT3 signalling pathway by BA or *S. aureus* administration.

Discussion

AI is the second most common form of anaemia worldwide. Pathophysiologically, AI is associated with elevated cytokine levels, iron trapped in iron stores, iron restricted erythropoiesis and hypoferremia. The current manuscript reveals for the first time that hepatocyte-specific *Alk3* deficiency partly protects mice from development of AI. The iron restricted diet fed prior to the experiment prevented development of the iron overload phenotype in *Alk3*[fl/fl]; *Alb-Cre* mice. After BA injection, these *Alk3*[fl/fl]; *Alb-Cre* mice presented higher Hb levels, serum iron levels, transferrin saturation, MCV, and MCH compared to BA injected control mice. In contrast, the inflammatory response to BA administration was not altered by hepatocyte-specific *Alk3* deficiency as indicated by comparably elevated granulocytes and cytokine levels. BM erythropoiesis was equally suppressed in control and *Alk3*[fl/fl]; *Alb-Cre* mice due to elevated cytokine levels. The data indicate that ALK3 was required for the cytokine mediated development of hypoferremia. The ALK3-hepcidin axis accounted with about one third to the development of AI. Therefore, ALK3 serves as a possible therapeutic target for AI.

Of note, the BA model used in this study cannot be compared to active bacterial infection, as heat-killed *Brucella abortus* bacteria do not replicate. Nevertheless, it is a well-known and frequently used model for AI that was previously used to investigate AI by Kim, Sasu, Kautz, Gardenghi and stated in a review by Fraenkel [15–17, 27, 28]. The typical pathophysiological development that leads to AI, an induction of hepcidin, is also caused by the BA injection after 6 h independent from iron restricted diet [16, 18].

The peptide hormone hepcidin has been reported to play an important role in development of AI [29]. Mice lacking hepcidin (*Hamp*-KO) fed an iron-deficient diet showed milder anaemia and faster recovery after BA administration compared to control mice [15, 16]. The IL-6/hepcidin signalling pathway plays a major role in the development of anaemia in an inflammatory condition. Steinbicker et al. demonstrated that the hepatocyte-specific deficiency of the BMP type I receptor ALK3 not only led to a suppression of basal hepcidin expression

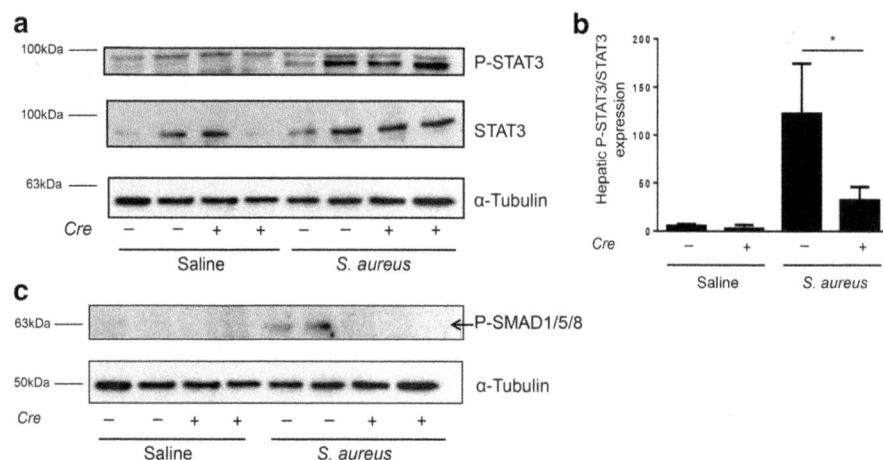

Fig. 9 Hepatic protein levels of STAT3 and SMAD1/5/8. Representative western blots (**a**) and quantitative analyses (**b**) of hepatic phospho-STAT3 and total-STAT3 protein expression from *Alk3*[fl/fl] (*Cre-*) and *Alk3*[fl/fl]; *Alb-Cre* (*Cre+*) mice 24 h after *S. aureus* administration. Two isoforms of phospho-STAT3 α and β (79/86 kDa) exist. Loading control is depicted by total STAT3 protein levels. **c** Hepatic protein expression of phospho-SMAD1/5/8, SMAD1, and α-tubulin from *Alk3*[fl/fl] (*Cre-*) and *Alk3*[fl/fl]; *Alb-Cre* (*Cre+*) mice 24 h after *S. aureus* administration

and iron overload (mice on a regular diet), but that ALK3 was required for the hepatic hepcidin mRNA induction by iron, BMP ligands and IL-6 [13, 30]. Based upon these findings, we investigated the effect of the hepatocyte-specific *Alk3* deficiency on the development of AI in a well described mouse model for AI [15–17]. Even with an abolished iron overload phenotype in *Alk3*^{fl/fl}; *Alb-Cre* mice fed an iron-restricted diet the hepatocyte-specific *Alk3* deficiency had a partially protective effect on the development of anaemia. The BMP type I receptor–SMAD-hepcidin signalling pathway contributed - as described in this manuscript - with about 30% to the development of anaemia in *Alk3*^{fl/fl}; *Alb-Cre* mice. Kim et al. and Gardenghi et al. reported for *Hamp*-KO and *IL-6*-KO mice similar findings with a protection of about 30% to the development of BA-induced anaemia [15, 16]. Pan et al. reported that *Smad4*-deficient mice developed severe anaemia with a decrease in their Hb levels by 70% compared to WT mice, which was not only due to hepcidin suppression in the liver, but due to blood loss caused by polyps in the stomach and colon of these mice [31]. *Alk3*^{fl/fl}; *Alb-Cre* mice displayed higher serum iron, Hb, transferrin saturation, MCV, and MCH levels compared to control mice after BA administration despite the iron-deficient diet.

This indicates that the lack of hepatic hepcidin expression in *Alk3*^{fl/fl}; *Alb-Cre* mice led to alterations in iron metabolism. An enhanced haemoglobinisation of RBCs contributed to the partial protection from anaemia.

Production of pro-inflammatory cytokines in inflammation triggers the development of anaemia via induction of hepcidin. In *Alk3*^{fl/fl}; *Alb-Cre* mice the induction of hepcidin was inhibited. BA administration led to an up-regulation of hepatic IL-6, TNF-α, and HO-1 mRNA levels in both, *Alk3*^{fl/fl} and *Alk3*^{fl/fl}; *Alb-Cre* mice, and higher SAA-1 mRNA levels in the latter. Granulocytosis indicates a chronic inflammation in both control and *Alk3* deficient mice. These data indicate that the inflammatory response was intact in both groups. The lack of early cytokine-induced hepcidin expression (after 6 h) might have caused the induction of SAA-1 mRNA levels in mice with hepatocyte-specific *Alk3* deficiency. In erythroferrone-deficient mice Kautz et al. not only observed a more severe AI upon BA administration (due to a lack of hepcidin suppression), but also lower SAA-1 levels accompanied by higher hepcidin levels [27]. Additionally, Pagani et al. observed higher SAA-1 levels after LPS administration in mice with iron-deficiency [32]. Pre-treatment with hepcidin or high serum levels such as in *Tmprss6*^{−/−} mice led to blunted inflammatory responses (and lower SAA-1 levels) [32]. Wang et al. reported that mice with hepatocyte-specific *Smad4* deficiency show a lack of hepcidin induction and display elevated SAA-1 levels upon IL-6 administration [9]. The results indicate that the lack of hepcidin and not iron

deficiency per se accounted for the elevated SAA-1 levels. These results are in line with the data presented in the current manuscript.

As expected, BA or *S. aureus* administration did not induce SMAD1/5/8 phosphorylation in mice with hepatocyte-specific *Alk3* deficiency. In control mice, *S. aureus*, but not BA application, led to an induction of SMAD1/5/8 phosphorylation. This might be due to the pronounced anaemia 14d after BA application. STAT3 phosphorylation was induced in control mice after BA or *S. aureus* administration. In mice with hepatocyte-specific *Alk3* deficiency, the induction was lower compared to *Alk3*^{fl/fl} mice. The data indicate that STAT3 phosphorylation requires intact BMP signalling.

The elevated hepatic ferroportin level and the protection from hypoferremia in hepatocyte-specific *Alk3* deficient mice indicate that the blunted BMP/SMAD signalling modulated the iron status in AI.

These results are in line with Ferga-Falzacappa et al., who determined the essential role of the SMAD binding element of the hepcidin promoter for hepcidin induction [10]. Furthermore Steinbicker et al. demonstrated that inhibition with the BMP type I receptor inhibitor LDN-193189 intraperitoneally, treated AI in wild-type mice [30]. Mayeur et al. reported that LDN-193189 given orally at a dose of 1 mg/kg to WT mice partially treated turpentine induced anaemia [33]. Taken together, the novel data of in vivo experiments of chronic inflammation in mice with and without hepatocyte-specific *Alk3* deficiency exposed to the BA and *S. aureus* model underline that ALK3 is the dominant BMP type I receptor of iron regulation in inflammation.

Conclusion

The current manuscript revealed in vivo for the first time that 1.) the previously described iron overload phenotype of hepatocyte-specific *Alk3* deficient mice could be blunted by iron restricted diet and, 2.) hepatocyte-specific *Alk3* deficient mice were protected against development of severe AI. The results of the chronic model of inflammation and AI support the findings of short term exposure to IL-6 in these mice, published previously [14]. ALK3 was essentially required for IL-6 and BA mediated hepcidin induction. As hypothesized previously in cell culture studies and short term experiments, the BA-AI in vivo experiment of chronic inflammation revealed that the BMP pathway with the dominant receptor ALK3 is essentially required for intact hepcidin induction by inflammation, the development of hypoferremia, and partly for the development of AI. The inflammatory IL-6-STAT3 pathway should not be seen as an independent pathway- it depends on an intact BMP pathway.

Additional files

Additional file 1: Experimental design. (a) Mice were fed an iron deficient diet since weaning and throughout the experiment. At the age of 12 weeks, female $Alk3^{fl/fl}$; Alb-Cre and Alk3$^{fl/fl}$ mice were intraperitoneally injected with 5×10^8 particles/mouse of heat-killed *Brucella abortus* (BA) or saline. Two weeks later blood and organs were collected. (b) 12 week old $Alk3^{fl/fl}$; Alb-Cre and $Alk3^{fl/fl}$ female mice fed a regular diet were intravenously inoculated with 1×10^6 colony forming units (CFUs) of *Staphylococcus aureus*. Twenty-four hours later blood and organs were collected. (TIFF 164 kb)

Additional file 2: Table S1. Semi-quantitative real-time PCR primer. (DOCX 15 kb)

Additional file 3: Raw data and analysis of the presented study. (XLSX 18 kb)

Additional file 4: Hepatocyte-specific *Alk3* deficiency resulted in suppressed liver Alk3 and hepcidin mRNA expression. Relative hepatic *Alk3* mRNA levels from $Alk3^{fl/fl}$ and $Alk3^{fl/fl}$; Alb-Cre 14 days after heat-killed *Brucella abortus* (BA) injection (*$P = 0.03$: $Alk3^{fl/fl}$ injected with saline [$n = 4$] vs $Alk3^{fl/fl}$; Alb-Cre saline [$n = 4$]; **$P = 0.004$: $Alk3^{fl/fl}$ injected with BA [$n = 6$] vs $Alk3^{fl/fl}$; Alb-Cre injected with BA [$n = 6$]. (TIFF 65 kb)

Additional file 5: Liver and spleen iron content from $Alk3^{fl/fl}$ and $Alk3^{fl/fl}$; Alb-Cre mice 14 days after BA challenge. (a) Liver iron content in $Alk3^{fl/fl}$ and $Alk3^{fl/fl}$; Alb-Cre mice 14 days after heat-killed *Brucella abortus* (BA) injection (*$P = 0.04$: $Alk3^{fl/fl}$; Alb-Cre injected with saline [$n = 4$] vs $Alk3^{fl/fl}$; Alb-Cre injected with BA [$n = 6$]). (b) Spleen iron content from $Alk3^{fl/fl}$ and $Alk3^{fl/fl}$; Alb-Cre mice 14 days after heat-killed *Brucella abortus* (BA) injection. (TIFF 82 kb)

Additional file 6: Hepatic ferritin expression in $Alk3^{fl/fl}$ and $Alk3^{fl/fl}$;Alb-Cre mice 14 days after BA challenge. Representative western blots (a) and quantitative analyses (b) of hepatic ferritin protein levels in $Alk3^{fl/fl}$ and $Alk3^{fl/fl}$; Alb-Cre mice 14 days after heat-killed *Brucella abortus* (BA) injection. As loading control α-tubulin expression is depicted. (TIFF 270 kb)

Additional file 7: Spleen and duodenum mRNA levels in $Alk3^{fl/fl}$ and $Alk3^{fl/fl}$;Alb-Cre mice 14 days after BA challenge. (a) Relative splenic ferroportin mRNA levels from $Alk3^{fl/fl}$ and $Alk3^{fl/fl}$; Alb-Cre 14 days after heat-killed *Brucella abortus* (BA) injection (*$P = 0.02$: $Alk3^{fl/fl}$ injected with saline [$n = 4$] vs $Alk3^{fl/fl}$ injected with BA [$n = 5$]; *$P = 0.03$: $Alk3^{fl/fl}$; Alb-Cre injected with saline [$n = 4$] vs $Alk3^{fl/fl}$; Alb-Cre injected with BA [$n = 4$]. (b) Relative splenic TfR1 mRNA levels (*$P = 0.01$: $Alk3^{fl/fl}$ injected with saline [$n = 4$] vs $Alk3^{fl/fl}$ injected with BA [$n = 6$]). (c) Relative duodenal ferroportin mRNA levels. The relative CT method was used to normalize the levels of target transcripts to 18S rRNA levels. (TIFF 103 kb)

Additional file 8: Immunofluorescence staining of ferroportin in the duodenum of $Alk3^{fl/fl}$ and $Alk3^{fl/fl}$; Alb-Cre mice. Ferroportin immunofluorescence staining of formalin fixed paraffin sections of the villosities of the duodenum with 20 times magnification. (Panel a) Control mice with nuclear (DAPI) and ferroportin (FITC) staining of a duodenal section. Cutout images merged (nuclear and ferroportin) and ferroportin (FITC) alone. (Panel b) Duodenal section of hepatocyte-specific *Alk3* deficient mice with cutout images merged (nuclear and ferroportin) and ferroportin (FITC) alone. White arrows highlight specific FPN staining. (TIFF 3601 kb)

Additional file 9: Supporting material and references. (DOCX 14 kb)

Additional file 10: Hepatic hepcidin mRNA levels, red blood cell count, spleen to bodyweight ratio, and hepatic erfe mRNA levels of $Alk3^{fl/fl}$; Alb-Cre mice and $Alk3^{fl/fl}$ mice. (a) Relative hepatic hepcidin mRNA levels compared to control mice fed a regular diet. The relative CT method was used to normalize the levels of target transcripts to 18S mRNA levels. (b) Red blood cell count from $Alk3^{fl/fl}$ and $Alk3^{fl/fl}$; Alb-Cre mice 14 days after heat-killed *Brucella abortus* (BA) injection (*$P = 0.01$: $Alk3^{fl/fl}$ injected with saline [$n = 4$] vs $Alk3^{fl/fl}$ injected with BA [$n = 6$]; *$P = 0.02$: $Alk3^{fl/fl}$; Alb-Cre injected with saline [$n = 4$] vs $Alk3^{fl/fl}$; Alb-Cre injected with BA [$n = 6$]). (c) Spleen to bodyweight ratio in $Alk3^{fl/fl}$ and $Alk3^{fl/fl}$; Alb-Cre mice 14 days after heat-killed *Brucella abortus* (BA) injection (*$P = 0.01$: $Alk3^{fl/fl}$ injected with saline [$n = 4$] vs $Alk3^{fl/fl}$ injected with BA [$n = 6$]; *$P = 0.01$: $Alk3^{fl/fl}$; Alb-Cre injected with saline [$n = 4$] vs $Alk3^{fl/fl}$; Alb-Cre injected with BA [$n = 6$]). (d) Relative hepatic erfe mRNA levels of $Alk3^{fl/fl}$ and $Alk3^{fl/fl}$; Alb-Cre mice 14 days after heat-killed *Brucella abortus* (BA) injection (*$P = 0.01$: $Alk3^{fl/fl}$; Alb-Cre injected with saline [$n = 4$] vs $Alk3^{fl/fl}$; Alb-Cre injected with BA [$n = 5$]). (TIFF 129 kb)

Abbreviations

AI: Anaemia of inflammation; Alk3: Activin receptor-like kinase; BMP: Bone morphogenetic protein; Cre: Cyclization recombination; Hb: Haemoglobin; IL: Interleukin; MCH: Mean corpuscular haemoglobin; MCV: Mean corpuscular volume; mRNA: Messenger RNA; SMAD: Small Mothers Against Decapentaplegic homolog; STAT: Signal transducer and activator of transcription; TNF-α: Tumor necrosis factor α

Acknowledgements

The authors thank Maria Eveslage, Institute of Biostatistics and Clinical Research, University of Muenster, Muenster, Germany, for assistance in statistical discussions. We thank Claudia Kemming from the Institute for Neuropathology, University of Muenster, Germany, for the assistance with the paraffin embedded sections of the duodenum.

Funding

This work was supported by grants from "Innovative Medical Research" Muenster Medical School, Muenster University (IMF ST 111206) and from the German Research Foundation (Deutsche Forschungsgemeinschaft) STE 1895/4–1 (AUS).

Authors' contributions

IG, NL, LT, VH, and AUS performed experiments; IG, LT, and AUS analysed results and prepared the Figures; NB, CF, TK, and CMT supported the experiments with advice and tools, and the manuscript with scientific discussions; AUS designed the research and IG and AUS wrote the manuscript. All authors read and approved the final manuscript.

Competing interests

The authors declare that they have no competing interests.

Author details

^{1}Department of Anaesthesiology, Intensive Care and Pain Medicine, University Hospital Muenster, Albert-Schweitzer Campus 1, Building A1, 48149 Muenster, Germany. ^{2}Department of Medicine A, Molecular Haematology and Oncology, University Hospital Muenster, 48149 Muenster, Germany. ^{3}Institute of Medical Microbiology, Jena University Hospital, 07747 Jena, Germany. ^{4}Department of Clinical Radiology, University Hospital Muenster, 48149 Muenster, Germany. ^{5}Institute for Neuropathology, University Hospital Muenster, 48149 Muenster, Germany. ^{6}Present Address: Department of Medicine V, Hematology, Oncology and Rheumatology, Heidelberg University Hospital, 69120 Heidelberg, Germany.

References

1. Andrews NC. Anemia of inflammation: the cytokine-hepcidin link. J Clin Invest. 2004;113(9):1251–3.
2. Nemeth E, Ganz T. Anemia of inflammation. Hematol Oncol Clin North Am. 2014;28(4):671–81. vi
3. Weiss G, Goodnough LT. Anemia of chronic disease. N Engl J Med. 2005; 352(10):1011–23.
4. Nemeth E, Tuttle MS, Powelson J, Vaughn MB, Donovan A, Ward DM, Ganz T, Kaplan J. Hepcidin regulates cellular iron efflux by binding to ferroportin and inducing its internalization. Science. 2004;306(5704):2090–3.
5. Goodnough LT, Nemeth E, Ganz T. Detection, evaluation, and management of iron-restricted erythropoiesis. Blood. 2010;116(23):4754–61.
6. Nemeth E, Rivera S, Gabayan V, Keller C, Taudorf S, Pedersen BK, Ganz T. IL-6 mediates hypoferremia of inflammation by inducing the synthesis of the iron regulatory hormone hepcidin. J Clin Invest. 2004;113(9):1271–6.
7. Verga Falzacappa MV, Vujic Spasic M, Kessler R, Stolte J, Hentze MW, Muckenthaler MU. STAT3 mediates hepatic hepcidin expression and its inflammatory stimulation. Blood. 2006;109(1):353–8.
8. Babitt JL, Huang FW, Wrighting DM, Xia Y, Sidis Y, Samad TA, Campagna JA, Chung RT, Schneyer AL, Woolf CJ, Andrews NC, Lin HY. Bone morphogenetic protein signaling by hemojuvelin regulates hepcidin expression. Nat Genet. 2006;38(5):531–9.
9. Wang RH, Li C, Xu X, Zheng Y, Xiao C, Zerfas P, Cooperman S, Eckhaus M, Rouault T, Mishra L, Deng CX. A role of SMAD4 in iron metabolism through the positive regulation of hepcidin expression. Cell Metab. 2005;2(6):399–409.

10. Verga Falzacappa MV, Casanovas G, Hentze MW, Muckenthaler MU. A bone morphogenetic protein (BMP)-responsive element in the hepcidin promoter controls HFE2-mediated hepatic hepcidin expression and its response to IL-6 in cultured cells. J Mol Med. 2008;86(5):531–40.

11. Morrell NW, Bloch DB, ten Dijke P, Goumans MJ, Hata A, Smith J, Yu PB, Bloch KD. Targeting BMP signalling in cardiovascular disease and anaemia. Nat Rev Cardiol. 2016;13(2):106–20.

12. Derwall M, Malhotra R, Lai CS, Beppu Y, Aikawa E, Seehra JS, Zapol WM, Bloch KD, Yu PB. Inhibition of bone morphogenetic protein signaling reduces vascular calcification and atherosclerosis. Arterioscler Thromb Vasc Biol. 2012;32(3):613–22. https://doi.org/10.1161/ATVBAHA.111.242594.

13. Steinbicker AU, Bartnikas TB, Lohmeyer LK, Leyton P, Mayeur C, Kao SM, Pappas AE, Peterson RT, Bloch DB, Yu PB, Fleming MD, Bloch KD. Perturbation of hepcidin expression by BMP type I receptor deletion induces iron overload in mice. Blood. 2011;118(15):4224–30.

14. Mayeur C, Lohmeyer LK, Leyton P, Kao SM, Pappas AE, Kolodziej SA, Spagnolli E, Yu B, Galdos RL, Yu PB, Peterson RT, Bloch DB, Bloch KD, Steinbicker AU. The type I BMP receptor Alk3 is required for the induction of hepatic hepcidin gene expression by interleukin-6. Blood. 2014;123(14):2261–8.

15. Gardenghi S, Renaud TM, Meloni A, Casu C, Crielaard BJ, Bystrom LM, Greenberg-Kushnir N, Sasu BJ, Cooke KS, Rivella S. Distinct roles for hepcidin and interleukin-6 in the recovery from anemia in mice injected with heat-killed Brucella abortus. Blood. 2014;123(8):1137–45.

16. Kim A, Fung E, Parikh SG, Valore EV, Gabayan V, Nemeth E, Ganz T. A mouse model of anemia of inflammation: complex pathogenesis with partial dependence on hepcidin. Blood. 2014;123(8):1129–36.

17. Sasu BJ, Cooke KS, Arvedson TL, Plewa C, Ellison AR, Sheng J, Winters A, Juan T, Li H, Begley CG, Molineux G. Antihepcidin antibody treatment modulates iron metabolism and is effective in a mouse model of inflammation-induced anemia. Blood. 2010;115(17):3616–24.

18. Lofruthe N, Gallitz I, Traeger L, Baumer N, Schulze I, Kuhlmann T, Muller-Tidow C, Steinbicker AU. Intravenous iron Carboxymaltose as a potential therapeutic in anemia of inflammation. PLoS One. 2016;11(7):e0158599.

19. Mishina Y, Hanks MC, Miura S, Tallquist MD, Behringer RR. Generation of Bmpr/Alk3 conditional knockout mice. Genesis. 2002;32(2):69–72.

20. Proctor RA, Christman G, Mosher DF. Fibronectin-induced agglutination of Staphylococcus Aureus correlates with invasiveness. J Lab Clin Med. 1984;104(4):455–69.

21. Bäumer N, Tickenbrock L, Tschanter P, Lohmeyer L, Diederichs S, Bäumer S, Skryabin BV, Zhang F, Agrawal-Singh S, Köhler G, Berdel WE, Serve H, Koschmieder S, Müller-Tidow C. Inhibitor of cyclin-dependent kinase (CDK) interacting with cyclin A1 (INCA1) regulates proliferation and is repressed by oncogenic signaling. J Biol Chem. 2011;286(32):28210–22.

22. Liu J, Zhang J, Ginzburg Y, Li H, Xue F, De Franceschi L, Chasis JA, Mohandas N, An X. Quantitative analysis of murine terminal erythroid differentiation in vivo: novel method to study normal and disordered erythropoiesis. Blood. 2013;121(8):e43–9.

23. Chen K, Liu J, Heck S, Chasis JA, An X, Mohandas N. Resolving the distinct stages in erythroid differentiation based on dynamic changes in membrane protein expression during erythropoiesis. Proc Natl Acad Sci U S A. 2009;106(41):17413–8.

24. Prince OD, Langdon JM, Layman AJ, Prince IC, Sabogal M, Mak HH, Berger AE, Cheadle C, Chrest FJ, Yu Q, Andrews NC, Xue QL, Civin CI, Walston JD,

Roy CN. Late stage erythroid precursor production is impaired in mice with chronic inflammation. Haematologica. 2012;97(11):1648–56.

25. Torrance JD, Bothwell TH. Tissue iron stores. In: Cook JD, editor. Methods in hematology. New York: Churchill Livingstone; 1980. p. 90–115.

26. Wang CY, Core AB, Canali S, Zumbrennen-Bullough KB, Ozer S, Umans L, Zwijsen A, Babitt JL. Smad1/5 is required for erythropoietin-mediated suppression of hepcidin in mice. Blood. 2017;130(1):73–83.

27. Kautz L, Jung G, Nemeth E, Ganz T. Erythroferrone contributes to recovery from anemia of inflammation. Blood. 2014;124(16):2569–74.

28. Fraenkel PG. Critical models for the anemia of inflammation. Blood. 2014;123(8):1124–5.

29. Nemeth E, Valore EV, Territo M, Schiller G, Lichtenstein A, Ganz T. Hepcidin, a putative mediator of anemia of inflammation, is a type II acute-phase protein. Blood. 2002;101(7):2461–3.

30. Steinbicker AU, Sachidanandan C, Vonner AJ, Yusuf RZ, Deng DY, Lai CS, Rauwerdink KM, Winn JC, Saez B, Cook CM, Szekely BA, Roy CN, Seehra JS, Cuny GD, Scadden DT, Peterson RT, Bloch KD, Yu PB. Inhibition of bone morphogenetic protein signaling attenuates anemia associated with inflammation. Blood. 2011;117(18):4915–23.

31. Pan D, Schomber T, Kalberer CP, Terracciano LM, Hafen K, Krenger W, Hao-Shen H, Deng C, Skoda RC. Normal erythropoiesis but severe polyposis and bleeding anemia in Smad4-deficient mice. Blood. 2007;110(8):3049–55.

32. Pagani A, Nai A, Corna G, Bosurgi L, Rovere-Querini P, Camaschella C, Silvestri L. Low hepcidin accounts for the proinflammatory status associated with iron deficiency. Blood. 2011;118(3):736–46.

33. Mayeur C, Kolodziej SA, Wang A, Xu X, Lee A, Yu PB, Shen J, Bloch KD, Bloch DB. Oral administration of a bone morphogenetic protein type I receptor inhibitor prevents the development of anemia of inflammation. Haematologica. 2015;100(2):e68–71.

19

The gastric H,K-ATPase in stria vascularis contributes to pH regulation of cochlear endolymph but not to K secretion

Hiromitsu Miyazaki[1,2,3], Philine Wangemann[2] and Daniel C. Marcus[1*]

Abstract

Background: Disturbance of acid–base balance in the inner ear is known to be associated with hearing loss in a number of conditions including genetic mutations and pharmacologic interventions. Several previous physiologic and immunohistochemical observations lead to proposals of the involvement of acid–base transporters in stria vascularis.

Results: We directly measured acid flux in vitro from the apical side of isolated stria vascularis from adult C57Bl/6 mice with a novel constant-perfusion pH-selective self-referencing probe. Acid efflux that depended on metabolism and ion transport was observed from the apical side of stria vascularis. The acid flux was decreased to about 40 % of control by removal of the metabolic substrate (glucose-free) and by inhibition of the sodium pump (ouabain). The flux was also decreased a) by inhibition of Na,H-exchangers by amiloride, dimethylamiloride (DMA), S3226 and Hoe694, b) by inhibition of Na,2Cl,K-cotransporter (NKCC1) by bumetanide, and c) by the likely inhibition of HCO_3/anion exchange by DIDS. By contrast, the acid flux was increased by inhibition of gastric H,K-ATPase (SCH28080) but was not affected by an inhibitor of vH-ATPase (bafilomycin). K flux from stria vascularis was reduced less than 5 % by SCH28080.

Conclusions: These observations suggest that stria vascularis may be an important site of control of cochlear acid–base balance and demonstrate a functional role of several acid–base transporters in stria vascularis, including basolateral H,K-ATPase and apical Na,H-exchange. Previous suggestions that H secretion is mediated by an apical vH-ATPase and that basolateral H,K-ATPase contributes importantly to K secretion in stria vascularis are not supported. These results advance our understanding of inner ear acid–base balance and provide a stronger basis to interpret the etiology of genetic and pharmacologic cochlear dysfunctions that are influenced by endolymphatic pH.

Keywords: Acid–base balance, Endolymph, Inner ear, Hydrogen ion secretion, Potassium secretion, Stria vascularis, Ion-selective self-referencing electrode

Background

Disturbance of acid–base balance in the inner ear is known to be associated with hearing loss in a number of conditions including genetic mutations (e.g., Pendred syndrome and hereditary distal renal tubular acidosis [1–4]) and pharmacologic interventions (e.g., acidic-vehicle drug delivery [5, 6]). Homeostasis of endolymphatic (luminal) pH by specific ion transporters in cochlear epithelial cells has been postulated and observed.

H^+ secretion by marginal cells of the stria vascularis was proposed based on observations of immunostaining of vH^+-ATPase near the apical membrane of the epithelial cells [3, 7]. H^+,K^+-ATPase [8] and Na^+,H^+ exchangers [9–11] have been immunolocalized to strial marginal cells and both Na^+,H^+ exchanger [12] and H^+-monocarboxylate transporter [13] activity have been observed. A counterbalancing secretion of HCO_3^- by apical pendrin (SLC26A4) in strial spindle cells, spiral prominence and outer sulcus cells is also critical to pH homeostasis and hearing [14].

The goal of the present study was to test the propositions that the stria vascularis secretes H^+ via vH^+-ATPase, and that the basolateral H^+,K^+-ATPase in strial marginal

* Correspondence: marcus@ksu.edu
[1]Department of Anatomy & Physiology, Cellular Biophysics Laboratory, Kansas State University, 228 Coles Hall, Manhattan, KS 66506-5802, USA
Full list of author information is available at the end of the article

cells provides a third K⁺ uptake pathway (in addition to the Na⁺,2Cl⁻,K⁺ cotransporter (NKCC1) and Na⁺,K⁺-ATPase) involved in K⁺ secretion. We demonstrate that the stria vascularis can indeed actively secrete H⁺, but via apical Na⁺,H⁺ exchange and not vH⁺-ATPase. The basolateral H⁺,K⁺-ATPase can contribute to this H⁺ secretory flux, but does not mediate a significant basolateral K⁺-uptake in parallel to the other two K⁺-secretory uptake pathways. Further, the apical Na⁺,H⁺ exchanger is poised to aid Na⁺ removal during pathological elevation of endolymphatic Na⁺. These results advance our understanding of inner ear acid–base balance by rejecting some prevailing concepts and by confirming others.

Methods

Tissue preparation

Adult C57Bl/6 mice of both genders were deeply anesthetized with 4 % tribromoethanol (0.014 ml/g body wt ip) and sacrificed by decapitation according to a protocol approved by the Kansas State University Institutional Animal Care and Use Committee (#2925). The handling of animals adhered to the ARRIVE guidelines. Stria vascularis (without spiral ligament) was microdissected from the cochlea. Stria vascularis was folded with the apical membrane to the outside of the loop and then mounted in a superfusion chamber on the stage of an inverted microscope and stabilized in the bath with a glass holding pipette.

Transepithelial hydrogen and potassium fluxes

K⁺ secretion by inner ear epithelia was measured by techniques well-established in this laboratory [15] and extended in this study to also measure H⁺ fluxes. Briefly, glass capillaries were pulled to a tip size of about 4 μm and silanized, filled with reference electrolyte (K⁺: 100 mM KCl in 0.2 % agar; pH: 500 mM KCl +20 mM hepes, pH 7.34 in 0.2 % agar), a short column of liquid ion exchanger (K⁺, potassium ionophore I-cocktail B: 50–100 μm column of Sigma-Fluka #99373; pH, hydrogen ionophore II: 20–30 μm column of Sigma-Fluka #95297) aspirated into the tip and the electrode was connected to an electrometer headstage via a Ag/AgCl wire in contact with the reference electrolyte. The ground was a Ag/AgCl wire connected to the bath via a 1 M KCl agar bridge.

The electrodes were first tested for a macroscopic slope of 50–60 mV/decade concentration change and then tested for their ability to detect a gradient near an artificial source (Fig. 1a). The artificial source was constructed from a glass pipette (~80 μm tip diameter) filled with 100 mM KCl or 2 mM H₂SO₄ solution at pH ~3.6 in 4 % agar, which permitted testing drugs for contributing any additional pH buffering or for interference with the liquid ion exchanger. The tip of the ion-selective electrode was positioned under visual control to within a few micrometers of the apical cell surface or the orifice of the artificial source. The electrode was then oscillated by linear translation stages via computer-controlled stepper motors a distance of 30 μm away from the tissue or source. The electrode signal was recorded at each of these two positions and the difference calculated at intervals of 6.8 s to obtain a representation of the relative flux of K⁺ or H⁺ [16]. This difference voltage was also obtained remote from the source (~500 μm) to establish the zero-flux baseline.

Tissues were fixed to the bottom of a microscope chamber and superfused with solutions at 37 °C. The superfusion solution reached both the apical and basolateral membranes of the marginal cells, since it was determined earlier that dissection of the stria from the spiral ligament compromises the integrity of the basal cell layer [17]. H⁺ flux was measured (Fig. 1b) in a weakly-buffered perilymph-like solution (below) to which transport inhibitors were added. Perfusion conditions were carefully adjusted to obtain the best compromise between good fluid exchange and maintenance of sufficient unstirred layer to establish a measureable concentration gradient near the tissue. Data are expressed as the difference in voltage of the ion-selective electrode across the 30 μm excursion or as the fraction (in %) of that voltage difference under test conditions compared to the value during the control period.

The bath solutions contained (in mM): 150 NaCl, 1.6 K₂HPO₄, 0.4 KH₂PO₄, 0.7 CaCl₂, 1.0 MgCl₂, 5 glucose, pH 7.4 (by NaOH). Measurements were made at 37 °C. Drugs were either pre-dissolved in DMSO [amiloride (Sigma A7410), HOE694 (3-methylsulfonyl-4-piperidino-benzoyl) guanidine methanesulfonate; gift from Dr. H-J. Lang), S3226 (3-[2-(3-guanidino-2-methyl-3-oxo-propenyl)-5-methyl]-N-isopropylidene-2-methyl-acrylamide; gift from Sanofi-Aventis Deutschland GmbH), dimethyla-miloride (DMA; Sigma A4562), ouabain (Sigma O3125), bumetanide (Sigma B3023), SCH28080 (Sigma S4443), DIDS (4,4'-Diisothiocyanatostilbene-2,2'-disulfonic acid; Sigma D3514)] and used at a final concentration of < =0.1 % DMSO or dissolved directly in bath solution [bafilomycin A1 (Sigma B1793)]. DMSO 0.1 % was also added to the control solution when it was used to dissolve the drug.

Tissues were superfused with the control bath solution (above) for at least 5 min to stabilize the preparation, followed by a 5-min first measurement period, then a 5 to 10 min experimental treatment period, followed by a second 5-min control period. Thirteen to 18 continuous digital samples were averaged near the end of the period prior to the experimental period and from a stable or early quasi-stable time period, typically 3 to 5 min post solution change. When there was a slow secondary phase to the experimental response, an earlier quasi-

a

Probe

Artificial source

b

Probe

Stria vascularis

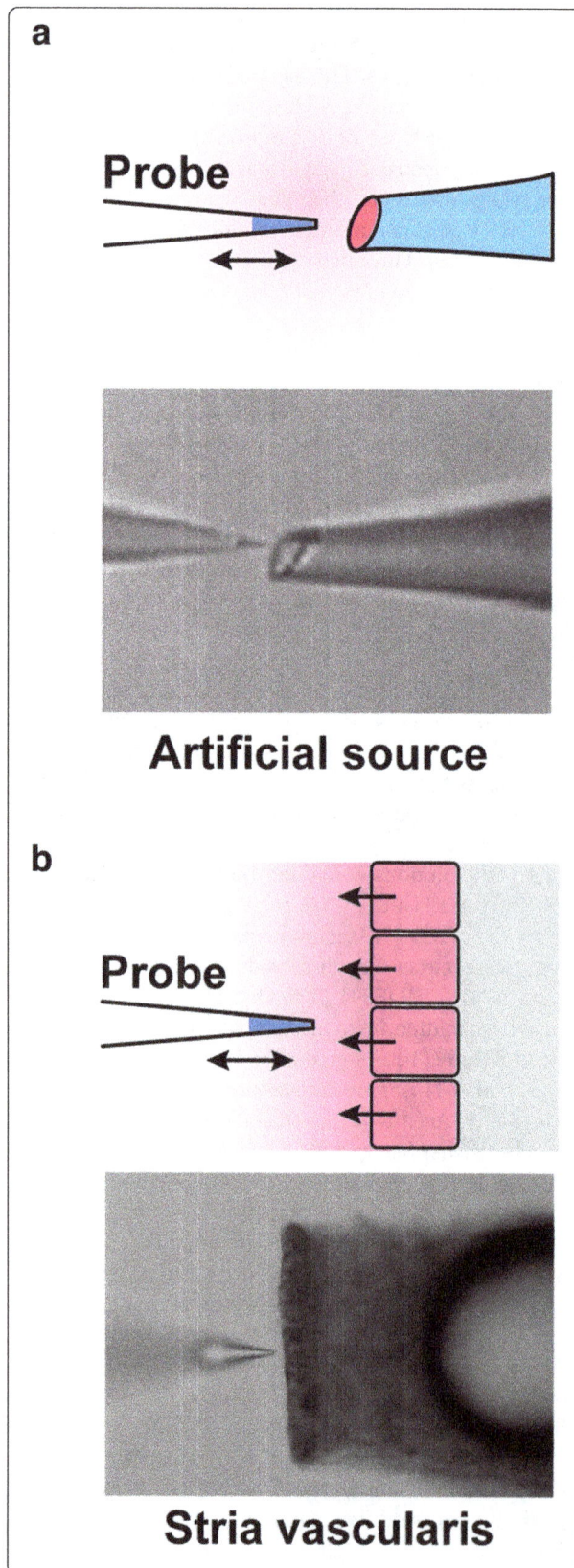

Fig. 1 Self-referencing ion-selective electrode method. The electrode (probe) tip oscillates a distance of about 30 μm (*double-headed arrow*). The mean position is first set remote from the source (about 500 μm away; not shown) and the difference signal from the oscillation is taken as zero. The oscillating probe is then set within several μm of the **a** artificial source or **b** epithelium, and the difference signal in the concentration gradient is taken as a relative measure of the ion flux. Changes in ion flux are monitored during bath perfusion of control and experimental solutions. (*Top panels*) diagram; (*Bottom panels*) photomicrographs of artificial and epithelial sources and adjacent probe. Liquid ion exchanger (selective for K^+ or H^+) is visible in the tip of the electrode

stable time period was chosen in order to minimize possible drift in the experiment or changes due to secondary effects from the experimental treatment [see Additional file 1].

Measurements from the experimental period were compared to the value from the prior period (time-control, glucose-free, ouabain, 50–200 μM bumetanide, DIDS, bafilomycin) or to the average of the two control periods when the response was clearly reversible (amiloride and its analogs, SCH28080, 1–10 μM bumetanide). Data are expressed as mean ± sem of the signal in μV or percent of the control, n = number of tissue samples [see Additional file 1].

Significance was determined by paired t-test and $P < 0.05$ was taken as a significant difference. Concentration-response data for SCH28080 and the NHE transport inhibitors were fitted to Michaelis-Menton kinetics using Origin software (OriginLab, Northampton, MA). The fits were made using the individual data points in order to avoid skewed weighting on the logarithmic scale and the best-fit curve then plotted with the average response at each concentration for clarity.

Results and discussion
Strial H^+ flux is linked to metabolism and Na^+,K^+-ATPase activity

H^+ flux was measured near the apical membrane of stria vascularis and the results were not significantly affected by the experimental protocol (Fig. 2a). A substantial H^+ flux was observed, as indicated by a mean voltage difference at the H^+-selective microelectrode of 32.6 ± 0.8 μV (n = 118) under control conditions. Both glucose-removal and inhibition of the basolateral Na^+,K^+-ATPase with ouabain (1 mM) reduced apical H^+ flux to 37.9 ± 0.6 % (n = 3) and to 39.7 ± 2.2 % (n = 3) of control values (Fig. 2b, c, d). These results are consistent with the interpretation 1) that strial H^+ flux requires metabolic energy and 2) that it depends on a transmembrane Na^+ gradient established by the Na^+-pump. The remaining ~40 % H^+ flux after removal of glucose may represent catabolism of other stored metabolic substrates, including glycogen or phosphocreatine, although glycogen stores in the stria

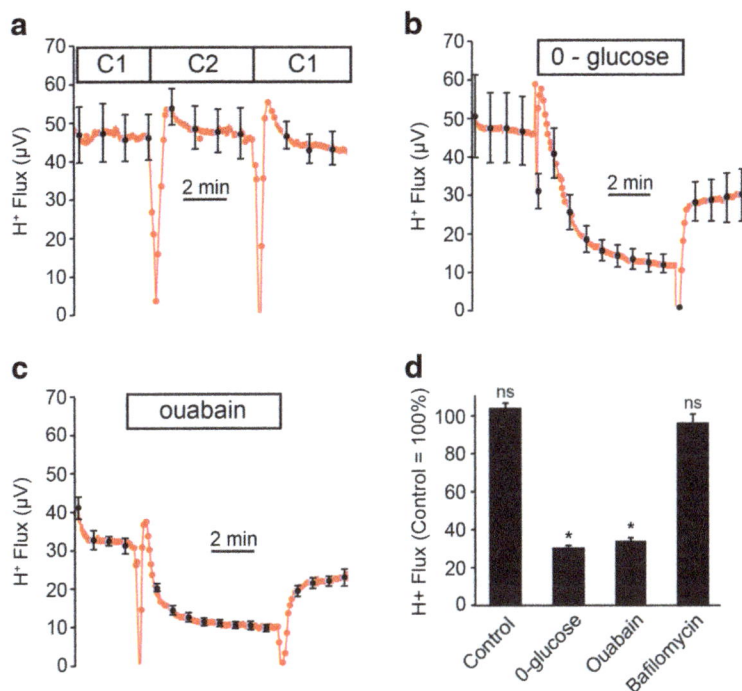

Fig. 2 H$^+$-flux from stria vascularis; control, glucose-free, ouabain and bafilomycin. **a** Summary traces ($N = 4$) of time-controls during perfusion of control bath solution in the absence of any experimental agents. Boxes labeled C1 and C2 are the perfusion times from two separate reservoirs of bath solution (see Methods for composition). **b** Summary traces ($N = 3$) of glucose-free (0-glucose) perfusion. **c** Summary traces ($N = 3$) of ouabain (1 mM) perfusion. **d** Bar graphs of steady state effects of time-control, glucose-free, ouabain and bafilomycin (1 µM; $N = 6$) perfusion. *, $P < 0.05$; ns, not significant. **a**, **b**, **c** Traces are the vertical averages of N experiments conducted with identical time-course. Standard error bars are indicated only at intervals for clarity; boxes show duration of the experimental period

vascularis are quite low compared to other inner ear structures [18]. The transport pathway of this remaining H$^+$ flux is not yet identified, but may be simple diffusion through H$^+$ channels [19] or through other integral membrane proteins [20].

The primary metabolic source of secreted acid is the unusually-high rate of CO_2 production from glucose, thought to be due to shunting of glycolysis through the hexose monophosphate pathway [21]. Strial metabolism occurs at a remarkably-high rate, similar to that of kidney [22]. The rate of O_2 consumption decreases by about half when the Na$^+$-pump is blocked by ouabain [22]. The coupling of O_2 respiration rate to CO_2 production with a respiratory quotient of 1.2 [21] predicts a drop of H$^+$ efflux by ouabain of a little more than half, which is consistent with our observation (above).

Strial H$^+$ flux is not carried by an apical vH$^+$-ATPase

The apical H$^+$ flux in the presence of 1 µM bafilomycin A1, a concentration that would produce a near maximal inhibition of H$^+$-ATPase, was not significantly different than under control conditions (Fig. 2d). This result demonstrates that H$^+$ flux is not mediated via an apical vH$^+$-ATPase and suggests that the immunostained vH$^+$-ATPase near the apical membrane of marginal cells [7]

is not contributing to H$^+$ efflux under our experimental conditions. It is conceivable that the immunostained vH$^+$-ATPase is in sub-apical vesicles [23].

Coupling of strial K$^+$ flux to H$^+$ flux

The effect of ouabain on H$^+$ flux (above) is consistent with a feedback of cellular ion transport to the rate of metabolism needed to power the transport. We evaluated specifically the primary ion transport function of stria (K$^+$ secretion) by inhibiting apical K$^+$ flux from strial marginal cells by blocking uptake of K$^+$ via the basolateral Na$^+$,2Cl$^-$,K$^+$ cotransporter with bumetanide (Fig. 3a, b). The average from all measurements of K$^+$ flux under control conditions was 5.6 ± 0.4 µV ($n = 28$). The IC$_{50}$ of bumetanide on K$^+$ flux in this series of experiments was 7×10^{-6} M, which is consistent with specific inhibition of NKCC1, and is similar to previous findings in vestibular dark cells and strial marginal cells [17, 24, 25]. Indeed, inhibition of K$^+$ secretion by bumetanide partially inhibited H$^+$ flux (Fig. 3d). This finding is consistent with the view that K$^+$ secretion is coupled to metabolic rate and thereby acid production and its subsequent efflux from the cells. The meaning of the observation that H$^+$ flux is reduced far more by ouabain than by bumetanide is not clear. These results are consistent

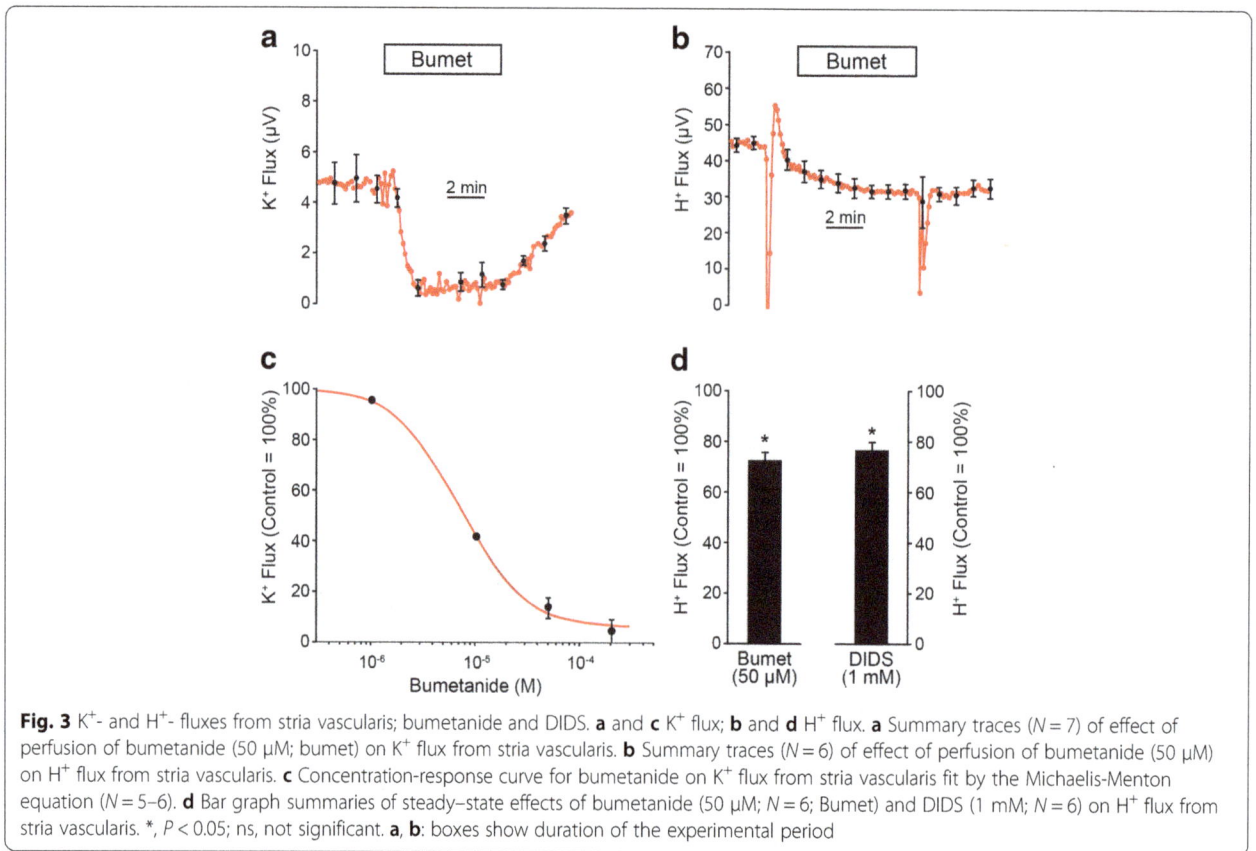

Fig. 3 K⁺- and H⁺- fluxes from stria vascularis; bumetanide and DIDS. **a** and **c** K⁺ flux; **b** and **d** H⁺ flux. **a** Summary traces ($N = 7$) of effect of perfusion of bumetanide (50 μM; bumet) on K⁺ flux from stria vascularis. **b** Summary traces ($N = 6$) of effect of perfusion of bumetanide (50 μM) on H⁺ flux from stria vascularis. **c** Concentration-response curve for bumetanide on K⁺ flux from stria vascularis fit by the Michaelis-Menton equation ($N = 5$–6). **d** Bar graph summaries of steady–state effects of bumetanide (50 μM; $N = 6$; Bumet) and DIDS (1 mM; $N = 6$) on H⁺ flux from stria vascularis. *, $P < 0.05$; ns, not significant. **a**, **b**: boxes show duration of the experimental period

with the notion that the Na⁺ pump energizes more processes than K⁺ secretion, such as the Na⁺,H⁺ exchangers (below) and/or other Na⁺-coupled transport [26].

We hypothesized that since reduction of metabolism (either by direct inhibition of metabolism or via inhibition of ion transport) lead to reduced apical H efflux, that stimulation of ion transport was expected to increase apical H efflux. DIDS stimulates K⁺ secretion through potentiation of apical KCNQ1/KCNE1 K⁺ channels [27] as well as its more-widely known inhibitory action on several types of Cl⁻-HCO₃⁻ transporters, including Slc26a4 [2, 28]. It was expected that if the primary action of DIDS were stimulation of K⁺ secretion, the metabolic rate would be increased and thereby increase the apical H⁺ flux. By contrast, it was observed that DIDS (1 mM), similar to bumetanide, reduced the H⁺ flux from strial marginal cells (Fig. 3d).

This result is inconsistent with our hypothesis and suggests that the primary effect of DIDS may be via its known inhibition of several anion transporters [28]. The drug target is not likely to be the Cl⁻,HCO₃⁻ exchanger Slc26a4, since Slc26a4 is not expressed in strial marginal cells, and even if HCO₃⁻ secretion by apical Slc26a4 in remote cells contributed to the net H⁺ flux recorded at the marginal cells, inhibition by DIDS would lead to an increase of net H⁺ flux, and not the observed decrease.

One could therefore speculate that there is normally a DIDS-sensitive basolateral HCO₃⁻ efflux (e.g., via NBCe1 as proposed in the proximal kidney tubule [28]) from strial marginal cells. Inhibition by DIDS of this putative basolateral HCO₃⁻ efflux would result in an accumulation of intracellular HCO₃⁻ which would be expected to slow down the hydrating reaction of CO₂ catalyzed by carbonic anhydrase, thereby reducing the available cytosolic H⁺ and apical H⁺ efflux, as observed. The unreacted CO₂ would diffuse passively across the basolateral membrane and be carried away in the blood (in vivo) or bath (in vitro). The actual mechanism remains unknown.

Strial H⁺ flux is carried by apical Na⁺,H⁺ exchangers

It was hypothesized that apical H⁺ efflux may be mediated by Na⁺,H⁺-exchangers (NHEs) in the apical membrane. Indeed, our results support the participation of NHEs in H⁺ secretion although the specific isoform(s) involved were not unambiguously determined. We found the apical H⁺ flux in strial marginal cells was reduced by several inhibitors of NHEs, including amiloride, dimethylamiloride (DMA), S3226 and Hoe694 (Fig. 4). The amiloride analogs employed here are more specific for the NHEs than is amiloride itself. Amiloride has additional inhibitory properties against the epithelial sodium channel (ENaC) and Na⁺,Ca²⁺-exchangers [29]. Dose–response

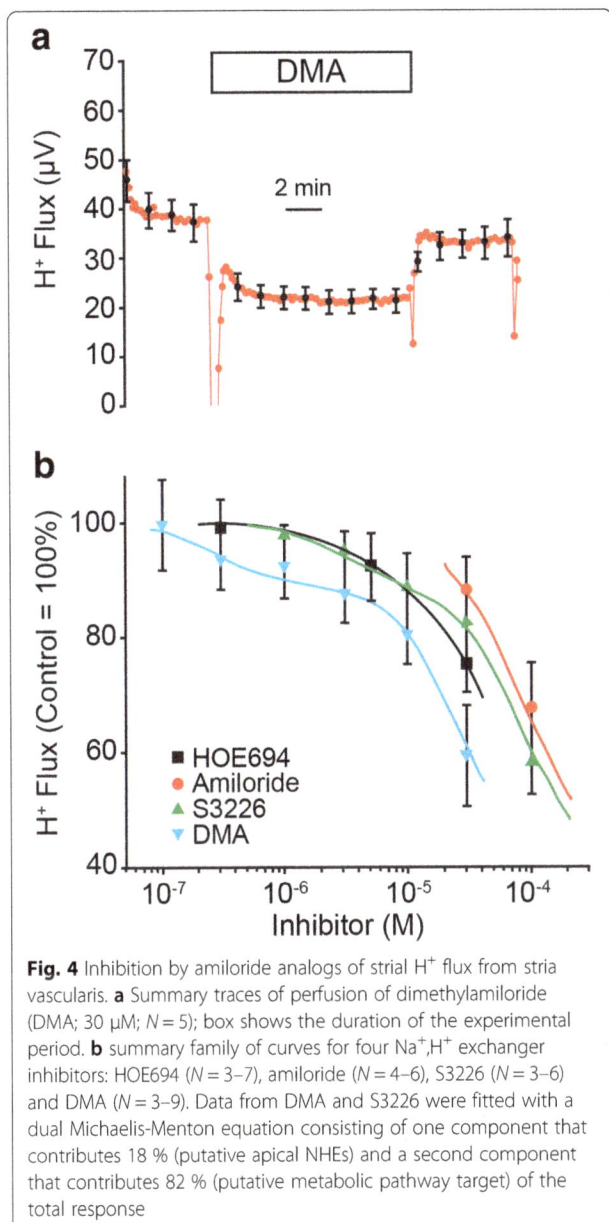

Fig. 4 Inhibition by amiloride analogs of strial H$^+$ flux from stria vascularis. **a** Summary traces of perfusion of dimethylamiloride (DMA; 30 μM; $N = 5$); box shows the duration of the experimental period. **b** summary family of curves for four Na$^+$,H$^+$ exchanger inhibitors: HOE694 ($N = 3$–7), amiloride ($N = 4$–6), S3226 ($N = 3$–6) and DMA ($N = 3$–9). Data from DMA and S3226 were fitted with a dual Michaelis-Menten equation consisting of one component that contributes 18 % (putative apical NHEs) and a second component that contributes 82 % (putative metabolic pathway target) of the total response

curves for DMA and S3226 were fitted by the Michaelis-Menton equation for two drug targets that contributed 18 % (high affinity) and 82 % (low affinity) of H$^+$ flux. The high affinity target had an IC$_{50}$ of 3×10^{-7} for DMA and 3×10^{-6} for S3226. The low affinity targets were taken to be in metabolic pathways rather than membrane transporters; interference with metabolism was shown to decrease the apical H$^+$ flux (e.g., removal of glucose, above). High concentrations of drugs (e.g., >100 μM) that are in equilibrium with a lipophilic chemical form (e.g., DIOA and NPPB) [30, 31], are able to integrate into mitochondrial membranes and interfere with ATP production.

Studies on NHE function have often been performed in cells which express multiple isoforms of NHE, which complicates the unambiguous identification of the active isoform(s). Other complicating factors include the strong dependence of the IC$_{50}$ of the amiloride analogs on extracellular [Na$^+$], making it difficult to compare specific IC$_{50}$ values for specific NHE isoforms in the literature derived under vastly different [Na$^+$] [29].

The greater sensitivity to DMA over S3226 found here is consistent with the H$^+$ flux being mediated by NHE2 [29]. NHE2 is expressed in other epithelial cells and can occur in either the apical [32] or basolateral membrane [33]. NHE2 mRNA transcripts were present in stria vascularis at age P10, determined by gene array (GEO Data set: GSE10587). Partial inhibition of the H$^+$ flux by the NHE3-specific inhibitor S3226 is consistent with NHE3 also mediating a part of the flux. Strong expression of NHE3 has been demonstrated in the apical membrane of strial marginal cells [9].

NHE1 activity has been identified in the basolateral membrane of vestibular dark cells (which are analogs of strial marginal cells in the vestibular labyrinth) [12], and transcripts of NHE1 were present in stria vascularis at age P10 (GEO Data set: GSE10587), but its contribution, if present, to the measurements here is clearly less than apical NHEs since all inhibitors caused decreases in the net flux. If basolateral NHE1 were the dominant target of any of these inhibitors at the concentrations used, the apical flux would have increased, as during inhibition of basolateral H$^+$ efflux via the H$^+$,K$^+$-ATPase (*vide infra*).

A transient decrease in Isc was observed in stria vascularis with apical perfusion of 500 μM amiloride [12]. The effect was smaller than seen with basolateral perfusion and previously interpreted as only leakage or diffusion to the basolateral side. However, the effect could be a direct inhibition of apical NHE and consequent cellular acidification via inhibited apical NHE activity, consistent with the present results.

NHE6 and NHE9 mRNA transcripts were also present in stria vascularis (GEO Data set: GSE10587). These isoforms occur predominantly in intracellular organelles, but have been observed occasionally in the plasma membrane of some cells [34].

Significance of NHE in apical membrane

The H$^+$ efflux observed in the present experiments in vitro were conducted under conditions that reveal and emphasize the presence of this transporter. That is, the difference in [Na$^+$] between the bath and marginal cell cytosol (Table 1) is sufficient to drive H$^+$ out of the cell, leading to the observed substantial H$^+$ secretion and to Na$^+$ absorption. However under normal in vivo conditions, the Na$^+$ difference is likely reversed in direction and larger than the outward H$^+$ difference (Table 1), assuming reasonable values for cytosolic pH and [Na$^+$].

Table 1 Estimated Na^+ and H^+ gradients across apical membrane of strial marginal cells

	[H$^+$],e-b (nM)	[H$^+$],c (nM)	[Na$^+$],e-b (mM)	[Na$^+$],c (mM)	R$_H$ (c/e-b)	R$_{Na}$ (e-b/c)	Direction of transport
In vitro	34 (pH 7.4)	63 (pH 7.2)	150	10	1.85	15	Na$^+$ in H$^+$ out
In vivo	32 (pH 7.5)	63 (pH 7.2)	1	10	1.95	0.1	Na$^+$ out H$^+$ in

[H$^+$], hydrogen ion concentration; [Na$^+$], sodium ion concentration; e-b, endolymph (in vivo) or bath (in vitro); c, cytosol; RH RNa, Ratio of H$^+$ and Na$^+$ concentrations between compartments; Direction of transport into or out of the cell across the apical membrane of strial marginal cells

The cytosolic values in Table 1 are taken from the accepted normative values in the literature that have been utilized for similar calculations on directions of transport in mammalian cells, for example cardiac cell Na^+, Ca^{2+} exchange and Na^+, H^+ exchange [35]. Even though there were some early estimates of intracellular Na^+ concentration in stria vascularis that were greater [36], a biochemical assay for Na^+, K^+-ATPase activity versus Na^+ concentration demonstrated a peak in activity at 10 mM [37], consistent with physiological control set to a normal level of 10 mM or less.

Therefore under normal homeostatic conditions, this apical membrane exchanger may actually provide a counterbalance to the primary Na^+ absorptive roles of Reissner's membrane, Claudius cells and outer sulcus cells [38–43]. Analogous push/pull transport systems of ion homeostasis for K^+ [17, 43] and for Ca^{2+} [2, 44–46] in endolymph have also been demonstrated. Although not highly active under normative conditions, the apical NHE is poised to respond to pathological increases in endolymphatic [Na^+], such as during vascular accidents that cause local ischemic anoxia [47, 48]. NHE therefore provides a controlled Na^+ "leak" into endolymph under normal homeostatic conditions and a Na^+ absorptive pathway during Na^+ loading of endolymph.

In addition, the H^+ flux from the lumen to the marginal cell cytosol (equivalent to HCO_3^- secretion) via NHE under normative conditions would augment the HCO_3^- secretory roles of strial spindle cells and spiral prominence/outer sulcus cells via the pendrin HCO_3^-/anion exchange activity [49].

Strial H$^+$ flux is carried by basolateral H$^+$,K$^+$ ATPase

Gastric H^+, K^+-ATPase (consisting of a heterodimer of HKalpha1 and HKbetaG subunits) is expressed in the basolateral membrane of strial marginal cells [8] and its transport function can be inhibited by SCH28080 but not ouabain, in contrast to the colonic H^+, K^+-ATPase, which is inhibited by ouabain but completely insensitive to SCH28080 [50]. We found that SCH28080 increased apical H^+ flux from strial marginal cells (Fig. 5).

The measurements were made over a concentration range of 10^{-11} to 10^{-7} M ($N = 3$–7), with maximal effect of 17.1 % increase and the EC$_{50}$ of SCH28080 was 1.9×10^{-9} M. This exquisite sensitivity is about 2 orders of magnitude better than for inhibition of this ATPase in isolated gastric glands, while the IC$_{50}$ of the ATPase by the protonated species of SCH28080 is about 1.5×10^{-8} M [51, 52], which is consistent with specific inhibition of this ion pump. By contrast, it was found by Shibata et al that a full decrease of endocochlear potential from vascular or perilymphatic perfusion of SCH28080 occurred at 3 and at 1 mM, respectively [8]. Our observed increase in H^+ flux suggests that blocking basolateral H^+ efflux from the marginal cells re-directed the flux through the apical membrane. An increased apical flux during SCH28080 perfusion also implies an elevated cytosolic [H^+] to drive this transport.

Strial K$^+$ flux is NOT carried by basolateral H$^+$,K$^+$ ATPase

It was proposed that the basolateral H^+, K^+-ATPase contributes to transepithelial K^+ secretion by taking up K^+ in parallel to the recognized action of the basolateral $Na^+, 2Cl^-, K^+$ cotransporter [8]. SCH28080 at a virtually maximal dose (10^{-8} M) decreased the apical K^+ flux in strial marginal cells by less than 5 % (Fig. 5). In order to determine whether this small decrease was physiologically relevant or if it only represented a small but consistent drift in that series of experiments, the sensitivity of this test was increased by first reducing the apical K^+ flux with a maximal dose (200 µM) of bumetanide. The residual K^+ flux in the presence of bumetanide was not significantly greater than zero and there was no significant difference by addition of SCH28080 (10^{-8} M). These data demonstrate that H^+, K^+-ATPase contributes no more than a minuscule fraction to K^+ secretion and that H^+, K^+-ATPase therefore does not provide an alternative route in the basolateral membrane for K^+ uptake to the normative route via the $Na^+, 2Cl^-, K^+$ cotransporter.

The report of a decrease in endocochlear potential in response to SCH28080 was ascribed to an inhibition of basolateral H^+, K^+-ATPase and a putative drop in basolateral K^+ uptake into strial marginal cells and consequently a drop in electrogenic K^+ transport [8]. The present results argue against this interpretation. It is also unlikely that the effect on EP is mediated by changes in marginal cell cytosolic pH or extracellular pH. As described above, the marginal cells possess both apical and basolateral NHEs that could respond to increased cytosolic acid and the KCNQ1/KCNE1 K^+ channel in

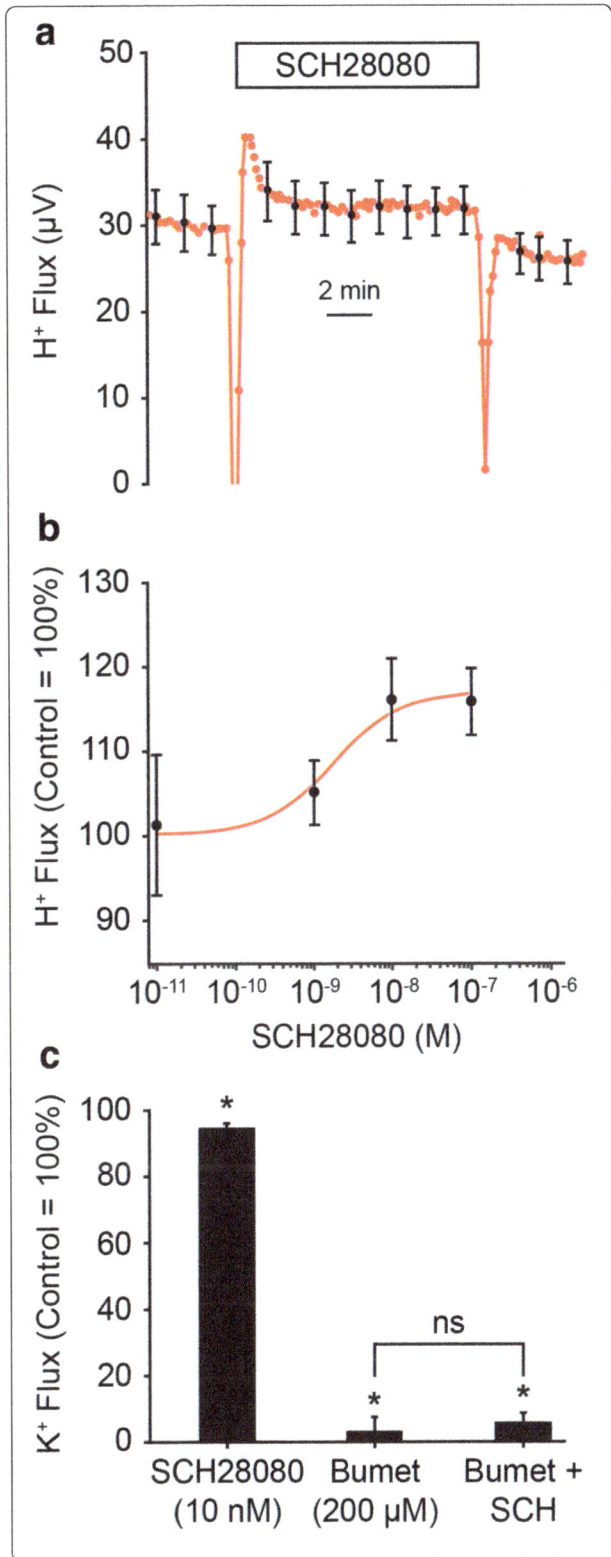

Fig. 5 Effects of inhibition of gastric H+,K+-ATPase on H+- and K+-fluxes from stria vascularis. **a** Summary traces ($N = 7$) of effect on H+ flux of perfusion of SCH28080 (10 nM). Box shows the duration of the experimental period. **b** Concentration-response curve ($N = 3–7$) for stimulation of strial H+-flux by SCH28080. Data fit by the Michaelis-Menton equation. **c** Small inhibition of K+ flux from stria vascularis by SCH28080 (10 nM; $N = 7$)) and absence of effect (SCH, SCH28080) after inhibition of K+ flux by bumetanide (200 µM; $N = 6$; bumet). *, $P < 0.05$; ns, not significant

the apical membrane of these cells is relatively insensitive to cytosolic acidification in the physiological range [53]. In addition, the KCNJ10 K+ channel of the neighboring intermediate cells is also relatively insensitive to changes in extracellular pH [54].

Conclusions

We have developed a technique for the recording of transepithelial H+ and K+ flux during continuous perfusion of isolated inner ear tissues at 37 °C and applied it to the investigation of pH homeostatic mechanisms in the cochlea (Fig. 6). Several long-standing questions about the mechanisms underlying cochlear pH homeostasis were resolved. 1) The basolateral H+/K+-ATPase

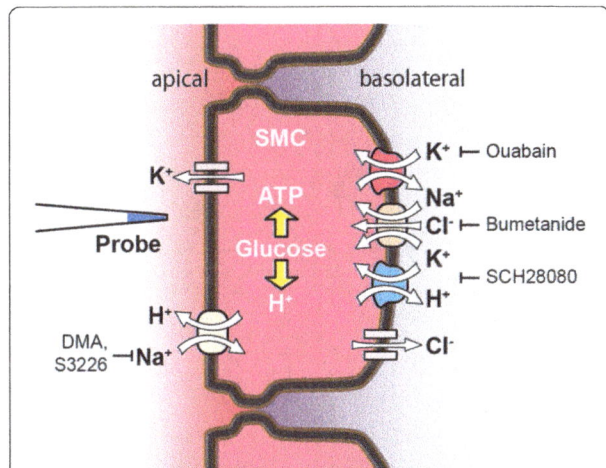

Fig. 6 Cell model of H+ and K+ secretion by strial marginal cells in the cochlea. Transepithelial secretion of K+ is mediated by uptake of K+ from the basolateral side of the strial marginal cells (SMC) via the Na+,K+-ATPase and the Na+,2Cl−,K+-cotransporter (NKCC1). The contribution to K+ flux by the gastric H+,K+-ATPase is minimal. K+ transport from the cytosol into endolymph is mediated by KCNQ1/KCNE1 K+ channels in the apical membrane. Metabolically-generated acid exits the cell via the basolateral gastric H+,K+-ATPase and the apical Na+,H+-exchangers. Apical membrane H+ exit is increased when the basolateral H+,K+-ATPase is inhibited and the H+ flux re-routed to the apical membrane. Cl− that was taken up into the cytosol via the Na+,2Cl−,K+-cotransporter is recycled across the basolateral membrane via the ClC-K/barttin Cl− channels. Additional putative acid/base transporters, such as basolateral DIDS-sensitive HCO3− efflux via NBCe1, are not shown

of strial marginal cells was earlier posited to contribute importantly to the cellular uptake of K^+ and the subsequent secretion across the apical membrane. Our measurements did not support that proposition, but did demonstrate its significant contribution to basolateral H^+ flux and its coordination with apical H^+ flux. 2) The vH^+-ATPase previously found near the apical membrane of strial marginal cells was posited to contribute importantly to apical H^+ secretion . Our measurements did not support that proposition. 3) Apical membranes of strial marginal cells were previously shown to express the Na^+, H^+ exchanger NHE3 and stria vascularis also expressed mRNA of NHE1, NHE2, NHE6 and NHE9. Our measurements support a functional H^+ flux from one or more apical Na^+, H^+ exchangers. These results advance our understanding of inner ear acid–base balance and provide a stronger basis to interpret the etiology of genetic and pharmacologic cochlear dysfunctions that are influenced by endolymphatic pH.

Abbreviations
DIDS, 4,4'-Diisothiocyanatostilbene-2,2'-disulfonic acid; DMA, dimethylamiloride; DMSO, dimethylsulfoxide; HOE694, (3-methylsulfonyl-4-piperidinobenzoyl) guanidine methanesulfonate; S3226, (3-[2-(3-guanidino-2-methyl-3-oxo-propenyl)-5-methyl]-N-isopropylidene-2-methyl-acrylamide

Acknowledgments
We thank Donald G. Harbidge and Joel D. Sanneman for their excellent technical support.

Funding
This work was supported by NIH grants R01-DC00212 (DCM), P20-RR017686 (DCM) and R01-DC01098 (PW) and by the College of Veterinary Medicine, Kansas State University.

Authors' contributions
HM contributed to the design and analysis of experiments, development of the modifications to the methodology and collected the experimental data. PW and DM contributed to the design and analysis of experiments, development of the modifications to the methodology and writing of the manuscript. All authors read and approved the final manuscript.

Competing interests
The authors declare that they have no competing interests.

Author details
[1]Department of Anatomy & Physiology, Cellular Biophysics Laboratory, Kansas State University, 228 Coles Hall, Manhattan, KS 66506-5802, USA. [2]Deparment of Anatomy & Physiology, Cell Physiology Laboratory, Kansas State University, 228 Coles Hall, Manhattan KS 66506-5802, USA. [3]Department of Otolaryngology-Head and Neck Surgery, Tohoku University Graduate School of Medicine, Sendai 980-8574, Japan.

References
1. Everett LA, Glaser B, Beck JC, Idol JR, Buchs A, Heyman M, Adawi F, Hazani E, Nassir E, Baxevanis AD, Sheffield VC, Green ED. Pendred syndrome is caused by mutations in a putative sulphate transporter gene (PDS). Nat Genet. 1997;17:411–22.
2. Wangemann P, Nakaya K, Wu T, Maganti RJ, Itza EM, Sanneman JD, Harbidge DG, Billings S, Marcus DC. Loss of cochlear HCO_{3-} secretion causes deafness via endolymphatic acidification and inhibition of Ca^{2+} reabsorption in a Pendred syndrome mouse model. Am J Physiol Renal Physiol. 2007;292:F1345–53.
3. Karet FE, Finberg KE, Nelson RD, Nayir A, Mocan H, Sanjad SA, Rodriguez-Soriano J, Santos F, Cremers CW, Di Pietro A, Hoffbrand BI, Winiarski J, Bakkaloglu A, Ozen S, Dusunsel R, Goodyer P, Hulton SA, Wu DK, Skvorak AB, Morton CC, Cunningham MJ, Jha V, Lifton RP. Mutations in the gene encoding B1 subunit of H^+-ATPase cause renal tubular acidosis with sensorineural deafness. Nat Genet. 1999;21:84–90.
4. Stover EH, Borthwick KJ, Bavalia C, Eady N, Fritz DM, Rungroj N, Giersch AB, Morton CC, Axon PR, Akil I, Al-Sabban EA, Baguley DM, Bianca S, Bakkaloglu A, Bircan Z, Chauveau D, Clermont MJ, Guala A, Hulton SA, Kroes H, Li VG, Mir S, Mocan H, Nayir A, Ozen S, Rodriguez-Soriano J, Sanjad SA, Tasic V, Taylor CM, Topaloglu R, Smith AN, Karet FE. Novel ATP6V1B1 and ATP6V0A4 mutations in autosomal recessive distal renal tubular acidosis with new evidence for hearing loss. J Med Genet. 2002;39:796–803.
5. Ikeda K, Morizono T. The preparation of acetic acid for use in otic drops and its effect on endocochlear potential and pH in inner ear fluid. Am J Otolaryngol. 1989;10:382–5.
6. Tanaka F, Whitworth CA, Rybak LP. Influence of pH on the ototoxicity of cisplatin: a round window application study. Hear Res. 2003;177:21–31.
7. Stankovic KM, Brown D, Alper SL, Adams JC. Localization of pH regulating proteins H^+ATPase and Cl^-/HCO_3^- exchanger in the guinea pig inner ear. Hear Res. 1997;114:21–34.
8. Shibata T, Hibino H, Doi K, Suzuki T, Hisa Y, Kurachi Y. Gastric type H+, K+-ATPase in the cochlear lateral wall is critically involved in formation of the endocochlear potential. Am J Physiol Cell Physiol. 2006;291:C1038–48.
9. Bond BR, Ng LL, Schulte BA. Identification of mRNA transcripts and immunohistochemical localization of Na/H exchanger isoforms in gerbil inner ear. Hear Res. 1998;123:1–9.
10. Goto S, Oshima T, Ikeda K, Takasaka T. Expression and localization of the Na^+-H^+ exchanger in the guinea pig cochlea. Hear Res. 1999;128:89–96.
11. Ikeda K, Sunose H, Takasaka T. Involvement of Na^+-H^+ exchange in intracellular pH recovery from acid load in the stria vascularis of the guinea-pig cochlea. Acta Otolaryngol (Stockh). 1994;114:162–6.
12. Wangemann P, Liu J, Shiga N. Vestibular dark cells contain the Na^+/H^+ exchanger NHE-1 in the basolateral membrane. Hear Res. 1996;94:94–106.
13. Shimozono M, Scofield MA, Wangemann P. Functional evidence for a monocarboxylate transporter (MCT) in strial marginal cells and molecular evidence for MCT1 and MCT2 in stria vascularis. Hear Res. 1997;114:213–22.
14. Kim HM, Wangemann P. Epithelial cell stretching and luminal acidification lead to a retarded development of stria vascularis and deafness in mice lacking pendrin. PLoS One. 2011;6, e17949.
15. Marcus DC, Shipley AM. Potassium secretion by vestibular dark cell epithelium demonstrated by vibrating probe. Biophys J. 1994;66:1939–42.
16. Sunose H, Liu J, Shen Z, Marcus DC. cAMP increases K^+ secretion via activation of apical I_{sK}/KvLQT1 channels in strial marginal cells. Hear Res. 1997;114:107–16.
17. Wangemann P, Liu J, Marcus DC. Ion transport mechanisms responsible for K^+ secretion and the transepithelial voltage across marginal cells of stria vascularis in vitro. Hear Res. 1995;84:19–29.
18. Thalmann R, Miyoshi T, Kusakari J, Ise I. Normal and abnormal energy metabolism of the inner ear. Otolaryngol Clin North Am. 1975;8:313–33.
19. DeCoursey TE. Voltage-gated proton channels: molecular biology, physiology, and pathophysiology of the H(V) family. Physiol Rev. 2013;93:599–652.
20. Wang X, Horisberger JD. A conformation of Na^+-K^+ pump is permeable to proton. Am J Physiol Cell Physiol. 1995;268:C590–5.
21. Marcus DC, Thalmann R, Marcus NY. Respiratory quotient of stria vascularis of guinea pig in vitro. Arch Otorhinolaryngol. 1978;221:97–103.
22. Marcus DC, Thalmann R, Marcus NY. Respiratory rate and ATP content of stria vascularis of guinea pig in vitro. Laryngoscope. 1978;88:1825–35.
23. White PN, Thorne PR, Housley GD, Mockett B, Billett TE, Burnstock G. Quinacrine staining of marginal cells in the stria vascularis of the guinea-pig cochlea: a possible source of extracellular ATP? Hear Res. 1995;90:97–105.

The gastric H,K-ATPase in stria vascularis contributes to pH regulation of cochlear endolymph...

247

24. Marcus DC, Marcus NY, Greger R. Sidedness of action of loop diuretics and ouabain on nonsensory cells of utricle: a micro-Ussing chamber for inner ear tissues. Hear Res. 1987;30:55–64.

25. Marcus NY, Marcus DC. Potassium secretion by nonsensory region of gerbil utricle in vitro. Am J Physiol. 1987;253:F613–21.

26. Krishnamurthy H, Piscitelli CL, Gouaux E. Unlocking the molecular secrets of sodium-coupled transporters. Nature. 2009;459:347–55.

27. Shen Z, Liu J, Marcus DC, Shiga N, Wangemann P. DIDS increases K$^+$ secretion through an IsK channel in apical membrane of vestibular dark cell epithelium of gerbil. J Membr Biol. 1995;146:283–91.

28. Parker MD, Boron WF. The divergence, actions, roles, and relatives of sodium-coupled bicarbonate transporters. Physiol Rev. 2013;93:803–959.

29. Masereel B, Pochet L, Laeckmann D. An overview of inhibitors of Na(+)/H(+) exchanger. Eur J Med Chem. 2003;38:547–54.

30. Pondugula SR, Kampalli SB, Wu T, De Lisle RC, Raveendran NN, Harbidge DG, Marcus DC. cAMP-stimulated Cl- secretion is increased by glucocorticoids and inhibited by bumetanide in semicircular canal duct epithelium. BMC Physiol. 2013;13:6.

31. Wangemann P, Wittner M, Di SA, Englert HC, Lang HJ, Schlatter E, Greger R. Cl(-)-channel blockers in the thick ascending limb of the loop of Henle. Structure activity relationship. Pflugers Arch. 1986;407 Suppl 2:S128–41.

32. Tse CM, Levine SA, Yun CH, Montrose MH, Little PJ, Pouyssegur J, Donowitz M. Cloning and expression of a rabbit cDNA encoding a serum-activated ethylisopropylamiloride-resistant epithelial Na$^+$/H$^+$ exchanger isoform (NHE-2). J Biol Chem. 1993;268:11917–24.

33. Soleimani M, Singh G, Bizal GL, Gullans SR, McAteer JA. Na+/H+ exchanger isoforms NHE-2 and NHE-1 in inner medullary collecting duct cells. Expression, functional localization, and differential regulation. J Biol Chem. 1994;269:27973–8.

34. Hill JK, Brett CL, Chyou A, Kallay LM, Sakaguchi M, Rao R, Gillespie PG. Vestibular hair bundles control pH with (Na$^+$, K$^+$)/H$^+$ exchangers NHE6 and NHE9. J Neurosci. 2006;26:9944–55.

35. Murphy E, Eisner DA. Regulation of intracellular and mitochondrial sodium in health and disease. Circ Res. 2009;104:292–303.

36. Marcus DC, Marcus NY, Thalmann R. Changes in cation contents of stria vascularis with ouabain and potassium-free perfusion. Hear Res. 1981;4:149–60.

37. Kuijpers W, Bonting SL. Studies on (Na + -K+)-activated ATPase. XXIV. Localization and properties of ATPase in the inner ear of the guinea pig. Biochim Biophys Acta. 1969;173:477–85.

38. Yoo JC, Kim HY, Han KH, Oh SH, Chang SO, Marcus DC, Lee JH. Na(+) absorption by Claudius' cells is regulated by purinergic signaling in the cochlea. Acta Otolaryngol. 2012;132 Suppl 1:S103–8.

39. Kim SH, Marcus DC. Regulation of sodium transport in the inner ear. Hear Res. 2011;280:21–9.

40. Yamazaki M, Kim KX, Marcus DC. Sodium selectivity of Reissner's membrane epithelial cells. BMC Physiol. 2011;11:4.

41. Kim SH, Kim KX, Raveendran NN, Wu T, Pondugula SR, Marcus DC. Regulation of ENaC-mediated sodium transport by glucocorticoids in Reissner's membrane epithelium. Am J Physiol Cell Physiol. 2009;296:C544–57.

42. Lee JH, Marcus DC. Endolymphatic sodium homeostasis by Reissner's membrane. Neuroscience. 2003;119:3–8.

43. Marcus DC, Chiba T. K$^+$ and Na$^+$ absorption by outer sulcus epithelial cells. Hear Res. 1999;134:48–56.

44. Yamauchi D, Raveendran NN, Pondugula SR, Kampalli SB, Sanneman JD, Harbidge DG, Marcus DC. Vitamin D upregulates expression of ECaC1 mRNA in semicircular canal. Biochem Biophys Res Commun. 2005;331:1353–7.

45. Yamauchi D, Nakaya K, Raveendran NN, Harbidge DG, Singh R, Wangemann P, Marcus DC. Expression of epithelial calcium transport system in rat cochlea and vestibular labyrinth. BMC Physiol. 2010;10:1.

46. Wood JD, Muchinsky SJ, Filoteo AG, Penniston JT, Tempel BL. Low endolymph calcium concentrations in deafwaddler2J mice suggest that PMCA2 contributes to endolymph calcium maintenance. J Assoc Res Otolaryngol. 2004;5:99–110.

47. Scherer EQ, Yang J, Canis M, Reimann K, Ivanov K, Diehl CD, Backx PH, Wier WG, Strieth S, Wangemann P, Voigtlaender-Bolz J, Lidington D, Bolz SS. Tumor necrosis factor-alpha enhances microvascular tone and reduces blood flow in the cochlea via enhanced sphingosine-1-phosphate signaling. Stroke. 2010;41:2618–24.

48. Sellick PM, Johnstone BM. Changes in cochlear endolymph Na$^+$ concentration measured with Na$^+$ specific microelectrodes. Pflugers Arch. 1972;336:11–20.

49. Wangemann P, Itza EM, Albrecht B, Wu T, Jabba SV, Maganti RJ, Lee JH, Everett LA, Wall SM, Royaux IE, Green ED, Marcus DC. Loss of KCNJ10 protein expression abolishes endocochlear potential and causes deafness in Pendred syndrome mouse model. BMC Med. 2004;2:30.

50. Codina J, DuBose Jr TD. Molecular regulation and physiology of the H+, K+ -ATPases in kidney. Semin Nephrol. 2006;26:345–51.

51. Briving C, Andersson BM, Nordberg P, Wallmark B. Inhibition of gastric H$^+$/K$^+$-ATPase by substituted imidazo[1,2-a]pyridines. Biochim Biophys Acta. 1988;946:185–92.

52. Wallmark B, Briving C, Fryklund J, Munson K, Jackson R, Mendlein J, Rabon E, Sachs G. Inhibition of gastric H+, K + -ATPase and acid secretion by SCH 28080, a substituted pyridyl(1,2a)imidazole. J Biol Chem. 1987;262:2077–84.

53. Unsold B, Kerst G, Brousos H, Hubner M, Schreiber R, Nitschke R, Greger R, Bleich M. KCNE1 reverses the response of the human K+ channel KCNQ1 to cytosolic pH changes and alters its pharmacology and sensitivity to temperature. Pflugers Arch. 2000;441:368–78.

54. Xu H, Cui N, Yang Z, Qu Z, Jiang C. Modulation of kir4.1 and kir5.1 by hypercapnia and intracellular acidosis. J Physiol Lond. 2000;524(Pt 3):725–35.

20

Disulfide high mobility group box-1 causes bladder pain through bladder Toll-like receptor 4

Fei Ma[1,2], Dimitrios E. Kouzoukas[1,3,6], Katherine L. Meyer-Siegler[4], Karin N. Westlund[1,2], David E. Hunt[1] and Pedro L. Vera[1,2,5*]

Abstract

Background: Bladder pain is a prominent symptom in several urological conditions (e.g. infection, painful bladder syndrome/interstitial cystitis, cancer). Understanding the mechanism of bladder pain is important, particularly when the pain is not accompanied by bladder pathology. Stimulation of protease activated receptor 4 (PAR4) in the urothelium results in bladder pain through release of urothelial high mobility group box-1 (HMGB1). HGMB1 has two functionally active redox states (disulfide and all-thiol) and it is not known which form elicits bladder pain. Therefore, we investigated whether intravesical administration of specific HMGB1 redox forms caused abdominal mechanical hypersensitivity, micturition changes, and bladder inflammation in female C57BL/6 mice 24 hours post-administration. Moreover, we determined which of the specific HMGB1 receptors, Toll-like receptor 4 (TLR4) or receptor for advanced glycation end products (RAGE), mediate HMGB1-induced changes.

Results: Disulfide HMGB1 elicited abdominal mechanical hypersensitivity 24 hours after intravesical (5, 10, 20 μg/150 μl) instillation. In contrast, all-thiol HMGB1 did not produce abdominal mechanical hypersensitivity in any of the doses tested (1, 2, 5, 10, 20 μg/150 μl). Both HMGB1 redox forms caused micturition changes only at the highest dose tested (20 μg/150 μl) while eliciting mild bladder edema and reactive changes at all doses. We subsequently tested whether the effects of intravesical disulfide HMGB1 (10 μg/150 μl; a dose that did not produce inflammation) were prevented by systemic (i.p.) or local (intravesical) administration of either a TLR4 antagonist (TAK-242) or a RAGE antagonist (FPS-ZM1). Systemic administration of either TAK-242 (3 mg/kg) or FPS-ZM1 (10 mg/kg) prevented HMGB1 induced abdominal mechanical hypersensitivity while only intravesical TLR4 antagonist pretreatment (1.5 mg/ml; not RAGE) had this effect.

Conclusions: The disulfide form of HMGB1 mediates bladder pain directly (not secondary to inflammation or injury) through activation of TLR4 receptors in the bladder. Thus, TLR4 receptors are a specific local target for bladder pain.

Keywords: HMGB1, TLR4, RAGE, bladder pain, abdominal mechanical hypersensitivity, urothelium

Background

Common causes of bladder pain are bacterial infection, painful bladder syndrome/interstitial cystitis (PBS/IC) and cancer. Bladder pain in the absence of infection or bladder pathology is a feature of PBS/IC patients, along with increased frequency and urgency [1]. However, common rodent models of bladder pain usually produce significant bladder injury and inflammation [2, 3].

Cyclophosphamide (CYP)-induced cystitis (a widely used chemical model) elicits severe bladder inflammation and urothelial damage along with significantly decreased abdominal mechanical threshold [4, 5]. Interestingly, CYP-induced bladder pain (abdominal mechanical hypersensitivity) was blocked by systemic administration of a high-mobility group box 1 protein (HMGB1) neutralizing antibody or a HMGB1 receptor antagonist without changing CYP-induced inflammation [5].

---

* Correspondence: pedro.vera@va.gov
[1]Research and Development, Lexington Veterans Affairs Medical Center, 1101 Veterans Drive, Room C-327, Lexington, Kentucky 40502, USA
[2]Department of Physiology, University of Kentucky, Lexington, Kentucky, USA
Full list of author information is available at the end of the article

HMGB1 is a ubiquitous and abundant non-histone nuclear chromatin-binding protein and a damage-associated molecular pattern molecule. HMGB1 is actively secreted in response to inflammatory signals, acting as a pro-inflammatory molecule in addition to its passive release from necrotic cells in various organs [6]. The extracellular activities of HMGB1 depend on the redox state of HMGB1 resulting in activation of different HMGB1 receptors. Physical/chemical trauma to tissues or organs results in the release of all-thiol (all-reduced) HMGB1, which binds to receptor for advanced glycation end products (RAGE) and potentiates chemotaxis [7]. During inflammation, all-thiol HGMB1 may be oxidized to the disulfide form of HGMB1, which then binds to Toll-like receptor 4 (TLR4) to induce cytokine production [7]. It is likely that both redox forms contribute to inflammation resulting from tissue damage. HMGB1 is a key player in the extracellular environment as a pro-inflammatory molecule and is also gaining prominence as a mediator in pain processing [6, 8].

We recently reported that activation of urothelial protease activated receptor 4 (PAR4) elicits bladder pain in mice without causing overt bladder inflammation [9]. In this model, PAR4 activation results in release of urothelial macrophage migration inhibitory factor (MIF) [9] and HMGB1 [10] along with abdominal mechanical hypersensitivity, representative of bladder pain. Systemic pretreatment with MIF antagonist prevented urothelial HMGB1 release [9] and abdominal mechanical hypersensitivity caused by intravesical PAR4-activating peptide (PAR4-AP) [9]. Moreover, systemic administration of a HMGB1 inhibitor also blocked abdominal mechanical hypersensitivity caused by intravesical PAR4-AP [10]. This indicates that HMGB1 signaling is involved in PAR4-induced bladder pain. However, it is still not known which redox form of HMGB1 is responsible for bladder pain and the type or location of the HMGB1 receptor mediating the effect. The current study utilized two redox forms of HMGB1 and receptor-specific antagonists in a rodent model of bladder pain without inflammation to explore the etiology of bladder pain.

Methods

Animals

All animal experiments were approved by the Lexington Veterans Affairs Medical Center Institutional Animal Care and Use Committee (VER-11-016-HAF) and performed according to the guidelines of the National Institutes of Health.

Disulfide or all-thiol HMGB1 treatment by intravesical instillation

13 – 17 week-old female C57BL/6 (SPF, 20-25 g, Jackson Laboratory, Bar Harbor, ME) were accommodated in ventilated animal housing with 14/10 light/dark cycle. Isoflurane-anesthetized mice were transurethrally catheterized (PE10, 11 mm length) and drained of urine. Disulfide HMGB1, all-thiol HMGB1 (1, 2, 5, 10 and 20 μg; 150 μl, HMGBiotech S.r.l., Milano, Italy) or vehicle control groups (PBS; 150 μl) (3-6/group) were randomly instilled into the bladder lumen and held for 1 hour [9, 10]. In other experiments mouse groups were pretreated with TLR4 antagonist TAK-242 (30 min prior) [11], or RAGE antagonist FPS-ZM1 (15 min prior) [12], either intraperitoneally (TAK-242, 3 mg/kg; FPS-ZM1, 10 mg/kg) or intravesically (TAK-242, 1.5 mg/ml; FPS-ZM1, 5 mg/ml). Then 10 μg disulfide HMGB1 was instilled and held for 1 hour as described.

Abdominal mechanical hypersensitivity test

Abdominal mechanical hypersensitivity was tested in instilled mice as previously described [10]. Briefly, von Frey filaments of ascending bending force (0.008, 0.020 0.040, 0.070 g) were pressed to the lower abdominal region in trials of 10 before (baseline) and 24 hours after HMGB1 instillation. Positive response was defined as any one of three behaviors: 1) licking the abdomen, 2) flinching/jumping, or 3) abdomen withdrawal. Mice responding more than 30% to the weakest filament (0.008 g) during baseline testing were excluded from the study.

Awake mice were tested for abdominal mechanical hypersensitivity and micturition changes 24 hours after bladder instillation.

Voided Stain on Paper (VSOP): micturition volume and frequency

Micturition volume and frequency were measured in mice using VSOP method [13]. Briefly, mice were gavaged with water (50 μl/g body weight) to induce diuresis, then placed in a plastic enclosure and allowed to move freely. Filter paper was placed under each mouse to collect urine during a 2-hour observation period. Micturition volumes were determined by linear regression using a set of known volumes. Micturition frequency was defined as the number of micturition within 2 hours.

Histology

Bladders were removed under anesthesia, fixed in 10% formalin, embedded in paraffin for histology and mice were euthanized at the end of the experiment.

Paraffin sections (5 μm) were processed for routine hematoxylin and eosin (H&E) staining. H&E stained sections were evaluated by a pathologist blinded to the experimental treatment and scored separately for edema and inflammation according to the following scale: 0 = no edema; no infiltrating cells; 1 = mild submucosal edema; occasional inflammatory cells; 2 = moderate edema; several inflammatory cells; 3 = frank edema, vascular congestion; many inflammatory cells [10].

Statistical analyses

Changes in positive response frequency (%) to von Frey stimulation at baseline and 24 hours after treatment were evaluated using a within subject 2-way (Time x Filament Strength) ANOVA. When the Time factor (pre vs. post) was significant, differences at each filament strength were compared (pre vs. post) using t-tests with a multiple comparison adjustment (Holm-Sidak) [14]. Single t-tests (mean = 0) were performed for the histological scores.

All data are presented as mean ± SE [14], with statistical differences of $p \leq 0.05$ considered significant. All statistical analyses were performed using R [15].

Results

HMGB1 redox form elicits abdominal mechanical hypersensitivity

We measured responses to von Frey filaments applied to the abdominal/perineal area at baseline (before) and 24 hours after bladder HMGB1 instillation of either disulfide HMGB1 or all-thiol HMGB1 (1, 2, 5, 10 and 20 μg). Intravesical vehicle control, 1 or 2 μg of disulfide HMGB1 did not cause any abdominal mechanical hypersensitivity 24 hours after instillation (Fig. 1a-c). Figure 1d shows that 5 μg (n = 5) of disulfide HMGB1 resulted in significant mechanical hypersensitivity of abdominal/perineal area only with the highest filament tested (0.07 g; Fig. 1d). Higher doses of disulfide HMGB1 10 (n = 6) or 20 μg (n = 3) significantly increased von Frey responses compared to baseline for all filaments tested (Fig. 1e, f). In contrast, intravesical all-thiol HMGB1 did not cause any change in abdominal mechanical hypersensitivity for any of the doses tested (Fig. 1g-k).

Micturition changes after HMGB1 bladder instillation

Table 1 shows micturition volume and frequency changes after different doses of either disulfide or all-thiol HMGB1. Only the highest dose of disulfide and all-thiol HMGB1 (20 μg, n = 3) resulted in a significant decrease in volume (141 ± 7 μl, 177 ± 24 μl) compared to vehicle control treated group (n = 5; 301 ± 39 μl). This dose of disulfide or all-thiol HMGB1 also increased micturition frequency (7.3 ± 0.7, 4.7 ± 0.3 vs 3.0 ± 0.4 of PBS). Lower doses of disulfide or all-thiol HMGB1 had no effect on these two micturition parameters (Table 1).

Histological changes

H&E stained bladder sections from mice that received different doses of disulfide HMGB1, all-thiol HMGB1 or vehicle control (PBS) were examined by a pathologist

blinded to the treatment and scored for inflammation and edema changes (Table 2). Intravesical installation of vehicle control did not produce any inflammation or edema (Table 2). Disulfide or all-thiol HMGB1 at doses < 20 μg did not produce any inflammation while minimal inflammation (not statistically significant) was observed after 20 μg of either disulfide or all-thiol HMGB1. Either disulfide or all-thiol HMGB1 at all doses tested induced minimal to mild bladder edema and stromal reactive changes in some mice (reactive submucosal fibrosis with lamina propria expansion, Fig. 2d, Table 2), not statistically significant compared to vehicle control (Fig. 2a).

Effect of TLR4 and RAGE antagonism on disulfide HMGB1 induced hypersensitivity

We chose the first dose of disulfide HMGB1 that showed significantly increased abdominal mechanical sensitivity across all von Frey filaments (10 μg; Fig. 3a) without inflammation to test the effect of specific HMGB1 receptor antagonism. Pretreatment with specific TLR4 (TAK-242) or RAGE (FPS-ZM1) antagonists was used to investigate which receptor signaling mechanism was activated by intravesical disulfide HMGB1 resulting in increased abdominal mechanical hypersensitivity.

Intravesical pretreatment with TAK-242 (TLR4 antagonist; 75 μg in 50 μl PBS, n = 4) prior to bladder instillation completely blocked abdominal mechanical hypersensitivity induced by disulfide HMGB1 for all the filaments (Fig. 3b). No difference was detected between pre and post disulfide HMGB1 instillation (F = 0.028). On the other hand, disulfide HMGB1-induced abdominal mechanical hypersensitivity was not blocked when FPS-ZM1 (RAGE antagonist; 250 μg, n = 6) was infused into the bladder before disulfide HMGB1 bladder instillation (Fig. 3d). There were still significant differences between pre and post disulfide HMGB1 instillation for all von Frey filaments (Fig. 3d).

Systemic (intraperitoneally) treatment with either TLR4 antagonist TAK-242 (3 mg/kg, 30 min pretreatment, n = 5) [11] or RAGE antagonist FPS-ZM1 (10 mg/kg, 15 min pretreatment, n = 3) [12] before intravesical infusion of disulfide HMGB1 (10 μg) prevented HMGB1-induced abdominal mechanical hypersensitivity (Fig. 3c, e).

Pretreatment of TLR4 and RAGE antagonists on micturition and histology

Intravesical disulfide HMGB1 (10 μg) did not change micturition volume or frequency (Table 1). No micturition changes were observed in groups pre-treated with TLR4 and RAGE antagonists either intraperitoneally (TLR4: 274 ± 42 in volume, 4.0 ± 0.7 in frequency;

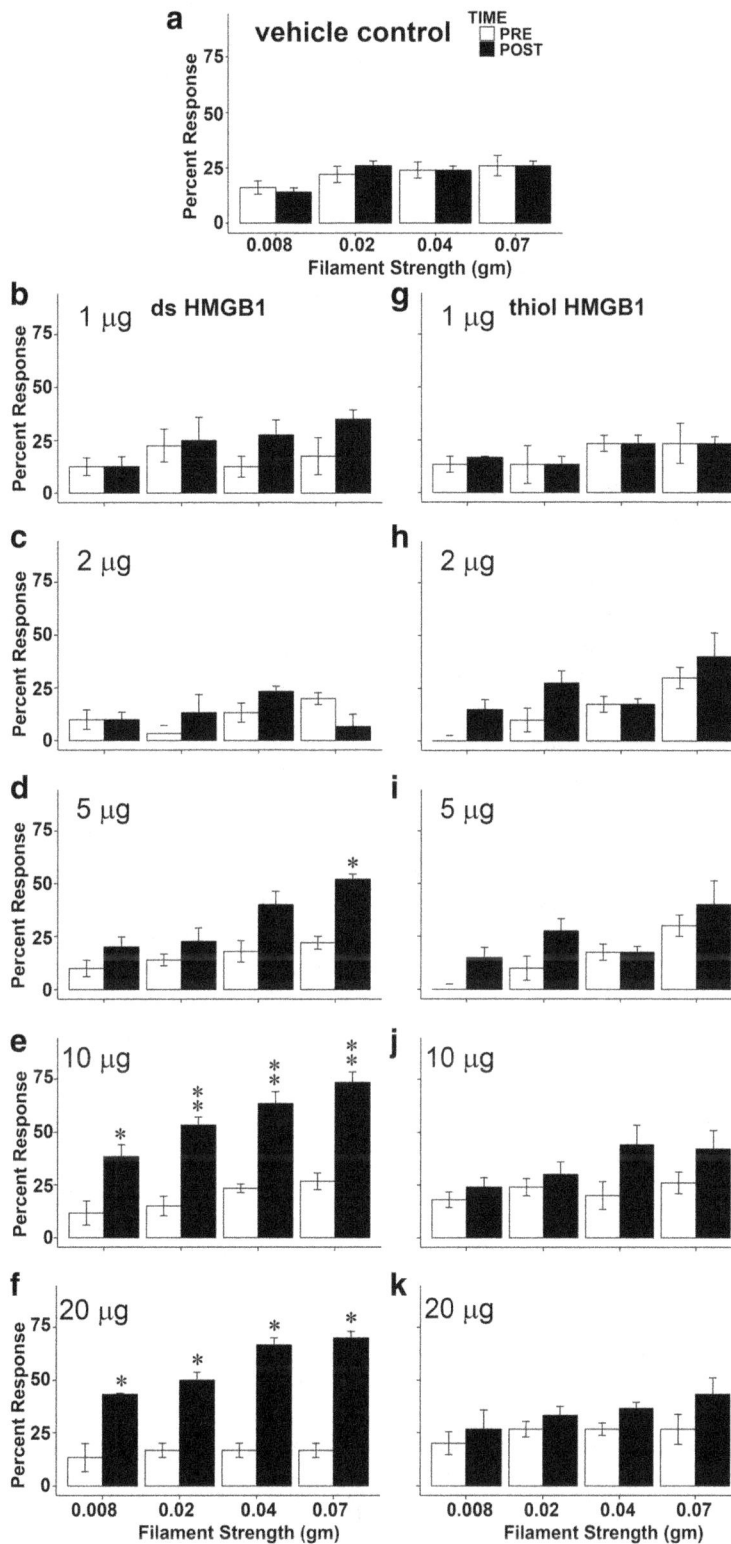

Fig. 1 Disulfide and all-thiol HMGB1 dose response effects on abdominal mechanical thresholds. (**a**) vehicle control, (**b**) 1 µg (n = 4) and (**c**) 2 µg (n = 3) disulfide HMGB1 did not affect abdominal mechanical threshold. (**d**) 5 µg (n = 5) disulfide HMGB1 significantly increased abdominal sensitivity using a 0.07 g filament. (**e**) 10 µg (n = 6) and (**f**) 20 µg (n = 3) disulfide HMGB1 significantly induced abdominal hypersensitivity using all four von Frey filaments. None of the all-thiol HMGB1 doses (**g**) 1 µg (n = 3), (**h**) 2 µg (n = 3), (**i**) 5 µg (n = 4), (**j**) 10 µg (n = 5) and (**k**) 20 µg (n = 3) changed abdominal mechanical sensitivity. *$p < 0.05$, **$p < 0.01$ compared with pre-instillation

Table 1 Effects of intravesical disulfide and all-thiol HMGB1 on mouse micturition

Dose (µg)	ds HMGB1		all-thiol HMGB1	
	Volume (µl)	Freq	Volume (µl)	Freq
0	301 ± 39.3	3.0 ± 0.4	301 ± 39.3	3.0 ± 0.4
1	288 ± 20.1	3.5 ± 0.6	230 ± 9.2	4.3 ± 0.7
2	359 ± 13.9	2.0 ± 0.0	240 ± 79.8	5.3 ± 1.7
5	255 ± 36.8	3.2 ± 0.9	267 ± 35.0	4.3 ± 0.9
10	264 ± 25.5	4.1 ± 1.0	214 ± 15.8	4.0 ± 0.8
20	141 ± 7.3*	7.3 ± 0.7*	177 ± 23.7*	4.7 ± 0.3*

0 = vehicle control
*$p < 0.05$ compared with 0 µg disulfide HMGB1

RAGE: 214 ± 37 in volume, 4.0 ± 0.6 in frequency) or intravesically (TLR4: 231 ± 16.9 in volume, 4.0 ± 0.5 in frequency; RAGE: 221 ± 19.4 in volume, 4.8 ± 0.3 in frequency) followed by intravesical disulfide HMGB1 when compared to disulfide HMGB1 instillation only group (264 ± 25.5 in volume; 4.0 ± 1.0 in frequency).

Pretreatment, either i.p. or intravesically, with TLR4 or RAGE antagonist did not elicit bladder inflammation (score = 0). Pretreatment with HMGB1 antagonist (i.p. or intravesical) followed by intravesical disulfide HMGB1 (10 µg/150) also showed minimal increases (not statistically significant) in edema (TAK 242, i.p, score = 0.13 ± 0.13; intravesical, score = 0; FPS-ZM1, i.p., score = 0, intravesical, score = 0.08 ± 0.08) compared to vehicle control (score = 0) or compared to intravesical disulfide (10 µg/150 µl alone; 0.5 ± 0.22) (Fig. 2b, c, e, f).

Discussion

We recently reported that intravesical activation of urothelial PAR4 receptors resulted in release of urothelial HMGB1, which mediated bladder pain [10]. Release of urothelial adenosine triphosphate (ATP) and activation of transit receptor potential vanilloid 1 (TRPV1) are well-described mechanisms of bladder pain [16–19]. Whether HMGB1 elicits bladder pain through ATP and/or TRPV1 remains to be investigated.

Table 2 Effects of intravesical disulfide and all-thiol HMGB1 on mouse bladder histology

Dose (µg)	Inflammation		Edema	
	ds HMGB1	all-thiol HMGB1	ds HMGB1	all-thiol HMGB1
0	0	0	0	0
1	0	0	0.4 ± 0.2	1.3 ± 0.7
2	0	0	0.7 ± 0.7	0.7 ± 0.3
5	0	0	0	1.0 ± 0.6
10	0	0	0.2 ± 0.2	0.9 ± 0.5
20	0.3 ± 0.3	0.3 ± 0.3	1.0 ± 1.0	0.7 ± 0.7

0 = vehicle control

The present study extends our earlier findings since we clearly demonstrate that HMGB1 infused into the bladder is capable of inducing abdominal mechanical hypersensitivity (an indirect index of bladder pain). Furthermore, the redox state of HMGB1 is important since only intravesical disulfide HMGB1 but not the all-thiol (reduced) form induced abdominal mechanical hypersensitivity.

We also examined physiological and histological changes in response to different doses and different redox forms of HMGB1 infused intravesically. Changes in micturition parameters were only observed with the highest dose of disulfide and all-thiol HMGB1 (20 µg; decreased micturition volume and increased frequency) whereas none of the lower doses had any effect on micturition (Table 1). In terms of histological changes, only the highest dose tested (20 µg) of either disulfide or all-thiol HMGB1 was able to elicit minimal bladder inflammation (Table 2), while minimal to mild bladder edema and subtle stromal reactive changes were present with all doses of either disulfide or all-thiol HMGB1. These histological findings are consistent with our previous publication that HMGB1 mediates bladder pain without overt bladder inflammation [10]. Similarly, intraplantar injection of HMGB1 at 10 and 20 µg caused paw withdrawal latency decrease as well as edema but only 20 µg HMGB1 elicited mild inflammation in hind paw [20]. Furthermore, our findings that disulfide HMGB1 mediates bladder pain in a model with no overt bladder inflammation extend the findings of Tanaka et al [5] who found that systemic HMGB1 antagonists could prevent bladder pain after chemical (cyclophosphamide) injury of the bladder but did not affect inflammatory changes in this chemical cystitis model.

Recent studies implicate HMGB1 in mediating pain both at the organ level and at the central nervous system level (for a review see Kato J & Svensson CI) [6]. Pain hypersensitivity was elicited when HMGB1 was injected into sciatic nerve and anti-HMGB1 treatment alleviated mechanical allodynia after injury, but the nociceptive signaling pathway is still unclear [21]. Thrombomodulin (HMGB1 sequester) treatment alleviates intraplantar injection HMGB1 induced mechanical hypersensitivity, indicating HMGB1's peripheral effect in nociception [20]. As an endogenous inflammatory mediator, HMGB1 influences adjacent neurons and glia, which contributes to the development of neuropathic pain states [21]. One report showed an increase in HMGB1 re-distribution into cytoplasm of sensory neurons in dorsal root ganglion in a model of tibial nerve injury induced neuropathic pain [22]. In this model, systemic application of glycyrrhizin, a HMGB1 blocker, reversed the neuropathic pain [22]. TLR4 and RAGE receptors were shown to be

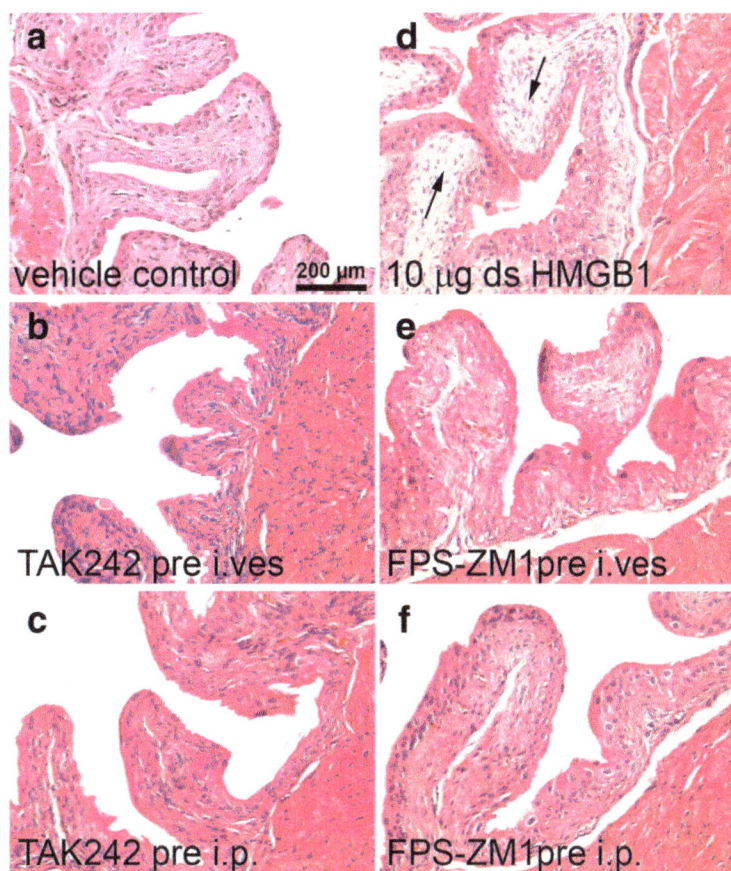

Fig. 2 Bladder histology after disulfide HMGB1 and pretreatment with intravesical or intraperitoneal HMGB1 receptor antagonists. (**a**) Intravesical vehicle control instillation (n = 5), (**b**) intravesical TAK242 (n = 4), (**c**) intraperitoneal TLR4 antagonist TAK242 (n = 5), (**d**) 10 μg disulfide HMGB1 induced submucosal fibrosis with lamina propria expansion (black arrows) (n = 6), (**e**) intravesical FPS-ZM1 pretreatment (n = 6) or (**f**) intraperitoneal RAGE antagonist FPS-ZM1 (n = 3)

mediating nociception differentially in peripheral tissue and nervous system while HMGB1 redox forms recognize their receptors respectively [11, 23–27]. TLR4 downregulation in spinal glial cells attenuates mechanical allodynia in a rat model of trinitrobenzene sulfonic acid induced chronic pancreatitis [28]. On the other hand, RAGE mRNA and protein were increased in dorsal root ganglia after tibial nerve injury and RAGE inhibition by neutralizing antibody reversed the pain related behavior [29]. There is also evidence that systemic or intrathecal HMGB1 neutralizing antibody or a specific antagonist can alleviate pain mediated by TLR4 or RAGE receptors, suggesting central effect of TLR4 and RAGE receptors [8, 20].

Two strategies were used in the current study to identify the HMGB1 receptor mediating the disulfide HMGB1-induced abdominal mechanical hypersensitivity. A dose of disulfide HMGB1 (10 μg) that produced no inflammation and only minimal edema was chosen for the intravesical infusion. Systemic pretreatment with either a TLR4 (TAK-242) or a RAGE

(FPS-ZM1) antagonist blocked abdominal mechanical hypersensitivity induced by disulfide HMGB1. Since both of these antagonists cross the blood-brain barrier [12, 30], the effect may be due to antagonism of central TLR4 or RAGE receptors and these receptors mediate pain in other models [24, 25]. We applied antagonists intravesically to determine whether and which of these receptors mediated the effect of disulfide HMGB1 at the organ level. TLR4 and RAGE receptors are found in the urothelium [26, 31] and sacral DRGs [29, 32] also contain TLR4 and RAGE although whether they innervate the bladder is not known. Intravesical pretreatment with TLR4 antagonist prevented hypersensitivity caused by disulfide HMGB1 while RAGE antagonist did not. Taken together, these findings indicate that TLR4 receptors at the organ level are responsible for the abdominal mechanical hypersensitivity induced by bladder infusion of disulfide HMGB1.

Our results also indicate that RAGE receptors modulate the effects of intravesical infusion of

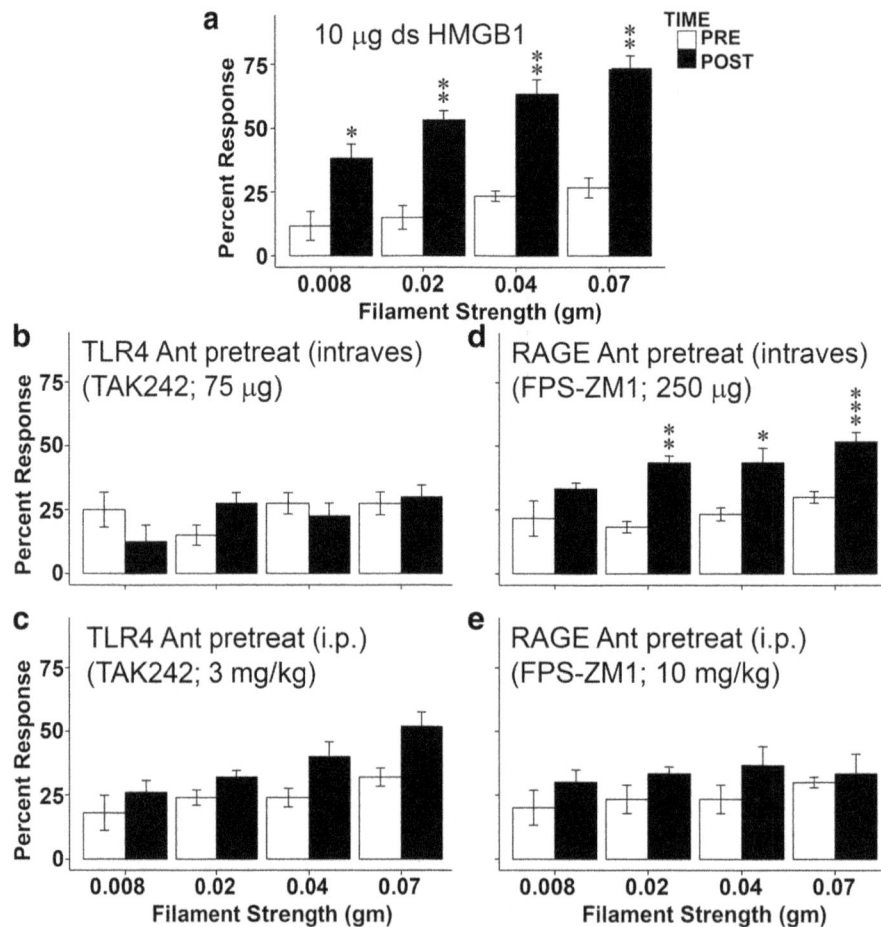

Fig. 3 TLR4 or RAGE antagonist pretreatment prevented abdominal mechanical hypersensitivity induced disulfide HMGB1. (**a**) 10 µg disulfide HMGB1 significantly increased abdominal mechanical sensitivity (percent responses) using all four von Frey filaments (n = 6). (**b**) Intravesical TLR4 antagonist TAK242 blocked disulfide HMGB1 induced abdominal hypersensitivity (n = 4). (**c**) Intraperitoneal TAK242 reduced mechanical hypersensitivity induced by 10 µg disulfide HMGB1 (n = 5). (**d**) Intravesical infusion of RAGE antagonist PSF-ZM1, however, did not affect abdominal mechanical hypersensitivity induced by disulfide HMGB1 (n = 6). (**e**) Intraperitoneal injection of PSF-ZM1 prevented disulfide HMGB1 induced mechanical hypersensitivity (n = 3). *$p < 0.05$, **$p < 0.01$, ***$p < 0.001$ Twenty-four hours post-instillation compared with pre-instillation

HMGB1 by acting not at the organ (i.e. bladder level) but possibly at the central nervous system level, since systemic administration was effective in blocking abdominal mechanical hypersensitivity. This agrees with the observation by Tanaka, et al. [5] that systemic administration of an antibody to HMGB1 or a RAGE inhibitor blocked cyclophosphamide- induced bladder pain. In contrast, we show that a systemic TLR4 antagonist administered systemically prevented disulfide HMGB1-induced bladder pain while Tanaka reported that a systemic TLR4 inhibitor had no effect on CYP-induced bladder pain [5]. This discrepancy may be due to the different method used to elicit bladder pain. Disulfide HMGB1 resulted in only minimal histological changes in the bladder while CYP is a strong chemical irritant that results in severe inflammation and hemorraghic cystitis [4].

PBS/IC is a condition characterized by bladder pain (or discomfort), frequency and urgency with unclear etiology [33] and in the absence of obvious bladder pathology [34]. Our current findings showed that disulfide HMGB1 elicited pain may account for bladder pain observed in the absence of inflammation. We realize that our model using intravesical infusion of substances (PAR4-AP; HMGB1) at doses that cause pain without accompanying micturition or inflammation changes, focus only on one aspect of PBS/IC, namely pain, without addressing increased frequency and urgency commonly seen in PBS/IC. Still these rodent models are useful because they are capable of eliciting bladder pain as a primary effect and not secondary to significant injury and inflammation. As such, they are useful tools in investigating the physiology of bladder pain in health and disease.

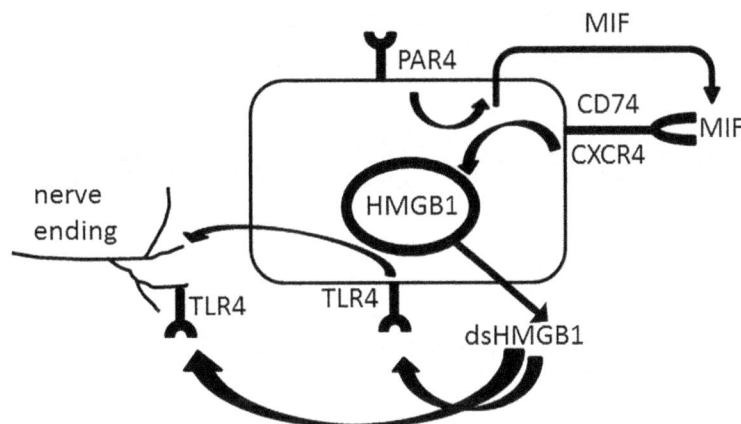

Fig. 4 Role of HMGB1 in PAR4 induced bladder pain. Activation of PAR4 receptors on urothelial cells elicits release of urothelial macrophage migration inhibitory factor (MIF). MIF binds to urothelial MIF receptors (CD74/CXCR4) to mediate release of urothelial HMGB1. Disulfide HMGB1 (ds HMGB1) may bind to TLR4 receptors in urothelium and/or nerve terminal innervating the bladder to mediate bladder pain

It is possible that urine proteases, already elevated in PBS/IC patients, activate urothelial PAR4 receptors to release MIF into the urine [35, 36]. MIF, in turn, activates urothelial MIF receptors to elicit HMGB1 release. Oxidation of HMGB1 in the extracellular space [6] or in the urine results in disulfide HMGB1 that binds to either urothelial TLR4 receptors to induce further signaling resulting in bladder pain or may bind directly to the mucosa or possible to elicit bladder pain (Fig. 4). This schema remains to be validated in the clinical condition in future studies.

Conclusions

We previously showed that activation of urothelial PAR4 receptors results in release of MIF and HMGB1 increasing abdominal mechanical hypersensitivity without bladder inflammation. We now report that HMGB1 infused directly into the bladder is capable to elicit mechanical hypersensitivity and this effect is produced by the disulfide isoform of HMGB1. Lastly, this effect is mediated by TLR4 receptors in the bladder and can also be modulated by systemic (presumably central) RAGE receptors. Neutralizing bladder MIF, MIF receptors, HMGB1 or antagonism of bladder TLR4 or systemic RAGE receptors may be potential specific and localized targets for bladder pain relief.

Abbreviations

ATP: Adenosine triphosphate; CYP: Cyclophosphamide; H&E: Hematoxylin and eosin; HMGB1: High mobility group box-1; MIF: Macrophage migration inhibitory factor; PAR4: Protease activated receptor 4; PAR4-AP: PAR4-activating peptide; PBS: Phosphate buffered saline; PBS/IC: Bladder pain syndrome/interstitial cystitis; RAGE: Receptors for advanced glycation endproducts; TLR4: Toll- like receptor 4; TRPV1: Transit receptor potential vanilloid 1; VSOP: Voided stain on paper

Acknowledgements

This material is the result of work supported with resources and the use of facilities at the Lexington (Kentucky) Veterans Affairs Medical Center. Judy Glass and Xiu Xu provided excellent technical assistance.

Authors'contributions

FM, DEK, KLMS, KNW, DEH and PLV conceived and carried out the experiments, performed the statistical analyses, drafted the manuscript, edited the manuscript and approved the final manuscript.

Competing interests

The authors declare that there are no competing interests.

Author details

[1]Research and Development, Lexington Veterans Affairs Medical Center, 1101 Veterans Drive, Room C-327, Lexington, Kentucky 40502, USA. [2]Department of Physiology, University of Kentucky, Lexington, Kentucky, USA. [3]Saha Cardiovascular Research Center, University of Kentucky, Lexington, Kentucky, USA. [4]Department of Natural Sciences, St. Petersburg College, St. Petersburg, Florida, USA. [5]Department of Surgery, University of Kentucky, Lexington, Kentucky, USA. [6]Present Address: Department of Molecular Pharmacology and Therapeutics, Loyola University Chicago, Maywood, Illinois, USA.

References

1. Warren JW, Brown V, Jacobs S, Horne L, Langenberg P, Greenberg P. Urinary tract infection and inflammation at onset of interstitial cystitis/painful bladder syndrome. Urology. 2008;71(6):1085–90.
2. Westropp JL, Buffington CA. In vivo models of interstitial cystitis. J Urol. 2002;167(2 Pt 1):694–702.
3. Olivar T, Laird JM. Cyclophosphamide cystitis in mice: behavioural characterisation and correlation with bladder inflammation. Eur J Pain. 1999; 3(2):141–9.
4. Vera PL, Iczkowski KA, Howard DJ, Jiang L, Meyer-Siegler KL. Antagonism of macrophage migration inhibitory factor decreases cyclophosphamide cystitis in mice. Neurourol Urodyn. 2010;29(8):1451–7.
5. Tanaka J, Yamaguchi K, Ishikura H, Tsubota M, Sekiguchi F, Seki Y, Tsujiuchi T, Murai A, Umemura T, Kawabata A. Bladder pain relief by HMGB1 neutralization and soluble thrombomodulin in mice with cyclophosphamide-induced cystitis. Neuropharmacology. 2014;79:112–8.
6. Kato J, Svensson CI. Role of extracellular damage-associated molecular pattern molecules (DAMPs) as mediators of persistent pain. Prog Mol Biol Transl Sci. 2015;131:251–79.

7. Agalave NM, Svensson CI. Extracellular high-mobility group box 1 protein (HMGB1) as a mediator of persistent pain. Mol Med. 2014;20:569–78.
8. Nakamura Y, Morioka N, Abe H, Zhang FF, Hisaoka-Nakashima K, Liu K, Nishibori M, Nakata Y. Neuropathic pain in rats with a partial sciatic nerve ligation is alleviated by intravenous injection of monoclonal antibody to high mobility group box-1. PLoS One. 2013;8(8):e73640.
9. Kouzoukas DE, Meyer-Siegler KL, Ma F, Westlund KN, Hunt DE, Vera PL. Macrophage Migration Inhibitory Factor Mediates PAR-Induced Bladder Pain. PLoS One. 2015;10(5):e0127628.
10. Kouzoukas DE, Ma F, Meyer-Siegler KL, Westlund KN, Hunt DE, Vera PL. Protease-activated receptor 4 induces bladder pain through high mobility group box-1. PLoS One. 2016;11(3):e0152055.
11. Belcher JD, Chen C, Nguyen J, Milbauer L, Abdulla F, Alayash AI, Smith A, Nath KA, Hebbel RP, Vercellotti GM. Heme triggers TLR4 signaling leading to endothelial cell activation and vaso-occlusion in murine sickle cell disease. Blood. 2014;123(3):377–90.
12. Deane R, Singh I, Sagare AP, Bell RD, Ross NT, LaRue B, Love R, Perry S, Paquette N, Deane RJ, et al. A multimodal RAGE-specific inhibitor reduces amyloid beta-mediated brain disorder in a mouse model of Alzheimer disease. J Clin Invest. 2012;122(4):1377–92.
13. Sugino Y, Kanematsu A, Hayashi Y, Haga H, Yoshimura N, Yoshimura K, Ogawa O. Voided stain on paper method for analysis of mouse urination. Neurourol Urodyn. 2008;27(6):548–52.
14. Cousineau D. Confidence intervals in within-subject designs: A simpler solution to Loftus and Masson's method. Tutorials in Quantitative Methods for Psychology. 2005;1(1):42–5.
15. Core Team: R: A Language and Environment for Statistical Computing. R Foundation for Statistical Computing 1993.
16. Sui G, Fry CH, Montgomery B, Roberts M, Wu R, Wu C. Purinergic and muscarinic modulation of ATP release from the urothelium and its paracrine actions. Am J Physiol Renal Physiol. 2014;306(3):F286–98.
17. Shiina K, Hayashida KI, Ishikawa K, Kawatani M. ATP release from bladder urothelium and serosa in a rat model of partial bladder outlet obstruction. Biomed Res. 2016;37(5):299–304.
18. Coelho A, Wolf-Johnston AS, Shinde S, Cruz CD, Cruz F, Avelino A, Birder LA. Urinary bladder inflammation induces changes in urothelial nerve growth factor and TRPV1 channels. Br J Pharmacol. 2015;172(7):1691–9.
19. Gonzalez EJ, Merrill L, Vizzard MA. Bladder sensory physiology: neuroactive compounds and receptors, sensory transducers, and target-derived growth factors as targets to improve function. Am J Physiol Regul Integr Comp Physiol. 2014;306(12):R869–78.
20. Tanaka J, Seki Y, Ishikura H, Tsubota M, Sekiguchi F, Yamaguchi K, Murai A, Umemura T, Kawabata A. Recombinant human soluble thrombomodulin prevents peripheral HMGB1-dependent hyperalgesia in rats. Br J Pharmacol. 2013;170(6):1233–41.
21. Shibasaki M, Sasaki M, Miura M, Mizukoshi K, Ueno H, Hashimoto S, Tanaka Y, Amaya F. Induction of high mobility group box-1 in dorsal root ganglion contributes to pain hypersensitivity after peripheral nerve injury. Pain. 2010; 149(3):514–21.
22. Feldman P, Due MR, Ripsch MS, Khanna R, White FA. The persistent release of HMGB1 contributes to tactile hyperalgesia in a rodent model of neuropathic pain. J Neuroinflammation. 2012;9:180.
23. Agalave NM, Larsson M, Abdelmoaty S, Su J, Baharpoor A, Lundback P, Palmblad K, Andersson U, Harris H, Svensson CI. Spinal HMGB1 induces TLR4-mediated long-lasting hypersensitivity and glial activation and regulates pain-like behavior in experimental arthritis. Pain. 2014;155(9):1802–13.
24. Li X, Yang H, Ouyang Q, Liu F, Li J, Xiang Z, Yuan H. Enhanced RAGE expression in the dorsal root ganglion may contribute to neuropathic pain induced by spinal nerve ligation in rats. Pain Med. 2016;17(5):803–12.
25. Ma YQ, Chen YR, Leng YF, Wu ZW. Tanshinone IIA downregulates HMGB1 and TLR4 expression in a spinal nerve ligation model of neuropathic pain. Evidence-based complementary and alternative medicine : eCAM. 2014; 2014:639563.
26. Roundy LM, Jia W, Zhang J, Ye X, Prestwich GD, Oottamasathien S. LL-37 induced cystitis and the receptor for advanced glycation end-products (RAGE) pathway. Adv Biosci Biotechnol. 2013;4(8B):1–8.
27. Yamasoba D, Tsubota M, Domoto R, Sekiguchi F, Nishikawa H, Liu K, Nishibori M, Ishikura H, Yamamoto T, Taga A, et al. Peripheral HMGB1-induced hyperalgesia in mice: Redox state-dependent distinct roles of RAGE and TLR4. J Pharmacol Sci. 2016;130(2):139–42.
28. Wang YS, Li YY, Wang LH, Kang Y, Zhang J, Liu ZQ, Wang K, Kaye AD, Chen L. Tanshinone IIA attenuates chronic pancreatitis-induced pain in rats via downregulation of HMGB1 and TRL4 expression in the spinal cord. Pain Physician. 2015;18(4):E615–28.
29. Allette YM, Due MR, Wilson SM, Feldman P, Ripsch MS, Khanna R, White FA. Identification of a functional interaction of HMGB1 with receptor for advanced glycation End-products in a model of neuropathic pain. Brain Behav Immun. 2014;42:169–77.
30. Hua F, Tang H, Wang J, Prunty MC, Hua X, Sayeed I, Stein DG. TAK-242, an antagonist for Toll-like receptor 4, protects against acute cerebral ischemia/ reperfusion injury in mice. J Cereb Blood Flow Metab. 2015;35(4):536–42.
31. Song J, Bishop BL, Li G, Duncan MJ, Abraham SN. TLR4-initiated and cAMP-mediated abrogation of bacterial invasion of the bladder. Cell Host Microbe. 2007;1(4):287–98.
32. Due MR, Piekarz AD, Wilson N, Feldman P, Ripsch MS, Chavez S, Yin H, Khanna R, White FA. Neuroexcitatory effects of morphine-3-glucuronide are dependent on Toll-like receptor 4 signaling. J Neuroinflammation. 2012;9:200.
33. Kim HJ. Update on the pathology and diagnosis of interstitial cystitis/ bladder pain syndrome: a review. Int Neurourol J. 2016;20(1):13–7.
34. Fry CH, Vahabi B. The role of the mucosa in normal and abnormal bladder function. Basic Clin Pharmacol Toxicol. 2016;119 Suppl 3:57–62.
35. Boucher W, el-Mansoury M, Pang X, Sant GR, Theoharides TC. Elevated mast cell tryptase in the urine of patients with interstitial cystitis. Br J Urol. 1995; 76(1):94–100.
36. Kuromitsu S, Yokota H, Hiramoto M, Morita S, Mita H, Yamada T. Increased concentration of neutrophil elastase in urine from patients with interstitial cystitis. Scand J Urol Nephrol. 2008;42(5):455–61.

21

Adiponectin is required for maintaining normal body temperature in a cold environment

Qiong Wei[1,2†], Jong Han Lee[1,3†], Hongying Wang[4,5†], Odelia Y. N. Bongmba[1], Chia-Shan Wu[4], Geetali Pradhan[1], Zilin Sun[2], Lindsey Chew[6], Mandeep Bajaj[7], Lawrence Chan[7], Robert S. Chapkin[4], Miao-Hsueh Chen[1] and Yuxiang Sun[1,4,8*]

Abstract

Background: Thermogenic impairment promotes obesity and insulin resistance. Adiponectin is an important regulator of energy homeostasis. While many beneficial metabolic effects of adiponectin resemble that of activated thermogenesis, the role of adiponectin in thermogenesis is not clear. In this study, we investigated the role of adiponectin in thermogenesis using adiponectin-null mice ($Adipoq^{-/-}$).

Methods: Body composition was measured using EchoMRI. Metabolic parameters were determined by indirect calorimetry. Insulin sensitivity was evaluated by glucose- and insulin- tolerance tests. Core body temperature was measured by a TH-8 temperature monitoring system. Gene expression was assessed by real-time PCR and protein levels were analyzed by Western blotting and immunohistochemistry. The mitochondrial density of brown adipose tissue was quantified by calculating the ratio of mtDNA:total nuclear DNA.

Results: Under normal housing temperature of 24 °C and ad libitum feeding condition, the body weight, body composition, and metabolic profile of $Adipoq^{-/-}$ mice were unchanged. Under fasting condition, $Adipoq^{-/-}$ mice exhibited reduced energy expenditure. Conversely, under cold exposure, $Adipoq^{-/-}$ mice exhibited reduced body temperature, and the expression of thermogenic regulatory genes was significantly reduced in brown adipose tissue (BAT) and subcutaneous white adipose tissue (WAT). Moreover, we observed that mitochondrial content was reduced in BAT and subcutaneous WAT, and the expression of mitochondrial fusion genes was decreased in BAT of $Adipoq^{-/-}$ mice, suggesting that adiponectin ablation diminishes mitochondrial biogenesis and altered mitochondrial dynamics. Our study further revealed that adiponectin deletion suppresses adrenergic activation, and down-regulates β3-adrenergic receptor, insulin signaling, and the AMPK-SIRT1 pathway in BAT.

Conclusions: Our findings demonstrate that adiponectin is an essential regulator of thermogenesis, and adiponectin is required for maintaining body temperature under cold exposure.

Keywords: Adiponectin, Thermogenesis, Brown adipose tissue, Beige cells, Cold exposure

* Correspondence: Yuxiang.Sun@tamu.edu
†Equal contributors
[1]USDA/ARS Children's Nutrition Research Center, Department of Pediatrics, Baylor College of Medicine, Houston, TX 77030, USA
[4]Department of Nutrition and Food Science, Texas A&M University, 214D Cater-Mattil; 2253 TAMU, College Station, TX 77843, USA
Full list of author information is available at the end of the article

Background

Adiponectin is a 30 kDa protein hormone secreted by adipocytes; it has high concentrations (0.5–30 mg/ml) in the circulation, and displays a wide range of metabolically beneficial effects [1–7]. Several lines of evidence show that adiponectin is involved in lipid metabolism [3, 4]. In insulin-resistant mouse models, adiponectin treatment improves insulin sensitivity [5, 6]. Clinical studies also reveal a correlation between circulating adiponectin and insulin sensitivity; and adiponectin levels are lower in obese humans compared to normal-weight subjects [1, 6, 7]. These findings suggest that adiponectin might be a promising candidate for prevention/treatment of metabolic syndrome and insulin resistance.

There are two types of adipose tissues: energy-storing white adipose tissue (WAT) and energy-burning brown adipose tissue (BAT). WAT is the main organ for long-term energy storage in mammals. In WAT, lipids are stored as triglycerides under positive energy balance, and fatty acids are released as metabolic fuel under negative energy balance [8, 9]. In contrast, BAT is primarily responsible for non-shivering thermogenesis, which converts fat into heat. Thermogenesis is vital in maintaining normal body temperature, which is crucial for the cellular functions of all cells in the body. BAT is a key protective mechanism for preventing hypothermia [10, 11]. In addition to BAT, there are brown-like adipocytes in subcutaneous WAT, aka brite/beige cells, which also possess thermogenic properties [8, 11, 12]. Emerging evidence reveals that non-shivering thermogenesis is linked to energy expenditure in healthy adult humans [13–16], and thermogenic activation improves glucose homeostasis [17–20]. Uncoupling protein 1 (UCP-1) is a key mitochondrial regulator of thermogenesis. Upon activation, UCP-1 dissipates the transmembrane proton gradient to generate heat [21]. It is important to note that the UCP-1 ablation in mice failed to display an obesogenic phenotype under normal laboratory housing temperature (18–22 °C), but animals became obese under thermoneutral temperature (30 °C) when thermal stress is eliminated [22]. This new revelation indicates that housing temperature has profound effects on metabolism.

It has been reported that cold exposure increases adiponectin levels [23, 24]. Acute cold exposure in rodents activates both non-shivering and shivering thermogenesis by activating the sympathetic nervous system (SNS) [25]. Cold exposure increases UCP-1 expression, as well as UCP-1 activity in BAT and subcutaneous WAT [26]. Although many beneficial metabolic effects of adiponectin phenocopy that of thermogenic activation [1–7], the effect of adiponectin on thermogenesis remains controversial. Two recent studies show opposite effects of adiponectin on thermogenesis [27, 28]. In the current study, we investigated the effects of adiponectin on thermogenic regulation using $Adipoq^{-/-}$ mice, which have normal body weight and insulin sensitivity [29]. Initial characterization of these $Adipoq^{-/-}$ mice showed minimal phenotype under unchallenged conditions [29]; subsequent studies revealed these mice have hepatic steatosis and mitochondrial dysfunction, and are prone to liver injuries [30]. Insulin levels have profound effects on thermogenesis [31–34], and thermogenic impairment has been shown to be associated with insulin resistance [35]. This line of $Adipoq^{-/-}$ mice with normal insulin sensitivity would allow us to investigate the metabolic effects of adiponectin independent from body weight and insulin action. In the current study, we used this $Adipoq^{-/-}$ mouse line to investigate the thermogenic effect of adiponectin.

We studied the core body temperature and expression of the genes involved in thermogenesis and mitochondrial dynamics in BAT and subcutaneous WAT under conditions of normal housing temperature (24 °C), negative energy balance (24 h fasting), and 4 °C cold exposure. Our results indicate that adiponectin plays an important role in thermoregulation. We found that adiponectin is required for sustaining body temperature under energy-deficient and cold challenged conditions, also adiponectin activates thermogenesis to enhance lipid metabolism to protect against hypothermia.

Methods
Animals

The $Adipoq^{-/-}$ mice were previously reported; they have been backcrossed to C57BL/6 J for at least 10 generations (with >99% C57BL/6 J background) [29]. Age-matched littermate male WT ($n = 6$–10) and $Adipoq^{-/-}$ ($n = 6$–10) mice were used in the studies. Animals were housed under normal housing temperature (24 ± 1 °C) with 12 h light/dark cycle (6 AM to 6 PM), and given free access to chow and water. All experiments were approved by the Institutional Animal Care and Use Committee (IACUC) of Baylor College of Medicine.

Body composition and indirect calorimetry

Whole-body composition (fat and lean mass) of mice was measured by an Echo MRI-100 whole-body composition analyzer (Echo Medical Systems, Houston, TX), following manufacturer's instructions as previously described [36]. Metabolic parameters were obtained by using Comprehensive Laboratory Animal Monitoring System (CLAMS) of Columbus Instruments (Columbus, OH). To minimize the confounding effects of stress, mice (6 WT, 6 $Adipoq^{-/-}$) were individually caged for 1 week and then placed in metabolic cages for at least 4 days prior to the indirect calorimetry testing. After 24 h of acclimatization in the calorimetry chambers, indirect calorimetry data were collected for 48 h. Energy expenditure was normalized to lean body mass [37]. Locomotor activity was measured using infrared beams to count the number of beam breaks during the recording period. Resting metabolic rate (RMR) was determined on the final day in the metabolic cages. Mice were fasted from 6 AM when the light was on, and RMR was calculated using the three lowest energy expenditure data points between 10 am and 2 pm as we previously described [36, 38].

Insulin tolerance test (ITT) and glucose tolerance test (GTT)

The insulin tolerance tests (ITT) were carried out with WT ($n = 6$) and $Adipoq^{-/-}$ ($n = 7$) male mice. Blood glucose concentration was measured using OneTouch Ultra blood glucose meter and test strips (LifeScan). For ITT, mice were *i.p.* injected with human insulin (Eli Lilly) at a dose of 1.0 U/kg of body weight following a 6 h of fasting period in the morning. Blood glucose was assessed at 0, 30, 60, 90 and 120 min after injections. For glucose tolerance tests (GTT), mice were *i.p.* injected with glucose at a dose of 2.0 g/kg body weight following a 18 h overnight fasting. The blood glucose was measured at 0, 15, 30, 60 and 120 min after injection.

Core body temperature measurement

To investigate the effects of acute cold exposure on body temperature, mice (10 WT, 9 $Adipoq^{-/-}$) were caged individually in a 4 °C cold room for 6 h with free access to food and water. Rectal temperature of the mice was measured using a TH-8 temperature monitoring system (Physitemp, Clifton, NJ). The probe was lubricated with petroleum jelly and then gently inserted into the rectum of the mice to a depth of approximately 1.5–2 cm, stabilized temperature was subsequently recorded.

Quantification of mitochondrial density of BAT

The mitochondrial density was assessed as we previously described [39]. Briefly, fresh interscapular BAT was homogenized in 1 mL isolation buffer (300 mM sucrose, 1 mM EDTA, 5 mM MOPS, 5 Mm KH_2PO_4, 0.01% BSA, pH 7.4), centrifuged at 800 g for 10 min at 4 °C, and then the pellet of nuclei was saved. The supernatant was subsequently further centrifuged at 8000 g for 10 min at 4 °C, with the resulting pellet saved as the mitochondrial fraction. Nuclear DNA was extracted using the standard phenol/chloroform method. PCR was performed to amplify the 162-nt region of the mitochondrial NADH dehydrogenase subunit 4 genes. The PCR product was purified using the high-pure PCR template preparation kit (Roche, Indianapolis, IN). The nuclear DNA and the amplified PCR products were quantified using a NanoDrop spectrophotometer (ND-1000 Thermo Scientific, Waltham, MA). The ratio of mtDNA:total DNA was then calculated.

Real-time PCR

Total RNA of tissues was isolated using TRIzol Reagent (Invitrogen, Carlsbad, CA). RNA was treated with DNase and run on agarose gels to validate RNA quality. The cDNA was synthesized from 500 ng RNA using the SuperScript III First-Strand Synthesis System (Invitrogen, Carlsbad, CA). Real-time PCR was performed on a Bio-Rad q-PCR machine using the SYBR Green PCR Master Mix, according to the protocol provided by the manufacturer. The expression was normalized by 18 s. Primers of genes used are available upon request.

Western blot analysis

Tissue was sonicated in 1X RIPA Buffer (20 mM Tris-HCl [pH 7.5], 150 mM NaCl, 1 mM Na_2EDTA, 1 mM EGTA, 1% NP-40, 1% sodium deoxycholate, 2.5 mM sodium pyrophosphate, 1 mM b-glycerophosphate, 1 mM Na_3VO_4,1 µg/ml leupeptin) containing complete Phosphatase Inhibitor Cocktail (PhosSTOP) and Protease Inhibitor Cocktail (Roche Inc.). Protein concentrations were determined using BCA (bicinchoninic acid) Protein Assay kit (Pierce, Rockford, IL). Protein (20 µg) was separated and transferred to a polyvinylidene difluoride membrane. Membranes were blocked in Tris-buffered saline with TWEEN° 20 (TBS-T, 50 mM Tris-HCl [pH 7.5–8.0], 150 mM NaCl, and 0.1% Tween 20) in 5% non-fat milk for 1 h at room temperature, and incubated overnight at 4 °C with phosphorylated and total AMPK (p-AMPK and t-AMPK) from Cell Signaling Technology (1:1000 in 3% BSA). Pierce ECL Western Blotting Substrate was used to detect the specific proteins. Densitometry analyses were performed using NIH ImageJ software.

Immunohistochemistry

Immunohistochemistry was performed as described [40, 41]. Briefly, tissue slides of BAT and inguinal fat were dewaxed in xylene, rehydrated in ethanol (100%, then 95%, ethanol washes) and rinsed in PBS. A heat-induced antigen retrieval step with Citric Acid Based Antigen Unmasking Solution (Vector laboratories, Burlingame, CA) was used to unmask antigens. To block endogenous peroxidases, slides were incubated in 3% H_2O_2 for 30 min at room temperature and then rinsed in PBS. Before primary antibody was applied, slides were soaked in blocking solution (containing 5% sheep serum, 0.2% BSA, and 0.1% Triton X-100 in PBS) for 1 h at room temperature. The following antibodies were used: rabbit-anti UCP-1 (1:50; Abcam) and mouse- anti mitochondria (1:25; Abcam). All antibody staining was performed at 4 °C overnight, followed by incubation with 1:1000 diluted anti-biotin secondary antibody (Vector Laboratories) for 45 min at room temperature. Slides were developed using a DAB kit (Vector Laboratories) and imaged using a DS-Fi1 camera connected to a Nikon E80i stereomicroscope. Images were processed using Nikon imaging software, NIS Elements RA3.2.

Data analysis

Statistical analysis was performed using Two-way ANOVA or one-way ANOVA followed by Tukey's post-hoc analysis. Data were presented as Mean ± SEM; $P < 0.05$ considered statistically significant.

Results

Body composition and insulin sensitivity

The body weights of $Adipoq^{-/-}$ mice were not different from that of their WT controls (Fig. 1a). There was a slight trend of increase of total fat mass in $Adipoq^{-/-}$ mice, but it did not reach statistical significance (Fig. 1b). $Adipoq^{-/-}$

mice had normal fasting blood glucose and insulin levels (data not shown). There was no difference in glucose response during GTT (Fig. 1c). Similarly, there was no difference detected in ITT (Fig. 1d).

Metabolic characterization

We next examined the metabolic profiles of $Adipoq^{-/-}$ mice using Comprehensive Laboratory Animal Monitoring System (CLAMS). Our data showed no difference in total daily food consumed by $Adipoq^{-/-}$ mice compared with WT mice (Fig. 1e), indicating that adiponectin ablation has no effect on total daily energy intake. To further assess whether there were difference in physical activity, we analyzed spontaneous locomotor activity. The locomotor activity was not changed under either ad lib. Fed or fasted conditions (Fig. 1f). The resting metabolic rate

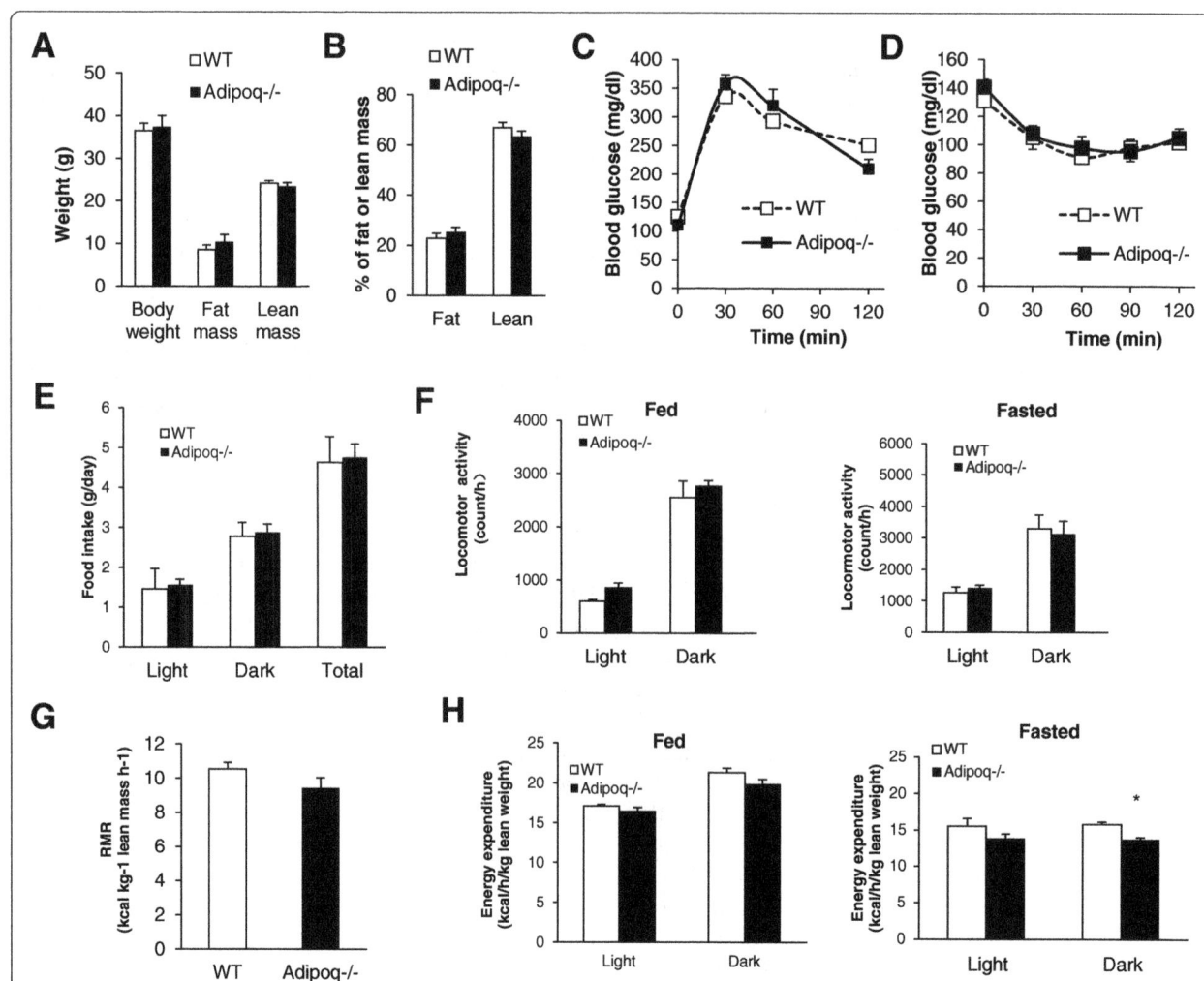

Fig. 1 $Adipoq^{-/-}$ mice show similar body composition, insulin sensitivity and metabolic profile under normal housing conditions. **a** Body weight, fat and lean mass. **b** Body composition of fat and lean. **c, d** Glucose tolerance tests (GTT) and Insulin tolerance tests (ITT) at 6-months of age. Calorimetry analysis of 5-month old male WT and $Adipoq^{-/-}$ mice: (**e**) Daily food intake, (**f**) Physical activity under *ad. lib*-fed and fasted conditions. **g** Resting metabolic rate (RMR) normalized by lean mass, and (**h**) Energy expenditure normalized by lean mass under *ad. lib*-fed and fasted conditions. $n = 6–7.$*$P < 0.05$, WT vs. $Adipoq^{-/-}$ mice

(RMR) was similar between WT and Adipoq$^{-/-}$ mice (Fig. 1g), which implies that the basal metabolic rate was unaffected. While Adipoq$^{-/-}$ mice exhibited no difference in energy expenditure under normal ad lib. Fed condition (Fig. 1h), the mice showed significantly reduced energy expenditure under fasting condition during the dark cycle (Fig. 1h).

Core body temperature during cold exposure

To assess the thermogenic phenotype of Adipoq$^{-/-}$ mice, mice were challenged with 4 °C cold exposure for 6 h. We measured the rectal temperature (as readout of core body temperature) every 2 h during the cold exposure. The rectal temperature of Adipoq$^{-/-}$ mice was significantly lower than that of WT mice during cold exposure, and the difference became more pronounced under prolonged cold exposure, i.e., the temperature difference between WT and Adipoq$^{-/-}$ mice increased from 0.03 °C at 0 h to 3.70 °C after 6 h of cold exposure (Fig. 2).

Expression of thermogenic genes in BAT in response to cold challenge

To understand the underlying molecular mechanisms of adiponectin-mediated thermogenesis, BAT was collected from WT and Adipoq$^{-/-}$ mice immediately following a 6 h cold exposure. There was no difference in total BAT weight or BAT/body weight ratio between WT and Adipoq$^{-/-}$ mice (Fig. 3a). The expression of thermogenic regulator UCP-1 was significantly decreased in BAT of Adipoq$^{-/-}$ mice compared to WT mice, while the

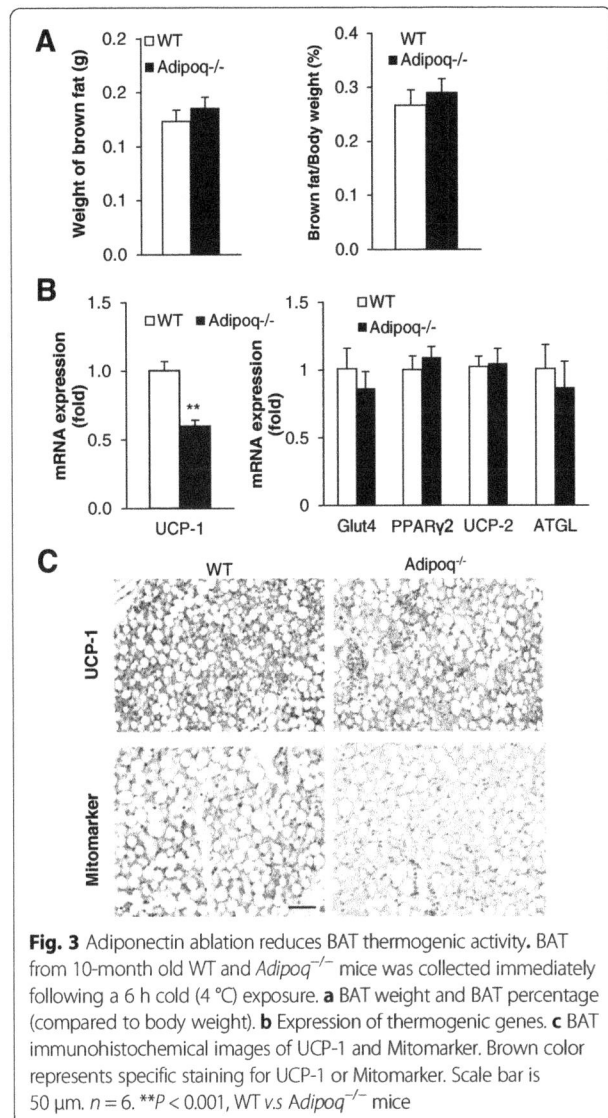

Fig. 3 Adiponectin ablation reduces BAT thermogenic activity. BAT from 10-month old WT and Adipoq$^{-/-}$ mice was collected immediately following a 6 h cold (4 °C) exposure. **a** BAT weight and BAT percentage (compared to body weight). **b** Expression of thermogenic genes. **c** BAT immunohistochemical images of UCP-1 and Mitomarker. Brown color represents specific staining for UCP-1 or Mitomarker. Scale bar is 50 μm. $n = 6$. **$P < 0.001$, WT v.s Adipoq$^{-/-}$ mice

expression of glucose uptake regulator (Glut4), adipogenic regulator (PPARγ2), fat utilization regulator (UCP-2), and lipolytic enzyme (ATGL) was unchanged (Fig. 3b). We also detected reduced UCP1 protein in BAT of Adipoq$^{-/-}$ mice (Additional file 1: Figure S1). Consistently, immunohistochemistry analysis showed that the immunostainings of UCP-1 and Mitomarker were lower in BAT of Adipoq$^{-/-}$ mice compared to WT mice (Fig. 3c). The reduced body temperature in Adipoq$^{-/-}$ mice under cold exposure indicates that adiponectin deficiency suppresses BAT thermogenesis.

Mitochondrial function is determined by mitochondrial biogenesis and mitochondrial dynamics [42]. To determine whether adiponectin deletion affected mitochondrial biogenesis in BAT, we analyzed mitochondrial density by measuring the ratio of mitochondrial DNA:nuclear DNA. Mitochondrial density of BAT from Adipoq$^{-/-}$ mice was lower than that of WT mice (Fig. 4a),

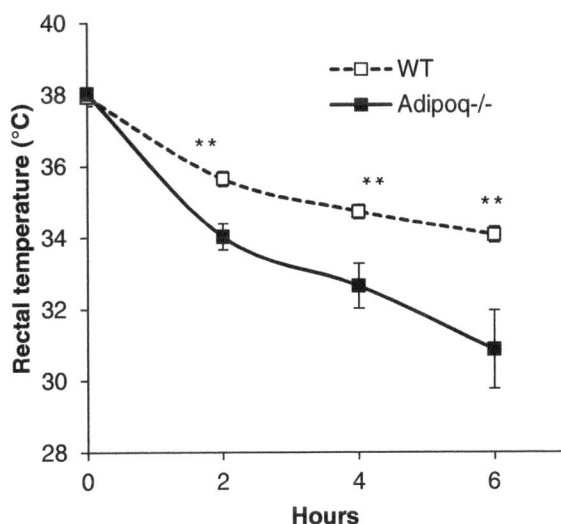

Fig. 2 Adipoq$^{-/-}$ mice are sensitive to cold exposure. Ten-month old male mice were individually caged at 4 °C and provide with free access to food and water. Rectal temperature was recorded every 2 h. $n = 9-10$. **$P < 0.001$, WT vs. Adipoq$^{-/-}$ mice

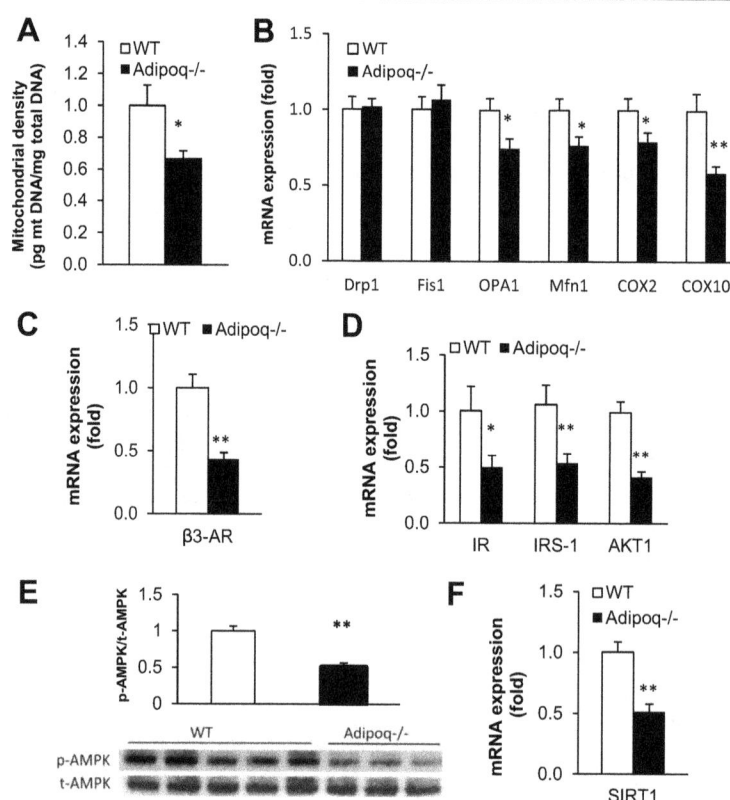

Fig. 4 Adiponectin ablation reduces the thermogenic capacity of mitochondria in BAT. BAT from male 10-month old WT and *Adipoq*$^{-/-}$ mice were collected after a 6 h of 4 °C cold exposure. **a** Quantification of mitochondrial density. **b** Expression of mitochondrial dynamic genes. **c, d** Expression of putative adiponectin-mediated thermogenic regulators. **e** Representative Western blots of AMPK activation in BAT from WT and *Adipoq*$^{-/-}$ mice. p-AMPK for phosphorylated AMPA; t-AMPK for total AMPK. **f** Expression of SIRT1, a downstream target of AMPK. $n = 6$. *$P < 0.05$, **$P < 0.001$ WT vs. *Adipoq*$^{-/-}$ mice

indicative of reduced mitochondrial biogenesis. Mitochondrial dynamics is another crucial component that controls mitochondrial function and cell survival [43–45]. Mitochondrial dynamics consist of the processes of the 'joining event' of fusion and the 'dividing event' of fission; the balance between fusion and fission is essential for the maintenance of normal mitochondrial function [44]. Fusion is mediated by mitofusins (Mfns) and optic atrophy gene 1 (OPA1); fission is mediated by dynamin-related protein 1 (Drp1) and fission 1 (Fis1) protein. To study mitochondrial dynamics of BAT, we analyzed key regulatory genes for mitochondrial dynamics and subunits of mitochondrial respiratory chain complexes. While the expression of mitochondrial fission genes (Drp1 and Fis1) in BAT of *Adipoq*$^{-/-}$ mice was unchanged, the expression of mitochondrial fusion genes (OPA1 and Mfns) was significantly decreased (Fig. 4b). Consistent with the decreased thermogenic function, the expression of the subunits of mitochondrial respiratory chain complexes IV (COX-2 and COX10) were decreased in *Adipoq*$^{-/-}$ mice (Fig. 4b).

Potential regulators and signaling pathways mediating the thermogenic effect of adiponectin

To further study the molecular mechanisms mediating thermogenic impairment induced by adiponectin deficiency, we investigated the expression of β3-adrenergic receptor (β3-AR). β3-AR expression was decreased in BAT of *Adipoq*$^{-/-}$ mice (Fig. 4c), suggesting reduced adrenergic activation. Insulin signaling in BAT is activated by cold stress [46] and insulin signaling mediator AKT (also known as "protein kinase B", PKB) has been linked to mitochondrial biogenesis [47, 48]. We assessed insulin signaling in BAT by studying the expression of key regulators of insulin signaling: insulin receptor (IR), insulin receptor substrate 1 (IRS-1) and AKT. In line with the reduced thermogenic phenotype, the expression of IR, IRS-1 and AKT1 in BAT of *Adipoq*$^{-/-}$ mice were significantly decreased in BAT of *Adipoq*$^{-/-}$ mice (Fig. 4d). We also detected reduced IRS1 protein in BAT of *Adipoq*$^{-/-}$ mice (Additional file 1: Figure S1). Adiponectin, AMP-activated protein kinase (AMPK) and sirtuin 1 (SIRT1) signaling have been suggested to promote mitochondrial biogenesis in muscle [49–51]. To determine whether AMPK and SIRT1 mediate the mitochondrial effect of adiponectin on BAT, we examined the activity of AMPK and the expression of SIRT1. Adiponectin ablation decreased phosphorylated AMPK (Fig. 4e) and downregulated SIRT1 (Fig. 4f) in BAT of $Adipoq^{-/-}$ mice.

The expression of thermogenic genes in subcutaneous WAT in response to cold stress

"Beige" adipocytes in subcutaneous WAT have been shown to possess thermogenic activity similar to classic BAT [11]. The weight ratio of subcutaneous WAT to total body weight was significantly higher in $Adipoq^{-/-}$ mice than WT mice (Fig. 5a). Similar to that of BAT,

UCP-1 expression in inguinal fat was decreased in coldchallenged $Adipoq^{-/-}$ mice, while the expression of Glut4, PPARγ2, UCP2 and ATGL were unchanged (Fig. 5b). Consistently, immunohistochemical analysis showed that UCP-1 and Mitomarker were significantly lower in WAT of $Adipoq^{-/-}$ mice than that of WT mice (Fig. 5c). However, unlike BAT, the mitochondrial dynamic genes (OPA1, Mfns, COX-2) were unchanged, while the expression of the mitochondrial respiratory chain complexes IV gene (COX-2) was decreased (Fig. 5d). Similar to BAT, adiponectin ablation decreased phosphorylated AMPK (Fig. 5e) and the expression of adrenergic receptor β3-AR and SIRT1 in subcutaneous (inguinal) fat in $Adipoq^{-/-}$ mice (Fig. 5f).

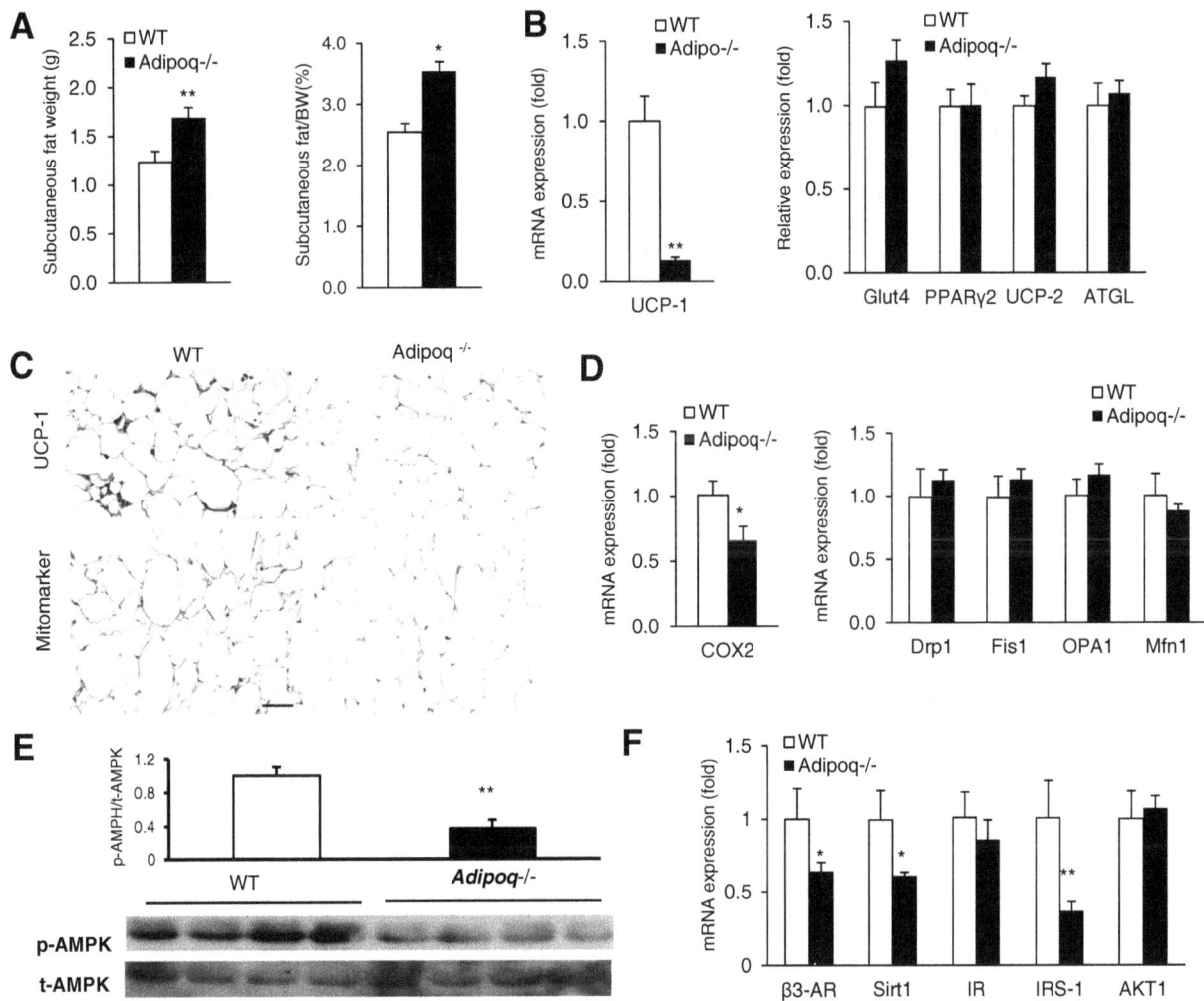

Fig. 5 Adiponectin ablation reduces thermogenic activity in subcutaneous fat. Subcutaneous (inguinal) fat from 10-month old WT and $Adipoq^{-/-}$ mice was collected after 6 h following 4 °C cold exposure. a Subcutaneous fat weight and percentage ratio compared to body weight (BW). b Expression of thermogenic genes. c Immunohistochemical images of the UCP-1 and Mitomarker in inguinal fat. Scale bar is 50 μm. d Expression of mitochondrial dynamic genes. e Representative Western blots of AMPK activation in inguinal fat of WT and $Adipoq^{-/-}$ mice. p-AMPK for phosphorylated AMPA; t-AMPK for total AMPK. f Expression of regulators potentially involved in adiponectin-mediated thermogenesis. n = 6. *P < 0.05, **P < 0.001 WT vs. $Adipoq^{-/-}$

Discussion

Non-shivering thermogenesis in BAT and "beige" adipocytes in subcutaneous WAT dissipates energy as heat to protect against hypothermia, that may protect against obesity [15]. Our findings reveal that adiponectin ablation exacerbates thermogenic dysfunction under cold stress, exhibiting reduced thermogenesis and impaired ability to maintain body temperature. Our study indicates that adiponectin plays a crucial role in thermogenesis under fasting and cold stress conditions. Specifically, our data show that adiponectin-ablated mice have normal thermoregulation at regular housing temperature and ad lib. Fed condition, but exhibit thermogenic impairment under fasting and cold condition. Thus, adiponectin is not required for thermogenic regulation under normal feeding and housing environment, but is required for heat production and body temperature maintenance under negative energy balance and cold exposure. Our data show that the rectal temperature of $Adipoq^{-/-}$ mice was significantly lower than that of WT mice under acute cold exposure, which decreased drastically with the length of cold exposure. It has been reported that cold exposure (4 °C for 12–24 h) reduces serum adiponectin in mice [52]. In accordance with our findings, another group recently reported that chronic cold exposure induces adiponectin accumulation in visceral fat, which in turn stimulates thermogenic activation [27]. A recent report has shown that beige adipose tissue fails to produce appreciable thermogenic activation in response to chronic cold [53]. So even though changes in thermogenic genes and protein were detected in both BAT and sub-WAT of adiponectin null mice, the thermogenic phenotype we observed is likely primarily due to BAT. Opposite from our finding, using a different adiponectin knockout mouse line with severe insulin resistance, Qiao et al. reported that adiponectin deficiency increases thermogenesis under cold stress [28]. It is known that insulin level and insulin sensitivity affects thermogenesis [32–34]. We intentionally used the $Adipoq-/-$ mouse line with no insulin resistance in our study. The different thermogenic phenotypes observed in these 2 different adiponectin-null models could be due to differences in insulin sensitivity status. In addition, study by Qiao et al. was conducted in young mice (2 months old); our study was conducted in older mice (10 months of age). It is know there is significant thermogenic decline in aging, and adiponectin level is positively correlated with aging [54]. Thus, the age difference may also contribute to the differential thermogenic phenotypes. Our findings collectively suggest that adiponectin is responsive to both acute and chronic cold insults, it is required to maintain body temperature under cold exposure, and it may be used to treat hypothermia. It is well documented that adiponectin has many beneficial metabolic effects, many of which phenocopy that of thermogenic activation [1–7]. Our finding that adiponectin deletion impairs thermogenesis is in agreement with the thermo-protective effect of exogenous adiponectin. Thermogenesis is affected not only by the cold, it is also affected by food intake (thermic effect of food). Also, the normal animal housing condition temperature (24 °C) is lower than the thermoneutral temperature (~30 °C) for mice [55]. For future studies, it would be interesting to study the fasted mice under thermoneutrality.

UCP-1 is a key regulator of thermogenesis, which allows protons to enter the mitochondrial matrix and dissipate energy as heat [9]. UCP-1 is the hallmark regulator which mediates cold-induced non-shivering thermogenesis [56]. We detected decreased UCP-1 mRNA expression in BAT and subcutaneous fat of $Adipoq^{-/-}$ mice under cold exposure, indicating that adiponectin-mediated thermoregulation is mediated through UCP-1. Thermogenic function of brown/beige adipocytes is determined by content and functional capacity of mitochondria [44]. While mitochondrial content is determined by mitochondrial biogenesis, mitochondrial function is controlled by mitochondrial structure integrity and dynamics. We detected a lower mitochondrial DNA content ratio in the BAT of $Adipoq^{-/-}$ mice after cold exposure, implying reduced mitochondrial biogenesis. Several studies show abnormal mitochondrial structure in obese and type 2 diabetic patients [57, 58]. Interestingly, while expression of mitochondrial fusion genes was decreased in the BAT of $Adipoq^{-/-}$ mice, the expression of fission genes were unchanged. The imbalance between fusion and fission in the BAT of $Adipoq^{-/-}$ mice can lead to mitochondrial fragmentation, and the impairment of mitochondrial dynamics can lead to mitochondrial dysfunction. In agreement with the reduced mitochondrial biogenesis and impaired mitochondrial dynamics, the expression of mitochondrial subunit genes of mitochondrial respiratory chain complexes IV (COX-2 and COX10) was decreased in BAT of $Adipoq^{-/-}$ mice, further supporting reduced thermogenic capacity [30]. COX-2 is known to be encoded by mtDNA [59]. We observed reduced expression of COX-2 in BAT of $Adipoq^{-/-}$ mice, which is consistent with the reduced mitochondrial DNA detected in BAT of $Adipoq^{-/-}$ mice, supporting reduced mitochondrial biogenesis. Our data demonstrate that Adiponectin deficiency decreases mitochondrial biogenesis and impairs dynamics, thereby attenuating thermogenic activity.

Activation of adrenergic signaling via β3-adrenergic receptor (β3-AR) is essential for thermogenic activation in brown adipocytes [52]. It has been reported that peripheral administration of adiponectin increases β3-AR expression in BAT of mice and rectal temperature [60]. We found that β3-AR is decreased in BAT and subcutaneous WAT of *Adipoq*$^{-/-}$ mice after cold exposure. Thus, the thermogenic phenotype of *Adipoq*$^{-/-}$ mice is likely linked to β-adrenergic activation. The β-adrenergic signaling in brown adipocytes can be activated centrally via sympathetic nerve activity (SNA), or peripherally by circulating adiponectins. Masaki et al. reported that peripheral, not central, adiponectin administration increases SNA and UCP1 expression in the BAT, and elevates rectal temperature [61]. Hui et al. recently reported that adiponectin directly induces browning of subcutaneous adipose tissues by promoting M2 macrophage proliferation [27]. Thus, we believe that the phenotype we see in adiponectin KO is primarily taken place at the adipocyte level. Thermogenic defects are associated with insulin resistance in BAT [35], and cold stress has been shown to stimulate the insulin-signaling pathway in BAT to improve glucose homeostasis and insulin sensitivity [32, 62]. Our data show that the insulin signaling in BAT was suppressed in *Adipoq*$^{-/-}$ mice after cold exposure, which suggests that adiponectin deficiency impairs the insulin sensitivity of brown adipocytes, which may lead to the suppression of thermogenic activity.

It has been reported that adiponectin activates AMPK-SIRT1 to regulate mitochondrial biogenesis and insulin sensitivity in muscle [49]. Similarly, it has been suggested that adiponectin, via SIRT1 and AMPK, regulates lipid metabolism in liver [50]. It has been reported that adipocyte AMPK is required for acute BAT-mediated thermogenesis [63], and that there is cross-talk between insulin signaling and AMPK signaling pathway [64]. AKT and AMPK activity is activated by cold exposure in BAT, and the activation of insulin signaling and AMPK are linked to enhanced UCP1 activity and thermogenic activation [65, 66]. Indeed, we found that adiponectin ablation suppresses AMPK activity in adipose tissues, and reduces expression of SIRT1 in BAT and subcutaneous fat in *Adipoq*$^{-/-}$ mice. Our data reveal that adiponectin ablation suppresses the AMPK-SIRT1 pathway, which may subsequently reduce mitochondrial biogenesis and suppress thermogenic function. Thus it is likely that adiponectin regulates thermogenic activity in BAT through different mechanisms: suppressing adrenergic activation of β3-AR, inhibiting insulin signaling, and/or deactivating the AMPK-SIRT1 pathway (Fig. 6).

Conclusions

Our data demonstrate that adiponectin regulates thermogenesis in BAT and subcutaneous fat under cold exposure. Adiponectin-associated thermogenesis is not essential under normal housing temperature and *ad.lib* feeding condition, but is required for fasting and cold-challenged conditions. Adiponectin is required for maintaining body temperature in cold environment. Moreover, our data reveals that adiponectin ablation attenuates thermogenic signaling, reduces mitochondrial biogenesis and impairs mitochondrial dynamics, possibly by suppressing insulin signaling and the AMPK-SIRT1 pathway in BAT. Therefore, adiponectin is an important thermogenic regulator under energy deficit and cold environment, and adiponectin may serve as an effective therapeutic agent for hypothermia.

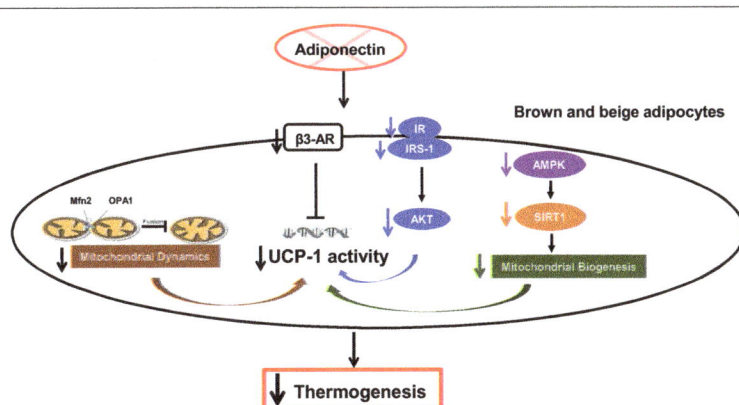

Fig. 6 A Schematic diagram of adiponectin-mediated thermogenic regulation in *brown* and *"beige"* adipocytes. Our data suggest that adiponectin may regulate thermogenesis in brown adipocytes via the following 4 independent and complementary cellular/molecular mechanisms: 1) Ablation of adiponectin decreases β3-AR expression, which directly inhibits UCP-1 gene expression and activity. 2) Ablation of adiponectin inhibits insulin signaling, which may reduce UCP-1 activity. 3) Ablation of adiponectin suppresses the signaling pathway of AMPK-SIRT1, which may in turn result in reduced mitochondrial biogenesis. 4) Ablation of adiponectin impairs mitochondrial dynamics in BAT, which may contribute to thermogenic dysfunction. Collectively, adiponectin ablation diminishes thermogenic activation by decreasing adrenergic activation, and impairing mitochondrial biosynthesis and/or dynamics, thus suppressing thermogenesis in *brown* and *"beige"* adipocytes

Abbreviations

$Adipoq^{-/-}$: Adiponectin-null mice; AMPK: AMP-activated protein kinase; BAT: Brown adipose tissue; Drp1: Dynamin-related protein 1; Fis1: Fission 1 protein; Glut4: Glucose uptake regulator; GTT: Glucose tolerance tests; IR: Insulin receptor; IRS-1: Insulin receptor substrate 1; ITT: Insulin tolerance tests; Mfns: Mitofusins; OPA1: Optic atrophy gene 1; RMR: Resting metabolic rate; SIRT1: Sirtuin 1; SNS: Sympathetic nervous system; UCP-1: Uncoupling protein 1; UCP-2: Fat utilization regulator; WAT: Subcutaneous white adipose tissue; β3-AR: β3-adrenergic receptor

Acknowledgments

We sincerely appreciate the excellent technical support of Ms. Lagina M. Nosavanh. Measurements of body composition, food intake and balance were performed in the Mouse Metabolic Research Unit at the USDA/ARS Children's Nutrition Research Center, Baylor College of Medicine. The authors acknowledge the expert assistance of Mr. Firoz Vohra and the MMRU Core Director, Dr. Marta Fiorotto. We also thank Ms. Aselin Puthenpurail at Texas A&M University and Mr. Michael R. Honig at Houston's Community Public Radio Station KPFT for their excellent editorial assistance.

Funding

This work was supported by the USDA National Institute of Food and Agriculture - Hatch grant 1,010,840 and CRIS grant 3092-5-001-059 (YS), American Heart Association grants 12IRG9230004 and 14GRNT18990019 (YS), American Diabetes Association #1–15-BS-177 (YS), and partly supported by NIH P30 DK56338 and 1T32HD071839.

Authors' contributions

QW, JHL, HW, OYNB, CSW, GP, and MHC. conducted research and analyzed data; QW, JHL, MHC and YSwrote the paper; LC, edited the manuscript; ZS and RSC consulted the study and proofread the manuscript; MB and LC provided the mice and edited the manuscript. YS has primary responsibility for final content. All authors read and approved the final manuscript.

Competing interests

The authors declare no competing interests.

Author details

[1]USDA/ARS Children's Nutrition Research Center, Department of Pediatrics, Baylor College of Medicine, Houston, TX 77030, USA. [2]Division of Endocrinology, Zhongda hospital, Southeast University, Nanjing, Jiangsu Province, People's Republic of China210002. [3]College of Pharmacy, Gachon University, Incheon 21936, South Korea. [4]Department of Nutrition and Food Science, Texas A&M University, 214D Cater-Mattil; 2253 TAMU, College Station, TX 77843, USA. [5]Laboratory of Lipid & Glucose Metabolism, The First Affiliated Hospital of Chongqing Medical University, Chongqing, Sichuan province, People's Republic of China400016. [6]Institute of Biosciences and Technology, Houston, TX 77030, USA. [7]Department of Medicine, Baylor College of Medicine, Houston, TX 77030, USA. [8]Huffington Center on Aging, Baylor College of Medicine, Houston, TX, USA.

References

1. Arita Y, Kihara S, Ouchi N, Takahashi M, Maeda K, Miyagawa J, Hotta K, Shimomura I, Nakamura T, Miyaoka K, et al. Paradoxical decrease of an adipose-specific protein, adiponectin, in obesity. Biochem Biophys Res Commun. 1999;257:79–83.
2. Bajaj M, Suraamornkul S, Piper P, Hardies LJ, Glass L, Cersosimo E, Pratipanawatr T, Miyazaki Y, DeFronzo RA. Decreased plasma adiponectin concentrations are closely related to hepatic fat content and hepatic insulin resistance in pioglitazone-treated type 2 diabetic patients. J Clin Endocrinol Metab. 2004;89:200–6.
3. Karbowska J, Kochan Z. Role of adiponectin in the regulation of carbohydrate and lipid metabolism. J Physiol Pharmacol. 2006;57(Suppl 6):103–13.
4. Liu Q, Yuan B, Lo KA, Patterson HC, Sun Y, Lodish HF. Adiponectin regulates expression of hepatic genes critical for glucose and lipid metabolism. Proc Natl Acad Sci U S A. 2012;109:14568–73.
5. Yamauchi T, Kamon J, Waki H, Terauchi Y, Kubota N, Hara K, Mori Y, Ide T, Murakami K, Tsuboyama-Kasaoka N, et al. The fat-derived hormone adiponectin reverses insulin resistance associated with both lipoatrophy and obesity. Nat Med. 2001;7:941–6.
6. Haluzik M. Adiponectin and its potential in the treatment of obesity, diabetes and insulin resistance. Curr Opin Investig Drugs. 2005;6:988–93.
7. Pajvani UB, Scherer PE. Adiponectin: systemic contributor to insulin sensitivity. Curr Diab Rep. 2003;3:207–13.
8. Walden TB, Hansen IR, Timmons JA, Cannon B, Nedergaard J. Recruited vs. nonrecruited molecular signatures of brown, "brite", and white adipose tissues. Am J Physiol Endocrinol Metab. 2012;302:E19–31.
9. Cannon B, Nedergaard J. Brown adipose tissue: function and physiological significance. Physiol Rev. 2004;84:277–359.
10. Lee P, Swarbrick MM, Ho KK. Brown adipose tissue in adult humans: a metabolic renaissance. Endocr Rev. 2013;34:413–38.
11. Wu J, Bostrom P, Sparks LM, Ye L, Choi JH, Giang AH, Khandekar M, Virtanen KA, Nuutila P, Schaart G, et al. Beige adipocytes are a distinct type of thermogenic fat cell in mouse and human. Cell. 2012;150:366–76.
12. Schulz TJ, Huang P, Huang TL, Xue R, McDougall LE, Townsend KL, Cypess AM, Mishina Y, Gussoni E, Tseng YH. Brown-fat paucity due to impaired BMP signalling induces compensatory browning of white fat. Nature. 2013;495:379–83.
13. Townsend KL, Tseng YH. Brown fat fuel utilization and thermogenesis. Trends Endocrinol Metab. 2014;25:168–77.
14. Nedergaard J, Cannon B. The changed metabolic world with human brown adipose tissue: therapeutic visions. Cell Metab. 2010;11:268–72.
15. Cannon B, Nedergaard J. Metabolic consequences of the presence or absence of the thermogenic capacity of brown adipose tissue in mice (and probably in humans). Int J Obes. 2010;34(Suppl 1):S7–16.
16. Townsend KL, Tseng YH. Of mice and men: novel insights regarding constitutive and recruitable brown adipocytes. Int J Obes Suppl. 2015;5:S15–20.
17. Sidossis LS, Porter C, Saraf MK, Borsheim E, Radhakrishnan RS, Chao T, Ali A, Chondronikola M, Mlcak R, Finnerty CC, et al. Browning of subcutaneous white adipose tissue in humans after severe adrenergic stress. Cell Metab. 2015;22:219–27.
18. Chondronikola M, Volpi E, Borsheim E, Porter C, Annamalai P, Enerback S, Lidell ME, Saraf MK, Labbe SM, Hurren NM, et al. Brown adipose tissue improves whole-body glucose homeostasis and insulin sensitivity in humans. Diabetes. 2014;63:4089–99.
19. Shinoda K, Luijten IH, Hasegawa Y, Hong H, Sonne SB, Kim M, Xue R, Chondronikola M, Cypess AM, Tseng YH, et al. Genetic and functional characterization of clonally derived adult human brown adipocytes. Nat Med. 2015;21:389–94.
20. Chondronikola M, Volpi E, Borsheim E, Porter C, Saraf MK, Annamalai P, Yfanti C, Chao T, Wong D, Shinoda K, et al. Brown adipose tissue activation is linked to distinct systemic effects on lipid metabolism in humans. Cell Metab. 2016;23:1200–6.
21. Rousset S, Alves-Guerra MC, Mozo J, Miroux B, Cassard-Doulcier AM, Bouillaud F, Ricquier D. The biology of mitochondrial uncoupling proteins. Diabetes. 2004;53(Suppl 1):S130–5.
22. Feldmann HM, Golozoubova V, Cannon B, Nedergaard J. UCP1 ablation induces obesity and abolishes diet-induced thermogenesis in mice exempt from thermal stress by living at thermoneutrality. Cell Metab. 2009;9:203–9.
23. Imbeault P, Depault I, Haman F. Cold exposure increases adiponectin levels in men. Metabolism. 2009;58:552–9.
24. Jankovic A, Korac A, Buzadzic B, Otasevic V, Stancic A, Vucetic M, Markelic M, Velickovic K, Golic I, Korac B. Endocrine and metabolic signaling in retroperitoneal white adipose tissue remodeling during cold acclimation. J Obes. 2013;2013:937572.
25. Nedergaard J, Golozoubova V, Matthias A, Asadi A, Jacobsson A, Cannon B. UCP1: the only protein able to mediate adaptive non-shivering thermogenesis and metabolic inefficiency. Biochim Biophys Acta. 2001;1504:82–106.
26. Puerta M, Abelenda M, Rocha M, Trayhurn P. Effect of acute cold exposure on the expression of the adiponectin, resistin and leptin genes in rat white and brown adipose tissues. Horm Metab Res. 2002;34:629–34.
27. Hui X, Gu P, Zhang J, Nie T, Pan Y, Wu D, Feng T, Zhong C, Wang Y, Lam KS, Xu A. Adiponectin enhances cold-induced Browning of subcutaneous

adipose tissue via promoting M2 macrophage proliferation. Cell Metab. 2015;22:279–90.

28. Qiao L, Yoo H, Bosco C, Lee B, Feng GS, Schaack J, Chi NW, Shao J. Adiponectin reduces thermogenesis by inhibiting brown adipose tissue activation in mice. Diabetologia. 2014;57:1027–36.

29. Ma K, Cabrero A, Saha PK, Kojima H, Li L, Chang BH, Paul A, Chan L. Increased beta -oxidation but no insulin resistance or glucose intolerance in mice lacking adiponectin. J Biol Chem. 2002;277:34658–61.

30. Zhou M, Xu A, Tam PK, Lam KS, Chan L, Hoo RL, Liu J, Chow KH, Wang Y. Mitochondrial dysfunction contributes to the increased vulnerabilities of adiponectin knockout mice to liver injury. Hepatology. 2008;48:1087–96.

31. Menendez JA, Atrens DM. Insulin and the paraventricular hypothalamus: modulation of energy balance. Brain Res. 1991;555:193–201.

32. Rothwell NJ, Saville ME, Stock MJ. Role of insulin in thermogenic responses to refeeding in 3-day-fasted rats. Am J Phys. 1983;245:E160–5.

33. Rothwell NJ, Stock MJ. Insulin and thermogenesis. Int J Obes. 1988;12:93–102.

34. Felig P. Insulin is the mediator of feeding-related thermogenesis: insulin resistance and/or deficiency results in a thermogenic defect which contributes to the pathogenesis of obesity. Clin Physiol. 1984;4:267–73.

35. Mercer SW, Trayhurn P. Effects of ciglitazone on insulin resistance and thermogenic responsiveness to acute cold in brown adipose tissue of genetically obese (ob/ob) mice. FEBS Lett. 1986;195:12–6.

36. Lin L, Saha PK, Ma X, Henshaw IO, Shao L, Chang BH, Buras ED, Tong Q, Chan L, McGuinness OP, Sun Y. Ablation of ghrelin receptor reduces adiposity and improves insulin sensitivity during aging by regulating fat metabolism in white and brown adipose tissues. Aging Cell. 2011;10:996–1010.

37. Lin L, Lee JH, Bongmba OY, Ma X, Zhu X, Sheikh-Hamad D, Sun Y. The suppression of ghrelin signaling mitigates age-associated thermogenic impairment. Aging (Albany NY). 2014;6:1019–32.

38. Lee JH, Lin L, Xu P, Saito K, Wei Q, Meadows AG, Bongmba OY, Pradhan G, Zheng H, Xu Y, Sun Y. Neuronal deletion of Ghrelin receptor almost completely prevents diet-induced obesity. Diabetes. 2016;65:2169–78.

39. Lin L, Sun Y. Thermogenic characterization of ghrelin receptor null mice. Methods Enzymol. 2012;514:355–70.

40. DH Y, Ware C, Waterland RA, Zhang J, Chen MH, Gadkari M, Kunde-Ramamoorthy G, Nosavanh LM, Shen L. Developmentally programmed 3' CpG island methylation confers tissue- and cell-type-specific transcriptional activation. Mol Cell Biol. 2013;33:1845–58.

41. Nosavanh L, DH Y, Jaehnig EJ, Tong Q, Shen L, Chen MH. Cell-autonomous activation of hedgehog signaling inhibits brown adipose tissue development. Proc Natl Acad Sci U S A. 2015;112:5069–74.

42. Jastroch M, Withers KW, Taudien S, Frappell PB, Helwig M, Fromme T, Hirschberg V, Heldmaier G, McAllan BM, Firth BT, et al. Marsupial uncoupling protein 1 sheds light on the evolution of mammalian nonshivering thermogenesis. Physiol Genomics. 2008;32:161–9.

43. Liesa M, Shirihai OS. Mitochondrial dynamics in the regulation of nutrient utilization and energy expenditure. Cell Metab. 2013;17:491–506.

44. Westermann B. Mitochondrial fusion and fission in cell life and death. Nat Rev Mol Cell Biol. 2010;11:872–84.

45. Su B, Wang X, Zheng L, Perry G, Smith MA, Zhu X. Abnormal mitochondrial dynamics and neurodegenerative diseases. Biochim Biophys Acta. 1802;2010:135–42.

46. Wang X, Wahl R. Responses of the insulin signaling pathways in the brown adipose tissue of rats following cold exposure. PLoS One. 2014;9:e99772.

47. Valverde AM, Arribas M, Mur C, Navarro P, Pons S, Cassard-Doulcier AM, Kahn CR, Benito M. Insulin-induced up-regulated uncoupling protein-1 expression is mediated by insulin receptor substrate 1 through the phosphatidylinositol 3-kinase/Akt signaling pathway in fetal brown adipocytes. J Biol Chem. 2003;278:10221–31.

48. Santos RX, Correia SC, Alves MG, Oliveira PF, Cardoso S, Carvalho C, Duarte AI, Santos MS, Moreira PI. Insulin therapy modulates mitochondrial dynamics and biogenesis, autophagy and tau protein phosphorylation in the brain of type 1 diabetic rats. Biochim Biophys Acta. 1842;2014:1154–66.

49. Iwabu M, Yamauchi T, Okada-Iwabu M, Sato K, Nakagawa T, Funata M, Yamaguchi M, Namiki S, Nakayama R, Tabata M, et al. Adiponectin and AdipoR1 regulate PGC-1alpha and mitochondria by ca(2+) and AMPK/SIRT1. Nature. 2010;464:1313–9.

50. Shen Z, Liang X, Rogers CQ, Rideout D, You M. Involvement of adiponectin-SIRT1-AMPK signaling in the protective action of rosiglitazone against alcoholic fatty liver in mice. Am J Physiol Gastrointest Liver Physiol. 2010;298:10.

51. Handa P, Maliken BD, Nelson JE, Morgan-Stevenson V, Messner DJ, Dhillon BK, Klintworth HM, Beauchamp M, Yeh MM, Elfers CT, et al. Reduced adiponectin signaling due to weight gain results in nonalcoholic steatohepatitis through impaired mitochondrial biogenesis. Hepatology. 2014;60:133–45.

52. Imai J, Katagiri H, Yamada T, Ishigaki Y, Ogihara T, Uno K, Hasegawa Y, Gao J, Ishihara H, Sasano H, Oka Y. Cold exposure suppresses serum adiponectin levels through sympathetic nerve activation in mice. Obesity (Silver Spring). 2006;14:1132–41.

53. Labbe SM, Caron A, Chechi K, Laplante M, Lecomte R, Richard D. Metabolic activity of brown, "beige" and white adipose tissues in response to chronic adrenergic stimulation in male mice. Am J Physiol Endocrinol Metab. 2016;311:E260–8.

54. Miller KN, Burhans MS, Clark JP, Howell PR, Polewski MA, DeMuth TM, Eliceiri KW, Lindstrom MJ, Ntambi JM, Anderson RM. Aging and caloric restriction impact adipose tissue, adiponectin, and circulating lipids. Aging Cell. 2017;16:497–507.

55. Abreu-Vieira G, Xiao C, Gavrilova O, Reitman ML. Integration of body temperature into the analysis of energy expenditure in the mouse. Mol Metab. 2015;4:461–70.

56. Golozoubova V, Cannon B, Nedergaard J. UCP1 is essential for adaptive adrenergic nonshivering thermogenesis. Am J Physiol Endocrinol Metab. 2006;291:E350–7.

57. Bach D, Pich S, Soriano FX, Vega N, Baumgartner B, Oriola J, Daugaard JR, Lloberas J, Camps M, Zierath JR, et al. Mitofusin-2 determines mitochondrial network architecture and mitochondrial metabolism. A novel regulatory mechanism altered in obesity. J Biol Chem. 2003;278:17190–7.

58. Parone PA, Da Cruz S, Tondera D, Mattenberger Y, James DI, Maechler P, Barja F, Martinou JC. Preventing mitochondrial fission impairs mitochondrial function and leads to loss of mitochondrial DNA. PLoS One. 2008;3:e3257.

59. Capaldi RA. Structure and function of cytochrome c oxidase. Annu Rev Biochem. 1990;59:569–96.

60. Maeda N, Shimomura I, Kishida K, Nishizawa H, Matsuda M, Nagaretani H, Furuyama N, Kondo H, Takahashi M, Arita Y, et al. Diet-induced insulin resistance in mice lacking adiponectin/ACRP30. Nat Med. 2002;8:731–7.

61. Masaki T, Chiba S, Yasuda T, Tsubone T, Kakuma T, Shimomura I, Funahashi T, Matsuzawa Y, Yoshimatsu H. Peripheral, but not central, administration of adiponectin reduces visceral adiposity and upregulates the expression of uncoupling protein in agouti yellow (ay/a) obese mice. Diabetes. 2003;52:2266–73.

62. Gasparetti AL, de Souza CT, Pereira-da-Silva M, Oliveira RL, Saad MJ, Carneiro EM, Velloso LA. Cold exposure induces tissue-specific modulation of the insulin-signalling pathway in Rattus Norvegicus. J Physiol. 2003;552:149–62.

63. Mottillo EP, Desjardins EM, Crane JD, Smith BK, Green AE, Ducommun S, Henriksen TI, Rebalka IA, Razi A, Sakamoto K, et al. Lack of Adipocyte AMPK exacerbates insulin resistance and hepatic Steatosis through Brown and Beige adipose tissue function. Cell Metab. 2016;24:118–29.

64. Hardie DG. AMPK–sensing energy while talking to other signaling pathways. Cell Metab. 2014;20:939–52.

65. Mulligan JD, Gonzalez AA, Stewart AM, Carey HV, Saupe KW. Upregulation of AMPK during cold exposure occurs via distinct mechanisms in brown and white adipose tissue of the mouse. J Physiol. 2007;580:677–84.

66. Labbe SM, Mouchiroud M, Caron A, Secco B, Freinkman E, Lamoureux G, Gelinas Y, Lecomte R, Bosse Y, Chimin P, et al. mTORC1 is required for Brown adipose tissue recruitment and metabolic adaptation to cold. Sci Rep. 2016;6:37223.

22

Renal effects of angiotensin II in the newborn period: role of type 1 and type 2 receptors

Angela E. Vinturache[*] and Francine G. Smith

Abstract

Background: Evidence suggests a critical role for the renin-angiotensin system in regulating renal function during postnatal development. However, the physiological relevance of a highly elevated renin-angiotensin system early in life is not well understood, nor which angiotensin receptors might be involved. This study was designed to investigate the roles of angiotensin receptors type 1 (AT1R) and type 2 (AT2R) in regulating glomerular and tubular function during postnatal development.

Methods: The renal effects of the selective antagonist to AT1R, ZD 7155 and to AT2R, PD 1233319 were evaluated in two groups of conscious chronically instrumented lambs aged ~ one week ($N = 8$) and ~ six weeks ($N = 10$). Two experiments were carried out in each animal and consisted of the assessment of renal variables including glomerular and tubular function, for 30 min before (Control) and 60 min after infusion of ZD 7155 and PD 123319, respectively. Statistical significance was determined using parametric testing (Student t-test, analysis of variance ANOVA) as appropriate.

Results: ZD 7155 infusion was associated with a significant decrease in glomerular filtration rate and filtration fraction at one but not six weeks; urinary flow rate decreased significantly in older animals, whereas sodium excretion and free water clearance were not altered. There was an age-dependent effect on potassium handling along the nephron, potassium excretion decreasing after ZD 7155 infusion in younger but not in older lambs. PD 123319 had no significant effects on glomerular filtration rate and tubular function in either age group.

Conclusions: These results provide evidence to support an important role for AT1Rs in mediating the renal effects of angiotensin II during postnatal maturation in conscious developing animals. In contrast to a role for AT2Rs later in life, there appears to be no role for AT2Rs in influencing the renal effects of Angiotensin II in the postnatal period.

Keywords: Newborn, Kidney, Angiotensin receptor type 1, Angiotensin receptor type 2, Angiotensin II, Electrolytes, Development

Background

The marked adaptive changes in renal function, including renal perfusion pressure, glomerular filtration [4, 35] and tubular function [5, 7, 10, 22, 24, 25, 44], at the time of birth may be mediated through complex temporal and spatial alterations in the level of expression and functionality of various factors, among which the renin-angiotensin system (RAS) may play a major role. All RAS components are highly expressed in numerous tissues and organs including the developing kidney of the fetus and the newborn and decrease gradually over the first months in an age-dependent manner (reviewed by Chen et al. (2004) [15]. Studies in mice, rats, sheep, swine and humans have shown that the expression and distribution of the angiotensin receptors (ATRs), type 1 (AT1R) and type 2 (AT2R), is developmentally regulated: A shift in the expression of ATRs subtypes occurs within the kidney, including the renal vasculature, from the AT2Rs, which predominate during fetal life, to AT1Rs whose expression is low in early gestation and increases

* Correspondence: aevintur@ucalgary.ca
Department of Physiology & Pharmacology; Alberta Children's Hospital Research Institute for Child and Maternal Health, Cumming School of Medicine, University of Calgary, 3330 Hospital Drive, NW, Calgary, AB T2N 4N1, Canada

with age to be the predominant receptor subtype expressed in the adult [1, 2, 6, 20, 49, 50, 63]. Previous studies from us in lambs [56] and from others in developing swine [6], human and simian kidney [63] support the dogma of altered intra-renal expression of ATRs genes with maturation.

Although strong evidence suggests the integrity of the AT1R signalling pathway is a pre-requisite for normal renal development [15, 28], the physiological effects mediated by activation of AT1Rs and/or AT2Rs during ontogeny are not well characterized [58].

Previous studies have shown that during the first six weeks of postnatal life, the pressor and vasoconstrictor effects of Angiotensin II (Ang II) are mediated through exclusive activation of AT1Rs in conscious chronically instrumented lambs [59]. Neonatal treatment with ACE inhibitors or AT1Rs antagonists produces irreversible renal anomalies and alters glomerular and tubular function in the newborn of several species, including the human [21, 26, 27, 37, 40, 43]. To date, however, the physiological relevance of renal AT2Rs during postnatal maturation is not known.

Therefore, the present study aims to address this gap in knowledge and investigate the roles of AT2Rs in regulating renal function in the developing kidney. Based on the anatomical evidence, we hypothesised that, under physiologic conditions, AT2Rs are more important in regulating renal function in the newborn, whereas AT1Rs predominantly regulate glomerular and tubular function later in life. To this end, we measured the responses to administration of selective antagonists to AT1Rs, ZD 7155, and to AT2Rs, PD123319, on various parameters of glomerular and tubular function in two groups of conscious chronically instrumented lambs aged ~ one week, newborns, and later in life, ~six weeks after birth.

Methods
Animals, maintenance and diet
Experiments were carried out in two age groups of conscious, chronically instrumented lambs: newborn lambs, aged ~ one week (8 ± 1 days; 7.4 ± 0.2 kg body weight; $N = 8$), and older animals, aged ~ six weeks (41 ± 1 days; 14.8 ± 0.1 kg body weight; $N = 10$). The choice of age reflects age-dependent major physiological changes that we have previously documented regarding baseline systemic and renal haemodynamics [21, 47], circulating levels of Ang II [39, 42], and the responsiveness of the systemic vasculature to vasoactive agents [45, 51].

Lambs were obtained from a local source (Woolfitt Acres, Olds, Alberta) and housed with their mothers in individual pens in the *vivarium* of the Health Science Center except during surgery, training and experiments. Lambs were allowed to suckle *ad libitum*. The lactating

ewes were provided with equilibrated diet of proteins, fat, crude fibers, minerals and vitamins and tap water *at libitum*.

All surgical and experimental procedures from this study were carried out with the approval of the Animal Care Committee at the University of Calgary, in accordance with the "Guide to the Care and Use of Experimental Animals" provided by the Canadian Council on Animal Care.

Surgical procedures
Surgery was performed on lambs using aseptic techniques as previously described [46, 59]. Following induction of isoflurane anaesthesia, catheters were inserted into left and right femoral arteries and veins (Tygon Microbore Tubing CO., USA) and advanced to the level of abdominal aorta and inferior vena cava, respectively for later infusion of drugs and fluids, arterial sampling and pressure measurements during experiments. Through a midline abdominal incision, the bladder was exposed and a catheter (adapted from a feeding tube, Medi-Craft Ltd., Malton, Ontario, Canada) was inserted directly across the bladder wall to be used for measurements of urinary flow rate and urine sample collection during experiments. A left flank incision exposed the left kidney and a pre-calibrated ultrasonic flow transducer (size 3-6S, Transonic Systems Inc., NY, USA) was placed around the renal artery for continuous measurements of renal blood flow during experiments. The incisions were closed and all catheters tunneled subcutaneously to exit the animal on the left and right flanks and secured inside pockets in a lamb body jacket (Lomir Inc., Montreal, Canada).

After surgery, animals were allowed to recover from the effects of anaesthesia and surgery inside a Shor-Line intensive care unit for small animals (Schroer Manufacturing Company, Kansas, USA) with adjustable temperature and oxygen supply. Lambs were returned to the ewe and closely monitored until suckling resumed. Antibiotic, Excenel° (Ceftriofur) 2.2 mg/kg, (Pfizer, Kirkland, QC, Canada), was administered intramuscularly prior to surgery and at 24 h intervals for the following 48 h. For at least four days of recovery after surgery, the lambs were trained for approximately one hour each day to rest comfortably in a supportive sling in the laboratory environment.

Experimental details
On the day of an experiment, each animal was transported to the laboratory and placed in the supportive sling. At least 60 min were allowed for the animal to become accustomed to its surroundings, during which a pre-warmed intravenous (I.V.) infusion of 5 % dextrose in 0.9 % sodium chloride administered at a rate of $4.17 \text{ mL} \cdot \text{kg}^{-1} \cdot \text{h}^{-1}$ through the right femoral venous catheter was initiated and continued for the duration of the study in order to assist fluid and electrolyte balance.

During this time the bladder was allowed to drain. A priming dose of lithium chloride was injected slowly (over ten seconds) 30 min before starting the experiments as a bolus injection of 200 $\mu m \cdot kg^{-1}$ for later determination of proximal tubular Na^+ reabsorption, as previously described [54, 55]. The left femoral venous and arterial catheters were connected to pressure transducers (Model P23XL, Statham, West Warwick RI, USA) for monitoring venous and arterial pressures, respectively. The flow transducer placed around the renal artery was connected to a flow meter (T101, Transonics Systems, Ithaca, NY) for measurement of renal blood flow (RBF). Haemodynamic variables were recorded onto a polygraph (Model 7, Grass Technologies, Astro-Med Inc., West Warwick, RI, USA) and simultaneously digitized at 200 Hz using the data acquisition and analysis software package, PolyVIEW™ (AstroMed Inc., Grass Technologies, Astro-Med Inc., West Warwick, RI, USA).

Two experiments were conducted in random order in each animal at 48 h intervals and consisted of a control period for 30 min (Control) followed by I.V. infusion for 60 min of either the angiotensin receptor antagonist, ZD 7155 (experiment one) or PD 123319 (experiment two) (Tocris Bioscince, Tocris Cookson Inc, Ellisville, MO, USA). Both drugs were administered as an I.V. infusion of 70 $\mu g \cdot kg^{-1} \cdot h^{-1}$ following an I.V. bolus of 100 $\mu g \cdot kg^{-1}$ using an infusion pump (Microinfusion pump MI 60-1B, World Precision Instruments, Sarasota, Fl, USA). These doses were carefully selected from previous dose–response experiments [14].

Urine was collected continuously and sampled at 30 min intervals. At the end of each collection period, urinary flow rate (V) was recorded and urine samples stored at –70 °C for later measurement of urinary electrolytes (Na^+, K^+, Li^+, Cl^-), urinary creatinine concentration and urinary osmolality (UOsm). At the midpoint of each 30 min urinary collection, blood samples (3.5 mL) were removed from the femoral arterial catheter. Whole blood (0.5 mL) was used for immediate measurement of haematocrit (Hct) using a microhaematocrit centrifuge (Clay Adams, Parsippany, NJ, USA). The remainder was placed into a chilled heparinised tube and immediately centrifuged; the supernatant was removed and stored at –70 °C for later measurement of the plasma concentrations of electrolytes (Na^+, K^+, Cl^-), plasma creatinine concentration and plasma osmolality. The volume of blood drawn was replaced with equal volumes of 5 % dextrose in 0.9 % NaCl to minimise the haemodynamic effects of sampling.

At the end of the experiments, lambs were euthanised with a lethal dose of barbiturate. The placement of the catheters was verified and the zero offset of the flow transducer was measured. Both kidneys were removed, examined grossly, and weighed to normalise measurements between the two age groups.

Analytical procedures

Urinary and plasma electrolytes (Na^+, K^+, Li^+, Cl^-), were measured on thawed samples by ion chromatography (IC 680, Methrom AG, Herisau, Switzerland). Urinary and plasma osmolalities were measured using a micro-osmometer (2430 Multi-OSMETTE™, Precision Systems Inc., Natic, MA, USA). Creatinine concentrations in urine and plasma were measured using a commercially available creatinine assay kit (QuantiChrom Creatinine assay kit, BioAssays Systems, Hayward, CA). Electrolyte concentrations in urine and plasma were used to calculate excretion rates, clearances, and reabsorptions. Creatinine measurements in urine and plasma were used to estimate glomerular filtration rate. Osmolality measurements in urine and plasma were used to calculate osmolar clearances and tubular water handling.

Data handling and analyses

Renal plasma flow (RPF) was calculated using the formula: RPF (mL/min) = [1 - (RBF x Hct)]. GFR was estimated as creatinine clearance: GFR = (UCr x V)/PCr. Filtration fraction (FF) was determined as GFR/RPF. Clearances of electrolytes (X) were calculated as follows: CX = (UX x V)/PX, where U and P refers to urinary and plasma concentrations of the electrolyte X and V is urinary flow rate. Fractional reabsorption (FR) of electrolytes was calculated from the ratio of electrolyte clearance to GFR: FRx (%) = [1- (CX/GFR)] x100. Proximal tubular Na^+ reabsorption was assumed equal to fractional Li^+ clearance (CLi/GFR). Free water clearance was calculated as the difference between urinary flow rate (V) and osmolar clearance. The ratio of urinary Na^+ concentration to urinary K^+ (UNa/UK) as well as the transtubular K^+ gradient (TTKG) were also calculated (TTKG = (UK/PK)/(UOsm/POsm), where UOsm/POsm is the ratio of UOsm to POsm and UK and PK are concentration of K^+ in urine and respectively plasma).

Renal haemodynamic variables and parameters of renal function were normalized per gram kidney weight to allow comparisons between the two different age groups since kidney weights were different at one and six weeks (Table 1).

Statistical analyses

Data were tested for normal distribution before statistical procedures were applied. Student's unpaired t-test was used to compare baseline measurements between the two groups. Two-way analysis of variance (ANOVA) procedures for repeated measures over time with factors age and treatment followed by Holm Sidak multiple comparisons were appropriate were used to compare the effects of the treatments between the groups. The Bonferroni correction was used to adjust for multiple comparisons. Significance was accepted

Table 1 Baseline demographic, haemodynamics, plasma and renal variables in conscious lambs

	One week	Six weeks
Animal characteristics		
Sample size, n	8	10
Sex	3♀/5♂	7♀/3♂
Age, days	8 (1)	41 (1)*
Kidney weight, g	62.9 (15.1)	80.6 (7.7)*
Baseline haemodynamics		
MAP, mmHg	72 (7)	77 (5)*
RBF, $mL \cdot g^{-1} \cdot min^{-1}$	1.7 (0.6)	4.0 (1.6)*
RVR, $mmHg \cdot g^{-1} \cdot min^{-1}$	44.7 (16.6)	19.1 (7.2)*
Baseline renal variables		
RPF, $mL \cdot g^{-1} \cdot min^{-1}$	1.07 (0.33)	5.60 (2.01)*
GFR, $mL \cdot g^{-1} \cdot min^{-1}$	0.39 (0.16)	0.37 (0.20)
FF, %	39.2 (22.8)	18.24 (11.6)*
V, $\mu L \cdot g^{-1} \cdot min^{-1}$	4.6 (1.5)	4.9 (3.4)
CH_2O, $\mu L \cdot g^{-1} \cdot min^{-1}$	−3.7 (2.8)	−8.3 (5.2)*
POsm, $mOsm/kgH_2O$	303 (9)	301 (8)
UOsm, $mOsm/kgH_2O$	627 (201)	835 (289)*
COsm, $\mu L \cdot g^{-1} \cdot min^{-1}$	7.9 (3.4)	10.6 (3.5)*
Plasma concentrations		
PNa, $mmol \cdot L^{-1}$	143.2 (5.5)	144.8 (9.3)
PK, $mmol \cdot L^{-1}$	3.5 (0.3)	3.7 (0.4)
PCl, $mmol \cdot L^{-1}$	65.4 (2.4)	64.7 (3.5)
Urinary excretion rates		
UNaV, $\mu mol \cdot g^{-1} \cdot min^{-1}$	0.05 (0.06)	0.05 (0.03)
UKV, $\mu mol \cdot g^{-1} \cdot min^{-1}$	0.51 (0.26)	0.84 (0.23)*
UClV, $\mu mol \cdot g^{-1} \cdot min^{-1}$	0.13 (0.12)	0.16 (0.11)
UNa/UK	0.07 (0.05)	0.08 (0.05)
TTKG	17.8 (6.9)	16.7 (3.1)
Renal clearances		
CNa, $\mu L \cdot g^{-1} \cdot min^{-1}$	0.2 (0.1)	1.1 (0.6)*
CCl, $\mu L \cdot g^{-1} \cdot min^{-1}$	2.0 (1.9)	2.4 (1.4)
CK, $mL^{-1} \cdot min^{-1}$	0.15 (0.1)	0.63 (0.3)*

Values are presented as mean (SD). *$p < 0.05$ six weeks compared with one week

MAP mean arterial pressure, *RBF* renal blood flow, *RVR* renal vascular resistance, *GFR* glomerular filtration rate, *RPF* renal plasma flow, *FF* filtration fraction, *V* urinary flow rate, *PX* plasma concentration of electrolyte X, *UXV* urinary excretion rate of electrolyte X, *CX* clearance of electrolyte X, *UNa/UK* urine Na^+ to K^+ ratio, *TTKG* transtubular K^+ gradient, *UOsm* urinary osmolality, *COsm* clearance of osmoles, *CH₂O* free water clearance

at the 95 % confidence interval. Data analysis was carried out using IBM SPSS statistical software (IBM SPSS Statistics for Windows, version 20.0, IBM Corp., Armonk, NY). All data were expressed as mean ± SD.

Results
Baseline parameters
The demographic characteristics and baseline variables of the two groups of lambs are presented in Table 1. Resting renal haemodynamics variables were significantly different between the groups; RVR was lower, whereas RBF was at higher at six weeks than at one week. There were no significant differences in baseline GFR when normalized per kidney weight between the two age groups. RPF and UOsm were significantly lower whereas FF was higher at one week as compared to six weeks. UKV and UClV were similar in both age groups, while CK and CNa were higher at six weeks.

Renal effects of the AT1R antagonist, ZD 7155
Infusion of ZD 7155 significantly altered systemic and renal haemodynamics variables in one and six week old lambs. As shown in Additional file 1: Table S1, arterial pressure fell by approximately 10 % within 10 min of infusion in both age groups of lambs, from 73 ± 6 mmHg to 63 ± 6 mmHg in one week old lambs and from 77 ± 5 to 69 ± 5 mmHg in six weeks old lambs ($p < 0.001$). Within 10 min of ZD 7155 infusion, RVR decreased in both age groups, whereas RBF increased from 4.1 ± 1.8 to 5.0 ± 2.1 $ml \cdot min^{-1} \cdot g^{-1}$ ($p < 0.001$) in older lambs and did not change in younger ones.

After ZD 7155 infusion, RPF increased in six but not in one week old lambs, from 5.7 ± 2.2 to 6.5 ± 2.5 $ml \cdot min^{-1} \cdot g^{-1}$ ($p = 0.018$). There was an age-dependent effect of ZD 7155 on GFR (F = 3.911, $p = 0.031$), which decreased in one week old lambs from 0.43 ± 0.13 $ml \cdot min^{-1} \cdot g^{-1}$ to 0.24 ± 0.18 $ml \cdot min^{-1} \cdot g^{-1}$ ($p = 0.010$). ZD 7155 did not significantly alter GFR in older lambs, although GFR tended to decline in this group as well, albeit to a lesser extent (from 0.43 ± 0.19 $ml \cdot min^{-1} \cdot g^{-1}$ to 0.37 ± 0.16 $ml \cdot min^{-1} \cdot g^{-1}$) (Fig. 1). Following the changes in RPF and GFR, ZD 7155 elicited age-dependent effects on FF (F = 5.889, $p = 0.009$). FF decreased from 48 ± 25 to 30 ± 26 % ($p = 0.002$) at one week and from 20 ± 10 to 12 ± 8 % at six weeks ($p = 0.145$) (Fig. 1).

Whereas UNaV was not influenced by the ZD 7155 treatment in either age group (Fig. 2), effects on K^+ excretion were age-dependent (F = 8.391, $p = 0.001$): ZD 7155 significantly decreased UKV in younger animals, from 0.62 ± 0.32 to 0.28 ± 0.22 $\mu mol \cdot min^{-1} \cdot g^{-1}$ but not in older ones (Fig. 2). This was accompanied by a decrease in TTKG by almost 30 % in younger lambs ($p < 0.001$) (Table 2). There was a trend towards an increase in the UNa/UK ratio after ZD 7155 infusion at one week but not six weeks ($p = 0.08$). There were no significant effects of the AT1R antagonist on Na^+ and K^+ reabsorption rates or CK in both groups of lambs (Table 2). CNa was altered by the infusion of ZD 7155 in an age-dependent manner: CNa increased in six but not one week old lambs (F = 28.577, $p < 0.001$).

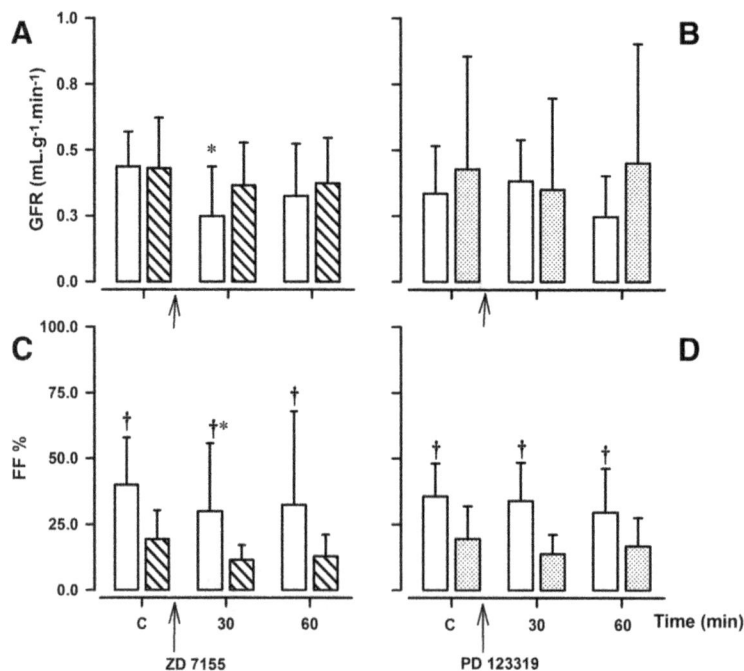

Fig. 1 Effects of ATR antagonists, ZD 7155 and PD 123319, on glomerular function in conscious lambs. Effects of ATR antagonists, ZD 7155 and PD 123319 on glomerular filtration rate (GFR; panel **a** and **b**), and filtration fraction (FF; panel **c** and **d**) in conscious lambs aged ~ one week (*open bars*) and ~ six weeks (*closed bars*) measured before (Control, **c**) and for 60 min after intravenous infusion of ZD 7155 (panels **a** and **c**, *striped line bars*) or PD 123319 (panels **b** and **d**, *gray shaded bars*). *$p < 0.001$ compared to C; †$p < 0.05$ compared to one week

V fell by ~ 50 % within 60 min of ZD 7155 infusion in older lambs ($p = 0.006$). Similar, there was a trend for V to decrease in younger animals; however, this did not reach statistical significance ($p = 0.058$) (Fig. 2).

There were also age-dependent effects of ZD 7155 treatment on UOsm (F = 27.721, $p < 0.001$) and COsm

(F = 7.267, $p = 0.017$). UOsm increased in six but not one week old lambs after 60 min of AT1R antagonist infusion ($p = 0.004$) (Fig. 2), whereas COsm decreased in one week old lambs ($p < 0.001$) (Table 2). There were no effects of ZD 7155 on CH2O or the UOsm/POsm ratio in either age group.

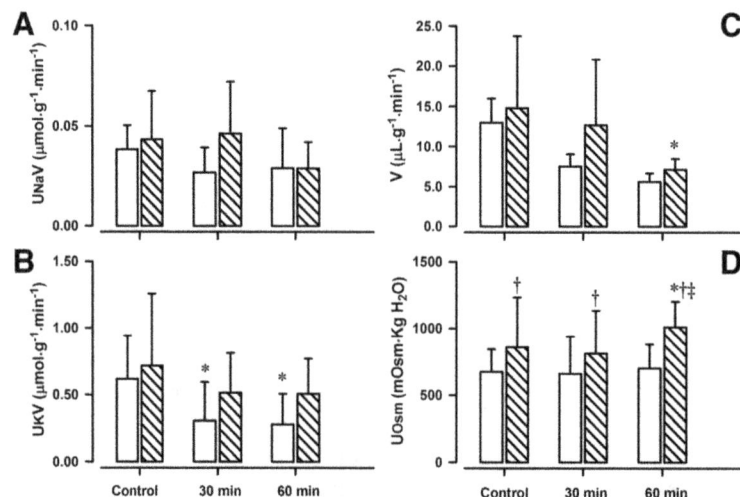

Fig. 2 Effects of AT1R antagonist, ZD 7155 on tubular function in conscious lambs. Effects of AT1R antagonist, ZD 7155, on urinary Na$^+$ excretion rate (UNaV, panel **a**), urinary K$^+$ excretion rate (UKV, panel **c**), urinary flow rate (V, panel **b**), and urine osmolality (UOsm, panel **d**) in conscious lambs aged ~ one week (*open bars*) and ~ six week (*closed, striped line bars*) measured before (Control, **c**) and for 60 min after intravenous infusion of ZD 7155. *$p < 0.001$ compared to **c**; †$p < 0.05$ compared to one week

Table 2 Tubular effects of the AT1R antagonist ZD 7155 in conscious lambs

Variable	One week			Six weeks		
	Control	30 min	60 min	Control	30 min	60 min
CNa ($\mu L \cdot g^{-1} \cdot min^{-1}$)	0.24 ± 0.05	0.18 ± 0.08	0.21 ± 0.16	0.90 ± 0.52**	0.94 ± 0.42**	0.62 ± 0.29**,*
FRNa %	99.93 ± 0.03	99.90 ± 0.08	99.73 ± 0.60	99.90 ± 0.12	99.84 ± 0.23	99.89 ± 0.12
PRNa %	78.3 ± 8.8	81.8 ± 9.1	84.1 ± 10.8	70.4 ± 19.1**	69.4 ± 21.1**	70.1 ± 15.6**
DRNa %	21.7 ± 8.8	18.1 ± 9.1	15.6 ± 10.6	29.5 ± 19.1**	30.6 ± 21.6**	29.8 ± 15.6**
CK ($mL \cdot g^{-1} \cdot min^{-1}$)	0.18 ± 0.10	0.09 ± 0.08	0.09 ± 0.07	0.64 ± 0.34**	0.45 ± 0.16**	0.39 ± 0.16**
FRK %	59.2 ± 17.1	66.0 ± 16.3	64.3 ± 23.7	56.7 ± 18.9	53.5 ± 14.3	57.0 ± 26.0
UNa/UK	0.08 ± 0.03	0.15 ± 0.13	0.12 ± 0.10	0.07 ± 0.04	0.10 ± 0.09	0.10 ± 0.10
TTKG	21 ± 7	17 ± 4*	16 ± 2*	17 ± 3	16 ± 3	16 ± 2**
CCl ($\mu L \cdot g^{-1} \cdot min^{-1}$)	2.0 ± 1.0	1.2 ± 0.9	0.9 ± 0.5*	2.2 ± 1.0	2.5 ± 1.7	2.6 ± 1.5
FRCl %	99.51 ± 0.24	99.46 ± 0.33	99.31 ± 0.92*	99.29 ± 0.39	99.62 ± 1.82	99.15 ± 0.49**
COsm ($\mu L \cdot g^{-1} \cdot min^{-1}$)	8.9 ± 1.3	4.6 ± 3.3*	4.2 ± 1.4*	10.1 ± 3.1	8.5 ± 3.3**	8.2 ± 1.9**
UOsm/POsm	1.9 ± 0.5	2.2 ± 0.8	2.2 ± 0.6	2.8 ± 1.2	2.7 ± 1.1	3.1 ± 1.2
CH$_2$O ($\mu L \cdot g^{-1} \cdot min^{-1}$)	-5.1 ± 1.4	-3.1 ± 2.9	-2.3 ± 1.2	-6.9 ± 2.8	-5.7 ± 2.8	-5.6 ± 2.4**

Data are mean ± SD. *$p < 0.05$ compared to C; **$p < 0.05$ compared to one week old lambs

CX clearance of electrolyte X, FRX fractional reabsorption of electrolyte X, PRX proximal reabsorption of electrolyte X, DRX distal reabsorption of electrolyte X, UNa/UK urine Na$^+$ to K$^+$ ratio, TTKG transtubular K$^+$ gradient, UOsm urinary osmolality, COsm clearance of osmoles, CH$_2$O free water clearance

Renal effects of PD 123319

The AT2R antagonist, PD 123319 had no significant effects on systemic and renal haemodynamics in either group of animals (Additional file 1: Table S1). There were also no changes in RPF, GFR or FF after infusion of PD 123319 (Fig. 1) in either age group. Also, no changes were observed in urine production (Fig. 3) and electrolyte excretion rates of Na$^+$, K$^+$, (Fig. 3) and Cl$^-$ (Table 3) after PD 123319 at one and six weeks. PD 123319 infusion did not alter reabsorption rates and clearances of electrolytes, urine osmolality nor osmolar clearance (Table 3).

Administration of ATRs antagonists, ZD 7155 and PD 123319, had no significant effects on plasma Na$^+$, K$^+$ and Cl$^-$ concentration, nor did it influence plasma osmolality in either of the age groups (Additional file 2: Table S2).

Discussion

The present study, exploring the potential roles of Ang II receptors type 1, AT1Rs and type 2, AT2Rs in

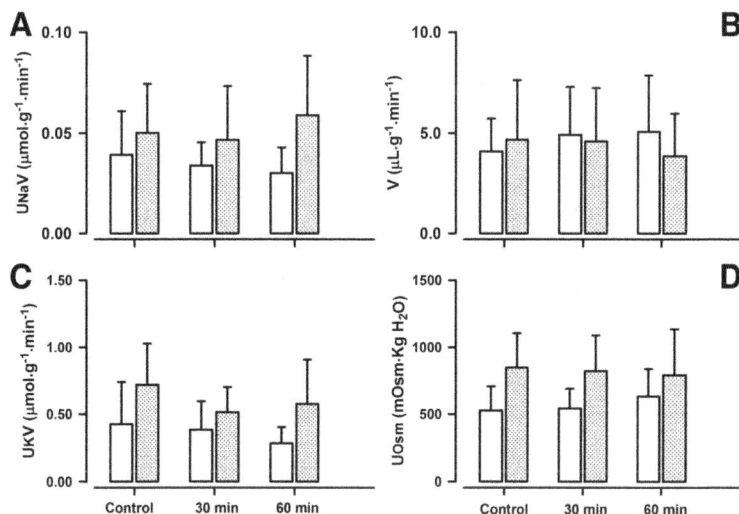

Fig. 3 Effects of AT2R antagonist PD 123319 on tubular function in conscious lambs. Effects of AT2R antagonist, PD 123319 on urinary Na$^+$ excretion rate (UNaV, panel **a**), urinary K$^+$ excretion rate (UKV, panel **c**), urinary flow rate (V, panel **b**), and urine osmolality (UOsm, panel **d**) in conscious lambs aged ~ one week (*open bars*) and ~ six week (*closed, gray shaded bars*) measured before (Control, **c**) and for 60 min after intravenous infusion of ZD 7155. *$p < 0.001$ compared to **c**; †$p < 0.05$ compared to one week

Table 3 Tubular effects of the AT2R antagonist PD 123319 in conscious lambs

Variable	One week			Six weeks		
	Control	30 min	60 min	Control	30 min	60 min
CNa (μL $\cdot$ g^{-1} $\cdot$ min^{-1})	0.14 ± 0.08	0.23 ± 0.18	0.36 ± 0.44	1.2 ± 0.6**	1.0 ± 0.5**	1.4 ± 1.2**
FRNa %	99.89 ± 0.13	99.85 ± 0.22	99.75 ± 0.30	99.88 ± 0.09	99.86 ± 0.13	99.86 ± 0.14
PRNa %	78.8 ± 11.2	80.1 ± 8.8	77.9 ± 8.3	67.0 ± 20.3**	67.4 ± 20.2**	72.7 ± 21.0**
DRNa %	21.1 ± 11.1	19.8 ± 8.7	21.9 ± 8.1	35.9 ± 19.0**	35.5 ± 18.8**	29.5 ± 20.8**
CK (mL $\cdot$ g^{-1} $\cdot$ min^{-1})	0.11 ± 0.10	0.12 ± 0.06	0.09 ± 0.03	0.62 ± 0.28**	0.47 ± 0.12**	0.42 ± 0.18**
FRK %	66.7 ± 16.2	66.7 ± 15.9	62.1 ± 16.2	52.8 ± 27.6	47.3 ± 24.3	68.1 ± 16.7
UNa/UK	0.07 ± 0.05	0.09 ± 0.06	0.14 ± 0.14	0.09 ± 0.05	0.11 ± 0.09	0.10 ± 0.09
TTKG	15 ± 5	15 ± 5	13 ± 5	17 ± 3	14 ± 2*	13 ± 4*
CCl (μL $\cdot$ g^{-1} $\cdot$ min^{-1})	2.1 ± 2.1	2.5 ± 2.0	2.1 ± 2.0	2.7 ± 1.8	2.4 ± 1.6	2.8 ± 1.5
FRCl %	99.42 ± 0.39	99.45 ± 0.42	99.30 ± 0.66	99.97 ± 0.02	99.97 ± 0.02	99.97 ± 0.02
COsm (μL $\cdot$ g^{-1} $\cdot$ min^{-1})	7.2 ± 3.9	8.1 ± 4.2	7.4 ± 2.8	10.9 ± 3.7	11.4 ± 3.2	11.1 ± 5.4
UOsm/POsm	1.7 ± 0.5	1.7 ± 0.5	2.0 ± 0.7	2.4 ± 0.7	2.8 ± 0.9	2.1 ± 0.7
CH$_2$O (mL $\cdot$ g^{-1} $\cdot$ min^{-1})	−3.2 ± 2.7	−3.2 ± 2.4	−2.6 ± 2.1	−7.5 ± 3.3**	−7.1 ± 1.9**	−5.7 ± 3.7

Data are mean ± SD. *$p < 0.05$ compared to C; **$p < 0.05$ six weeks compared to one week
V urinary flow rate, *CX* clearance of electrolyte X, *FRX* fractional reabsorption of electrolyte X, *PRX* proximal reabsorption of electrolyte X, *DRX* distal reabsorption of electrolyte X, *UNa/UK* urine Na$^+$ to K$^+$ ratio, *TTKG* transtubular K$^+$ gradient, *UOsm* urinary osmolality, *COsm* clearance of osmoles, *CH$_2$O* free water clearance

regulating renal function during postnatal maturation, provides new information on the renal effects of ATRs during the newborn period as follows: i) glomerular ultrafiltration is regulated by Ang II through activation of AT1Rs in an age-dependent manner; ii) production of urine is modulated by activation of AT1Rs predominantly later in life; iii) AT1Rs mediate the effects of Ang II of K$^+$ handling along the nephron in an age-dependent manner; iv) AT2Rs alone do not appear to mediate any of the glomerular and tubular effects of Ang II in the newborn period. Therefore, our current findings provide new evidence that, early in life, in conscious animals, Ang II regulates both, glomerular and tubular function through predominant activation of AT1Rs but not AT2Rs.

To our knowledge, no previous studies have explored the roles of ATRs in regulating kidney function in newborns in the conscious, undisturbed state. To date, the evidence is limited to the roles of AT1Rs and comes from studies in anaesthetised newborns animals. For instance, in anaesthetised newborn rabbits, the AT1R antagonist, losartan, elicits dose-dependent systemic and glomerular responses [40]. In neonatal rats, chronic subcutaneous administration of DuP 753 decreased arterial pressure but left GFR unchanged [16]. Intra-renal infusion of the AT1R antagonist A-81988, increased RBF in three weeks old piglets, while the effects on glomerular function were similar in young and adult anaesthetised pigs [52]. This is in contrast with transient effect of the selective AT1R antagonist, ZD 7155 on GFR only in newborns lambs observed in the current experiments in conscious lambs. The differences in responses to AT1R

inhibition may be a consequence of selectivity, dose and mode of administration of the drugs (systemic vs. intrarenal), or related to variability in terms of age, renal maturation (level of expression and localization of the receptors within kidney regions in different species), as well as the experimental setting (anaesthetised vs. conscious). Anaesthesia has been shown to activate the RAS and it is conceivable that, in the anaesthetised animals, the RAS is up-regulated to levels much higher than that of conscious newborn animals.

Based on the distinct pattern of ATRs distribution in the developing kidney in several species, including porcine, ovine and primate kidney [6, 29, 30, 41, 49, 56, 57, 61, 63], we hypothesised that immediately after birth activation of AT2Rs may contribute to the adaptation of glomerular function in the immediate newborn period. This was not the case. Our study shows that endogenous Ang II effects on glomerular function are mediated entirely through activation of AT1Rs, likely through a predominant effect on efferent arterioles, with no apparent role for AT2Rs. Nonetheless, the contribution of AT2R in regulating vasomotor activity of the intrarenal vasculature cannot be ruled out at this time and remains to be elucidated.

The intriguing observation that the decline of GFR after ZD 7155 was not sustained in newborn lambs despite the continued inhibition of AT1Rs, also lends support to the concept of redundant mechanisms that are, most likely, already in place at birth. Thus, the newborn kidney is probably able to mobilise additional vasoactive factors to maintain glomerular filtration. For example, AT1R inhibition may have revealed the role of other vasoactive factors, such as prostaglandins, bradykinin, or nitric oxide. Previously, we have reported that the renal haemodynamic effects of nitric oxide are regulated by Ang II through activation of both ATRs [57, 60] in an age-dependent manner, with AT2Rs being a more important regulator of renal haemodynamics in the newborn and AT1Rs more predominant later in life [57]. Also, pre-treatment with the cyclooxygenase inhibitor, indomethacin, augments the pressor response to Ang II and modulates the vasomotor effect of Ang II in response to infusion of the nitric oxide inhibitor, L-NAME, thus removing endogenously produced nitric oxide [23]. Taken together, these findings may suggest that AT2Rs may not need to be recruited to assist in regulating glomerular function in the face of the numerous vasodilators already present.

In adulthood, the effects of Ang II in regulating sodium transport within the kidney, ranging from natriuresis to antinatriuresis are mediated through multiple receptors, including AT1Rs and AT2Rs. Much less is known about Ang II contribution to Na^+ handling in newborn mammals [29, 32, 53]. For example, in adult animals, in which the RAS is activated by dietary salt restriction, treatment with ACE inhibitors elicits a robust increase in water and electrolyte excretion [12, 36]. Therefore, we anticipated that, in newborn lambs, in which the RAS is also activated [9, 34], there would be a significant increase in water and electrolyte excretion after ATRs inhibition. We also predicted that AT2Rs, which are the predominant type of ATRs expressed within the kidney after birth, may play a predominant role in water and electrolyte handling in the newborn. This was not the case. Effects of Ang II on renal handling of water and electrolytes appeared rather to be mediated predominantly through activation of AT1Rs in an age-dependent manner, whereas AT2Rs do not appear to regulate water and salt handling along the nephron in developing animals.

The decrease in K^+ excretion in young animals reported in the present study may be due to inhibition of aldosterone secretion through a feedback mechanism at the adrenal gland level, or by inhibition of possible direct regulatory mechanisms of Ang II on K^+ channels along the collecting duct. The decrease in the flow of tubular fluid in this age group may have contributed to a fall in K^+ secretion and, therefore, a reduction in K^+ excretion rate. Absence of significant changes in the UNa/UK ratio may suggest that aldosterone levels may not have been altered after ATRs inhibition. Further studies are needed to explore more in depth the effects of ATRs inhibition on aldosterone activity in newborn.

Our findings are in keeping with observations of the renal effects of the AT1R antagonist losartan in adult, salt-depleted animals, in which the RAS is also activated,

similar to newborn lambs in the present experiments [3, 8, 17, 19, 62]. For instance, in sodium-depleted anaesthetised adult rats, AT1R antagonists decreased GFR, urine and electrolytes excretion [16, 33], whereas in sodium-depleted conscious and anaesthetised adult dogs, AT1R antagonists increased GFR and elicited a significant increase in urine volume and urinary sodium excretion rate [8, 18, 31]. However, in this species, AT2R inhibition antagonized the vasoconstrictor effects of exogenous Ang II and induced an increase in urine flow and free water formation, suggesting a functional role for AT2Rs in water handling by the adult kidney [18, 31]. Other studies in adult animals have shown a role for AT2R in mediating vasodilation, natriuresis and diuresis [11, 38], albeit these effects were revealed in anesthetised animals, in conditions of RAS activation and AT1Rs inhibition. As such, an age-dependent functional role for AT2R in renal homeostasis awaits confirmation.

Strengths and limitations

There are several limitations to our study: i) Due to the technical limitations of surgery and postoperative recovery, the effects of ATRs activation immediately after birth, especially within the first few days after birth could not be evaluated; ii) The sample size in this study was predetermined in order to identify significant changes in arterial pressure [13, 59]. Heterogeneity in study designs and lack of power calculations in most of the previous reports that investigated the effects of ATRs in newborns, offered limited information for sample size calculation in our study; iii) For some of the physiologic variables studied, a trend in changes was observed that did not reach statistical significance. This may be altered if the group sizes were considerably larger although our previous evaluations of renal function in these two age groups have revealed significant differences with similar sample sizes [39, 48]; iv) We were not able to describe the continuum of changes in ATRs functions from one to six weeks after birth, thus we could not determine the postnatal age at which the changes in the activity of ATRs occur. On the other hand, as opposed to the previous studies in fetal animals, which provide only a snapshot of the ATRs function at one gestational age, our study evaluated renal effects of ATRs antagonists at two different stages of postnatal development, thus providing an insight into the physiological changes of renal function that occur with the process of maturation and transition to adulthood. Furthermore, our study was conducted in conscious animals, trained to the laboratory environment, and, therefore, the findings represent physiological conditions.

Conclusions

In summary, the present observations provide evidence for a more important role for Ang II through AT1Rs in governing renal function during the critical period of postnatal development and adaptation to extra-uterine life. AT1Rs are the predominant effectors of Ang II mediated renal effects throughout postnatal maturation, whereas the physiological functions of AT2R in modulating the kidney have not been elucidated. Additional studies are warranted to explore potential roles of the AT2Rs in modulating AT1R-mediated renal responses during ontogeny.

Abbreviations

AngII: angiotensin II; AT1R: angiotensin receptor type 1; AT2R: angiotensin receptor type 2; CH2O: free water clearance; COsm: clearance of osmoles; CX: clearance of electrolyte X; DRX: distal reabsorption of electrolyte X; FF: filtration fraction; FRX: fractional reabsorption of electrolyte X; GFR: glomerular filtration rate; MAP: mean arterial pressure; Osm: osmolality; PRX: proximal reabsorption of electrolyte X; PX: plasma concentration of electrolyte X; RAS: renin-angiotensin system; RBF: renal blood flow; RPF: renal plasma flow; RVR: renal vascular resistance; TTKG: transtubular K+ gradient; UNa/UK: urine Na$^+$ to K$^+$ ratio; UOsm: urinary osmolality; UXV: urinary excretion rate of electrolyte X; V: urinary flow rate.

Competing interests

The authors declare that they have no competing interests.

Authors' contributions

AV conceived, designed and carried out the experiments, participated in animal care and instrumentation, performed the analytical and statistical analyses, and drafted the manuscript. FG conceived the principle of the study, participated in its design and coordination and edited the manuscript. Both authors read and approved the final manuscript.

Acknowledgements

This work was supported by an Operating Grant provided by the Canadian Institutes for Health Research. At the time of these studies, AEV was a doctoral candidate supported by the CIHR Training Program in Genetics, Child Development, and Health, Queen Elizabeth II, and Faculty of Graduate Studies graduate awards. The authors gratefully acknowledge Dr. Wei Qi and Mrs. Lucy Yu for technical assistance with the animals.

References

1. Aguilera G, Kapur S, Feuillan P, Sunar-Akbasak B, Bathia AJ. Developmental changes in angiotensin II receptor subtypes and AT1 receptor mRNA in rat kidney. Kidney Int. 1994;46:973–9.
2. Allen AM, Zhuo J, Mendelsohn FA. Localization of angiotensin AT1 and AT2 receptors. JASN. 1999;10 Suppl 11:S23–9.
3. Andersen JL, Sandgaard NCF, Bie P. Volume expansion during acute angiotensin II receptor (AT1) blockade and NOS inhibition in conscious dogs. Am J Physiol Regul Integr Comp Physiol. 2002;282:R1140–8.
4. Aperia A, Broberger O, Elinder G, Herin P, Zetterstrom R. Postnatal development of renal function in pre-term and full-term infants. Acta Paediatr Scand. 1981;70:183–7.
5. Aperia A, Herin P, Lundin S, Melin P, Zetterstrom R. Regulation of renal water excretion in newborn full-term infants. Acta Paediatr Scand. 1984;73:717–21.
6. Bagby SP, LeBard LS, Luo Z, Ogden BE, Corless C, McPherson ED, Speth RC. ANG II AT(1) and AT(2) receptors in developing kidney of normal microswine. Am J Physiol Renal Physiol. 2002;283:F755–64.
7. Berry LM, Ikegami M, Woods E, Ervin MG. Postnatal renal adaptation in preterm and term lambs. Reprod Fertil Dev. 1995;7:491–8.
8. Bovee KC, Wong PC, Timmermans PB, Thoolen MJ. Effects of the nonpeptide angiotensin II receptor antagonist DuP 753 on blood pressure and renal functions in spontaneously hypertensive PH dogs. Am J Hypertens. 1991;4:327S–33.
9. Broughton Pipkin F, Lumbers ER, Mott JC. Birth and angiotensin II-like activity in lambs. J Physiol. 1972;226:109P–10.
10. Bueva A, Guignard JP. Renal function in preterm neonates. Pediatric Res. 1994;36:572–7.
11. Carey RM, Padia SH. Angiotensin AT2 receptors: control of renal sodium excretion and blood pressure. Trends Endocrinol Metab. 2008;19:84–7.
12. Carmines PK, Rosivall L, Till MF, Navar LG. Renal hemodynamic effects of captopril in anesthetized sodium-restricted dogs. Relative contributions of prostaglandin stimulation and suppressed angiotensin activity. Renal Physiol. 1983;6:281–7.
13. Chappellaz ML, Smith FG. Dose-dependent systemic and renal haemodynamic effects of angiotensin II in conscious lambs: role of angiotensin AT1 and AT2 receptors. Exp Physiol. 2005;90:837–45.
14. Chappellaz ML, Smith FG. Systemic and renal hemodynamic effects of the AT1 receptor antagonist, ZD 7155, and the AT2 receptor antagonist, PD 123319, in conscious lambs. Pflugers Arch. 2007;453:477–86.
15. Chen Y, Lasaitiene D, Friberg P. The renin-angiotensin system in kidney development. Acta Paediatr Scand. 2004;181:529–35.
16. Chevalier RL, Thornhill BA, Belmonte DC, Baertschi AJ. Endogenous angiotensin II inhibits natriuresis after acute volume expansion in the neonatal rat. Exp Physiol. 1996;270:R393–7.
17. Clark KL, Hilditch A, Robertson MJ, Drew GM. Effects of dopamine DA1-receptor blockade and angiotensin converting enzyme inhibition on the renal actions of fenoldopam in the anaesthetized dog. J Hypertens. 1991;9:1143–50.
18. Clark KL, Robertson MJ, Drew GM. Role of angiotensin AT1 and AT2 receptors in mediating the renal effects of angiotensin II in the anaesthetized dog. Br J Pharmacol. 1993;109:148–56.
19. Cogan MG, Xie MH, Liu FY, Wong PC, Timmermans PB. Effects of DuP 753 on proximal nephron and renal transport. Am J Hyperten. 1991;Suppl 4:315S–20.
20. Cox BE, Rosenfeld CR. Ontogeny of vascular angiotensin II receptor subtype expression in ovine development. Pediatric Res. 1999;45:414–24.
21. de Wildt SN, Smith FG. Effects of the angiotensin converting enzyme (ACE) inhibitor, captopril, on the cardiovascular, endocrine, and renal responses to furosemide in conscious lambs. Can J Physiol Pharmacol. 1997;75:263–70.
22. Drukker A, Guignard J. Renal aspects of the term and preterm infant: a selective update. Curr Opin Pediatr. 2002;14:175–82.
23. Ebenezar KK, Wong AK, Smith FG. Haemodynamic responses to angiotensin II in conscious lambs: role of nitric oxide and prostaglandins. Pflugers Arch. 2012;463:399–404.
24. Gruskin AB, Edelmann Jr CM, Yuan S. Maturational changes in renal blood flow in piglets. Pediatr Res. 1970;4:7–13.
25. Guignard JP. Renal function in the newborn infant. Pediatr Clin North Am. 1982;29:777–90.
26. Guron G, Nilsson A, DiBona GF, Sundelin B, Nitescu N, Friberg P. Renal adaptation to dietary sodium restriction and loading in rats treated neonatally with enalapril. Am J Physiol. 1997;273:R1421–9.
27. Guron G, Nilsson A, Leyssac PP, Sundelin B, Friberg P. Proximal tubular function in adult rats treated neonatally with enalapril. Acta Physiol Scand. 1998;164:99–106.
28. Guron G, Sundelin B, Wickman A, Friberg P. Angiotensin-converting enzyme inhibition in piglets induces persistent renal abnormalities. Clin Exp Pharmacol Physiol. 1998;25:88–91.
29. Hill KJ, Lumbers ER. Renal function in adult and fetal sheep. J Dev Physiol. 1988;10:149–59.
30. Kakuchi J, Ichiki T, Kiyama S, Hogan BL, Fogo A, Inagami T, Ichikawa I. Developmental expression of renal angiotensin II receptor genes in the mouse. Kidney Int. 1995;47:140–7.
31. Keiser JA, Bjork FA, Hodges JC, Taylor Jr DG. Renal hemodynamic and excretory responses to PD 123319 and losartan, nonpeptide AT1 and AT2 subtype-specific angiotensin II ligands. J Pharm Exp Ther. 1992;262:1154–60.
32. Kleinman LI. Renal sodium reabsorption during saline loading and distal blockade in newborn dogs. Am J Physiol. 1975;228:1403–8.
33. Macari D, Bottari S, Whitebread S, De Gasparo M, Levens N. Renal actions of the selective angiotensin AT2 receptor ligands CGP 42112B and PD 123319 in the sodium-depleted rat. Eur J Pharmacol. 1993;249:85–93.

34. Mott JC. The place of the renin-angiotensin system before and after birth. Br Med Bull. 1975;31:44–50.

35. Nakamura KT, Matherne GP, McWeeny OJ, Smith BA, Robillard JE. Renal hemodynamics and functional changes during the transition from fetal to newborn life in sheep. Pediatric Res. 1987;21:229–34.

36. Navar LG, Jirakulsomchok D, Bell PD, Thomas CE, Huang WC. Influence of converting enzyme inhibition on renal hemodynamics and glomerular dynamics in sodium-restricted dogs. Hypertension. 1982;4:58–68.

37. Nilsson AB, Friberg P. Acute renal responses to angiotensin-converting enzyme inhibition in the neonatal pig. Pediatr Nephrol. 2000;14:1071–6.

38. Padia SH, Howell NL, Siragy HM, Carey RM. Renal angiotensin type 2 receptors mediate natriuresis via angiotensin III in the angiotensin II type 1 receptor-blocked rat. Hypertension. 2006;47:537–44.

39. Patel A, Smith FG. Renal haemodynamic effects of B2 receptor agonist bradykinin and B2 receptor antagonist HOE 140 in conscious lambs. Exp Physiol. 2000;85:811–7.

40. Prevot A, Mosig D, Guignard JP. The effects of losartan on renal function in the newborn rabbit. Pediatric Res. 2002;51:728–32.

41. Ratliff BB, Sekulic M, Rodebaugh J, Solhaug MJ. Angiotensin II regulates NOS expression in afferent arterioles of the developing porcine kidney. Pediatric Res. 2010;68:29–34.

42. Robillard JE, Smith FG, Segar JL, Guillery EN, Jose PA. Mechanisms regulating renal sodium excretion during development. Pediatr Nephrol. 1992;6:205–13.

43. Robillard JE, Weismann DN, Gomez RA, Ayres NA, Lawton WJ, VanOrden DE. Renal and adrenal responses to converting-enzyme inhibition in fetal and newborn life. Am J Physiol. 1983;244:R249–56.

44. Robillard JE, Weismann DN, Herin P. Ontogeny of single glomerular perfusion rate in fetal and newborn lambs. Pediatric Res. 1981;15:1248–55.

45. Sener A, Smith FG. Acetylcholine chloride and renal hemodynamics during postnatal maturation in conscious lambs. J Appl Physiol. 1999;87:1296–300.

46. Sener A, Smith FG. Dose-dependent effects of nitric oxide synthase inhibition on systemic and renal hemodynamics in conscious lambs. Can J Physiol Pharmacol. 1999;77:1–7.

47. Sener A, Smith FG. Nitric oxide modulates arterial baroreflex control of heart rate in conscious lambs in an age-dependent manner. Am J Physiol Heart Circ Physiol. 2001;280:H2255–63.

48. Sener A, Smith FG. Glomerular and tubular responses to N(G)-nitro-L-arginine methyl ester are age dependent in conscious lambs. Am J Physiol Regul Integr Comp Physiol. 2002;282:R1512–20.

49. Shanmugam S, Corvol P, Gasc JM. Ontogeny of the two angiotensin II type 1 receptor subtypes in rats. Am J Physiol. 1994;267:E828–36.

50. Shanmugam S, Lenkei ZG, Gasc JM, Corvol PL, Llorens-Cortes CM. Ontogeny of angiotensin II type 2 (AT2) receptor mRNA in the rat. Kidney Int. 1995;47:1095–100.

51. Smith FG, Abraham J. Renal and renin responses to furosemide in conscious lambs during postnatal maturation. Can J Physiol Pharmacol. 1995;73:107–12.

52. Solhaug MJ, Wallace MR, Granger JP. Nitric oxide and angiotensin II regulation of renal hemodynamics in the developing piglet. Pediatric Res. 1996;39:527–33.

53. Spitzer A. The role of the kidney in sodium homeostasis during maturation. Kidney Int. 1982;21:539–45.

54. Thomsen K, Olesen OV. Renal lithium clearance as a measure of the delivery of water and sodium from the proximal tubule in humans. Am J Med Sci. 1984;288:158–61.

55. Thomsen K, Schou M, Steiness I, Hansen HE. Lithium as an indicator of proximal sodium reabsorption. Pflugers Arch. 1969;308:180–4.

56. Vinturache AE, Qi W, Smith FG. Age dependent expression of angiotensin II receptors in the ovine kidney. FASEB J. 2009;23:606.2.

57. Vinturache AE, Smith FG. Angiotensin receptors modulate the renal hemodynamic effects of nitric oxide in conscious newborn lambs. Physiol Rep. 2014;2:5. doi:10.14814/phy2.12027.

58. Vinturache AE, Smith FG. Angiotensin type 1 and type 2 receptors during ontogeny: cardiovascular and renal effects. Vascul Pharmacol. 2014;63:145–54.

59. Vinturache AE, Smith FG. Do angiotensin type 2 receptors modulate haemodynamic effects of type 1 receptors in conscious newborn lambs? Vascul Pharmacol. 2014;63:145–54.

60. Wehlage SJ, Smith FG. Nitric oxide and angiotensin II regulate cardiovascular homeostasis and the arterial baroreflex control of heart rate in conscious lambs. J Renin Angiotensin Aldosterone Syst. 2011;13:99–106.

61. Wintour EM, Alcorn D, Butkus A, Congiu M, Earnest L, Pompolo S, Potocnik SJ. Ontogeny of hormonal and excretory function of the meso- and metanephros in the ovine fetus. Kidney Int. 1996;50:1624–33.

62. Wong PC, Price Jr WA, Chiu AT, Duncia JV, Carini DJ, Wexler RR, Johnson AL, Timmermans PB. In vivo pharmacology of DuP 753. Am J Hypertens. 1991;4:288S–98.

63. Zoetis T, Hurtt ME. Species comparison of anatomical and functional renal development. Birth Defects Res B Dev Reprod Toxicol. 2003;68:111–20.

Permissions

The contributors of this book come from diverse backgrounds, making this book a truly international effort. This book will bring forth new frontiers with its revolutionizing research information and detailed analysis of the nascent developments around the world.

We would like to thank all the contributing authors for lending their expertise to make the book truly unique. They have played a crucial role in the development of this book. Without their invaluable contributions this book wouldn't have been possible. They have made vital efforts to compile up to date information on the varied aspects of this subject to make this book a valuable addition to the collection of many professionals and students.

This book was conceptualized with the vision of imparting up-to-date information and advanced data in this field. To ensure the same, a matchless editorial board was set up. Every individual on the board went through rigorous rounds of assessment to prove their worth. After which they invested a large part of their time researching and compiling the most relevant data for our readers.

The editorial board has been involved in producing this book since its inception. They have spent rigorous hours researching and exploring the diverse topics which have resulted in the successful publishing of this book. They have passed on their knowledge of decades through this book. To expedite this challenging task, the publisher supported the team at every step. A small team of assistant editors was also appointed to further simplify the editing procedure and attain best results for the readers.

Apart from the editorial board, the designing team has also invested a significant amount of their time in understanding the subject and creating the most relevant covers. They scrutinized every image to scout for the most suitable representation of the subject and create an appropriate cover for the book.

The publishing team has been an ardent support to the editorial, designing and production team. Their endless efforts to recruit the best for this project, has resulted in the accomplishment of this book. They are a veteran in the field of academics and their pool of knowledge is as vast as their experience in printing. Their expertise and guidance has proved useful at every step. Their uncompromising quality standards have made this book an exceptional effort. Their encouragement from time to time has been an inspiration for everyone.

The publisher and the editorial board hope that this book will prove to be a valuable piece of knowledge for researchers, students, practitioners and scholars across the globe.

Contributors

Daniel A Beard and Muriel Mescam
Center for Computational Medicine, Biotechnology and Bioengineering Center, Department of Physiology, Medical College of Wisconsin, Milwaukee, WI, USA

Hernan P Fainberg, Cyril Rauch, and Alison Mostyn
School of Veterinary Medicine and Science, University of Nottingham, Sutton Bonington Campus, Leicestershire LE12 5RD, UK

Michael E Symonds
Early Life Nutrition Research Unit, Academic Child Health, School of Clinical Sciences, University Hospital, The University of Nottingham, Nottingham NG7 2UH, UK

Kayleigh L Almond
Early Life Nutrition Research Unit, Academic Child Health, School of Clinical Sciences, University Hospital, The University of Nottingham, Nottingham NG7 2UH, UK
Current address: Primary Diets, Melmerby Industrial state, Melmerby, Ripon, North Yorkshire HG4 5HP, UK

Dongfang Li
School of Biosciences, The University of Nottingham, Sutton Bonington Campus, Leicestershire LE12 5RD, UK

Paul Bikker
Schothorst Feed Research, PO Box 533, 8200 AM Lelystad, The Netherlands. Current address: Wageningen UR Livestock Research, PO Box 338, 6700 AH Wageningen, The Netherlands

Sven M Jørgensen and Aleksei Krasnov
Nofima, Ås, Norway

Vicente Castro
Nofima, Ås, Norway

Institute of Animal Sciences, Norwegian University of Life Sciences (UMB), Ås, Norway.
AVS Chile S.A., Puerto Varas, Chile.

Harald Takle
Nofima, Ås, Norway
AVS Chile S.A., Puerto Varas, Chile
Nofima, Ås, Norway

Ståle J Helland
Institute of Animal Sciences, Norwegian University of Life Sciences (UMB), Ås, Norway
Aquaculture Protein Centre, CoE, Ås, Norway
Nofima, Ås, Norway

Barbara Grisdale-Helland
Aquaculture Protein Centre, CoE, Ås, Norway
Nofima, Ås, Norway

Jan Helgerud
Norwegian University of Science and Technology, Faculty of Medicine, Trondheim, Norway

Guy Claireaux
Université de Bretagne Occidentale, LEMAR, Unité de Physiologie Fonctionnelle des Organismes Marins, Ifremer, Plouzané, France

Anthony P Farrell
Faculty of Land and Food Systems, and Department of Zoology, University of British Columbia, Vancouver, BC, Canada

Mardi S Byerly
Department of Physiology, Johns Hopkins University School of Medicine, Baltimore, MD, USA
Department of Neuroscience, Johns Hopkins UniversitySchool of Medicine, Baltimore, MD, USA
Center for Metabolism and Obesity Research, Johns Hopkins University School of Medicine, Baltimore, MD, USA

G William Wong
Department of Physiology, Johns Hopkins University School of Medicine, Baltimore, MD, USA
Center for Metabolism and Obesity Research, Johns Hopkins University School of Medicine, Baltimore, MD, USA

Roy D Swanson
Department of Neuroscience, Johns Hopkins UniversitySchool of Medicine, Baltimore, MD, USA

Seth Blackshaw
Department of Neuroscience, Johns Hopkins UniversitySchool of Medicine, Baltimore, MD, USA
Department of Neurology, Johns Hopkins University School of Medicine, Baltimore, MD, USA
Department of Ophthalmology, Johns Hopkins University School of Medicine, Baltimore, MD, USA
Center for High-Throughput Biology, Johns Hopkins University School of Medicine, Baltimore, MD, USA
Institute for Cell Engineering, Johns Hopkins University School of Medicine, Baltimore, MD, USA

Eleni Apostolidou, Efrosyni Paraskeva and Paschalis-Adam Molyvdas
Department of Physiology, University of Thessaly Medical School, Larissa, Biopolis 41110, Greece

Chrissi Hatzoglou
Department of Physiology, University of Thessaly Medical School, Larissa, Biopolis 41110, Greece
Department of Respiratory Medicine, University of Thessaly Medical School, University Hospital of Larissa, Larissa, Biopolis 41110, Greece

Konstantinos Gourgoulianis
Department of Respiratory Medicine, University of Thessaly Medical School, University Hospital of Larissa, Larissa, Biopolis 41110, Greece.

Olessia Kroupa, Evelina Vorrsjö, Gunilla Olivecrona and Thomas Olivecrona
Department of Medical Biosciences/ Physiological Chemistry, Umeå University, Umeå SE-90187, Sweden

Stefan K Nilsson
Department of Medical Biosciences/ Physiological Chemistry, Umeå University, Umeå SE-90187, Sweden Present address: Department of Medicine, University of Gothenburg, Gothenburg SE-405 30, Sweden.

Rinke Stienstra, Frits Mattijssen and Sander Kersten
Nutrition, Metabolism and Genomics group, Division of Human Nutrition, Wageningen University, Wageningen 6700EV, The Netherlands

Peter Joseph Durcan, Johannes D Conradie and Kathryn Helen Myburgh
Department of Physiological Science, Stellenbosch University, Private Bag X1 Matieland, 7602 Stellenbosch, South Africa.

Mari Van deVyver
Division of Endocrinology, Department of Medicine, Stellenbosch University, Tygerberg, South Africa

Kanishk Sharma, Kyle Laster, Mohamed Hersi, Christina Torres and Thomas J Lukas
Department of Molecular Pharmacology and Biological Chemistry, Northwestern University, Chicago, IL 60611, USA

Calvin Wu
Department of Molecular Pharmacology and Biological Chemistry, Northwestern University, Chicago, IL 60611, USA
Department of Biological Sciences, University of North Texas, Denton, TX 76203, USA
Department of Speech and Hearing Sciences, University of North Texas, Denton, TX 76203, USA

Ernest J Moore
Department of Molecular Pharmacology and Biological Chemistry, Northwestern University, Chicago, IL 60611, USA
Department of Speech and Hearing Sciences, University of North Texas, Denton, TX 76203, USA

Danielle L Ippolito, John A Lewis and Jonathan D Stallings
The United States Army Center for Environmental Health Research, Environmental Health Program, Bldg. 568 Doughten Drive, Fort Detrick, Frederick, MD 21702-5010, USA

Chenggang Yu
Biotechnology High Performance Computing Software Applications Institute, Frederick, MD 21702-5010, USA

Lisa R Leon
Thermal Mountain Medicine Division, US Army Research Institute of Environmental Medicine, Natick, MA 01760-5007, USA

Satyanarayana R Pondugula, Suresh B Kampalli, Tao Wu, Nithya N Raveendran, Donald G Harbidge and Daniel C Marcus
Dept. Anatomy and Physiology, Cellular Biophysics Laboratory, Kansas State University, Manhattan, KS 66506, USA

Robert C De Lisle
Dept. Anatomy and Cell Biology, University of Kansas Medical Center, Kansas City, KS 66160, USA.
Vincent Jonchère, Aurélien Brionne, Joël Gautron and Yves Nys
INRA, UR83 Recherches Avicoles, F-37380, Nouzilly, France

Erica E. Alexeev and Bo Lönnerdal
Department of Nutrition, University of California, Davis, CA 95616, USA

Ian J. Griffin
Department of Pediatrics, University of California, Davis Medical Center, Sacramento, CA 95817, USA

Alexey E Lebedev and Vladimir V Galatenko
Moscow State University, Leninskie Gory, Moscow 119991, Russia

Alexander G Tonevitsky
Moscow State University, Leninskie Gory, Moscow 119991, Russia
The Institute of General Pathology and Pathophysiology, Russian Academy of Medical Sciences, Baltiiskaya str. 8, Moscow 125315, Russia

Maxim U Shkurnikov
The Institute of General Pathology and Pathophysiology, Russian Academy of Medical Sciences, Baltiiskaya str. 8, Moscow 125315, Russia

Diana V Maltseva, Timur R Samatov and Dmitry A Sakharov
SRC Bioclinicum, Ugreshskaya str 2/85, Moscow 115088, Russia

Asghar Abbasi and Hinnak Northoff
Institute of Clinical and Experimental Transfusion Medicine (IKET), University of Tübingen, Otfried-Müller-str. 4/1, Tübingen 72076, Germany

Anatoly I Grigoriev
Institute for Biomedical Problems, Russian Academy of Sciences, Khoroshevskoe road 76a, Moscow, 123007, Russia

Rakel Nyrén, Evelina Vorrsjö, Thomas Olivecrona and Gunilla Olivecrona
Department of Medical Biosciences/ Physiological Chemistry, Umeå University, Umeå, Sweden

Chuchun L Chang
Institute of Human Nutrition, College of Physicians and Surgeons, Columbia University, New York, NY, USA

Per Lindström and Anastasia Barmina
Department of Integrative Medical Biology (IMB), Umeå University, Umeå, Sweden

Yusuf Ali and Lisa Juntti-Berggren
The Rolf Luft Research Center for Diabetes and Endocrinology, Karolinska Institutet, Stockholm, Sweden

André Bensadoun
Division of Nutritional Science, Cornell University, Ithaca, NY, USA

Stephen G Young
Department of Medicine, David GeffenSchool of Medicine, University of California, Los Angeles, CA, USA

Benjamin Vandendriessche, An Goethals, Alba Simats and Peter Brouckaert
Inflammation Research Center, VIB, 9052 Ghent, Belgium
Department of Biomedical Molecular Biology, Ghent University, 9000 Ghent, Belgium

Evelien Van Hamme
Bio Imaging Core, Inflammation Research Center, VIB, 9052 Ghent, Belgium

Anje Cauwels
Inflammation Research Center, VIB, 9052 Ghent, Belgium
Department of Biomedical Molecular Biology, Ghent University, 9000 Ghent, Belgium
Cytokine Receptor Lab - Department of Medical Protein Research, VIB, 9000 Ghent, Belgium

Anna P Malykhina and Qi Lei
Department of Surgery, Division of Urology, University of Pennsylvania School of Medicine, Glenolden, PA 19036-2307, USA

Chris S Erickson and Miles L Epstein
Department of Neurosciences, University of Wisconsin-Madison, Madison, WI 53706, USA

Marcia R Saban, Carole A Davis and Ricardo Saban
Department of Physiology, College of Medicine, Urinary Tract Physiological Genomics Laboratory, University of Oklahoma Health Sciences Center (OUHSC), 800 Research Parkway, Room 410, Oklahoma City, OK 73104, USA

Caroline Mwendwa Kijogi
Department of Molecular Microbiology and Immunology, Division of Immunology, Graduate School of Biomedical Sciences, Nagasaki University, Nagasaki, Japan
Institute of Tropical Medicine and Infectious Diseases-KEMRI (ITROMID-KEMRI), Nairobi, Kenya

Christopher Khayeka-Wandabwa
African Population and Health Research Center (APHRC), P.O. Box 10787-00100, Nairobi, Kenya
Institute of Tropical Medicine and Infectious Diseases-KEMRI (ITROMID-KEMRI), Nairobi, Kenya

Keita Sasaki, Yoshimasa Tanaka, Hiroshi Kurosu, Hayato Matsunaga and Hiroshi Ueda
Department of Pharmacology and Therapeutic Innovation, Graduate School of Biomedical Sciences, Nagasaki University, Nagasaki, Japan

Inka Gallitz, Niklas Lofruthe, Lisa Traeger and Andrea U. Steinbicker
Department of Anaesthesiology, Intensive Care and Pain Medicine, University Hospital Muenster, Albert-Schweitzer Campus 1, Building A1, 48149 Muenster, Germany

Nicole Bäumer
Department of Medicine A, Molecular Haematology and Oncology, University Hospital Muenster, 48149 Muenster, Germany

Carsten Müller-Tidow
Department of Medicine A, Molecular Haematology and Oncology, University Hospital Muenster, 48149 Muenster, Germany
Present Address: Department of Medicine V, Hematology, Oncology and Rheumatology, Heidelberg University Hospital, 69120 Heidelberg, Germany

Verena Hoerr
Institute of Medical Microbiology, Jena University Hospital, 07747 Jena, Germany
Department of Clinical Radiology, University Hospital Muenster, 48149 Muenster, Germany

Cornelius Faber
Department of Clinical Radiology, University Hospital Muenster, 48149 Muenster, Germany

Tanja Kuhlmann
Institute for Neuropathology,University Hospital Muenster, 48149 Muenster, Germany

Daniel C. Marcus
Department of Anatomy and Physiology, Cellular Biophysics Laboratory, Kansas State University, 228 Coles Hall, Manhattan, KS 66506-5802, USA

Hiromitsu Miyazaki
Department of Anatomy and Physiology, Cellular Biophysics Laboratory, Kansas State University, 228 Coles Hall, Manhattan, KS 66506-5802, USA
Deparment of Anatomy and Physiology, Cell Physiology Laboratory, Kansas State University, 228 Coles Hall, Manhattan KS 66506-5802, USA
Department of Otolaryngology-Head and Neck Surgery, Tohoku University Graduate School of Medicine, Sendai 980-8574, Japan

Philine Wangemann
Deparment of Anatomy and Physiology, Cell Physiology Laboratory, Kansas State University, 228 Coles Hall, Manhattan KS 66506-5802, USA.

David E. Hunt
Research and Development, Lexington Veterans Affairs Medical Center, 1101 Veterans Drive, Room C-327, Lexington, Kentucky 40502, USA.

Fei Ma and Karin N. Westlund
Research and Development, Lexington Veterans Affairs Medical Center, 1101 Veterans Drive, Room C-327, Lexington, Kentucky 40502, USA
Department of Physiology, University of Kentucky, Lexington, Kentucky, USA

Pedro L. Vera
Research and Development, Lexington Veterans Affairs Medical Center, 1101 Veterans Drive, Room C-327, Lexington, Kentucky 40502, USA
Department of Physiology, University of Kentucky, Lexington, Kentucky, USA
Department of Surgery, University of Kentucky, Lexington, Kentucky, USA

Dimitrios E. Kouzoukas
Research and Development, Lexington Veterans Affairs Medical Center, 1101 Veterans Drive, Room C-327, Lexington, Kentucky 40502, USA
Saha Cardiovascular Research Center, University of Kentucky, Lexington, Kentucky, USA
Present Address: Department of Molecular Pharmacology and Therapeutics, Loyola University Chicago, Maywood, Illinois, USA

Katherine L. Meyer-Siegler
Department of Natural Sciences, St. Petersburg College, St. Petersburg, Florida, USA

Odelia Y. N. Bongmba, Geetali Pradhan and Miao-Hsueh Chen
USDA/ARS Children's Nutrition Research Center, Department of Pediatrics, Baylor College of Medicine, Houston, TX 77030, USA

Yuxiang Sun
USDA/ARS Children's Nutrition Research Center, Department of Pediatrics, Baylor College of Medicine, Houston, TX 77030, USA
Department of Nutrition and Food Science, Texas A&M University, 214D Cater-Mattil; 2253 TAMU, College Station, TX 77843, USA
Huffington Center on Aging, Baylor College of Medicine, Houston, TX, USA

Qiong Wei
USDA/ARS Children's Nutrition Research Center, Department of Pediatrics, Baylor College of Medicine, Houston, TX 77030, USA

Division of Endocrinology, Zhongda hospital, Southeast University, Nanjing, Jiangsu Province, People's Republic of China210002

Zilin Sun
Division of Endocrinology, Zhongda hospital, Southeast University, Nanjing, Jiangsu Province, People's Republic of China210002

Jong Han Lee
USDA/ARS Children's Nutrition Research Center, Department of Pediatrics, Baylor College of Medicine, Houston, TX 77030, USA
College of Pharmacy, Gachon University, Incheon 21936, South Korea

Robert S. Chapkin and Chia-Shan Wu
Department of Nutrition and Food Science, Texas A&M University, 214D Cater-Mattil; 2253 TAMU, College Station, TX 77843, USA.

Hongying Wang
Department of Nutrition and Food Science, Texas A&M University, 214D Cater-Mattil; 2253 TAMU, College Station, TX 77843, USA
Laboratory of Lipid and Glucose Metabolism, The First Affiliated Hospital of Chongqing Medical University, Chongqing, Sichuan province, People's Republic of China400016

Lindsey Chew
Institute of Biosciences and Technology, Houston, TX 77030, USA

Mandeep Bajaj and Lawrence Chan
Department of Medicine, Baylor College of Medicine, Houston, TX 77030, USA

Angela E. Vinturache and Francine G. Smith
Department of Physiology and Pharmacology; Alberta Children's Hospital Research Institute for Child and Maternal Health, Cumming School of Medicine, University of Calgary, 3330 Hospital Drive, NW, Calgary, AB T2N 4N1, Canada

Index